Immunologic Concepts in Transfusion Medicine

Immunologic Concepts in Transfusion Medicine

Edited by

ROBERT W. MAITTA, MD, PHD
Department of Pathology
University Hospitals Cleveland Medical Center
Case Western Reserve University School of Medicine
Cleveland, Ohio, United States

ELSEVIER

Immunologic Concepts in Transfusion Medicine

Copyright © 2020 Elsevier Inc. All rights reserved.

ISBN: 978-0-323-67509-3

Notices

Publisher: Dolores Meloni
Acquisition Editor: Robin R Carter
Editorial Project Manager: Pat Gonzalez
Production Project Manager: Poulouse Joseph
Cover Designer: Alan Studholme

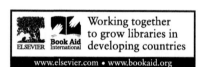

Working together to grow libraries in developing countries

www.elsevier.com • www.bookaid.org

List of Contributors

Tahmeena Ahmed, MBBS
Clinical Assistant Professor of Pathology
Department of Pathology
Stony Brook Medicine
Stony Brook University Medical Center
Stony Brook, NY, United States

Esther Babady, PhD, D(ABMM)
Associate Attending
Laboratory Medicine
Memorial Sloan Kettering Cancer Center
New York, NY, United States

Director of Clinical Operations
Clinical Microbiology Service
Memorial Sloan Kettering Cancer Center
New York, NY, United States

Ian L. Baine, MD, PhD
Department of Pathology
Mount Sinai School of Medicine
New York, NY, United States

Assistant Professor
Department of Pathology
Mount Sinai School of Medicine
New York, NY, United States

Nicholas Brown, PhD
Assistant Director
Transplant Immunology and Immunogenetics
    Laboratory
Pathology
University of Chicago
Chicago, IL, United states

Sally A. Campbell-Lee, MD
Director
Transfusion Medicine and Clinical Pathology
Associate Department Head
Associate Professor
Department of Pathology
University of Illinois at Chicago
Chicago, IL, United States

Meghan Delaney, DO, MPH
Division Chief
Pathology & Laboratory Medicine
Director
Transfusion Medicine at Children's National
    Medical Center

Associate Professor
Pathology & Pediatrics
George Washington University Health Sciences
Washington DC, United States

Robert A. DeSimone, MD
Assistant Professor of Pathology and Laboratory
    Medicine
Assistant Director of Transfusion Medicine
    and Cellular Therapy
Weill Cornell Medicine/New York Presbyterian
    Hospital
New York, NY, United States

Michelle L. Erickson, MD, MBA
Chair and Medical Director
Pathology and Laboratory Medicine York Hospital
WellSpan Health
York, PA, United States

Magali J. Fontaine, MD, PhD
Director of Transfusion Services
Associate Professor of Pathology and Medicine
University of Maryland School of Medicine
Baltimore MD, United States

Melissa R. George, DO, FCAP, FASCP
Medical Director
Transfusion Medicine Pathology
Penn State Health Hershey Medical Center
Hershey, PA, United States

Interim Chair
Associate Professor
Pathology
Penn State Health Hershey Medical Center
Hershey, PA, United States

Ruchika Goel, MD, MPH
Assistance Professor of Internal Medicine and Pediatrics
Division of Hematology/Oncology
Simmons Cancer Institute at SIU SOM

Medical Director
Mississippi Valley Regional Blood Center
Springfield, IL, United States

Adjunct Asst. Professor of Pathology
Div. of Transfusion Medicine

School of Medicine
Johns Hopkins University
Baltimore, MD, United States

Ian M. Harrold, MD
Resident Physician
Pathology and Laboratory Medicine
Penn State Health
Hershey, PA, United States

Hong Hong, MD, PhD
Assistant Attending Physician
Department of Lab Medicine
Memorial Sloan Kettering Cancer Center
New York, NY, United States

Jingmei Hsu, MD, PhD
Assistant Professor
Department of Medicine
Division of Hematology & Oncology/Bone Marrow
    and Hematopoietic Stem Cell Transplantation
Weill Cornell Medicine/New York Presbyterian
    Hospital
New York, NY, United States

Emily J. Larkin, BSc
Research Assistant
Department of Pathology
University of Maryland School of Medicine
Baltimore MD, United States

Kathleen M. Madden, MD
Department of Pathology
University of New Mexico
Albuquerque, NM, United States

Robert W. Maitta, MD, PhD
Department of Pathology
University Hospitals Cleveland Medical Center
Case Western Reserve University School of Medicine
Cleveland, OH, United States

Yupo Ma, MD, PhD
Professor of Pathology
Department of Pathology
Stony Brook Medicine
Stony Brook University Medical Center
Stony Brook, NY, United States

Faisal Mukhtar, MBBS, MD, FCAP, FASCP
Co-Medical Director Transfusion Services
Clinical Assistant Professor
Department of Pathology
University of Florida Health
Gainesville, FL, United States

J. Peter R. Pelletier, MD, FCAP, FASCP
Medical Director Transfusion Services
Clinical Associate Professor
Department of Pathology
Immunology and Laboratory Medicine
Department of Anesthesia
University of Florida Health
Gainesville, Florida, United States

Melissa Pessin, MD, PhD
Chair
Department of Laboratory Medicine
Memorial Sloan Kettering Cancer Center
New York, NY, United States

Huy P. Pham, MD, MPH
Department of Pathology
Keck School of Medicine of the University of Southern
    California
Los Angeles, CA, United States

Sabrina Ewa Racine-Brzostek, MD, PhD
New York Blood Center

Transfusion Medicine
New York Blood Center
New York, NY, United States

Transfusion Medicine and Cellular Therapy
Weill Cornell Medicine
New York, NY, United States

Jay S. Raval, MD
Associate Professor
Pathology
University of New Mexico
Albuquerque, NM, United States

Hollie M. Reeves, DO
Assistant Medical Director of Transfusion Medicine
Blood Bank and Apheresis Center
Department of Pathology
University Hospitals Cleveland Medical Center
Cleveland, Ohio, United States

Assistant Professor of Pathology
Case Western Reserve University School of Medicine
Cleveland, Ohio, United States

Alex B. Ryder, MD, PhD
Assistant Professor
Pediatrics
University of Tennessee Health Science Center
Memphis, TN, United States

Assistant Professor
Pathology and Laboratory Medicine
University of Tennessee Health Science Center
Memphis, TN, United States

Medical Director
Transfusion Services and Clinical Laboratory
Le Bonheur Children's Hospital
Memphis, TN, United States

Lisa Senzel, MD, PhD
Clinical Associate Professor of Pathology
Department of Pathology
Stony Brook Medicine
Stony Brook University Medical Center
Stony Brook, NY, United States

Kristin Stendahl, MD
Department of Laboratory Medicine
Yale University School of Medicine
New Haven, CT, United States

Christopher A. Tormey, MD
Department of Laboratory Medicine
Yale University School of Medicine
New Haven, CT, United States

Associate Professor
Laboratory Medicine
Yale University School of Medicine
New Haven, CT, United States

Medical Director of the Transfusion Service
Yale-New Haven Hospital
New Haven, CT, United States

Pathology & Laboratory Medicine Service
VA Connecticut Healthcare System
West Haven, CT, United States

Ljiljana V. Vasovic, MD
Assistant Professor
Pathology and Laboratory Medicine

Associate Director of Cellular Therapy
Assistant Director of Transfusion Medicine

Weill Cornell Medicine/New York Presbyterian
 Hospital
New York, NY, United States

Chief of Clinical Pathology and Transfusion Medicine
NewYork-Presbyterian/Lower Manhattan Hospital
New York, NY, United States

Geoffrey D. Wool, MD, PhD
Interim Director
Blood Bank
Pathology
University of Chicago
Chicago, IL, United States

Yan Zheng, MD, PhD
Assistant Member
Pathology
St. Jude Children's Research Hospital
Memphis, TN, United States

Preface

Immunology and Transfusion Medicine are two disciplines that obligate many of us in medicine to take sides and specialize in one or the other. Exemplifying this, I trained on the first but found my medical niche on the latter. Nevertheless, just like an impressionist painting in which you are challenged to see the significance or relationship between strokes up close, if you step back the picture comes into focus. This is what contributors who have worked on this book wish to bring to the attention of our readers. Both disciplines, though distinct and complex in their own right, intersect in many areas which helps to understand when complications due to transfusion occur. Without a doubt, blood and its components when used appropriately provide support to patients when they are most vulnerable, including during extensive blood losses. In these settings transfusions provide the needed support to attempt to restore or ameliorate the disrupted hemodynamic steady state that patients need as they fight a given presentation. However, the closeness of immunologic responses and transfusion practice requires we step back and bring into the open a better understanding of the role that immunity plays upon blood exposure.

Blood is a tissue and as such is made of a diverse array of cells, some of which have functions that are helpful to patients requiring transfusions while others do not. For example, platelet transfusions provide the ability to slow down or stop bleeding, but this represents just one of the many known functions of platelets. These additional functions can lead to release of mediators that potentially affect the recipient. Likewise, red blood cell transfusions provide oxygen-carrying capacity but they also undergo changes during storage which in a susceptible recipient may lead to unforeseen adverse events. However, it needs to be emphasized that blood is safer today not only through expanded testing and donor deferrals, but also through the recognition decades ago of the potential harmful effects caused by leukocytes still present in the blood component in the recipient which resulted in the push for universal leukoreduction. These changes have curtailed many of those adverse events reported 30 years ago but complications secondary to transfusion still occur, though with less frequency.

Some of us see transfusion as an exposure to a very large dose of antigenic determinants which can affect the intended recipient; it is with this long-earned respect for blood that we set forth presenting these topics. Therefore, those of us contributing to this book have written chapters which review what is known of a particular concept in Transfusion Medicine in which immunological responses play an essential role. Utilizing a careful and thorough discussion of basic science and clinical evidence, the text goes over those important elements in each of the selected topics discussing blood exposure in the context of what is known immunologically. To bring all readers up to date the book begins with a refresher of basic descriptive immunology and soon moves to concepts such as TRALI, transfusion reactions, alloimmunization, TRIM, complications to transplantation, HLA-incompatibility, responses in adults versus neonate/pediatric patients and more, even including state-of-the-art topics such as polyclonal/monoclonal therapies and CAR T. We encourage readers to see these chapters as our effort to increase levels of awareness of blood usage and use what is learned from what is described to continue to make transfusions safer.

Robert W. Maitta, MD, PhD
Department of Pathology
University Hospitals Cleveland Medical Center
Case Western Reserve University School of Medicine

Contents

CHAPTER 1

A Focused Review of Basic Immunology Concepts

IAN L. BAINE, MD, PHD • CHRISTOPHER A. TORMEY, MD

INTRODUCTION

The field of transfusion medicine is unique and complex, as it is one of the few areas of medicine solely focused on a single organ. Yet as the field has developed over the past 200 or so years, drawing upon experiences in the combat, emergency medical, surgical, and general hospital inpatient settings, it has become abundantly clear that there is much more to the field than simply transfusing blood. From the earliest Nobel prize-winning experiments of Landsteiner at the turn of the 20th century demonstrating the fundamental ABO blood groups to the identification of the RhD antigen by Landsteiner and Wiener in the 1940s, to the development of RhoGAM, to modern-day practices of molecular genotyping for Rh and other antigens, the practice of transfusing blood and blood components has always been grounded in basic immunology.[1] Moreover, the very word "compatible" when used in the context of transfusion medicine refers to *immunologic* compatibility with the recipient of the transfusion. In this sense, blood and blood component transfusion shares much in common with solid organ and bone marrow transplantation; many of the same immunologic considerations must be addressed.[2-4]

Antibody-mediated rejection, cell-mediated rejection, and HLA and other minor histocompatibility antigen haplotypes should all be incorporated into a transfusion plan to ensure maximal therapeutic benefit while minimizing patient risk and preserving future transfusion/transplant compatibility.[5-7] Therefore, before exploring the immunology of transfusion medicine specifically, a basic and simplified immunology primer is useful to better understand the mechanisms underlying certain types of transfusion reactions, the formation of alloantibodies to red blood cells (RBCs) and platelets, as well as more complex events such as rejection or tolerance of hematopoietic stem cell transplants. We will begin with a basic overview of the relevant cells that comprise innate and adaptive immune systems, then discuss how antigens are presented to the adaptive immune system. We will then focus on the cellular and humoral arms of the immune systems, concentrating mainly on how they work together to promote humoral responses. We will also briefly touch on the role of the complement cascade in this context as well. We will then examine the concept of immunologic memory, focusing on primary versus secondary or "recall" immune responses, and conclude with a very brief overview of immunotolerance and its potential role in transfusion. Note that this brief overview chapter assumes some knowledge of basic immunology, and represents a review of basic concepts with a transfusion medicine focus. The reader is referred to any of several excellent Immunology and Molecular Biology textbooks for a more generalized and comprehensive review.[8-10]

Antigens and Immunogens

Throughout all arms of the immune system, the overarching theme is that of recognition of foreign molecular patterns (termed antigens) by its cells, followed by a series of reactions designed to produce a neutralizing effect on the source of that foreign substance; the antigens that elicit an immune response are termed "immunogenic" antigens or immunogens. More specifically, the specific portion of a peptide or carbohydrate complex that is recognized and responded to by immune cells is termed an epitope. If that description sounds a bit vague and overly generalized, it is because from a traditional standpoint, we think of the immune system as identifying and reacting to invading pathogens, and producing both cellular and humoral, or antibody-mediated responses directed against that pathogen. This would imply that the immune system somehow "knows" what antigens derive from pathogens and which do not, and selectively "chooses" to respond to

Immunologic Concepts in Transfusion Medicine. https://doi.org/10.1016/B978-0-323-67509-3.00001-9

pathogens. However, although the immune system demonstrates a remarkable degree of complexity in antigen recognition and response, it does not in any way possess "knowledge" of which peptides are pathogenic and which are benign. As we will expand upon in a bit, the cells of the innate immune system possess invariate surface receptors that recognize pathogen-*associated* molecular patterns (PAMPs), which is to say that they recognize *patterns* of certain types of carbohydrate residues, lipopolysaccharides, free nucleic acids, and other molecules that are *usually associated* with pathogens.[11–14] However, these cells cannot distinguish the presence of these patterns on a bacterium or virus from the same patterns on another nonpathogenic cell type. By contrast, cells of the adaptive immune system possess surface receptors of varying composition that recognize antigens either directly, or as they are presented to them by specialized "antigen-presenting" cells (APCs) such as macrophages, dendritic cells, and B cells. Similar to the innate immune system, these cells cannot distinguish between antigen recognition derived from a

pathogen versus the same (or a highly similar) one derived from other sources such as the person's own cells and tissues, or from other foreign sources, such as transfused cells or transplanted tissues. All of these points serve to underscore the main concept that the immune system as a whole can simply recognize and respond to antigens to which it has cognate receptors, and broadly speaking, can respond whether that antigen is derived from a pathogen, or other exogenous source (Fig. 1.1).

Innate and Adaptive Immunity

The immune system in humans can be broadly divided into two major branches, innate and adaptive, which comprise numerous cells and cell subsets. Evolutionarily speaking the innate immune system is far more ancient having evolved initially in organisms as simple as an Ameba, and is well developed in insects such as the fruit fly. Much of our initial understanding of innate immunity is based on studies involving *Drosophila*. By contrast, classicallydefined adaptive immunity is a

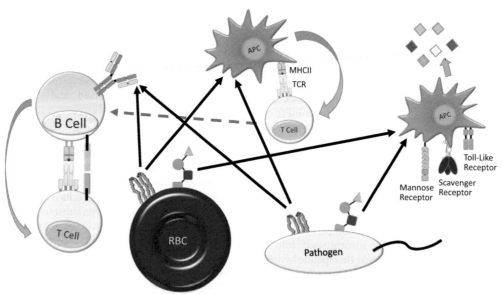

FIG. 1.1 Recognition of Antigen by the Cellular Immune System From Multiple Sources. Cells of the innate immune system such as professional antigen-presenting cells (APC) are capable of recognizing binding pathogen-associated molecular patterns (PAMPs) such as sequences of mannose-containing surface glycoproteins, lipopolysaccharide, and other pathogen-associated markers, indicated by the chain of colored shapes. Note that similar molecular patterns may be present on both pathogens as well as other sources such as RBCs; the innate immune system does not distinguish between the source of the molecular pattern. Similarly, homologous or shared protein antigens on the surface of pathogens or RBCs (blue arches) are recognized directly by B cells, or are processed and presented via MHC molecules by professional APCs in the setting of innate immune activation to T cells, which activate and assist in the development of T-dependent humoral immune responses. Similar tomolecular patterns, the adaptive immune system does not distinguish between sources of antigen.

feature of vertebrates, with mammals possessing its most evolved form. We will now provide a brief overview of the major cell types in the innate immune system, and broadly discuss basic functions, while maintaining a transfusion medicine-oriented focus. It is important to note that due to the immense complexity among immune cells, only a very brief overview is provided here; numerous subsets exist within each type of immune cell, with varying functions; differing subsets of the same type of cell can sometimes have counteracting or opposite functions even. Therefore, a more in-depth discussion of these cells can be found in any number of immunology textbooks.[9,10]

As mentioned earlier, innate immunity is generally characterized by cellular recognition of molecular "patterns" or "motifs" that are often present on pathogens such as lipopolysaccharides, mannose-containing carbohydrates, and single- and double-stranded free nucleic acids.[11-16] Generally, they exert their immune effects primarily through direct phagocytosis,[17] and the secretion of cytokines that promote inflammation and cellular immune activation. Critically, they also phagocytose antigens, "process" them intracellularly, and then present them to the adaptive immune system via specialized antigen presentation molecules. Thus, in addition to directly promoting immune response and pathogen killing in response to basic molecular pattern recognition, they also play a critical role in priming and activating the adaptive immune system.[18]

Recognition of pathogens via pattern receptors is a key feature of a class of innate immune cells known as "professional" APCs. These cells consist of two major types, macrophages and dendritic cells. Macrophages are myeloid-derived cells that originate from precursors in the bone marrow, and circulate in the peripheral blood as monocytes. Upon trafficking to tissues, they differentiate further into macrophages, where they provide local immune "surveillance," patrolling peripheral tissues for PAMPs such as mannose residues, complement bound to cells or antibodies, β-glucan residues, free nucleic acids, and others (Fig. 1.2) that they recognize via their numerous surface receptors. Similarly, dendritic cells are professional APCs derived from the myeloid lineage that patrol tissues in an immature state in which they recognize PAMPs via their various surface receptors.[18] Upon recognition of pathogens, both cell types undergo activation. In the case of macrophages, this results in an increase in phagocytic activity and

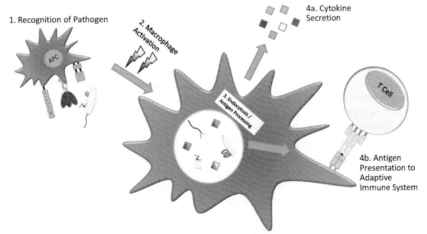

FIG. 1.2 **Innate Immune System Activation by Detection of Pathogen-Associated Molecular Patterns.** (1) Free-floating pathogens are encountered by surveilling APCs of the innate immune system, and various PAMPs are bound via surface receptors on the APC. (2) This binding induces an activating signal transduction cascade within the APC, leading to phagocytosis of the pathogen within endosomal compartments and fusion with lysosomes. (3) This results in the digestion and proteolysis of these pathogens, (4a) rendering the protein fragments of the pathogen amenable to presentation to the T cells via MHC molecules. (4b). A secondary effect of innate immune activation is the secretion of numerous proinflammatory cytokines such as IL1-β, TNF-α, IL-12, IFN-γ, and others. These cytokines serve to promote further immune activation at a distance as they diffuse outwards and activate nearby innate immune cells and further guide the differentiation of activating T cells into various subsets. Note that in this figure, the shape of the APC shown implies a cell such as a macrophage or dendritic cell. However, B cells also function as APCs as well, and serve a similar critical role in T-cell stimulation and T-dependent immune responses.

generation of proteolytic and oxidative enzymes. Italso induces secretion of proinflammatory and immune-stimulatory cytokines,[19] and increased presentation of antigens to cells of the adaptive immune system via specialized antigen-presenting molecules of the major histocompatibility complex (MHC) family, as well as increased surface expression costimulatory molecules such as CD80, CD86, and others that help to activate cells of the adaptive immune system (discussed later).[20] In the case of dendritic cells, these cells migrate to regional lymph nodes, where they too undergo a maturation process in which they largely increase their expression of MHC and costimulatory molecules to resident adaptive immune cells.[21]

From a transfusion medicine perspective, it is important to note that whatever the stimulus, once activated, these innate immune cells *indiscriminately* phagocytose surrounding material in their environment, including RBCs, which can then be presented to cells of the adaptive immune system. As we shall see, the adaptive immune system recognizes and reacts to *foreign* or *nonself* peptide and carbohydrate antigens, and generates cellular and humoral responses specifically directed against those antigens. If a transfused red cell expresses an antigen that is foreign to the recipient, it is possible that their innate immune cells willphagocytose these cells, present them to the adaptive immune system, and elicit a humoral response against antigens on the transfused red cells.[22,23]

By contrast, the adaptive immune system, comprised in humans of B and T lymphocytes primarily, serves the role of *selective* and *specific* identification of distinct and unique protein and carbohydrate sequences, termed antigens. The unique and defining feature of the adaptive immune system is its ability to adjust and tune the specificity of its response to a given antigen. Indeed, the adaptive immune system is "trained" to respond to various specific antigens as part of its activation, and displays the ability to "remember" antigens it has reacted to previously; this is termed "immunologic memory." These features are critical to protection of the host from pathogens; both of these concepts underlie the fundamental efficacy of vaccines, in which the patient's immune system is "trained" to protect against various pathogens that are exposed to the adaptive immune system via immunization.

However, despite its ability to generate antigen-specific responses, the adaptive immune system, like its innate counterpart, possesses no specific "knowledge" regarding the antigens to which it responds. It simply responds to antigens presented to it by APCs of the innate immune system. The adaptive immune system comprises two major classes of cells, B cells and T cells. Both are lymphocytes, derived from a common lymphoid progenitor in the bone marrow.[24] Both recognize antigen by means of surface-bound *variable* antigen receptors; B cells recognize free antigen by means of surface-bound immunoglobulin (Ig),[25] also termed the B-cell receptor (BCR), while T cells recognize antigen via their surface bound T-cell receptors (TCRs) when presented by specialized MHC antigen presentation molecules.[26,27] Both the BCR and TCR share the common feature of variability in their antigen recognition domain. This is achieved via a remarkable process of germline rearrangement of up to three different families of genes termed V, D, and J genes, that code for the portion of the BCR or TCR that actually binds antigen, termed the "variable" region.[28,29] The result is a BCR or TCR with a highly unique antigenic specificity (Fig. 1.3). Thus, while the B or T cell overall possesses a total of up to 84 combined V, D, and J genes, the combinatorial diversity made possible by this germline rearrangement process and additional steps that introduce further variability to the BCR or TCR, results in a staggering number of possible combinations. Furthermore, because the same process occurs simultaneously and independently on each of the two chains of the BCR (heavy and light chains) or TCR (α/γ and β/δ chains), the result is a theoretical diversity of 5×10^{13} and 1×10^{18} unique antigenic specificities for B and T cells, respectively.[30–32]

Now that we have established the major cellular players of the innate and adaptive immune systems in the context of antigen detection and recognition, we will discuss how antigens are presented to cells of the adaptive immune system, as this mechanism is what initially triggers an adaptive immune response. As mentioned previously, upon activation, cells of the innate immune system increase their phagocytosis of surrounding extracellular environmental particles, increase expression of their costimulatory surface molecules, and in some cases secrete proinflammatory cytokines that mediate a number of downstream effects including recruitment of additional innate immune cells such as neutrophils. In the background of this proinflammatory context, small peptide fragments derived from local phagocytosed particles are "presented" by specialized surface molecules termed MHC proteins, of which there are two major classes.

The Class I and Class II MHC molecules themselves are specialized molecules encoded by a 3Mb stretch of DNA on chromosome 6p21. The Class I MHC molecule comprises an α-chain containing three distinct domains, arranged in an L-shaped configuration, and

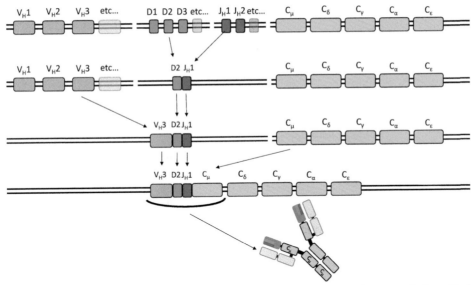

FIG. 1.3 **Germline Rearrangement of V, D, and J Segments to Produce the Complete Antigen-Binding Region of an Antigen Receptor.**   Gene segments coding for the variable region of the Ig heavy chain exist as sets of highly homologous copies for the "variable or V", "diversity or D", "joining or J", and "constant or C" regions over a relatively large distance across Chr14. Through a recombination process akin to a "mix-and-match buffet", the cell first selects one of the D and one of the J genes and excises the intervening DNA stretch to bring them adjacent to each other. The cell then selects one of the V_H gene copies, and combines it with the recentlyformed DJ segment, to create a VDJ gene segment, which codes for the complete antigen-recognition portion of the antigen receptor. In the case of Ig formation, the protein is then paired with the C_H region to form the Ig heavy chain, complete with the isotype-defining F_c region (IgM shown in this figure as an example). This figure focuses specifically on the Ig heavy chain, hence the V_H and J_H nomenclature and C regions, however the concepts and process is for the most part analogous for the Ig light chains, as well as for the α/β and γ/δ T-cell receptors (except that these combine with constant region genes for the TCR α, β, γ, or δ chains instead of Ig constant regions).

inserted into the cell membrane at one end. The α-chain associates with the β-2-microglobulin molecule, which provides stability to the MHC molecule. The antigenic peptide itself resides in an antigen-presentation "cleft" located at the juncture between the α1 and α2 domains (Fig. 1.4). By contrast, the Class II MHC molecule comprises two distinct chains, α and β, each inserted into the cell membrane and each containing two domains. The antigen-presentation cleft is located at the juncture between the α1 and β1 domains, which are at the distal end of the molecule (Fig. 1.4).[33]

Generally speaking, Class I molecules typically present peptides derived from *intracytosolic* sources such as endogenous self-peptides, as well as those derived from intracytosolic pathogens such as viruses. By contrast, Class II MHC molecules typically present peptides derived from *extracellular* sources that have been phagocytosed by the cell. After phagocytosis of extracellular objects, the antigen-presenting cell sequesters

them in a specialized organelle called a phagosome. Through a complex series of steps, the phagosome is fused with another organelle termed the lysosome, which contains numerous acidic hydrolases and other proteolytic enzymes that serve to break down the phagosomal contents into small peptide fragments.[34] Once extracellular peptides are digested in the phagolysosome into small fragments, they are then "loaded" into the antigen-presentation cleft of Class II MHC molecules where they remain anchored as the antigen:MHC II complex that is everted by the cell to the extracellular environment. There, it is exposed and ready to be detected by CD4+ T cells (Fig. 1.4). Although peptides presented by Class I MHC and the Class I molecule itself play a critical role in solid organ transplant compatibility and many other functions, the Class II MHC pathway is more important to understand in a transfusion medicine context, as antigens derived from transfused RBCs usually are generated by extracellular

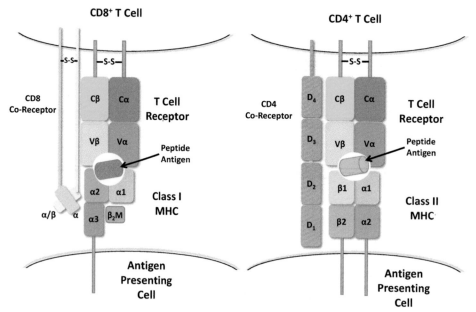

FIG. 1.4 Structure of MHC Class I and II Molecules, and Their Presentation of Peptide Antigens to T Cells. The MHC Class I molecule comprises three α domains in association with β₂-microglobulin, and presents peptide antigen in a specialized antigen-presentation pocket at the junction of the α1/α2 domains. Similarly, the MHC Class II molecule comprises α and β chains each with two domains, with the antigen-presentation pocket at the junction of the α1/β1 domains. MHC molecules present the peptide to α/β T cells, which recognize both the specific antigen, together with the MHC molecule itself via the antigen-recognition portion of the T-cell receptor (TCR), comprised the junction of variable regions of the α and β chains. Separately, the CD8 or CD4 coreceptors (for CD8⁺ or CD4⁺ T cells, respectively) stabilize and facilitate this interaction via binding to nonvariable, external faces of the Class I or II MHC molecules, respectively. This interaction, along with a costimulatory signal (see Fig. 6), induces a signal transduction cascade leading to T-cell activation and proliferation.

phagocytosis and processing in the endosome and lysosome.[35] They are then loaded and presented to CD4⁺ T cells via the Class II pathway. Class I MHC molecules present antigen to CD8⁺ T cells, while Class II MHC molecules present antigen to CD4⁺ T cells. Therefore, CD4⁺ T cells appear to be the primary driver of alloimmune responses to transfused RBCs.[36]

Immune Self-Tolerance

This process of antigen receptor formation is a requisite part of a B or T cells' maturation process, and occurs stochastically and without a priori guidance. This however raises the possibility of generating T cells that recognize epitopes present on an individual's own tissues, raising the possibility of an immune response to one's own antigens, a process clinically manifesting as autoimmunity.[37] Therefore, mechanisms have evolved in vertebrates to screen maturing B and T cells for so-

called "autoreactive" cells and cause them to be eliminated by inducing their death. After development of immature T cells from lymphoid precursors in bone marrow, they undergo an "education" process in which they traffic to the thymus, where they are exposed to a large variety of self-expressed peptides via specialized APCs in the epithelium of the thymic cortex and medulla. This accomplishes two goals. First, it ensures that maturing T cells only recognize antigen presented in the context of one's own specific isoform of MHC molecules. Second, and critical for the purposes of transfusion medicine, it ensures that developing T cells that react too strongly to self-antigens are deleted via apoptosis.[38] (Fig. 1.5).Autoreactive B cells are also capable of undergoing deletion through mechanisms such as apoptosis, or a process known as receptor editing, in which a secondary process of germline recombination results in an "edited" version of antigen

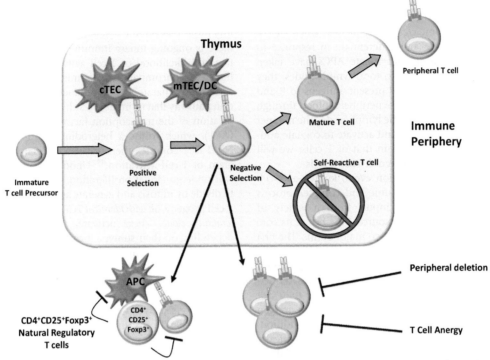

Thymus

cTEC

mTEC/DC

Peripheral T cell

Mature T cell

Immune Periphery

Immature
T cell Precursor

Positive
Selection

Negative
Selection

Self-Reactive T cell

APC

CD4+
CD25+
Foxp3+

CD4+CD25+Foxp3+
**Natural Regulatory
T cells**

Peripheral deletion

T Cell Anergy

FIG. 1.5 **Thymic Education of T Cells and Immune Self-tolerance.**   To prevent generalized autoimmunity, it is critically important to "educate" the T-cell repertoire not to react to self-proteins. This is accomplished through the process of central immune tolerance. T-cell precursors migrate from their place of origin in the bone marrow to the thymus, where they interact with specialized thymic epithelial cells in the cortex (cTEC) and medulla (mTEC) that through presentation of self-peptide-MHC complexes, impose a "goldilocks" effect on T-cell activation. This ensures that T cells released into the periphery tolerate self-MHC and self-proteins, while reacting to foreign MHC and to foreign antigens. Cells that are self-reactive are deleted centrally in the thymus via apoptosis. Rare self-reactive cells that manage to "escape" central tolerance induction can be regulated in the immune periphery through numerous mechanisms such as T-cell anergy induction, peripheral activation-induced deletion, or via dominant suppression by regulatory T cells (peripheral tolerance mechanisms are not discussed in this chapter).

specificity.[39] Thus, it establishes the important immunologic concept of self-tolerance; adaptive immune cells should only recognize and respond to epitopes that are not present on host tissues. This concept underlies the fundamental mechanisms of alloantibody formation to RBC antigens. In fact, the very term *allo* translates from Latin to mean "other," and in this context denotes nonself RBC antigens. Therefore, a patient's immune system only reacts to foreign antigens present on transfused red cells. It is important to emphasize that the differences in epitopes between self andnonself antigens does not need to be large. In fact differences as small as a single amino acid (sometimes differing in structure by as little as a single methyl or hydroxyl group on an amino acid's side chain!) are readily detected by B and T cells, and can render a highly

homologous antigen as foreign. This is directly applicable to transfusion medicine, as differences between alternate forms of RBC antigens, such as C and c, E and e, Jk^a and Jk^b, as well as numerous others often differ by just a single amino acid, yet are readily detected as foreign.[40]

Based on these fundamental immunology concepts of innate immune activation, antigen update, processing, and presentation via MHC molecules to adaptive immune cells, we can now transition to activation of the adaptive immune system, with a primary focus on humoral immune responses, as these are the primary type of immune response involved in RBC alloantibody formation. As we mentioned previously, individual B and T cells possess unique BCRs and TCRs, respectively, each of which is capable of binding to a different epitope. Each unique B or T cell, with its unique antigenic specificity is called as a "clone," a term whose significance will become clear subsequently, when we see how B cells activate and differentiate in response to antigenic stimulation. After innate APCs have taken up antigen and trafficked to local lymph nodes, they take up residence there and present antigens to B and T cells as they traffic from the peripheral blood through the cortex and medulla of the lymph node. The manner in which B cells recognize and activate to cognate antigens is slightly different from that of T cells; we will focus on T cells first, and then discuss B cells.

The initial T-cell activation event, known as T-cell "priming" is a highly dynamic and complex process with numerous signaling inputs from a variety of cellular and environmental sources,[41,42] but at its core can be (over)simplified into two major events. The first is the recognition of the unique antigen:MHC complex on the APC by the T cell's unique TCR. The predominant type of TCR comprises two distinct chains, termed Alpha and Beta, which form a heterodimer in the T-cell membrane. The $\alpha\beta$ TCR has evolved to detect antigen *only* when presented by the MHC molecule. In addition, as described previously, one's own T cells are typically educated to only respond to antigen presented by one's own MHC haplotype, and any nonself MHC molecules are considered as foreign antigens by the host immune system. The strength of this interaction between these 2 cells is tenuous, and depends on how "strongly" the TCR can bind to the antigen:MHC complex. Therefore, a coreceptor present on the T cell, either CD8 or CD4, binds a separate site on the external surface of the Class I or Class II MHC, respectively. This allows for sufficient contact time to take place in this antigen: MHC:TCR trimeric complex, and enables signal transduction via the tyrosine kinases associated with the transmembrane and intracytoplasmic domains of the TCR and associated CD3 molecules. The resulting tyrosine kinase cascade ultimately results in the nuclear translocation of the transcription factor nuclear factor of activated Tcells (NFAT), where it partners with other transcription factors. This signal, uncreatively termed "Signal 1" represents the first of two signals required for full T-cell activation. The second comes in the form of a so-called "costimulatory" signal termed (you guessed it...) "Signal 2". This signal is most commonly transmitted by the interaction between CD28 molecule on the T cell and either CD80 or CD86 on the APC. Although CD80 and CD86 are thought of as the predominant costimulatory molecules, there are a myriad of other such molecules in this family, with both T cell activating and inhibiting

roles; discussion of these is far beyond our scope here.[43] Keep in mind that increased levels of costimulatory molecules on APCs are typically only present when there is ongoing innate immune activation. Thus, the fate and likelihood of T-cell activation is inextricably linked to concomitant innate immune activation. This activates a separate and simultaneous signal transduction pathway that ultimately results in the nuclear translocation of the transcription factor activator protein 1 (AP1), which forms a heterodimer with NFAT. The NFAT:AP1 complex then drives a transcriptional program of T-cell activation.[44] Upon activation, a T cell will undergo clonal proliferation, that is, it will begin to divide by mitosis and generate an "army" of activated T-cell progeny, *all with identical TCR specificity to that of its founding clone.* These activated T cells themselves, depending on their subtype, begin to secrete immunomodulatory and immunoproliferative cytokines such as interleukin (IL)-2, IL-4, IL-5, IL-10, IL-12, IL-13, interferon (IFN)-γ, tumor necrosis factor (TNF)-α, and many others. They also begin to express their own costimulatory markers such as CD154 and others. In the case of CD4$^+$ helper T cells, this is crucial as CD154 will play a key role in activating subsequent B cells to produce immunoglobulin, and is critical in mouse models of RBC alloimmunization (Fig. 1.6).[36]

The process of B-cell activation is analogous in many ways to that of T-cell activation.[45] Similar toT cells, B cells are activated by the interaction of the unique BCR with the unique cognate antigen. However, different from the TCR, the BCR does not require a special antigen presentation molecule to bind fully, and can recognize free-floating antigen extracellularly. Binding of multiple identical BCRs on the surface of a B cell results in BCR "clustering" within the local cell membrane region, and brings the intracellular portions of the BCR, which contain associated signal transducing kinases, into proximity. This allows for initiation of the B-cell signaling cascade that results in B-cell activation, and is analogous to the "Signal 1" seen by T cells. This induces endocytosis of the bound antigen by the B cell, processing along the endosome/phagolysosome pathway, and processing into fragments for presentation by Class II MHC, as outline earlier.

T-Dependent and T-Independent B-Cell Activation

Different from T cells, Signal 1 alone is sufficient for activation of B cells, and can induce their clonal proliferation and secretion of antibodies, largely of the IgM class. This is accomplished by clustering of BCRs within the cell membrane sufficiently to allow

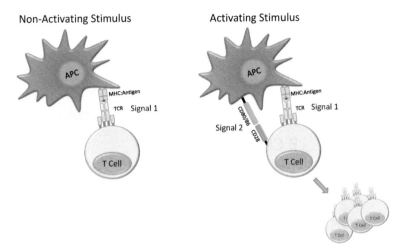

FIG. 1.6 Adaptive Immune Cells Rrequire two Signals to Fully Activate.   T-cell activation (shown here as example, analogous concepts apply to B cells) comprises two major signals. Signal 1is the interaction of the MHC:Antigen complex with the antigen-recognition domain of the TCR. This results in signal transduction within the T cell that ultimately leads to translocation of the protein NFAT into the T-cell nucleus. When this occurs in combination with Signal 2—the interaction of costimulatory ligands and receptors on the APC and T cell (CD80/86 and CD28 shown here as an example)—a second signal transduction cascade via the PI3 kinase/MAPK cascade results in the presence of the protein AP1 in the nucleus. NFAT and AP1 then combine to form a heterodimer, and function together as a transcription factor to promote a genetic program of T-cell activation that involves increased metabolism, secretion of cytokines, and a proliferative response.

transphosphorylation of their intracellular domains, and initiation of signal transduction. Alternatively, the Signal 2costimulus signal can be provided by the interaction of C3 complement-tagged antigens with the CD21-CD19-CD81 B-cell coreceptor complex on B cells, or signaling through the Toll-like receptor pathway, which initiates a second signal transduction cascade to promote B-cell activation in the absence of T cells. Because this situation does not involve T cells, it is known as a "T-independent" humoral response, and is generally In this situation, B cells activate and proliferate clonally, but are restricted to IgM production, and cannot undergo further fine-tuning of antibody affinity for the cognate antigen.[9]

However, because in many cases antigen presentation takes place in the lymph node where the B cells and T cells are clustered together, it is often the case that a local preprimed T cell will recognize the antigen being presented by the B cell. This allows interaction of CD154 (from the preprimed T cell) with CD40 on the B cell. This is known as "T-dependent" response because it involves "help" from CD4[+] T cells, and results in more robust B-cell activation. This interaction serves as a costimulatory "Signal 2" to the B cell, and allows it to not only clonally proliferate, but to also

undergo antibody isotype switching from the IgM class to other secreted isotypes such as IgG, IgA and others. Additionally, these B cells migrate to the germinal center of lymph nodes where they undergo a process known as somatic hypermutation.[46] In this process, an enzyme will randomly deaminate various cytosine residues in the rearranged immunoglobulin gene, resulting in the conversion of cytidine residues to uracil, and leads to C:G base pairing to convert to an A:T pairing. This random insertion of mutations allows B cells to select for even higher-affinity clones as the humoral response progresses, a process termed affinity maturation. Additionally, B-cell activation induces differentiation of proliferating B cells into long-lived "memory" B cells and plasma cells, whose specialized function is to secrete large amounts of antibody.[47] Again, because each of these differentiated B-cell progeny derived from the *clonal* expansion of the originally activated B cell, their antigenic specificity is virtually identical to that of the original clone (Fig. 1.7).

Immunologic Memory—Primary and Secondary Responses

A unique feature of the adaptive immune system is that of immunologic "memory." In the context of RBC

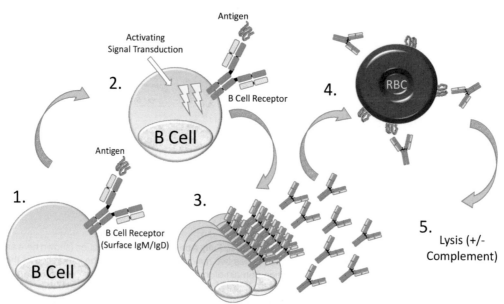

FIG. 1.7 **Simplified Overview of steps in RBC Antibody Production.** 1. The B cell recognizes RBC-specific antigen either as free-floating antigen or when bound to RBC membrane (not shown), via its B-cell receptor (BCR), which is surface-bound IgM or IgD. 2. After receiving activating signaling to cross an activation threshold via either sufficient binding avidity to antigen or via T-cell help, B cells activate. 3. Upon activation, B cells proliferate clonally and begin to differentiate into antibody-secreting plasma cells or long-lived memory B cells. Usually, B cells undergo class-switch recombination, causing secretion of IgG, and less commonly, IgA and IgE antibodies. Plasma cells generated from a single immune response secrete a specific clone of antibody that is unique to the antigen originally encountered by the B cell is Step 1. 4. These antibodies bind their specific "cognate" antigen on RBCs, causing either endocytosis by cells of the reticuloendothelial system in the spleen (not shown), or 5. Fixation of complement and intravascular RBC lysis. (Adapted from Maitta RW. *Clinical Principles of Transfusion Medicine*: Elsevier; 2018.)

transfusion, it is most straightforward to think of T-dependent responses as playing the major role in promoting the initial alloimmunization event. The ensuing humoral response is what is known as a "recall" or secondary immune response. This can be described as a more rapid and robust antigen-specific cellular and humoral immune response when an antigen is presented to the immune system *for the second time* after it has already been activated and primed once.[48] This is due to the aforementioned differentiation of B cells following the initial T-dependent activation response. A portion of activated B cells will differentiate into so-called "memory" B cells with a unique immunophenotypic profile ($CD19^+CD27^+sgM^-sIgD^-$).[49] These cells migrate to the bone marrow where they can reside for years, sometimes for the life of the host. When these memory B cells are exposed to a second stimulus of cognate antigen, they rapidly clonally proliferate, differentiate into plasma cells, and secrete high amounts of

antibody. Although the initial primary humoral immune response occurs on the order of days to weeks, a secondary response happens much more quickly, on the order of just a few days. This is the fundamental process underpinning the long-lived immunity provided by vaccination. Indeed, the use of chemical and biologic adjuvant materials as part of a vaccine formula is designed to induce a T-dependent antigen-specific primary response to the vaccine, providing long-lived immune protection against a specific pathogen.

This process can be visualized readily in a transfusion medicine context as well. When a patient that is antigen-negative for a specific RBC antigen (Kell for example) is transfused with Kell-positive RBCs, the patient does not immediately clear these RBCs from circulation. Rather, their immune system recognizes these Kell-bearing RBCs as foreign, and they develop a specific anti-Kell antibody over the course of several weeks, with a red cell screen typically becoming positive around

30 days following the initial immune priming event (in this case, RBC transfusion). If for some unfortunate reason, this patient is once again transfused with Kell-positive RBCs, even months to years later, the patient can much more rapidly produce anti-Kell antibodies as a secondary immune response, and the transfused RBCs will be cleared from circulation in just a few short days. Alternatively, if the antibody activates the complement cascade (described very briefly later), it can induce intravascular hemolysis of the transfused red cells, resulting in free hemoglobin release, resultant acute kidney injury and potential severe complications for the patient. This underscores just how powerful and rapid a secondary immune response can be.

Complement Cascade

Having discussed the processes of innate immune activation, the adaptive immune response, and the way in which the two are linked, we will now turn back briefly to an innate immune defense mechanism known as the complement system or cascade. The reason for discussing it at this point is because although the complement cascade's primary function is the binding and lysis of pathogens by quite literally poking holes in their cell membranes, it is activated in a transfusion medicine context by the prior binding of alloantibodies to the RBC membrane.[50] Therefore, a prior understanding of the process of RBC alloantibody formation was necessary. It should be noted that only a brief and grossly generalized overview of the complement cascade will be provided here with a transfusion medicine focus, with many important features glossed over for the sake of brevity. For a more in depth and complete picture of the complement cascade, its methods of activation, and roles in host defense, the reader is referred to any number of excellent immunology reference texts and review articles ([8–10,51]).

The complement system is a noncellular, innate immune defense mechanism that consists of enzymes synthesized by the liver that circulate in the blood in their inactive state. As part of the innate immune system, its role is to provide a biochemical means of direct enzymatic pathogen destruction. It is most often called as the complement "cascade" because like a cascading series of waterfalls or dominoes, its activation is initiated by the binding of enzymes most "upstream" in the pathway to either mannose residues commonly found on pathogens, or to antibodies that are bound to pathogen surfaces (or to RBC surfaces!). These in turn activate their downstream members of the cascade. At several points during the activation cascade, enzymatic heterocomplexes of complement cascade components create so-called "convertase" enzymes that serve to greatly amplify the effect of initial activation events to ultimately provide meaningful enzymatic killing of target cells.

Broadly speaking, there are three major pathways in which the complement cascade is initiated. One known as the "lectin" pathway, is initiated by the recognition of mannose residues common to many bacteria by Mannose-Binding Lectins. These in turn serve as scaffolding for the juxtaposition of the most upstream members of the complement cascade, which then activate downstream members. Another pathway is known as the "alternative" pathway, in which there is spontaneous deposition of complement proteins on the surfaces of cells, which left unchecked, initiates downstream members of the cascade. This process is kept in check in healthy individuals by a series of complement regulatory proteins such as Factors D, P, B, H and others. Underscoring the importance of this regulatory arm, mutations in these regulatory proteins underlie the pathophysiology of certain types of so-called nondiarrheal or "atypical" hemolytic uremic syndrome, which manifest as spontaneous unchecked complement-mediated intravascular hemolysis, and can be a cause of significant morbidity and mortality.[52] A third method of complement initiation is the so-called "classical" pathway, which is the primary applicable pathway for transfusion medicine purposes. In this pathway, bound IgG serves as the scaffolding by which the upstream members of the complement pathway, C1q, C1r, and C1s, form a complex and activate, initiating activation of the downstream elements of the pathway.

Importantly, similar to the coagulation cascade, all three complement initiation pathways result in a "final common pathway" of the cascade, by which a "membrane attack complex" is formed through polymerization of the C5b/C6/C7/C8/C9 proteins. This complex literally punches a hole through the membrane of the cell on which it forms, resulting in the leak of cytoplasmic contents, dysregulation of osmotic stability across the cell membrane, and cell rupture. In the context of transfusion medicine, this manifests as acute intravascular hemolysis, in which RBCs are burst while in circulation, releasing free hemoglobin and other intracellular components. This precipitates acute renal toxicity, and is the major cause of significant morbidity and mortality in transfused patients.

Antibody Responses to Red Blood Cell Antigens

From a transfusion medicine perspective, IgG class antibodies are generally directed against protein antigens, and react at physiologic body temperatures (approximately 37°C). Therefore, they are considered clinically significant when identified in a screen or antibody panel. In contrast to IgM antibodies, IgG class antibodies can fix complement to varying degrees, depending on subtype. IgG1 and IgG3 are notable for complement fixation, while IgG2 and IgG4 fix complement poorly[53,54] This is the main reason why ABO group antibodies are so highly clinically significant, as these antibodies comprise at least in part of IgM class antibodies with broad thermal amplitude reactivity.[54] By contrast, the major consideration regarding IgG alloantibodies in transfusion medicine is their ability to opsonize transfused RBCs and cause their removal from circulation by the recipient's spleen. Additionally, because of their monomeric state and relatively small size, they are able to readily cross the placenta in pregnant women and bind antigens on fetal RBCs, causing their destruction. This is the mechanism underlying immune-mediated hemolytic disease of the fetus and newborn.[55]

SUMMARY

The goal of this chapter has been to provide a cursory and transfusion-focused overview of basic immunologic concepts, to better frame subsequent discussions of RBC alloimmunization, transfusion during transplant support, platelet alloimmunization, hemolytic disease of the fetus/newborn, fetal/neonatal alloimmune thrombocytopenia, and certain types of immune-mediated transfusion reactions such as hemolytic and serologic reactions, TRALI, posttransfusion purpura, and others. Based on the concepts introduced in this chapter, we can better understand how upon transfusion, cells of the innate immune system as well as B cells phagocytose fragments of or entire transfused RBCs, and process their surface antigens into peptides that are presented via Class II MHC molecules on professional APCs and B cells to CD4$^+$ T cells. In cases of B-cell recognition of antigen alone, they activate and secrete largely IgM class antibodies, as part of a T-independent humoral response. Alternatively, these B cells can present to CD4$^+$ T cells, which recognize cognate antigen by means of their TCR, and activate to provide costimulatory help to B cells, inducing a T-dependent humoral immune response, in which B cells proliferate and class-switch

to secrete IgG class antibodies and other types. We have also discussed how B cells differentiate into long-lived plasma cells and memory B cells, thus providing a long-term immunologic "memory" to previouslyidentified antigens. Thus, when reexposed to that same antigen, a rapid and strong secondary or "recall" response occurs, and antigen-bearing transfused RBCs are rapidly cleared via antibody-dependent mechanisms. Finally, we closed with a brief look at the complement cascade, focusing on its role in RBC hemolysis and acute hemolytic transfusion reactions via antibody-dependent mechanisms. Hopefully, this chapter has provided a basis for better understanding the immunologic mechanisms behind the transfusion medicine concepts discussed in the coming chapters.

DISCLOSURE STATEMENT

The authors (ILB, CAT) have no direct financial interests in subject matter or materials discussed in this article/chapter.

REFERENCES

1. Hosoi E. Biological and clinical aspects of ABO blood group system. *J Med Investig*. 2008;55:174–182.
2. Heal JM, Liesveld JL, Phillips GL, Blumberg N. What would Karl Landsteiner do? The ABO blood group and stem cell transplantation. *Bone Marrow Transplant*. 2005;36:747–755.
3. Akkok CA, Seghatchian J. Immunohematologic issues in ABO-incompatible allogeneic hematopoietic stem cell transplantation. *Transfus Apher Sci*. 2018;57:812–815.
4. Jaramillo A, Ramon DS, Stoll ST. Technical aspects of oh crossmatching in transplantation. *Clin Lab Med*. 2018;38:579.
5. Forest SK, Hod EA. Management of the platelet refractory patient. *Hematol Oncol Clin N*. 2016;30:665.
6. Salama OS, Aladl DA, El Ghannam DM, Elderiny WE. Evaluation of platelet cross-matching in the management of patients refractory to platelet transfusions. *Blood Transfus-Italy*. 2014;12:187–194.
7. Patel SR, Zimring JC. Transfusion-induced bone marrow transplant rejection due to minor histocompatibility antigens. *Transfus Med Rev*. 2013;27:241–248.
8. Alberts BJA, Lewis J, et al. *Molecular Biology of the Cell*. 6th ed. New York, NY: Garland Science - Taylor & Francis; 2015.
9. Kenneth M, Murphy CW. *Janeway's Immunobiology*. 9th ed. New York, NY: Garland Science, Taylor & Francis Group; 2016.
10. Punt JSS, Jones PP, Owen JA. *Kuby Immunology*. 8th ed. New York, NY: WH Freeman MacMillan Learning; 2019.
11. Cerboni S, Gentili M, Manel N. Diversity of pathogen sensors in dendritic cells. *Adv Immunol*. 2013;120:211–237.

12. Platt AM, Mowat AM. Mucosal macrophages and the regulation of immune responses in the intestine. *Immunol Lett.* 2008;119:22–31.

13. Allavena P, Chieppa M, Monti P, Piemonti L. From pattern recognition receptor to regulator of homeostasis: the double-faced macrophage mannose receptor. *Crit Rev Immunol.* 2004;24:179–192.

14. Krieg AM. Signal transduction induced by immunostimulatory CpG DNA. *Springer Semin Immunopathol.* 2000;22:97–105.

15. Pashenkov MV, Murugina NE, Budikhina AS, Pinegin BV. Synergistic interactions between NOD receptors and TLRs: mechanisms and clinical implications. *J Leukoc Biol.* 2019;105:669–680.

16. Pelka K, De Nardo D. Emerging concepts in innate immunity. *Methods Mol Biol.* 2018;1714:1–18.

17. Rosales C, Uribe-Querol E. Phagocytosis: afundamental process in immunity. *BioMed Res Int.* 2017;2017:9042851.

18. Akira S, Uematsu S, Takeuchi O. Pathogen recognition and innate immunity. *Cell.* 2006;124:783–801.

19. Arango Duque G, Descoteaux A. Macrophage cytokines: involvement in immunity and infectious diseases. *Front Immunol.* 2014;5:491.

20. Mosser DM, Edwards JP. Exploring the full spectrum of macrophage activation. *Nat Rev Immunol.* 2008;8:958–969.

21. Sousa CRE. Activation of dendritic cells: translating innate into adaptive immunity. *Curr Opin Immunol.* 2004;16:21–25.

22. Straat M, van Bruggen R, de Korte D, Juffermans NP. Red blood cell clearance in inflammation. *Transfus Med Hemotherapy.* 2012;39:353–360.

23. Richards AL, Hendrickson JE, Zimring JC, Hudson KE. Erythrophagocytosis by plasmacytoid dendritic cells and monocytes is enhanced during inflammation. *Transfusion.* 2016;56:905–916.

24. Kondo M. Lymphoid and myeloid lineage commitment in multipotent hematopoietic progenitors. *Immunol Rev.* 2010;238:37–46.

25. Heesters BA, van der Poel CE, Das A, Carroll MC. Antigen presentation to B cells. *Trends Immunol.* 2016;37:844–854.

26. Cone RE. Molecular basis for T lymphocyte recognition of antigens. *Prog Allergy.* 1981;29:182–221.

27. Wang JH, Reinherz EL. Structural basis of T cell recognition of peptides bound to MHC molecules. *Mol Immunol.* 2002;38:1039–1049.

28. Hozumi N, Tonegawa S. Evidence for somatic rearrangement of immunoglobulin genes coding for variable and constant regions. *Proc Natl Acad Sci USA.* 1976;73:3628–3632.

29. Alt FW, Oltz EM, Young F, et al. VDJ recombination. *Immunol Today.* 1992;13:306–314.

30. Lieber M. Immunoglobulin diversity: rearranging by cutting and repairing. *Curr Biol.* 1996;6:134–136.

31. Zarnitsyna VI, Evavold BD, Schoettle LN, et al. Estimating the diversity, completeness, and cross-reactivity of the T cell repertoire. *Front Immunol.* 2013;4:485.

32. Nikolich-Zugich J, Slifka MK, Messaoudi I. The many important facets of T-cell repertoire diversity. *Nat Rev Immunol.* 2004;4:123–132.

33. Jones EY. MHC class I and class II structures. *Curr Opin Immunol.* 1997;9:75–79.

34. Xu H, Ren D. Lysosomal physiology. *Annu Rev Physiol.* 2015;77:57–80.

35. Ryder AB, Zimring JC, Hendrickson JE. Factors influencing RBC alloimmunization: lessons learned from Murine models. *Transfus Med Hemotherapy.* 2014;41:406–419.

36. Natarajan P, Liu D, Patel SR, et al. CD4 depletion or CD40L blockade results in antigen-specific tolerance in a red blood cell alloimmunization model. *Front Immunol.* 2017;8:907.

37. Theofilopoulos AN, Kono DH, Baccala R. The multiple pathways to autoimmunity. *Nat Immunol.* 2017;18:716–724.

38. Mouchess ML, Anderson M. Central tolerance induction. *Curr Top Microbiol Immunol.* 2014;373:69–86.

39. Nemazee D. Mechanisms of central tolerance for B cells. *Nat Rev Immunol.* 2017;17:281–294.

40. Reid ME, Lomas-Francis C, Olsson ML. *The Blood Group Antigen Factsbook.* 3rd ed. Amsterdam: Elsevier/AP; 2012.

41. Santana MA, Esquivel-Guadarrama F. Cell biology of T cell activation and differentiation. *Int Rev Cytol.* 2006;250:217–274.

42. Smith-Garvin JE, Koretzky GA, Jordan MS. T cell activation. *Annu Rev Immunol.* 2009;27:591–619.

43. Chen L, Flies DB. Molecular mechanisms of T cell co-stimulation and co-inhibition. *Nat Rev Immunol.* 2013;13:227–242.

44. Macian F. NFAT proteins: key regulators of T-cell development and function. *Nat Rev Immunol.* 2005;5:472–484.

45. Harwood NE, Batista FD. Early events in B cell activation. *Annu Rev Immunol.* 2010;28:185–210.

46. Chahwan R, Edelmann W, Scharff MD, Roa S. AIDing antibody diversity by error-prone mismatch repair. *Semin Immunol.* 2012;24:293–300.

47. Suan D, Sundling C, Brink R. Plasma cell and memory B cell differentiation from the germinal center. *Curr Opin Immunol.* 2017;45:97–102.

48. Farber DL, Netea MG, Radbruch A, et al. Immunological memory: lessons from the past and a look to the future. *Nat Rev Immunol.* 2016;16:124–128.

49. Sanz I, Wei C, Lee FE, Anolik J. Phenotypic and functional heterogeneity of human memory B cells. *Semin Immunol.* 2008;20:67–82.

50. Yazdanbakhsh K. Controlling the complement system for prevention of red cell destruction. *Curr Opin Hematol.* 2005;12:117–122.

51. Noris M, Remuzzi G. Overview of complement activation and regulation. *Semin Nephrol*. 2013;33:479—492.

52. Afshar-Kharghan V. Atypical hemolytic uremic syndrome. *Hematology Am Soc Hematol Educ Program*. 2016;2016: 217—225.

53. Stowell SR, Winkler AM, Maier CL, et al. Initiation and regulation of complement during hemolytic transfusion reactions. *Clin Dev Immunol*. 2012;2012:307093.

54. Flegel WA. Pathogenesis and mechanisms of antibody-mediated hemolysis. *Transfusion*. 2015;55(Suppl 2): S47—S58.

55. de Haas M, Thurik FF, Koelewijn JM, van der Schoot CE. Haemolytic disease of the fetus and newborn. *Vox Sang*. 2015;109:99—113.

CHAPTER 2

Methods of RBC Alloimmunization to ABO and Non-ABO Antigens, and Test Methodologies

KRISTIN STENDAHL, MD • CHRISTOPHER A. TORMEY, MD • IAN L. BAINE, MD, PHD

INTRODUCTION

Red blood cell (RBC) transfusions are a vital part of clinical patient care and can be a critical, life-saving procedure. According to Center for Disease Control and Prevention 2015 National Collection and Utilization Survey (NBCUS), 12,591,000 whole-blood derived and apheresis RBC units were collected and approximately 11,349,000 whole-blood derived and apheresis RBC units were transfused at acute care hospitals in the United States.[1] Blood transfusions only became routine procedures less than 100 years ago. The first successful transfusion of human blood to a patient occurred in 1818 by a British obstetrician, James Blundell, for treatment of postpartum hemorrhage.[2,3] The goal of this chapter is to provide readers with a basic foundation of blood group antigens, antibodies, and blood group systems. With this foundation, the process of RBC alloimmunization will be reviewed including various factors that impact the rate of alloimmunization as well as special considerations for populations at risk for high rates of alloimmunization. Lastly, a brief discussion of the most common testing methodologies as well as emerging molecular techniques will be reviewed.

BLOOD GROUP ANTIGENS

Blood group antigens are clinically important due to their ability to react with antibodies that are formed in antigen-negative individuals after exposure to antigen-positive RBCs either through transfusion or pregnancy with the potential to cause hemolytic transfusion reactions or hemolytic disease of the fetus and newborn (HDFN). The RBC membrane has 23 major antigens present on the extracellular surface that comprised both proteins and carbohydrates. The specificity of blood group antigen is determined either by oligosaccharide epitopes such as ABO antigens or by the amino acid sequence such as the Rh and Kell antigens. The variable RBC antigens arise due to polymorphisms in the genes encoding these proteins, such as single nucleotide polymorphisms, insertions/deletions, or gene rearrangements.[4,5] RBC antigens are involved in several functions including RBC membrane structural integrity, transport proteins, cell adhesion, ligand and/or microbe receptors, complement regulatory proteins, and numerous other functions.[6] Many of the antigens are integrated into the membrane of the red cell; however, others are soluble antigens that are adsorbed onto the surface of the red cell. The portions of the antigens that are recognized by the immune system are termed immunodominant epitopes. The immunodominant epitopes consist of linear stretches of sugars or amino acids, or of amino acids that are distant from each other in primary sequence, but assume a three-dimensional protein structure that brings the amino acid sequences near each other to form a "conformational" antigen (see Fig. 2.1).

For carbohydrate antigens, this usually is up to seven residues long, and most often involves the terminal nonreducing sugar. One important example of such an epitope is the A/B/H glycoprotein/glycolipid antigens. For protein antigens, there are two major groups on the RBC membrane, termed Type 1 and Type 2 proteins. Type 1 proteins pass through the cell membrane once (they resemble a "stick floating upright in water"), and therefore have a single extracellular domain, a single transmembrane domain, and a single intracellular domain. By contrast, Type 2 transmembrane proteins make multiple passes through the cell membrane (resembling the "Loch Ness Monster in a lake"). As such, they have multiple extracellular, intracellular,

Immunologic Concepts in Transfusion Medicine. https://doi.org/10.1016/B978-0-323-67509-3.00002-0

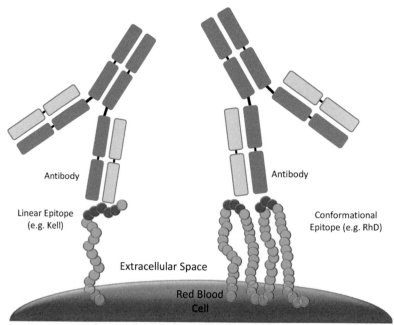

FIG. 2.1 Immunodominant Epitopes. (Adapted from Maitta RW. *Clinical Principles of Transfusion Medicine*. Elsevier; 2018.)

and transmembrane domains. Therefore, antibodies formed against a given protein may be directed against multiple extracellular loops of the same polypeptide chain, as it traverses in and out of the RBC membrane.

BLOOD GROUP ANTIBODIES AND THEIR RESPONSE TO RED BLOOD CELL ANTIGENS

RBC antibodies are classified as either alloantibodies, those produced by individuals against antigens that are not present on their RBC surface, or autoantibodies, those produced by individuals against antigens present on their own RBC surface. In addition, antibodies can be divided into two major categories, naturally occurring antibodies, those formed after exposure to environmental antigens that are similar to RBC antigens, and induced antibodies, those formed after an immune response to red cells through transfusion or pregnancy.

Naturally occurring antibodies, which are generally present at the time of birth or very early in life, arise either from exposure to environmental antigens that have similar structure to red cell antigens or spontaneously. Animal studies in the 1940s and 1950s by Landsteiner and Weiner showed that exposure to pathogens such as certain strains of *Escherichia coli*, which contain antigens similar to the group B RBC antigens resulted

in anti-B alloimmunization in mice who were never exposed to the B antigen directly.[8] This is likely due to cross-reactivity of anti-*Escherichia coli* antibodies with the B antigen, which has further been supported by findings in humans as well.[9–12] Examples of antibodies that are thought to arise spontaneously include those directed against the Rh-E antigen, as well as Lu[a], Di[a], and others.[13] In general, naturally occurring antibodies, whether due to exposure to an antigenic mimic or spontaneously, are formed against carbohydrate antigens (with the exception of anti-E). In addition, naturally occurring antibodies are predominantly IgM, but can contain at least a partial IgG component, with pure IgG antibodies being rare.[14]

Induced antibodies, such as those against the Rh-D, K, Jk, and Fy antigens are only produced after exposure to antigen-positive RBCs via transfusion or pregnancy. The alloimmune responses consist of a gradually forming, weak primary immune response followed by a rapid, strong secondary immune response, with the secondary response being responsible for the clinical manifestations of immunologic transfusion reactions. Studies using Rh-D alloimmunization as the model have demonstrated that alloantibodies are detected by standard serologic methods beginning at approximately 4 weeks after exposure, and reach maximum concentration between 6 and 10 weeks.[15] Studies using other antigens have also demonstrated that the kinetics of primary and secondary responses vary by antigen, but follow the same paradigm as that seen with Rh-D.[16] Consistent with our understanding of immunogenicity of antigens, there appears to be a minimum threshold model of exposure for RBC antigens, above which is sufficient to induce an alloantibody response, and below which does not.[17,18] Whether a recipient will respond or not and the degree to which the recipient will respond to allogeneic RBC exposure will vary based on numerous factors intrinsic to the RBC as well as the patient, which will be discussed later in this chapter.

BLOOD GROUP SYSTEMS

A blood group system consists of inherited RBC antigens defined by specific antibodies. There are over 30 blood group systems currently recognized, each encoded by individual genes.[19] The following discussion is limited to the most clinically relevant blood group systems, including ABO, Rh, Kell, Kidd, Duffy, and MNS blood group systems because of their association with clinically significant antibodies.

ABO Blood Group System

The ABO and H blood groups are the oldest and most important blood group system in transfusion medicine due to their high immunogenicity. The ABO system was originally discovered in 1900 by Austrian scientist, Karl Landsteiner, for which he later received the Nobel prize in 1930. Landsteiner used agglutination tests on glass slides to demonstrate the presence of groups A, B, and O (originally termed C) and later AB in 1902.[3]

The ABO antigens are carbohydrate antigens that are present not only on the surface of RBCs and other hematopoietic cells, but also on organ tissues throughout the body including the kidney, heart, and lung, thus are considered histocompatibility antigens for the purposes of organ transplantation. According to the central dogma of molecular biology, DNA is transcribed into RNA, which is subsequently translated to proteins. However, the ABO and H antigens are carbohydrates antigens attached to the terminal amino acid residues of multiple surface glycoproteins on tissues, including RBCs. The structural base on which both the A and B antigens are built is the H substance, also termed the O antigen. This represents an α1-2 linkage between the terminal galactose and an L-fucose sugar, catalyzed by the enzyme α-2-L-fucosyltransferase (H transferase), coded for by the H gene, an enzyme present in more than 99.99% of the general population. Once the H substance is formed, it can be further modified by the action of two other enzymes to produce either the A or B antigens. Rather than coding for the sugars themselves, the ABO genetic locus at 9q34 has three alternative major alleles, A, B and O, which codes for alternative forms of an enzyme that functions as glycosyltransferases. The alleles coding for A and B differ in just three critical amino acid residues G235S, L266M, and G268A.[20] These mutations determine the substrate specificity of the enzyme, and therefore determine the type of sugar that the enzyme will add to the H substance and the resulting antigen formed. The enzyme α-3-N-acetylgalactosaminyltransferase (A transferase), coded by the A allele, can transfer a single N-acetylgalactosamine (GlcNAc) in an α1-3 linkage to the terminal galactose to make the A antigen. Alternatively, the enzyme α1,3-galactosaminyl transferase (B transferase), coded by the B allele, transfers a galactose in a α1-3 linkage to the terminal galactose to make the B antigen. If both isoforms of the A and B genes code for nonfunctional forms of the aforementioned two enzymes, then neither modification is made to the terminal galactose, and the H substance remains untouched; it is then termed the O antigen (Fig 2.2). Conversely, if both of the genes are expressed, both the A and B chains will be produced, and the patient will have the phenotype of Group AB. If the genotype is AA or AO, the patient will express the A antigen only. Similarly, the patient will express the B antigen only with a BB or BO genotype. The genes coding for these varying glycosyltransferases, and thus, for the different A/B/O phenotypes, is present at varying frequencies in the U.S. population depending on ethnicity, as outlined in Table 2.1.

In addition to allelic variants that simply code for the A, B, or O forms of the glycosyltransferases, there are additional genetic mutations that can alter the level of catalytic activity of the enzyme giving rise to what is termed ABO "subgroups." Subgroups are distinguished by decreased amounts of A, B, or O (H) antigens on the RBC surface. This bears the most relevance for how it affects the enzyme responsible for the formation of the A antigen, as A-antigen subgroups are the most common. Review of the A-antigen subgroup will be the primary focus here, as other reference texts cover this topic more comprehensively.[21,22] In approximately 80% of individuals who express the A antigen, the α-3-N-acetylgalactosaminyltransferase has a relatively high level of enzymatic activity, resulting in the production of approximately 1×10^6 A antigens on the surface of a single RBC. This isoform of the enzyme, and its resulting high activity level, is termed A_1. By contrast, the

TABLE 2.1
Diversity of ABO Phenotypes in the United States

ABO Type	Caucasian (%)	Black (%)	Asian (%)	Hispanic (%)
O	45	50	40	56
A	40	28	28	31
B	11	20	25	10
AB	4	4	7	3

remaining 20% of individuals express a relatively ineffi-cient form of the α-3-N-acetylgalactosaminyltransferase enzyme, termed A_2, resulting in approximately 2×10^5 A antigens per RBC.[23] The difference between A_1 and A_2 is important, as individuals who express the A_2 pheno-type or A_2B phenotype are capable of making an anti-A_1 antibody. These individuals may demonstrate an anti-A on serological typing, potentially confounding results. Furthermore, this anti-A_1 can sometimes be reactive at 37°C, making it clinically significant. Therefore, A_2 pa-tients should only receive transfusions from O or A_2 do-nors, and A_2B patients should only be transfused with O, A_2, A_2B, or B donors. There are also numerous other isoforms of the enzyme that catalyzes A antigen

formation, including A_3, A_x, A_m, and A_{el}, the details of which are beyond the scope of this text .

The ABO antigens are present on RBCs as early as 5–6 weeks of gestation, and reach adult levels of expres-sion between 2 and 4 years old due to the increasing levels of branching with age in the precursor chains on which the ABO and H antigens are built. Critically important is the fact that antibodies to the A and/or B antigens form in children by 1 year old, even in the absence of deliberate exposure to these antigens; there-fore, ABO antibodies are considered naturally occurring antibodies. It is thought that these antibodies develop spontaneously due to exposure to environmental bacte-ria with antigens similar to the A and B antigens. Thus,

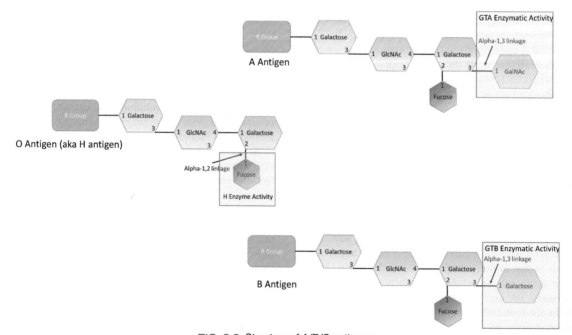

FIG. 2.2 Structure of A/B/O antigens.

natural anti-A and anti-B are likely antibodies to other antigens that cross-react with RBC ABO antigens.

The ABO blood group system is defined by the presence of A and B antigens on the RBC surface and anti-A and anti-B antibodies in the serum. Therefore, patients expressing A antigen will make anti-B antibodies, patients expressing B antigen will make anti-A antibodies, patients expressing O will express both anti-A and anti-B antibodies, as well as an additional third antibody that can react with either A or B, termed anti-A,B antibody. Patients expressing the AB phenotype will not make any anti-ABO antibodies, which is why their plasma is potentially valuable as universal donor units. Anti-A and anti-B antibodies are IgM class antibodies with a broad thermal amplitude, agglutinating cells most efficiently at around 25°C, but can also fix complement and lyse RBCs at 37°C. They cause rapid-onset acute intravascular hemolytic reactions, with associated complications that arise from such a reaction including thrombosis from free hemoglobin exposure and acute renal failure. The anti-A,B antibody formed by Type O patients is an IgG class antibody. Therefore, while anti-A and anti-B cannot cross the placenta in ABO-mismatched maternal–fetal scenarios, the IgG-class anti-A,B can, and in fact it is the most common cause of HDFN. Importantly though, it does not manifest as severely as other antigen mismatches such as anti-D or anti-K, and fetal anemia is often less severe or absent. Anti-A, anti-B, and anti-A,B antibodies are present at varying titers throughout life, but are always detectable, and do not demonstrate senescence.

Rh(D) Blood Group System

After the ABO blood group, the Rh blood group system is the second most antigenic and clinically important of all RBC antigens, with the D antigen being the most clinically important within this system. Alloantibodies to Rh antigens represent some of the most common alloantibodies identified, and are generally considered clinically significant. There is up to an 80% risk of alloantibody formation when Rh(D)-negative patients are exposed to D antigen-positive blood, which is responsible for the most severe forms of HDFN.[24,25]

More than 50 independent Rh antigens have been described with the most important clinically including D, C/c, and E/e. These five major Rh antigens were identified in the 1940s, including Rh-D, C/c, and E/e, with C/c and E/e being alternative alleles. By contrast, there is no alternative allele to the D antigen; it is either expressed or not expressed on the RBC surface. Originally, it was uncertain as to whether these antigens were coded for by a single gene (*RhDCE*) or by three

separate genes (*RhD*, *RhC*, and *RhE*), however, it was later discovered by Tippett in 1980s that all Rh antigens are coded for by two genes, *RhD* and *RhCE*, both located on chromosome 1.[26–28] *RhD* and *RhCE* are highly homogenous genes, each comprising 10 exons and separated from each other by approximately 30 kb.[29,30] The *RhD* gene encodes the D antigen, and the *RhCE* gene encodes the RhCE protein to produce the Cc and Ee antigens. The *RhD* and *RhCE* genes code for transmembrane proteins, each 417 amino acid residues in length, that are nearly identical in structure. Each protein makes 12 passes through the RBC membrane, resulting in six extracellular domains. Two point mutations in different extracellular loops of the RhCE protein, which result in two amino acid substitutions, S103P and P226A, differ between the C/c and E/e alleles, respectively.[13] The phenotypic frequencies of Rh antigen expression vary by ethnic background, and are listed in Table 2.2. A third gene, *RhAG*, located on chromosome 6, encodes for an Rh-associated glycoprotein (RhAG), which is needed for expression of Rh antigens.

As mentioned earlier, only the D allele (denoted by a capital D) can be expressed; a "d" allele does not exist; it is either deleted or mutated resulting in the silencing of its expression, which is denoted as a lowercase d when considering the genotype. Therefore, a patient's genotype can have one expressed copy of RhD (D/d), two expressed copies of RhD (D/D), or no expressed copies (d/d). Phenotypically, patients with either the D/D or D/d genotype will express the D antigen, and are said to be RhD+ ("Rh+"). In contrast, patient's with the d/d genotype will not express any D antigen on the RBC surface, and will be RhD− ("Rh−"). In contrast to the D allele, the C and E alleles are inherited like normal allelic variants as CE, cE, Ce, or ce, with both alleles of the *RhCE* gene being expressed. It should also be noted that advances in molecular sequencing of the Rh genes have identified at least 58 different Rh phenotypic variants, some of which may be clinically significant in certain scenarios, and that genetic recombination events can create novel hybrid genes between *RhD* and *RhCE*; discussion of both of these concepts is beyond the scope here.[21,31]

Using the foundation built in earlier chapters, we can expect that an RhD− patient who is transfused with RhD+ RBCs will form alloantibodies to the RhD antigen. Alloimmunization to the D antigen can occur to any of the extracellular loops or combination of loops that may function as linear or conformational epitopes. Numerous antigenic variants with at least 30 epitopes have been defined to date.[32,33] The antigenicity of the D antigen depends on its density on the transfused RBC. Patients may express the D antigen at a

TABLE 2.2
Rh Antigen Frequency Based on Ethnicity.

Rh Antigen	Caucasian (%)	Black (%)	Asian (%)	Hispanic (%)
D	85	92	99	93
C	68	27	93	71
E	29	22	39	41
c	80	96	47	64
e	98	98	96	81

much lower level; this is termed the "weak D" antigen.[34] Although the extracellular portions of the weak D antigen are the same as those in normal RhD+ patients, the weak D antigen results from numerous amino acid changes that result in impaired efficiency of protein insertion in the cell membrane and decreased stability of the RhD protein in the RBC membrane, resulting in reduced expression of D protein epitopes at the surface. Weak D patients may test as RhD-negative by serologic methods; however, if weak D RBCs are transfused into a truly RhD− patient, the patient may alloimmunize or experience a hemolytic transfusion reaction. Conversely, weak D patients who are pregnant with an RhD− fetus will not need Rh immune globulin (RhIg) prophylaxis, despite serologic negative testing. The most common weak D phenotype, RhD weak type 1, is the result of the nucleotide substitution $89T > G$.[35] Alternatively, another mechanism by which patients may express lower levels of D antigen a phenomenon known as C-*in trans*/Cipellini effect, in which patients with the C allele present *in trans* to the D gene (i.e., on the other copy of chromosome 1), express lower levels of D protein on the RBC surface.[21] These patients may also test serologically as RhD−; however, alloimmunization or hemolytic reactions can occur if their RBCs are transfused into true RhD− patients. Other forms of weak D expression exist such as D_{el}; however, discussion is beyond the scope of this text. Most important clinically is that blood donors who express even small amount of D antigen must be labeled Rh(D)+ to prevent alloimmunization to RhD− patients. As such, AABB Standards require that D-negative blood donors are tested for weak D.[36] In addition, women of childbearing age with RhD phenotyping suggestive of a possible weak D should undergo RhD genotyping, as weak D types 1, 2, or 3 do not need prophylactic RhIg during pregnancy and can receive RhD+ transfusions.

In addition to the weak D antigen, there is another variant known as the "partial D" antigen. Partial D antigen is formed by a hybrid gene rearrangement between the *RhD* and *RhCE*, resulting in a novel RhD-like protein that is missing certain residues in the extracellular portions of the protein, present in the normal RhD protein. As a result, the host is able to form antibodies against these missing residues, and can develop an anti-RhD alloantibody if transfused with RhD+ cells. Partial D antigen can be identified via extended anti-D serologic testing with a panel of anti-D reagents, or by molecular sequencing. Clinically, patients with partial D should be considered D-negative and blood donors with partial D should be considered D-positive.

The anti-C/c and anti-E/e antibodies are produced in response to different epitopes on the RhCE protein. Similar to RhD, the RhCE protein makes 12 passes through the RBC membrane, resulting in six extracellular domains. The C and c antigens differ by a single amino acid substitution, S103P, and the E and e antigens differ by P226A. As mentioned earlier, there are two alleles of RhCE, both of which are expressed. Hence, C/c/E/e antigen expression follows typical Mendelian rules of inheritance, but are codominantly expressed. Similar to RhD, there are several variants of RhCE, with a variant E antigen being the most common, however, still quite rare; these are discussed more fully in other resources.[22,37,38] Antibodies to the Rh system can be directed against the D, C/c, and E/e antigens, or any variants thereof. For the purposes of simplicity, we will only focus on anti-RhD (anti-D), anti-RhC/c (anti-C or c), and anti-Rh-E/e (anti-E or e).

The D antigen is the most immunogenic of the Rh system, with experimental studies showing up to an 85% alloimmunization rate.[25] Transfusion of even a portion of 1 unit of Rh-incompatible cells is adequate to elicit an antibody response. Interestingly, the remaining 15% of patients that do not form detectable anti-D antibodies upon first exposure are termed "nonresponders"; however, half of this group will eventually form an anti-D antibody upon subsequent exposure to Rh-incompatible cells. In addition, retrospective studies of D-negative patients who received numerous intraoperative D+ transfusions showed an alloimmunization rate of 95% when detected with enzyme-treated cells. Studies of patients who received fewer or a single unit show lower rates of alloimmunization, but still at significant rates, especially when "boosted" with a second antigen exposure 6 months later.[15,39,40] Interestingly, immunosuppressed patients make anti-D at relatively low rates, underscoring the role of the recipient's immune status at the time of antigen exposure. Anti-D antibodies can wane over a period of many years, but have been detected up to 38 years following exposure.[41] Nonetheless, even if the antibody is not detected by serologic methods, the patient will remain immunized to the D antigen for the remainder of their life.

Anti-D is an IgG class antibody, it can cross the placenta and cause a severe form of HDFN. Maternal formation of anti-D antibody can be seen as early as 2 months and as late 5 months, and does not form more rapidly if exposed multiple times. Although anti-D IgG_1 and IgG_3 subclasses have been demonstrated, anti-D generally does not fix complement efficiently, and more often results in a serologic transfusion reaction, with extravascular clearance of antigen-positive RBCs. Due to its IgG nature, anti-D is primarily detected via the indirect antiglobulin test (IAT), though some antisera can agglutinate RBCs directly. Formation of anti-D antibodies in patients has become increasingly rare due to the introduction of RhIg prophylaxis in the late 1960s combined with the standardized use of RhD typing to detect patients with weak D and partial D variants. RhIg acts by binding the RhD+ RBCs and shields them from immune recognition, thereby preventing the formation of anti-D. There are a few scenarios, however, that still pose a risk of alloimmunization. Pregnant women who receive inadequate prenatal care and fail to receive RhIg prophylaxis are at increased risk of forming anti-D antibodies. In addition, release of emergent Rh-incompatible units to trauma patient's presenting with massive bleeding can result in the formation of anti-D antibodies, although the rates of alloimmunization in this population are decreased as compared to healthy recipients.[42] Another more commonly encountered scenario is a Rh-D negative patient receiving platelet transfusions, which contain a small amount of contaminating RBCs. One study of immunosuppressed patients receiving "Rh-incompatible" platelet units showed that up to 8% of patients develop detectable anti-D, although other studies have demonstrated lower rates.[43–45] The formation of anti-D following platelet transfusion can be mitigated with the coadministration of RhIg as a prophylactic measure. In addition to blood transfusions, anti-D can form following solid organ transplantations with one study showing 5% incidence of anti-D formation after a renal transplant.[46]

Clinically significant IgG class antibodies directed against the C, c, E, and e antigens have all been documented. Of these, the anti-E antibody is the most common with an incidence of 19.4%,[47] however, virtually all cases are naturally occurring anti-E, making the E antigen a very weak antigen from the perspective of alloimmunization. Anti-C is the next most common antibody, with an incidence of less than 5% in a large study of over 18,700 transfused U.S. military veterans.[47] This study population was largely male, and therefore the incidence in the general population is likely slightly higher due to exposure through pregnancy. Anti-c, while rare, is notable because it is solely formed because of antigenic exposure; no natural forms of this antibody exists. Anti-e has been reported, although studies show the e antigen to be weakly immunogenic. Anti-e antibody, however, is clinically significant once formed.

Although most anti-Rh antibodies are alloreactive antibodies, resulting from antigen exposure via transfusion or pregnancy, well-documented cases of Rh-specific autoantibodies exist as well. By far, the most commonly encountered specificity is the auto-anti-E, which is characterized as a natural antibody, appearing in patients without transfusion, and in both pregnant and nulliparous women. Generally speaking, the auto-anti-E is clinically insignificant, as these antibodies are only detected via the IAT, and do not cause destruction of E-antigen positive RBCs at 37°C. Cold-reactive auto-anti-D IgG antibodies can be detected as well in up to 3% of patients in some studies; however, similar to the auto-anti-E, these antibodies are generally clinically insignificant, and only rare case reports exist of auto-anti-D antibodies reactive at 37°C. Auto-anti-C antibodies have also been characterized and are cold-reactive antibodies typically of the IgG class, and are not considered clinically significant.

Kell Blood Group System

The Kell blood group system, which consists of at least 34 antigens,[13] is the third most immunogenic, following the ABO and Rh systems. Compared to the RhD antigen, the K antigen is approximately 8–10 times less immunogenic. The Kell antigens are encoded by the *KEL* gene located on chromosome 7q33 and carried by the Kell glycoprotein, a 93-kd single-pass membrane protein. The following discussion will focus on the most frequently clinically encountered antigens including K, k, Kp[a], Kp[b], Js[a], and Js[b]. A comprehensive review of all antigens can be found in numerous texts.[21,22,48,49]

Within the Kell system, the K antigen, and its alternate allele k, is encountered the most frequently clinically. The K and k antigens are encoded by a single protein that differs only by a single amino acid substitution, T193M, which disrupts the motif for N-glycosylation and may explain for the high immunogenicity of the K antigen.[50] The K antigen is expressed in approximately 9% of whites and 1.5% of blacks, either in homozygous or heterozygous (Kk) forms. In contrast, the k antigen (also called as "Cellano") is present in nearly 100% of patients. Additional K alleles, also on 7q33, code for the closely related antigens Kp[a], Kp[b], Js[a], and Js[b]. The Kp[a] and Kp[b] antigens differ by single amino acid substitution, W281 and R281, respectively. Similarly, Js[a] and Js[b] antigens differ by single amino acid substitution, P597 and L597, respectively.[13]

After ABO and Rh antibodies, anti-K is the next most common alloantibody with an incidence ranging between 14% and 28%.[51,52] Studies have estimated the risk of forming an anti-K at 10% if an individual is transfused with at least 1 unit of K-antigen positive blood.[53,54] Similar to formation of anti-C antibodies, recipients who form anti-D antibodies are more likely to form anti-K antibodies as well, likely reflective of the general "responder" capability of the individual patient. Although anti-K antibodies are able to fix complement, they do so incompletely, and do not cause formation of the membrane attack complex. Nonetheless, anti-K is predominantly an IgG$_1$ class antibody, therefore, capable of causing severe hemolytic transfusion reactions. In addition, severe HDFN can occur in K-antigen positive fetuses due to the ability of the antibody to cross the placenta and clear fetal red cells from circulation as well as bind and destroy fetal erythrocytic precursors, which express the K antigen early in lineage development.[55–57] As a consequence, severe fetal anemia results due to suppressed fetal hematopoiesis. The frequency of anti-K in pregnant women is approximately 1/1000,[58,59] and the incidence of HDFN due to anti-K is estimated at 1/20,000. Different from other cases of maternal–fetal alloimmunization where the antibody titer correlates with the severity of fetal anemia, anti-K titers do not correlate with the degree of anemia. In the presence of maternal anti-K antibodies,

TABLE 2.3 Diversity of Kell Phenotypes by Ethnicity.		
Kell Phenotype	**Caucasian (%)**	**Black (%)**
K−k+	91	98
K + k+	9	2
K + k−	0.2	<1
Kp[a]−Kp[b]+	98	100
Kp[a] + Kp[b]+	2	<1
Js[a]−Js[b]+	<1	0
Js[a] + Js[b]+	100	80
Js[a] + Js[b]−	<1	19

the rate of hydrops or fetal death ranges from 15% to 38%.[60–64] Cell-free fetal DNA testing assays now exist to test fetal K genotype in pregnant mothers with a known anti-K. Although anti-K is by far the most prevalent and severe cause of HDNF, Js[a] and Js[b] and Kp[a] antibodies have also been associated with HDFN.

In contrast to anti-K, anti-k antibody is rare due to its status as a high-incidence antigen with expression in approximately 98% of patients. Conversely, the incidence of anti-k ranges from 0.005% of blacks, to up to 2% of whites in the United States.[22] Anti-Kp[a] and Kp[b] are also rare, as are anti-Js[a] and Js[b,] about 0.5% and 0.4%, respectively.[47] Similar to anti-K, they too are capable of mediating hemolytic transfusion reactions. The antigenic frequencies of the various Kell group antigens are outlined in Table 2.3.

Kidd Blood Group System

The Kidd blood group system consists of three antigens, Jk[a], Jk[b], and Jk3, encoded for by the *Slc14a1* gene located on chromosome 18q12. The Kidd protein is a 10-pass transmembrane protein, with five extracellular loops.[22] It is known to function as a urea transporter in the RBC membrane, transporting urea out of red cells as they pass through regions of high urea concentration thus preventing dehydration.[65]

The antigenic frequencies of the various Kidd group antigens are outlined in Table 2.4. Jk[a] and Jk[b] antigens are codominantly expressed and differ by the p.D280N polymorphism.[13] The Jk3 phenotype, which is present at an incidence of up to 1.4% in some Pacific Islander populations,[66] represents a null phenotype, where the individual has an unexpressed allele at the *Slc14a1* locus. This is most commonly due to a splice site mutation, or a p.S291P point mutation.[67]

TABLE 2.4 Diversity of Kidd Phenotypes by Ethnicity.			
Kidd Phenotype	Caucasian (%)	Black (%)	Asian (%)
$Jk^a + Jk^b-$	26	52	23
$Jk^a + Jk^b+$	50	40	50
Jk^a-Jk^b-	24	8	27

TABLE 2.5 Diversity of Duffy Phenotypes by Ethnicity.			
Duffy Phenotype	Caucasian (%)	Black (%)	Asian (%)
$Fy^a + Fy^b-$	20	10	81
$Fy^a + Fy^b+$	48	3	15
Fy^a-Fy^b+	32	20	4
Fy^a-Fy^b-	0	67	0

Most anti-Jk^a and Jk^b antibodies are IgG_1 and IgG_3, but $IgG_{2/4}$ and IgM components also exist. A large study of transfused U.S. veterans showed a frequency of 21% for anti-Jk^a antibody and approximately 1% for anti-Jk^b.[47] Two important features of anti-Jk^a and Jk^b antibodies are their ability to fully activate the complement cascade, resulting in delayed acute and serologic hemolytic transfusion reactions. The latter feature is due to their ability to fall to undetectable levels by conventional serologic methods just several months following alloimmunization, a phenomenon known as antibody evanescence. In addition, Jk^a and Jk^b antigens have a role as minor histocompatibility antigens in renal allografts due to the high concentration of the Jk antigens on renal medullary tissue. Studies have shown that mismatched renal allografts show a higher degree of cellular infiltration in early rejection.[68]

Duffy Blood Group System

There are five antigens in the Duffy system including Fy^a, Fy^b, Fy3, Fy5, and Fy6.[13] Antigens within the Duffy blood group system are coded by the *DARC* gene, which codes for the (CD234) receptor protein that binds inflammatory cytokines interleukin-8, monocyte chemotactic peptide (MCP-1), and melanoma growth stimulatory activity (MGSA).[69] The most commonly encountered antigens within the Duffy system are Fy^a and Fy^b, which are expressed codominantly and differ by the G42D polymorphism. Approximately two thirds of blacks in the United States express neither antigen, and some populations worldwide show 100% of people with a Fy^a-/Fy^b-phenotype. This is due to a mutation in the promoter of the *DARC* gene at the binding site of GATA-1, a transcription factor that drives Fy antigen transcription. The Fy antigen is still expressed on other tissue,[70] preventing alloantibody formation in these patients. Cases also exist where Fy^a and Fy^b antigens are missing due to deletions or other inactivating mutations; in these cases, Fy antigen expression is completely lost in all tissues, and these patients can form the anti-Fy3 or anti-Fy5 antibodies, which react with $Fy^{a/b}$ antigen positive RBCs. The antigenic frequencies of the various Duffy blood group antigens are outlined in Table 2.5.

Anti-Fy^a is present in about 30% of patients,[47] with anti-Fy^b being much less common. There appears to be a strong association between anti-Fy^a formation and the human leukocyte antigen (HLA) DRB1*04 allele, indicating that presentation of the Fy^a antigen may be dependent on a very specific antigen presentation configuration.[71] Anti-Fy^a and anti-Fy^b are predominantly IgG_1 class antibodies and are known to cause both acute and delayed hemolytic transfusion reactions, as well as HDFN.[72]

An association between *Plasmodium vivax* and *Plasmodium knowlesi* and patients with $Fy^{a/b}$ null phenotype is well known.[73,74] The Duffy glycoprotein is the receptor for the malarial parasite. It was discovered that the Fy antigens serve as a binding site and point of entry for these parasites into RBCs and patients with $Fy^{a/b}$ null phenotype were resistant to RBC infection. This may explain selective evolutionary pressure toward the $Fy^{a/b}$ null phenotype in malaria-endemic regions. Duffy antigens are destroyed by proteolytic enzymes, which is helpful in serologic methods to determine antibody specificity when multiple antibodies are under investigation.[21,75]

MNS Blood Group System

The MNSs system is notable for marked antigenic diversity; however, most of the variants are not clinically significant. There are over 46 different alleles currently identified within the blood group system. The antigens are encoded by *GYPA* and *GYPB* homologous genes located on chromosome 4. *GYPA* contains seven exons and encodes the glycophorin A (GPA) molecule; *GYPB* contains five exons and encodes the glycophorin B (GPB) molecule.[13,76] GPA and GPB are single-pass proteins that contain distinct intracellular, transmembrane, and extracellular domains, and serve as entry receptors for *Plasmodium falciparum*.[77,78] Glycophorin B also serves as a binding site for the C3b component of the complement cascade.

The MNS system is divided into the MN and Ss loci, the two major allelic loci of most frequent clinical significance. Both of these alleles follow Mendelian inheritance, and can be expressed codominantly making all possible permutations of M/N/S/s expression possible. The M and N antigens are expressed on GPA, while the S and s (and U) antigens are expressed on GPB, with the differences between M and N, and S and s, consisting of alterations in the terminal amino acid sequence of their respective proteins. The S-s- phenotype is rare, and found in approximately 1.5%; these individuals also lack the high incidence U antigen (100% whites, 99% blacks), and are capable of developing an alloantibody to the U antigen,[79] making it exceedingly difficult to obtain compatible units. Table 2.6 shows the frequency of MNS phenotypes by ethnicity.

Anti-M and anti-N alloantibodies are common, typically naturally occurring, cold-reactive antibodies, all of which are at least partly IgM class; auto-anti-M may be IgG alone. Up to 4% of infants and adults are found to have anti-M that is reactive at 37°C; therefore, anti-M is a clinically significant antibody.[47,80] Anti-M alloantibody has been demonstrated to form up to 12% of the time in the context of alloimmunization to other major alloantigens, such as RhD, indicating that the M antigen itself is not highly immunogenic. Although anti-M and anti-N do not bind complement or mediate intravascular hemolysis, there are case reports of delayed hemolytic reactions due to anti-M and anti-N, and therefore these antigens are still honored when providing compatible red cell units to patients. In addition, they are not implicated in HDFN as they are IgM class antibodies.

Anti-S and anti-s are typically IgG class antibodies that are reactive at 37°C, and can mediate both hemolytic transfusion reactions and HDFN. The high-incidence U antigen is a shared epitope of the S and s antigens; patients that are S-s- are therefore capable of alloimmunizing to U as well and forming a clinically significant anti-U, which can cause hemolytic reactions and HDFN.

ALLOIMMUNIZATION TO BLOOD GROUP ANTIGENS

Introduction

Although potentially life-saving, RBC transfusions are not without risks. One of the most clinically significant risks of transfusions is alloimmunization and its consequences. In 2015, hemolytic transfusion reactions due to non-ABO incompatibilities (14% of fatalities) and ABO incompatibilities (7.5% of fatalities) accounted for the third leading cause of transfusion-associated deaths in the United States, following transfusion-related acute lung injury and transfusion associated circulator overload.[81] Therefore, an understanding of factors that impact alloimmunization rates, patient populations at greatest risk, and mitigation strategies to prevent and minimize alloimmunization is critical for transfusion medicine physicians as well as clinicians.

RBC alloimmunization is the process of forming antibodies against nonself RBC antigens that occurs when an individual that lacks a particular antigen is exposed to the antigen through transfusion or pregnancy. Antigen exposure is necessary but not sufficient to trigger alloimmunization. There are numerous factors that are believed to impact whether an individual will alloimmunize. The main mechanism believed to underlie alloimmunization is the presentation of donor antigen peptides by APC to TCR on recipient CD4 T cells.

Factors that Impact Alloimmunization

Some patients alloimmunize rapidly to an initial exposure to antigen, while others respond poorly. Thus, patients can be classified as "responders" and "nonresponders," with those who do alloimmunize further classified as either a "strong" or "weak" responder to allogeneic RBCs. There are several factors that impact whether or not a patient will become alloimmunized, divided broadly into those related to the donor and recipient, those intrinsic to the RBC antigen, and those related to the transfused RBC unit.[82]

Donor and recipient factors include underlying disease state, degree of inflammation, number of previous transfusions, patient intrinsic "immune

TABLE 2.6 Diversity of MNS Phenotypes by Ethnicity.		
MNS Phenotype	**Caucasian (%)**	**Black (%)**
M + N−	30	25
M + N+	49	49
N−N+	21	26
S + s−	10	6
S + s+	42	24
S−s+	48	68
S−s−	0	2

responder" status, ethnicity, prior pregnancies, HLA haplotype, and others. Patient inflammatory status at the time of transfusion is believed to have a large impact on the rate of alloimmunization. For example, in patients with sickle cell disease (SCD), alloimmunization rates have been shown to be higher when patients receive a transfusion during an acute illness.[83] Other conditions with increased inflammation have also shown increased rates of alloimmunization such as inflammatory bowel disease and other chronic autoimmune diseases.[84] Patients HLA haplotype has also been correlated with alloimmunization. A study looking at the impact of HLA haplotype suggested that the HLA-DRB1*15 phenotype may predispose transfused recipients to the formation of multiple different RBC alloantibodies. Specifically, the study found that HLA-DRB*15 was present in approximately 40% of individuals possessing multiple antibodies versus in approximately 25% of individuals with a single antibody or control population.[85]

Factors intrinsic to the antigen include the immunogenicity and copy number of the antigen. The immunogenicity of an antigen is estimated based on the number of individuals that produce an alloimmune response to that particular antigen combined with the probability that they were exposed to that antigen, which is based on the frequency of the antigen in the donor population. The density or copy number of antigens on the surface of the RBC also varies between the different antigens and is thought to contribute to immunogenicity. Animal studies investigating the role of copy number in immune responses to transfused transgenic murine RBCs expressing human KEL glycoprotein showed that recipients transfused with RBCs expressing KEL antigen at a greater copy number where more likely to generate anti-KEL antibodies after a single transfusion compared to recipients transfused RBCs with a lower copy number.[86]

Factors related to the RBC unit include the age of the unit and method of unit preparation such as washing, volume reduction, leukoreduction, irradiation, among others. Studies looking at the effect of the age of the RBC unit on the potential for alloimmunization in general show no effect of aged RBC units on RhD alloimmunization.[87–89] One retrospective study evaluating the association between RBC unit age and alloimmunization rates in patients with SCD, however, found an association between age of the unit and risk of RBC antibody formation with an HR of 3.5 with units 7 days old and an HR of 9.8 with units 35 days old. Given that SCD patients are known to have a higher baseline risk for alloantibody formation, additional studies are needed to clarify whether this holds up for other patient populations, ideally factoring in patient disease and immune status.[90]

Other components of the overall blood transfusion process can contribute to potential alloimmunization including process errors that can occur during the manufacturing of the blood component, in which there is a breakdown in the process by which the correct compatible blood unit is matched to the correct patient. There are many steps in this, and can briefly be summarized as follows: collection of blood unit from correctly identified donor → testing of collected unit for ABO and Rh(D) antigens → correct labeling of the unit → duration and conditions of storage and transport of the unit → correct drawing and labeling of type and screen sample from the recipient → assuming unit is compatible by type and screen/crossmatch and antibody panel if needed, correct labeling of the unit with the intended transfusion recipient → transfusion of the unit within the allotted 4 hours upon exit from the blood bank. A breakdown in this process most commonly occurs in the clerical steps during which there is correct identification and labeling of patients, blood units, and type/screen samples, both at the collection center and at the transfusion center. Lookback studies determined that 0.25% of blood was administered to the wrong patient[91] and a large study of nearly 700,000 collected blood samples showed mislabeling in 1 out of every 165 samples. Newer additions to the process of collection/labeling, such as barcode scanner identification of both the patient and sample at the patient's bedside, will help to mitigate this source of error.

Alloimmunization in Select Populations
General hospital-based patients
Approximately 1%–3% of the general hospital-based patient population will form an alloantibody;[92–94] however, this data is based on retrospective analysis of patients at a single institution and thus alloimmunization rates are likely higher than these reports. Up to 7% of healthy adults in the general transfused population will form an alloantibody,[95] reflecting the overall relatively low frequency of transfusions. In contrast, patient populations who chronically receive numerous transfusions, including patients with hemoglobinopathies as well as patients with hematologic malignancies, are more likely to form alloantibodies.

Patients with hemoglobinopathies
Patients with SCD receive frequent transfusions, and alloimmunization in this population has critical clinical consequences including acute and delayed hemolytic

transfusion reactions, bystander hemolysis, delay in providing compatible blood, and HDFN. In addition, a recent study correlated RBC alloimmunization with overall worse survival in patients with SCD, with patients without alloimmunization showing life expectancies approximately a decade longer than did alloimmunized patients.[96] Studies have estimated the alloimmunization rate in children and adults with SCD to be up to 29% and 47%, respectively, when partial or extended Rh antigen matching is not performed.[97,98] The antibodies most prevalent in patients with SCD include those against Rh, K, and Jk^b antigens.[99] The high alloimmunization rates in SCD are thought to be due not only to the frequency of transfusions, but also to population-level discrepancies in the frequency of the Rh-system and K antigens. Therefore, many institutions will procure RhD/C/E and K-antigen matched units when transfusing SCD patients. Another related factor to the high alloimmunization rate in this population is the finding that patients with SCD have been shown to express unique variants of Rh-system antigens at a higher frequency than the general population, further complicating the identification of truly matched units.[100] This may account for more recent studies showing persistent alloimmunization in SCD patients even when receiving phenotypically D/C/E/K-matched units.[100] Future molecular RBC phenotyping and matching methods may address this important issue. In the case of SCD specifically, alloimmunization rates in children are lower than in adults, and studies have shown that alloimmunization rates are lower with RBC exposure via erythrocytapheresis as compared to simple transfusion.[101,102] Interestingly, a subset of patients with SCD never become alloimmunized despite chronic transfusions. The degree of chronic inflammation at the time of transfusion is postulated to play a role, in addition to differences in immunologic or genetic signatures in "responder" and "nonresponders" patients. Studies have shown that patients with SCD presenting with acute chest syndrome or vaso-occlusive crises were more likely to alloimmunize than nonacute SCD patients.[83,96]

β-Thalassemia is another condition in which chronic transfusions are necessary for disease management, typically beginning early in life. Several studies have investigated the rate of alloimmunization in patients with thalassemia showing a range from 5% to 48%,[103] with most antibodies directed against Rh or K antigens, although the overall rates vary depending on the region studied and the likely degree of donor/recipient phenotype mismatch. One study showed

approximately 21% of patients alloimmunizing after 6 years of transfusion (average 18 units/year), with drastically lower rates present in the group receiving D/C/E/K matched units (3.7%) as compared to RhD-only matched units (15.7%).[104–106]

Patients with hematologic malignancies

Patients with hematological disorders frequently require multiple transfusions placing this population at increased risk for alloimmunization. Several studies have investigated the rates alloimmunization in patients with various hematologic disorders. Studies investigating alloimmunization in patients with myelodysplastic syndrome (MDS) or MDS-related disorders and acute myeloid leukemia have shown rates ranging from 15% to 59%[107,108] and 3% to 16%,[108,109] respectively. Conversely, studies investigating the rate of alloimmunization in patients with lymphoid neoplasms have shown very lower rates of alloimmunization thought to be due to either underlying impaired immune function or the chemotherapy regimen. Studies have shown a 0% rate of alloimmunization in patients with acute lymphocytic leukemia and Hodgkin lymphoma.[108,110] Rates ranging from 2% to 3% have been demonstrated in patients with non-Hodgkin lymphomas and plasma cell neoplasms.[108]

Preventing and Managing Red Blood Cell Alloimmunization

Because the primary goal of the transfusion medicine service is to provide safe and effective blood components, the prevention of alloimmunization is essentially the chief safety role of the transfusion physician on a day-to-day basis. In addition to the short-term consequences of potential immune-mediated transfusion reactions and their sequelae, the long-term consequences of developing novel alloantibodies are significant as well. Depending on the nature of the alloantibody, it can moderately or severely restrict the available pool of compatible RBC units going forward for the patient, potentially prolonging the process of finding safe blood for transfusion in time-sensitive clinical situations such as acute chest syndrome in patients with SCD. These considerations are of particular importance for populations who require chronic lifelong transfusions such as patients with SCD or β-thalassemia major. Thus, preventing alloantibodies from forming in the first place or mitigating the dangers of existing alloantibodies would lead to decreased transfusion-associated morbidity and mortality.

Patient transfusion history

Because many alloantibodies evanesce over time, obtaining a complete, accurate transfusion history for a patient is of critical, as it may reveal an undetectable clinically significant alloantibody. It is common for patients to receive transfusions at more than one institution, and to date there is no national centralized transfusion database or alloantibody identification records, leaving only the patient's recollection as our best option for determining undetectable alloantibodies. One study of 100 patients undergoing hospital transfusion revealed a 64% prevalence of discrepancy in alloantibody records when comparing detection at the authors' institution and records obtained from other local and distant hospitals.[111] These data highlight the need for a centralized shared antibody database to ensure safe blood administration to patients.

RBC transfusion threshold

One method to prevent the formation or sequela of alloantibodies is the adoption of a restrictive transfusion strategy, thereby preventing patients from exposure to RBC antigens. Currently, there still remains variation in clinical practice on thresholds used to transfuse patients. Based on review of several randomized control studies, the AABB has issued clinical practice guidelines recommending a restrictive transfusion approach with a hemoglobin threshold of 7 g/dL for hospitalized adult patients who are hemodynamically stable and a value of 8 g/dL for patients undergoing cardiac or orthopedic surgery and patients with preexisting cardiovascular disease. In patients with acute coronary syndrome, severe thrombocytopenia, and chronic transfusion-dependent anemia a threshold of 7 g/dL is likely comparable to 8 g/dL; however, no randomized control data is available for this population.[112] According to the 2015 NBCUS, there has been a 13.9% decline in RBC transfusions in the United States compared to 2013, likely reflective in part due to this evidence supporting judicious use of blood components as well as increased awareness of appropriate transfusion thresholds.[1]

Antigen-matched red blood cells

An additional strategy to mitigate alloimmunization is to provide partially antigen-matched RBC units between the donor and recipient. Current guidelines[113] recommended that patients with SCD receive prophylactically matched RBCs for C/c, E/e, and K/k for reasons outlined previously. Currently, many institutions provide C/c, E/e, and K-antigen serologically matched units when transfusing patients with SCD. Currently, there

are no guidelines regarding providing phenotypically matched units beyond Rh(D) for patients with β-thalassemia. Studies, however, have shown lower rates of alloimmunization in patients with thalassemia receiving RBCs matched at ABO, Rh, and K (3.7%) compared with patients receiving RBCs matched at ABO and Rh(D) (22.6%).[114]

Leukoreduction

Leukoreduction is another method with potential to minimize RBC alloimmunization rates. Leukoreduction is the process of removing donor leukocytes from the RBC unit through a filter by action of size exclusion, with most of the RBCs and platelets passing through the filter and leukocytes remaining behind. In addition, adhesion between the filter and leukocytes further prevents leukocytes from passing through the filter. The process of leukoreduction can occur either at the time of blood component manufacturing, termed prestorage leukoreduction, or immediately before transfusion of the RBC unit, termed poststorage leukoreduction. There are approximately 5×10^8 leukocytes in one unit of RBCs before leukoreduction. After leukoreduction, this is decreased to at least 5×10^6 leukocytes or less per RBC unit.[115] In addition to removing leukocytes, leukoreduction also has been shown to remove proinflammatory mediators such as IL-1 and IL-8, reduce HLA antibody production, and prevent transmission of certain infectious agents. Studies investigating the role of leukoreduction for prevention of alloimmunization have shown mixed results with some studies showing clinical benefit and reduced rates of alloimmunization,[116] while others showing no benefit. Additional well-controlled studies are needed to clarify this further. In addition, it is thought that the timing of the leukoreduction processing may impact the number of leukocytes, cytokines, and other particles[117] and therefore the rate of alloimmunization.

TESTING METHODOLOGIES

The blood bank service performs various tests to ensure the safe administration of blood components to patients. This section will cover the most common immunohematologic tests performed by the transfusion medicine service for transfusion compatibility and antibody identification, including antibody screening, direct and indirect antiglobulin tests, red blood cell eluates, and minor antigen phenotyping. In addition, emerging molecular methods for genotyping will be briefly discussed.

Serological Typing Methods

In 1907, Ludvig Hektoen realized that the safety of transfusions might be improved by cross-matching blood between donors and patients. Reuben Ottenberg, subsequently performed the first blood transfusion using blood typing and cross-matching. Today, the transfusion service performs various tests including ABO and Rh typing, direct antiglobulin testing (DAT), and antibody detection and identification procedures in addition to others to provide the most effective, safe blood components to patients. In addition to pretransfusion testing, red blood cell phenotyping is used to screen blood donors and donor RBC units for select antigens and in prenatal testing to type fathers of mothers with alloantibodies that can cause fetal hemolysis.

ABO and Rh(D) antigens are the most important antigens for safe transfusion to avoid severe hemolytic complications; therefore, typing for these antigens is routinely performed for both transfusion recipients and blood donors. In 1947, it became standard practice to perform ABO blood-typing on each RBC unit. Typing for common minor blood group antigens is not typically performed; however, an antibody screen against selected antigens in the Rh, Kell, Kidd, Duffy, and MNS system is performed. Serologic typing is the most commonly used method of testing, which uses the principle of hemagglutination as the reaction end point. Hemagglutination is the recognition of red cell clumping because of antibody binding to antigen on the RBC surface when a patients' specimen, either plasma or RBCs, is mixed with a reagent. A scale of 0−4 + is used to grade the presence of hemagglutination, with 0 indicating no agglutination and 4 + indicating a strong agglutination reaction. Hemagglutination reactions can be read and interpreted either manually or by automated methods. Serologic typing methods offer the benefit of being inexpensive, rapid, and accurate for most blood donors and recipients. Various serologic typing methods to detect hemagglutination have been developed for compatibility testing including tube typing, gel typing, solid phase adherence, among others. Tube typing involves visualizing a red cell serum mixture macroscopically and looking for the presence of hemagglutination. Grading of the strength of hemagglutination reaction using this method is manually performed by technologist and therefore is somewhat subjective and requires extra time by technologist to interpret. Gel typing, in contrast, has the potential for automation in addition to increased sensitivity compared to tube typing. The gel test was first developed in 1985 by Dr. Yves Lapierre.[118]

In this method, RBCs interact with antibodies at the top of a column. RBCs are forced into dextran-acrylamide gel matrix by centrifugation and based on the principle of size exclusion, agglutinated RBCs are too large to go through the matrix, therefore remain at the top of the gel column while nonagglutinated RBCs move to the bottom of the gel column. The gel typing method requires less technologist time as the gel cards can be read either using automated equipment or manually. Moreover, the gel typing provides a more stable reaction endpoint that can be reviewed up to 3 days and more reproducible results compared to the tube typing method. The most recently developed method, solid phase typing, is a method in which antihuman globulin is immobilized onto a solid medium and the patient's serum is added, resulting in the binding to the F_c region of the patient's serum antibodies. Then, reagent red cells are added and incubated, and the reaction is centrifuged. A positive reaction constitutes the spreading of the RBCs in a "carpet" pattern across the well indicating binding of reagent to RBCs, whereas a negative reaction constitutes an RBC "button" at the bottom of the well after centrifugation. Solid phase tests have shown to be more sensitive than conventional tube methods[119] and can also be automated. Automation decreases the opportunity for human errors and allows personnel to perform other tasks. Modifications to these various standard serologic methods described earlier may be necessary in certain situations such as obtaining phenotypes in patients recently transfused; however, discussion of this topic is outside the scope of this text (Fig. 2.3).

When the blood bank service receives a request for a blood component transfusion, a type and screen is performed. The type refers to determining the patients ABO and Rh(D) status, and the screen refers to detecting and identifying RBC autoantibodies or alloantibodies in the patient's plasma or serum. A patient's ABO status is determined by performing a forward grouping (also called as front type) for the presence or absence of A or B antigens and a reverse grouping (also called as back type) for the presence of anti-A or anti-B antibodies in plasma. For most patients, the Rh(D) status is determined by testing for the presence or absence of Rh(D), with phenotyping for other non-Rh(D) antigens reserved for select populations at increased risk for alloimmunization. Various tests are used to identify autoantibodies and alloantibodies for the purpose of identifying clinically significant antibodies associated with hemolytic transfusion reactions and HDFN. These include the IAT, DAT, RBC panel tests, and RBC elution, which will be discussed later (Table 2.7).

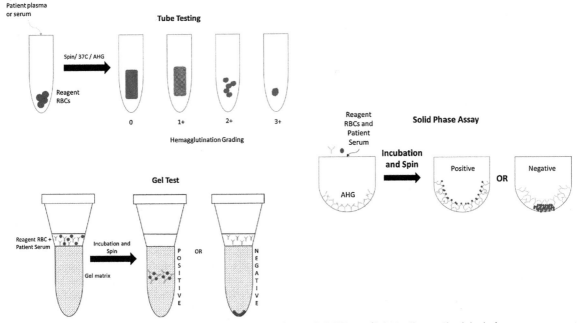

FIG. 2.3 Diagram of Tube (left), Gel (middle), and Solid Phase (right testing methodologies).

The purpose of the IAT is to identify possible antibodies by mixing patient plasma with various reagent screening cells expressing clinically significant non-ABO antigens. Antihuman globulin (AHG) is added to detect the presence of agglutination. A positive IAT will be followed up with an RBC antibody panel to determine the specific antibody or antibodies causing the positive IAT reaction. RBC panel assays are performed by mixing patients' plasma with several reagent screening cell lines.

The DAT (also known as the Direct Coombs test) is a two-step process used to determine whether antibody and/or complement bound is bound to the surface of RBCs. In the first step, a polyspecific reagent to detect IgG or C3 complement on the surface of RBCs is added to patient RBCs, either resulting in no agglutination (negative DAT) or agglutination (positive DAT). In the case of a positive DAT, AHG or anti-C3 is then added to determine if IgG (positive with addition of AHG) and/or C3 (positive with addition of anti-C3) is coating the surface of the RBC. Generally, a positive IgG DAT indicates a warm-reactive antibody and extravascular hemolysis, while a positive C3 DAT indicate a cold-reactive antibody and intravascular hemolysis. There are various reasons for a positive DAT result, however, the most clinically relevant is hemolysis. Examples of causes of false positive DATs include previous transfusion, RBC rouleaux, and certain drugs.

TABLE 2.7
ABO Typing.

REACTION WITH CELLS		REACTION WITH SERUM			INTERPRETATION
Anti-A	Anti-B	A1 cells	B cells	O cells	ABO group
0	0	+	+	0	O
+	0	0	+	0	A
0	+	+	0	0	B
+	+	0	0	0	AB

RBC elution studies are used to evaluate positive DATs with IgG reactivity to determine the specificity of antibody bound to the RBC surface. An acidic elution buffer is added to patient's antibody-coated RBCs, which causes the antibodies to dissociate from the surface of the RBCs. The resultant concentrated antibody eluate is mixed with reagent panel cells to determine the antibody specificity. Note that C3 positive DATs are typically associated with IgM antibodies, which are poorly eluted from the RBC surface.

Molecular Typing Methods

Although RBC phenotyping to evaluate antigen expression on the surface of RBCs has historically been performed using serologic methods, molecular typing has emerged in recent years as a potential alternative or supplemental method. Although serological typing involves directly determining a patient's phenotype, molecular typing involves indirectly predicting a patient's phenotype by genotype test. As discussed in the beginning of this chapter, most blood group antigens are inherited from single nucleotide gene polymorphisms via Mendelian inheritance. Molecular typing uses DNA methods to determine these polymorphisms and mutations controlling antigen expression to predict the antigen phenotype. Molecular typing is generally performed using genomic DNA extracted from whole blood or alternatively cellular samples. A polymerase chain reaction is used to amplify the region of interest with subsequent detection of sequence variations unique for the antigens.

Although not currently widely adapted, molecular typing is now offered at several blood centers and reference testing laboratories. In addition, select hospital blood banks are starting to offer limited molecular testing. There are particular situations in which molecular typing can be especially useful such as fetal genotyping for HDFN, molecular testing of fetal and paternal samples in pregnant women with clinically significant antibodies, follow-up for patients with positive DAT, recently transfused patients, identifying variant antigens such as weak and partial D, resolving serologic typing discrepancies, and identification and matching for Rh variants more commonly seen in SCD populations.

Molecular typing, however, is not without limitations and therefore for the time being is typically used in conjunction with serologic typing. Currently, molecular typing requires specialized equipment, trained personnel, and laboratory informatics platforms for processing results. In addition, because molecular testing only offers a prediction of the patient's likely phenotype based on polymorphisms, the patients' true phenotype may be different if various changes that impact the protein are not taken into consideration. Therefore, molecular typing results should be interpreted with caution and in conjunction with serologic typing results.

SUMMARY

In this chapter, we reviewed the most clinically significant blood group systems, as well as the various factors impacting alloimmunization. We hope that this chapter provided a basic understanding of the mechanism of RBC alloimmunization and the resulting clinical significance. Although many advances have been made in understanding factors that impact alloimmunization rates, much more work remains to understand the causes of differing alloimmunization rates observed between individuals. Lastly, we briefly covered the most common testing methodologies performed by the blood bank service including emerging molecular genotyping methods.

DISCLOSURE STATEMENT

The authors (KS, CAT, ILB) have no direct financial interests in subject matter or materials discussed in this article/chapter.

REFERENCES

1. Ellingson KD, et al. Continued decline in blood collection and transfusion in the United States-2015. *Transfusion.* 2017;57:1588−1598.
2. Greenwalt TJ. A short history of transfusion medicine. *Transfusion.* 1997;37(5):550−563.
3. Giangrande PL. The history of blood transfusion. *Br J Haematol.* 2000;110(4):758−767.
4. Storry JR, Olsson MR. Genetic basis of blood group diversity. *Br J Haematol.* 2004;126:759−771.
5. Daniels G. The molecular genetics of blood group polymorphism. *Hum Genet.* 2009;126:729−742.
6. Reid ME, Mohandas N. Red blood cell blood group antigens: structure and function. *Semin Hematol.* 2004;41(2): 93−117.
7. Maitta RW. *Clinical Principles of Transfusion Medicine.* Elsevier; 2018.
8. Wiener AS. Origin of naturally occurring hemagglutinins and hemolysins; a review. *J Immunol.* 1951;66(2): 287−295.
9. Drach GW, Reed WP, Williams Jr RC. Antigens common to human and bacterial cells: urinary tract pathogens. *J Lab Clin Med.* 1971;78(5):725−735.
10. Drach GW, Reed WP, Williams Jr RC. Antigens common to human and bacterial cells. II. *E. coli* O14, the common

Enterobacteriaceae antigen, blood groups A and B, and *E. coli* 086. *J Lab Clin Med.* 1972;79(1):38–46.

11. Springer GF, Horton RE. Blood group isoantibody stimulation in man by feeding blood group-active bacteria. *J Clin Investig.* 1969;48(7):1280–1291.

12. Wittels EG, Lichtman HC. Blood group incidence and *Escherichia coli* bacterial sepsis. *Transfusion.* 1986;26(6): 533–535.

13. Reid M, et al. *The Blood Group Antigens Factbook.* 3rd ed. Cambridge, Mass: Academic Press; 2012.

14. Chattoraj A, Gilbert Jr R, Josephson AM. Immunologic characterization of anti-H isohemagglutinins. *Transfusion.* 1968;8(6):368–371.

15. Samson D, Mollison PL. Effect on primary Rh immunization of delayed administration of anti-Rh. *Immunology.* 1975;28(2):349–357.

16. Redman M, Regan F, Contreras M. A prospective study of the incidence of red cell allo-immunisation following transfusion. *Vox Sang.* 1996;71(4):216–220.

17. Cohen F, et al. Mechanisms of isoimmunization. I. the transplacental passage of fetal erythrocytes in homospecific pregnancies. *Blood.* 1964;23:621–646.

18. Zipursky A, et al. The transplacental passage of foetal red blood-cells and the pathogenesis of Rh immunisation during pregnancy. *Lancet.* 1963;2(7306):489–493.

19. International Society of Blood Transfusion, R.C.I.a.B.G.T.h.w.i.o.w.-p.r.-c.-i.-a.-b.-g.-t.

20. Yamamoto F, et al. Molecular genetic basis of the histo-blood group ABO system. *Nature.* 1990;345: 229–233.

21. Fung MK, et al. *Technical Manual of the American Association of Blood Banks.* 18th ed. Bethesda, MD: American Association of Blood Banks (AABB); 2014.

22. Klein HG, Anstee DJ. *Mollison's Blood Transfusion in Clinical Medicine.* 12th ed. West Sussex, United Kingdom: John Wiley & Sons; 2014.

23. Hosoi E. Biological and clinical aspects of ABO blood group system. *J Med Investig.* 2008;55:174–182.

24. Pollack W, et al. Studies on Rh prophylaxis. II. Rh immune prophylaxis after transfusion with Rh-positive blood. *Transfusion.* 1971;11(6):340–344.

25. Urbaniak SJ, Robertson AE. A successful program of immunizing Rh-negative male-volunteers for anti-D production using frozen-thawed blood. *Transfusion.* 1981; 21(1):64–69.

26. Colin Y, Bailly P, Cartron JP. Molecular-genetic basis of Rh and Lw blood-groups. *Vox Sang.* 1994;67:67–72.

27. Colin Y, et al. Genetic basis of the RhD-positive and RhD-negative blood-group polymorphism as determined by Southern analysis. *Blood.* 1991;78(10):2747–2752.

28. Mouro I, et al. Molecular-genetic basis of the human Rhesus blood-group system. *Nat Genet.* 1993;5(1):62–65.

29. Flegel WA. Molecular genetics and clinical applications for RH. *Transfus Apher Sci.* 2011;44(1):81–91.

30. Westhoff CM. The structure and function of the Rh antigen complex. *Semin Hematol.* 2007;44(1):42–50.

31. Nardozza LM, et al. The molecular basis of RH system and its applications in obstetrics and transfusion medicine. *Rev Assoc Med Bras.* 1992;56(6):724–728, 2010.

32. Avent ND, et al. Site directed mutagenesis of the human Rh D antigen: molecular basis of D epitopes. *Vox Sang.* 2000;78(Suppl 2):83–89.

33. Scott ML, et al. Epitopes on Rh proteins. *Vox Sang.* 2000; 78(Suppl 2):117–120.

34. Agre PC, et al. A proposal to standardize terminology for weak D antigen. *Transfusion.* 1992;32(1):86–87.

35. Quraishy N, Sapatnekar S. Advances in blood typing. *Adv Clin Chem.* 2016;77:221–269.

36. Ooley PW, et al. *Standards for Blood Banks and Transfusion Services.* 30th ed. Bethesda: AABB; 2015.

37. Flegel WA. Molecular genetics of RH and its clinical application. *Transfus Clin Biol.* 2006;13(1–2):4–12.

38. Prisco Arnoni C, et al. RHCE variants inherited with altered RHD alleles in Brazilian blood donors. *Transfus Med.* 2016;26(4):285–290.

39. Mollison PL, et al. Suppression of primary RH immunization by passively-administered antibody. Experiments in volunteers. *Vox Sang.* 1969;16(4):421–439.

40. Woodrow JC, et al. Mechanism of Rh prophylaxis: an experimental study on specificity of immunosuppression. *Br Med J.* 1975;2(5962):57–59.

41. Stratton F. Rapid Rh-typing: a sandwich technique. *Br Med J.* 1955;1(4907):201–203.

42. Meyer E, Uhl L. A case for stocking O D+ red blood cells in emergency room trauma bays. *Transfusion.* 2015;55(4): 791–795.

43. Cid J, et al. Low frequency of anti-D alloimmunization following D+ platelet transfusion: the Anti-D Alloimmunization after D-incompatible Platelet Transfusions (ADAPT) study. *Br J Haematol.* 2015;168(4):598–603.

44. Goldfinger D, McGinniss MH. Rh-incompatible platelet transfusions–risks and consequences of sensitizing immunosuppressed patients. *N Engl J Med.* 1971; 284(17):942–944.

45. Weinstein R, et al. Prospective surveillance of D- recipients of D+ apheresis platelets: alloimmunization against D is not detected. *Transfusion.* 2015;55(6):1327–1330.

46. Quan VA, et al. Rhesus immunization after renal transplantation. *Transplantation.* 1996;61(1):149–150.

47. Tormey CA, Fisk J, Stack G. Red blood cell alloantibody frequency, specificity, and properties in a population of male military veterans. *Transfusion.* 2008;48(10): 2069–2076.

48. Daniels G, et al. International Society of Blood Transfusion Committee on terminology for red blood cell surface antigens: Macao report. *Vox Sang.* 2009;96(2): 153–156.

49. Daniels GL, et al. Terminology for red cell surface antigens. ISBT working party Oslo report. International Society of Blood Transfusion. *Vox Sang.* 1999;77(1):52–57.

50. Lee S, Wu X, Reid ME. Molecular basis of the Kell (K1) phenotype. *Blood.* 1995;85:912–916.

51. Grove-Rasmussen M. Routine compatibility testing: standards of the AABB as applied to compatibility tests. *Transfusion.* 1964;4:200–205.

52. Tovey GH. Preventing the incompatible blood transfusion. *Haematologia*. 1974;8(1–4):389–391.

53. Maurer C, Buttner J. [The frequency of irregular erythrocyte antibodies (author's transl)]. *Dtsch Med Wochenschr*. 1975;100(30):1567–1570, 1573.

54. Wiener AS, et al. Studies on immunization in man. III. Immunization experiments with pooled human blood cells. *Exp Med Surg*. 1955;13(4):347–352.

55. Daniels G, Green C. Expression of red cell surface antigens during erythropoiesis. *Vox Sang*. 2000;78(Suppl 2): 149–153.

56. Vaughan JI, et al. Inhibition of erythroid progenitor cells by anti-Kell antibodies in fetal alloimmune anemia. *N Engl J Med*. 1998;338(12):798–803.

57. Vaughan JI, et al. Erythropoietic suppression in fetal anemia because of Kell alloimmunization. *Am J Obstet Gynecol*. 1994;171(1):247–252.

58. Caine ME, Mueller-Heubach E. Kell sensitization in pregnancy. *Am J Obstet Gynecol*. 1986;154(1):85–90.

59. Mayne KM, Bowell PJ, Pratt GA. The significance of anti-Kell sensitization in pregnancy. *Clin Lab Haematol*. 1990; 12(4):379–385.

60. Bowman JM, et al. Maternal Kell blood group alloimmunization. *Obstet Gynecol*. 1992;79(2):239–244.

61. Frigoletto Jr FD. Anti-Kell and hydrops. *Am J Obstet Gynecol*. 1978;130(3):376.

62. Frigoletto FD, Davies IJ. Erythroblastosis fetalis with hydrops resulting from anti-Kell isoimmune disease. *Am J Obstet Gynecol*. 1977;127(8):887.

63. Goh JT, et al. Anti-Kell in pregnancy and hydrops fetalis. *Aust N Z J Obstet Gynaecol*. 1993;33(2):210–211.

64. Scanlon JW, Muirhead DM. Hydrops fetalis due to anti-Kell isoimmune disease: survival with optimal long-term outcome. *J Pediatr*. 1976;88(3):484–485.

65. Macey RI, Yousef LW. Osmotic stability of red cells in renal circulation requires rapid urea transport. *Am J Physiol*. 1988;254:669–674.

66. Woodfield DG, et al. The Jk(a-b-) phenotype in New Zealand polynesians. *Transfusion*. 1982;22(4):276–278.

67. Lawicki S, Covin RB, Powers AA. The Kidd (JK) Blood Group System. *Transfus MedRev*. 2017 Jul;31(3):165–172.

68. Rourk A, Squires JE. Implications of the Kidd blood group system in renal transplantation. *Immunohematology*. 2012;28(3):90–94.

69. Hadley TJ, Peiper SC. From malaria to chemokine receptor: the emerging physiologic role of the Duffy blood group antigen. *Blood*. 1997;89(9):3077–3091.

70. Rojewski MT, Schrezenmeier H, Flegel WA. Tissue distribution of blood group membrane proteins beyond red cells: evidence from cDNA libraries. *Transfus Apher Sci*. 2006;35(1):71–82.

71. Noizat-Pirenne F, et al. Relative immunogenicity of Fya and K antigens in a Caucasian population, based on HLA class II restriction analysis. *Transfusion*. 2006; 46(8):1328–1333.

72. Goodrick MJ, Hadley AG, Poole G. Haemolytic disease of the fetus and newborn due to anti-Fy(a) and the potential clinical value of Duffy genotyping in pregnancies at risk. *Transfus Med*. 1997;7(4):301–304.

73. Miller LH, et al. The resistance factor to Plasmodium vivax in blacks. The Duffy-blood-group genotype, FyFy. *N Engl J Med*. 1976;295(6):302–304.

74. Horuk R, et al. A receptor for the malarial parasite Plasmodium vivax: the erythrocyte chemokine receptor. *Science*. 1993;261(5125):1182–1184.

75. Meny GM. The Duffy blood group system: a review. *Immunohematology*. 2010;26:51–56.

76. Reid ME. MNS blood group system: a review. *Immunohematology*. 2009;25:95–101.

77. Li X, et al. Identification of a specific region of Plasmodium falciparum EBL-1 that binds to host receptor glycophorin B and inhibits merozoite invasion in human red blood cells. *Mol Biochem Parasitol*. 2012;183(1):23–31.

78. Wang HY, et al. Rapidly evolving genes in human. I. the glycophorins and their possible role in evading malaria parasites. *Mol Biol Evol*. 2003;20(11):1795–1804.

79. Issitt PD. Heterogeneity of anti-U. *Vox Sang*. 1990;58(1): 70–71.

80. Murakami J. MNSs blood group system and antibodies(anti-M, -N, -S and -S antibodies). *Nihon Rinsho*. 2010; 68(Suppl 6):743–747.

81. FDA/CBER. Fatalities Reported to FDA Following Blood Collection and Transfusion. Annual Summary for Fiscal Year 2015. %3ci%3e%3ca href= https://www. notifylibrary.org/sites/default/files/FDA%20Fatality% 20Report-2015.pdf. [cited 2019 March 10].

82. Hendrickson JE, Tormey CA. Understanding red blood cell alloimmunization triggers. *Hematology Am Soc Hematol Educ Program*. 2016;1:446–451.

83. Fasano RM, et al. Red blood cell alloimmunization is influenced by recipient inflammatory state at time of transfusion in patients with sickle cell disease. *Br J Haematol*. 2015;168(2):291–300.

84. Ryder AB, Hendrickson JE, Tormey CA. Chronic inflammatory autoimmune disorders are a risk factor for red blood cell alloimmunization. *Br J Haematol*. 2016; 174(3):483–485.

85. Schonewille H, et al. HLA-DRB1 associations in individuals with single and multiple clinically relevant red blood cell antibodies. *Transfusion*. 2014;54(8):1971–1980.

86. Hendrickson JE, et al. Development of a murine model of weak Kel: similarities to weak Rh(D). *Blood*. 2012;120: 842.

87. Dinardo CL, et al. Transfusion of older red blood cell units, cytokine burst and alloimmunization: a case-control study. *Rev Bras Hematol Hemoter*. 2015;37(5):320–323.

88. Lacroix J, et al. Age of transfused blood in critically ill adults. *N Engl J Med*. 2015;372(15):1410–1418.

89. Yazer MH, Triulzi DJ. Receipt of older RBCs does not predispose D-negative recipients to anti-D alloimmunization. *Am J Clin Pathol*. 2010;134(3):443–447.

90. Desai PC, et al. Alloimmunization is associated with older age of transfused red blood cells in sickle cell disease. *Am J Hematol*. 2015;90(8):691–695.

91. Baele PL, et al. Blood transfusion errors. A prospective survey by the Belgium SanGUIS group. *Vox Sang.* 1994; 66:117–121.
92. Winters JL, et al. RBC alloantibody specificity and antigen potency in Omsted county, Minnesota. *Transfusion.* 2001; 41:1413–1420.
93. Spielmann W, Seidl S. Prevalence of irregular red cell antibodies and their significance in blood transfusion and antenatal care. *Vox Sang.* 1974;26:551–559.
94. Hoeltge GA, et al. Multiple red cell transfusions and alloimmunization. Experience with 6996 antibodies detected in a total of 159,262 patients from 1985 to 1993. *Arch Pathol Lab Med.* 1995;119:42–45.
95. Ngoma AM, et al. Red blood cell alloimmunization in transfused patients in sub-Saharan Africa: a systematic review and meta-analysis. *Transfus Apher Sci.* 2016;54(2): 296–302.
96. Telen MJ, et al. Alloimmunization in sickle cell disease: changing antibody specificities and association with chronic pain and decreased survival. *Transfusion.* 2015; 55(6):1378–1387.
97. Aygun B, et al. Clinical significance of RBC alloantibodies and autoantibodies in sickle cell patients who received transfusions. *Transfusion.* 2002;42(1):37–43.
98. Josephson CD, et al. Transfusion in the patient with sickle cell disease: a critical review of the literature and transfusion guidelines. *Transfus Med Rev.* 2007;21(2):118–133.
99. Vichinsky EP, Earles A, Johnson RA. Alloimmunization in sickle-cell-anemia and transfusion of racially unmatched blood. *N Engl J Med.* 1990;322(23):1617–1621.
100. Chou ST, et al. High prevalence of red blood cell alloimmunization in sickle cell disease despite transfusion from Rh-matched minority donors. *Blood.* 2013;122(6): 1062–1071.
101. Michot JM, et al. Immunohematologic tolerance of chronic transfusion exchanges with erythrocytapheresis in sickle cell disease. *Transfusion.* 2015;55(2):357–363.
102. Wahl SK, et al. Lower alloimmunization rates in pediatric sickle cell patients on chronic erythrocytapheresis compared to chronic simple transfusions. *Transfusion.* 2012;52(12):2671–2676.
103. Matteocci A, Pierelli L. Red blood cell alloimmunization in sickle cell disease and in thalassaemia: current status, future perspectives and potential role of molecular typing. *Vox Sang.* 2014;106(3):197–208.
104. Azarkeivan A, et al. RBC alloimmunization and double alloantibodies in thalassemic patients. *Hematology.* 2015;20(4):223–227.
105. Azarkeivan A, et al. Blood transfusion and alloimmunization in patients with thalassemia: multicenter study. *Pediatr Hematol Oncol.* 2011;28(6):479–485.
106. Dhawan HK, et al. Alloimmunization and autoimmunization in transfusion dependent thalassemia major patients: study on 319 patients. *Asian J Transfus Sci.* 2014; 8(2):84–88.
107. Guelsin GA, Rodrigues C, Visentainer JE. Molecular matching for Rh and K reduces red cell alloimmunisation in patients with myelodysplastic syndrome. *Blood Transfus.* 2015;13(1):53–58.
108. Seyfried H, Walewska I. Analysis of immune response to red blood cell antigens in multitransfused patients with different diseases. *Mater Med Pol.* 1990;22(1): 21–25.
109. Blumberg N, Hael JM, Gettings KF. WBC reduction of RBC transfusions is associated with a decreased incidence of RBC alloimmunization. *Transfusion.* 2003;43(7): 945–952.
110. Blumberg N, Peck K, Ross K. Immune response to chronic red blood cell transfusion. *Vox Sang.* 1983;44(4): 212–217.
111. Unni N, et al. Record fragmentation due to transfusion at multiple health care facilities: a risk factor for delayed hemolytic transfusion reactions. *Transfusion.* 2014;54(1): 98–103.
112. Carson JL, et al. Clinical practice guidelines from the AABB: red blood cell transfusion thresholds and storage. *J Am Med Assoc.* 2016;316(19):2025–2035.
113. NIH N. *Evidence-based Management of Sickle Cell Disease: Expert Panel Report;* 2014. Available at: https://www.nhlbi.nih.gov/health-topics/evidence-based-management-sickle-cell-disease.
114. Spanos T, Karageorga M, Ladis V. Red cell alloantibodies in patients with thalassemia. *Vox Sang.* 1990;58(1): 50–55.
115. Jackman RP, et al. Leukoreduction and ultraviolet treatment reduces boht the magnitude and the duration of teh HLA antibody response. *Transfusion.* 2014;54: 672–680.
116. Ryder AB, Zimring JC, Hendrickson JE. Factors influencing RBC alloimmunization: lessons learned from murine models. *Transfus Med Hemotherapy.* 2014;41(6): 406–419.
117. Radwanski K, et al. The effects of red blood cell preparation method on in vitro markers of red blood cell aging and inflammatory response. *Transfusion.* 2013;53(12): 3128–3138.
118. Lapierre Y, et al. The gel test: a new way to detect red cell antigen-antibody reactions. *Transfusion.* 1990;30(2): 109–113.
119. Uthemann H, Poschmann A. Solid-phase antiglobulin test for screening and identification of red cell antibodies. *Transfusion.* 1990;30:114–116.

CHAPTER 3

Autoimmunity: Cold and Warm Autoantibodies and Autoimmune Hemolytic Anemia

EMILY J. LARKIN, BSC • MEGHAN DELANEY, DO, MPH • MAGALI J. FONTAINE, MD, PHD

INTRODUCTION

Red blood cell (RBC) autoantibody occurrence is a common finding during RBC typing and antibody screen in blood bank-based immunohematology laboratories. The rate of autoantibody formation in patients with RBC antibody screens is low at 0.17%. For most (80%) of those patients, these autoantibodies do not cause hemolysis and are often referred as silent autoantibodies.[1] Silent autoantibodies are often naturally occurring, have low affinity to self-antigens, and may play a role in initiating or suppressing biologic effects that are not always well determined. However, this chapter will focus on autoantibodies associated with autoimmune hemolytic anemia (AIHA).

AIHA is a disease in which autoantibodies bound to erythrocytes induce hemolysis. AIHA is a relatively rare disorder with an incidence of 1 in 90,000: 30% more common in females than males and in adults greater than 40 years old.[2] These autoantibodies are bound to self-erythrocyte antigens, characterized by a positive Coombs test, also referred as a direct antiglobulin test (DAT). Diagnostically, the temperature, at which the autoantibody is active in vitro, often classifies AIHA mimicking the in vivo environment causing clinical symptoms. Warm-reactive autoantibodies are implicated in most AIHA cases for both children and adults (~75% and ~90%, respectively) with the rest being classified as cold-reactive or mixed (i.e., both warm- and cold-reactive) antibodies.[3] AIHA can also be categorized based on etiology; primary or idiopathic AIHA comprises ~50% of cases while the other 50% of AIHA cases are secondary to malignancy, an autoimmune disease, or an infection.[3] The current understanding of the immune dysregulation associated with autoantibody formation, as well as the mechanism of

RBC destruction may vary depending on the type of AIHA and are reviewed later (Fig. 3.1). The clinical presentation and laboratory findings are discussed as well.

MECHANISM OF AUTOANTIBODY DEVELOPMENT

The pathophysiology of autoantibody formation is variable but is most often associated with a dysregulation of the normal humoral immune response resulting in a loss of tolerance to RBC self-antigens. The mechanism of the breakdown in B-cell tolerance may be due to a molecular mimicry, a lack of deletion of autoreactive B cells, or a polyclonal T- and/or B-cell activation. Either one of these can be triggered by a lymphoproliferative disorder, an infection, a medication or may be idiopathic. Autoantibodies in warm-type AIHA are IgG isotypes in 90% of cases, whereas cold-type AIHA are primarily associated with IgM class antibodies.

Idiopathic Warm-Type AIHA

The pathogenesis of idiopathic warm-type AIHA is commonly associated with autoimmunization following transfusion.[4,5] In a retrospective analysis of 717 patients type and screen results showing RBC autoantibodies, 200 patients (28%) had alloantibodies as well. The diagnosis of both auto- and alloantibodies occurred simultaneously in 73 of these following blood transfusions.[5] In a similar retrospective analysis by Young and colleagues, out of the 58,946 type and screen results reviewed, 2618 of these were positive; among these, 121 (4.6%) showed autoantibodies.[6] In the cohort of patients with autoantibodies, 41 out of 121 (34%) had both alloantibodies and warm autoantibodies and the remaining 80 (66%) had RBC

Immunologic Concepts in Transfusion Medicine. https://doi.org/10.1016/B978-0-323-67509-3.00003-2

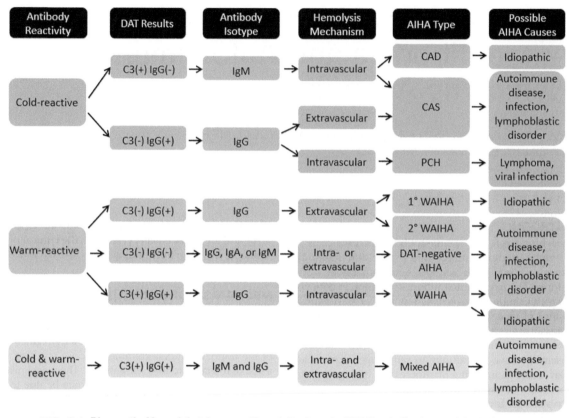

FIG. 3.1 Diagnostic Map of Autoimmune Hemolytic Anemia (AIHA).   Antibody reactivity indicated in AIHA can be broken down into cold-, warm-, and cold- and warm-reactive antibodies, which in turn dictate the results of the direct antiglobulin test (DAT). Based on the results of the DAT, antibody isotype class and subsequently hemolysis mechanism can be theorized. Serological results coupled with clinical findings allow physicians to identify the suspected type of AIHA indicated, as well as causes for the AIHA.

autoantibodies only. Similar to the study by Ahrens et al., a significant percentage (12 out of 41%, 25%) of these patients developed both allo- and autoantibodies in temporal association with a blood transfusion. Investigators posit that the mechanism of autoimmunization begins with immature, low affinity alloantibodies that bind to both alloantigens and host moieties. These alloantibodies then mature into autoantibodies capable of binding to host antigens.[5] It is also proposed that autoantibodies may form after blood transfusion because donor lymphocytes survive and recognize the host RBCs as foreign, producing alloantibodies that mimic autoantibodies.[7] This microchimerism, which may occur in pregnancy and autoimmune diseases, may induce autoantibody formation in idiopathic cases of AIHA. Kaminski and associates demonstrated that T lymphocytes from patients

who were repeatedly transfused developed cytotoxicity against autologous RBCs.[8] Similarly, Paglieroni et al. found, in a cohort study of sickle cell patients, that IgM levels and number of CD5[+] B cells (a precursor B-cell population that produces autoantibodies) were two times greater posttransfusion compared to pretransfusion values.[8] These IgM autoantibodies produced by CD5[+] B cells are polyclonal with low affinity to self-antigens as well as viral antigens, suggesting that therapeutic interventions targeting CD5[+] B cells dysregulation may improve RBC allo- and/or autoimmunization following allogeneic RBC transfusion.

Secondary Warm-Type AIHA

Lymphoproliferative disorders such as Hodgkin's disease, chronic lymphocytic leukemia, or non-Hodgkin's lymphoma, rather than infections, are the leading causes of secondary warm-type AIHA, resulting from an immune dysregulation and a loss of tolerance to RBC antigens.[9−11] Deviant expression of B-cell activating factor of the TNF family has been observed in a variety of autoimmune disorders, resulting in B-cell dysfunction and excess immunoglobulin production. A recent study by Zhao et al. reported increased BAFF serum levels in patients with secondary AIHA compared to healthy controls and to patients with idiopathic AIHA. BAFF serum levels were increased in patients with positive DAT for presence of IgG and complement fraction C3 on RBC surfaces, compared to control healthy patients. Patients with a positive DAT for IgG only, or for C3 only, did not have a significant increase in their BAFF serum levels.[10] These data suggest that BAFF targeted therapies may be considered in a very specific presentation of warm-type AIHA with positive DAT for both IgG and C3, but no such therapeutic trial has yet been reported.

Idiopathic Cold-Type AIHA

Idiopathic cold-type AIHA is also referred as cold agglutinin disease (CAD). Recent studies have uncovered genetic autoantibody features specific to CAD for the immunoglobulin heavy chain (IGH) and light chain that explain the heterogeneity of clinical presentation and disease activity. In a molecular analysis of heavy and light chains of cold agglutinins produced by patients with CAD, almost all patients displayed circulating monoclonal antibodies encoded by the IGH gene *V4-34*, a gene specific for antibody binding to I-antigen.[12] Furthermore, serological testing indicated that light chain immunoglobulin Kappa (IGK) was encoded by either the *IGKV3-20* or the *IGKV3-45* gene in 80% of patients, suggesting that the light chain also contributes to I antigen binding.[13,14] Interestingly, the homology of the complementarity-determining region 3 (CDR3) of *IGKV3-20* was highly conserved in younger patients. As both *IFHV4-34* and *IGKV3-20* genes encode antibodies that bind to infectious antigens,[15] this provides evidence that antigen selection is a primary cause of CAD, especially in younger patients. However, whether the antigen involved in the selection is I antigen or a related exogenous pathogen that triggers CAD is unknown.[16] Similarly, possible causative genetic mutations in CAD include mutations of the *KMT2D* and *CARD11* genes, leading to B-cell proliferation and autoantibody formation.[13] In all, CAD is an indolent lymphoproliferative B-cell disorder with unique mechanisms of dysregulated autoantibody formation and should be distinctly classified from other cold-type AIHA cases.

Secondary Cold-Type AIHA or Cold Agglutinin Disease

Secondary CAD, also known as cold agglutinin syndrome, is rarely due to a lymphoproliferative disorder as is warm-mediated AIHA. The formation of autoantibodies in CAD is more commonly transient and due to infections.[17,18] The best-known infections associated with CAD are mycoplasma pneumonia and Epstein–Barr virus (EBV) infection (i.e., infectious mononucleosis). In CAD associated with *Mycoplasma Pneumoniae*, a high titer of IgM agglutinins is identified in the patient's plasma, 2−3 weeks after the onset of the infection, sometime after resolution of the respiratory symptoms but in the presence of a sudden onset of severe symptomatic anemia. The formation of this IgM-mediated CAD is hypothesized to be a cross-reactive immune response to the mycoplasma antigen with I-antigen specificity. In CAD associated with EBV infection, the IgM agglutinin is cross-reactive with i-RBC antigen, and assumed to be due to a molecular mimicry with EBV surface antigens as well. However, other mechanisms of autoantibody formation in CAD have also been described such as a B-cell hypersensitivity to Toll-like receptor of macrophages, which leads to the activation of B cells through the B-cell receptor/Toll-like receptor (TLR) 7 and TLR9 interaction pathway. The end result is increased proliferation or differentiation of RBC autoantibody secreting cells and subsequent hemolysis.[19]

Paroxysmal Cold Hemoglobinuria

Despite being least common overall, comprising ∼2% of all AIHA cases, paroxysmal cold hemoglobinuria (PCH) was the first AIHA pathology to be recognized.[2] PCH was recognized first in the early 1900s because of the striking symptom of hemoglobinuria, with most cases associated with late or congenital syphilis. Donath and Landsteiner elucidated the pathophysiology of PCH, as a biphasic-reactive antibody (usually IgG) that sensitizes the RBC at cold temperatures, and then causes hemolysis as the temperature rises. Over 100 years later, today PCH is most commonly associated with Parvovirus infection in the pediatric population, with an autoantibody with anti-P specificity against the P antigen on the RBC surface. Other infections, such as infectious mononucleosis or mycoplasma pneumonia, have been less commonly reported to be associated with PCH. Studies of parvovirus inducing anti-P antibodies suggest that the interaction of the virus with the P antigen during infection alters the antigen in such a way that anti-P autoantibody formation is stimulated causing hemolysis.[20]

Atypical AIHA

Atypical AIHA cases present with both warm autoantibodies and cold agglutinins and are relatively rare. Due to the rarity of this condition and heterogeneity of presentation, no singular mechanism of autoantibody formation has been described. However, it is likely that patients with mixed AIHA form autoantibodies via mechanisms observed in both warm- and cold-type AIHA. Therefore, the proposed mechanisms of autoantibody formation in mixed AIHA include polyclonal T-cell and/or B-cell activation, errors in central or peripheral tolerance due to infections,[18] drugs,[21] or immunoregulatory disorders including lymphoproliferative conditions.

MECHANISMS/DETERMINANTS OF RED CELL DESTRUCTION

Mechanisms of red cell destruction in AIHA depend on the type of autoantibody and hence cause different clinical presentations requiring specialized treatment. The properties of RBC clearance depend on the ability of

the autoantibody to activate complement and/or the interaction of the autoantibody with macrophage Fc-receptors. Differences in macrophage Fc-receptor polymorphisms, overall phagocytic activity, expression of complement regulators, and presence of autoreactive natural killer cells have all been shown to influence clinical outcome in AIHA.[22] Here, we describe the main routes for erythrocyte destruction: Fc-mediated hemolysis, complement-mediated hemolysis, as well as other alternative proposed mechanisms for erythrocyte destruction (Figs. 3.2–3.4).

Extravascular Fc-Mediated Hemolysis and Other IgG-Driven Mechanisms

Most warm-mediated AIHA are associated with an IgG isotype binding to the RBC surface (Fig. 3.2). The antibody–RBC complex can form anywhere in the vasculature, and is subsequently susceptible to sequestration by mononuclear phagocytes, mainly macrophages, and destruction in the reticuloendothelial system. This immune red cell destruction occurs mainly in the spleen and liver, referred as extravascular

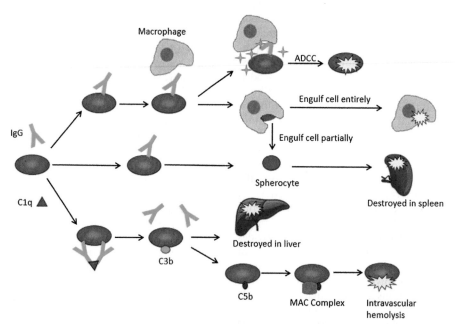

FIG. 3.2 IgG-mediated Hemolysis can Occur Through Three Main Mechanisms. After IgG binding, the Fc region of the antibody can be recognized by macrophages, which destroy the cell by antibody-dependent cellular cytotoxicity (ADCC) or phagocytosis (either complete or partial). Partially phagocytized cells are known as spherocytes and are destroyed completely in the spleen by macrophages along with intact IgG-bound red cells. The third and most rare form of IgG-mediated hemolysis involves the complement pathway. IgG antibodies spaced appropriately for C1q binding can initiate either the classical complement pathway, leading to extravascular hemolysis in the liver via complement protein C3b, or the alternative complement pathway, causing intravascular hemolysis via complement protein C5b and the recruited MAC attack complex.

destruction.[2] Macrophages express IgG receptors specific to the Fc portion of IgG molecules near the carboxyl terminus of the heavy chain.[23] Upon binding to the macrophages Fc receptor, IgG-sensitized red cells are either entirely engulfed by macrophages and destroyed or are only partially internalized, releasing smaller size RBCs called spherocytes. These smaller RBCs may circulate through the blood stream as spherocytes. Hence, spherocytes shown on the peripheral blood smear are indicative of Fc-mediated extravascular hemolysis.[24] Alternatively, lymphocytes are known to have receptors for IgG and complement and secrete lytic cytokines to induce hemolysis via antibody-dependent lymphocyte-mediated cytotoxicity (ADCC).[25,26] Braun et al. have identified a possible mediator of RBC phagocytosis in AIHA as stromal interaction molecule 1 (STIM1), an essential protein for Ca^{2+}-entry-mediated Fc-γ receptor activation.[27] Using a mouse model of AIHA, Braun et al. showed that pathogenic treatment of anti-RBC monoclonal IgG antibodies causes a significantly stronger hematocrit reduction in wild-type mice compared to STIM1$^{-/-}$ mice, indicating that STIM1 is a mediator of AIHA and that STIM1 deficiency is protective against IgG-induced anemia.[27] These findings may serve as a basis for the development of novel pharmacological agents to control or prevent AIHA targeted at these pathways.

Complement-Mediated Hemolysis

Most IgM and certain IgG isotypes (mostly IgG1 and IgG3) bind complement and cause intravascular hemolysis (Fig. 3.3). The IgG or IgM molecules complex with the RBC surface in the peripheral vasculature. The RBC-IgM/IgG complex then fixes complement protein 1q (C1q), initiating the complement pathway. C1 esterase activates C2 and C4 to form C3 convertase, which then cleaves C3 into C3a and C3b. IgM/IgG then detach and separate from the RBC, leaving C3b bound to the red cell surface. C3b-opsonized red cells are prone to extravascular hemolysis via phagocytic monocytes in the liver. Surviving C3b-bound erythrocytes can undergo an additional complement cleavage step to form C3d, a protein with protective properties against hemolysis that can be detected by a DAT. Alternatively, complement activation can also proceed past the C3 stage via the terminal complement pathway in which C3b cleaves C5 into C5a and C5b, initiating the formation of the membrane attack complex (MAC) with other accessory complement proteins (C6, C7, C8, and C9) to cause intravascular hemolysis. Interestingly, authors have shown that positive DAT with IgM only does not necessarily result in intravascular hemolysis, as the IgM coated RBC may also be removed extravascularly by macrophages through their C3 receptor (CR1 and CR3) (Fig. 3.4). If RBCs are sensitized with IgM only (no complement), these may survive normally because macrophages have no receptor for IgM.[28]

PCH, most often caused by transient viral or bacterial infections, is associated with an IgG autoantibody characterized by the Donath and Landsteiner (DL) test. The DL test should be considered in a patient with a DAT result due to C3 and presenting with hemoglobinemia, hemoglobinuria, or both; and no evidence of autoantibody in the serum or the eluate (bound to

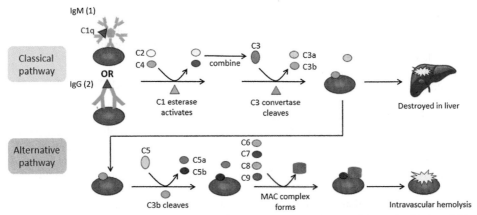

FIG. 3.3 Complement-mediated Intravascular Hemolysis. This is initiated through the fixation of C1q to the Fc portion of one IgM antibody or two adjacent IgG antibodies bound to red cells. Then, erythrocyte destruction can occur either through the classical pathway or through the alternative pathway, respectively, leading to extravascular and intravascular hemolysis.

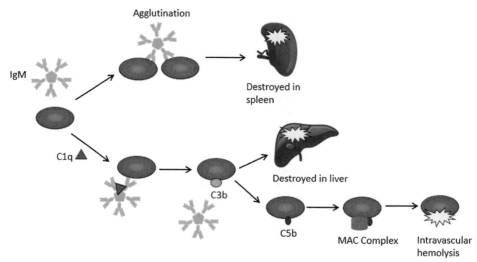

FIG.3.4 **IgM-mediated Extravascular Versus Intravascular Hemolysis.** This mainly occurs through two mechanisms. First, IgM antibodies can bridge the zeta potential of neighboring RBCs and cause agglutination. Agglutinated red cells are then rapidly removed from the vasculature and brought to the spleen for extravascular hemolysis via macrophages. Alternatively, IgM can initiate the complement pathway, which is the main method of erythrocyte destruction for cold-reactive IgM. After fixation of complement, erythrocyte destruction can occur via either the classical complement pathway leading to extravascular hemolysis in the liver or the alternative complement pathway causing intravascular hemolysis.

RBC surface). For the DL test, patient's serum tested should be separated from a freshly collected blood sample maintained at 37°C. The IgG antibodies responsible for PCH are biphasic: they bind to erythrocytes and fix complement (C1) at 4°C temperatures in the peripheral vasculature but then cause intravascular hemolysis when complement is activated at 37°C.

Other Possible Mechanisms

In addition to the classical Fc- and complement-mediated pathways of erythrocyte destruction, recent studies have also described alternative mechanisms of destruction. Aggregation of RBCs, themselves increases splenic sequestration and destruction in a complement-independent mechanism.[22] RBC distortion and subsequent aggregation can arise due to different complications, some of which may be antibody mediated. Erythrocytes coincubated with antibodies against glycophorin A (GPA), a sugar bearing transmembrane proteins abundantly present in erythrocyte membranes, induces an increase in membrane rigidity.[29] Researchers posited that this increase in membrane rigidity may be due to transmembrane signaling that occurs after glycophorin is bound, which then in turn causes the cytoplasmic portion of GPA to bind to the cytoskeletal network. Moreover, transient

reactions between antibody and erythrocyte may damage the integrity of the erythrocyte membrane and lead to hemolysis. Both anti-Pr IgM and anti-A IgG have been shown to directly induce red cell destruction through activation of cation channels leading to calcium entry and subsequent membrane destabilization.[22] Furthermore, lectins that bind to GPA cause an irreversible change in membrane permeability that persists even after lectin removal, which in turn causes an increase in phosphatidylserine to be expressed on the surface of RBCs, leading to increased clearance.[30]

CLINICAL AND LABORATORY EVALUATION
Clinical Evaluation

The clinical findings in patients with AIHA often correlate with the type of antibody and the mechanism of hemolysis (Fig. 3.1). Acute presentation with fever, back pain, and rapidly progressing anemia associated with jaundice and splenomegaly is usually associated with IgG warm-mediated AIHA. Cold-type AIHA following an infection usually has a more insidious onset with bone marrow compensation for hemolysis; symptoms are subtle until severe anemia develops. Chronic-type CAD presents with cold-induced circulatory symptoms ranging from slight acrocyanosis to Raynaud phenomena. PCH is similar clinically to cold-type AIHA, with intravascular hemolysis and hemoglobinuria.

Laboratory Evaluation

The laboratory evaluation is important in categorizing the type of antibody causing the hemolysis and subsequent treatment regimen. Some treatment options are ineffective against certain antibody types and reactivities (i.e., CAD patients unresponsive to steroid treatment) because different antibodies promote different mechanisms of erythrocyte destruction. Therefore, it is essential that the antibody type and reactivity is uncovered before any intervention so that the proper mode of hemolysis is addressed. The hemolytic event should be confirmed by showing evidence of anemia combined with increased hemoglobin degradation products. Elevation of lactate dehydrogenase (LDH) is a marker of hemolysis but is nonspecific, as elevation of LDH may be present in many kinds of tissue damage. On the other hand, elevation of bilirubin levels is a more specific marker of heme degradation. Elevation of direct bilirubin favors extravascular hemolysis, whereas indirect bilirubin rise combined with low haptoglobin (<14 g/dL) indicates an intravascular hemolysis. Other laboratory tests such as a high reticulocytosis can show indirect evidence of hemolysis, but can also be seen in other causes of anemia.

In the presence of hemolysis, the Coombs test or DAT should be performed to confirm the presence of an antibody on the surface of the RBC and if positive, an elution is performed. The elution consists of removing the antibody coating the patient's RBC and testing it against RBC reagent cells to determine the specificity of the antibody. Laboratory evidence that supports the diagnosis of warm AIHA is a positive DAT demonstrating an autoantibody reacting with all RBC screening reagent cells, including the patient's own cells. However, the diagnosis can only be confirmed with clinical evidence of AIHA. Indeed as described in the introduction, many of these autoantibodies are considered "silent" and never cause hemolysis. After confirming the presence of an autoantibody, transfusion medicine service providers must then determine the characteristics of the autoantibody on which the therapeutic management of the AIHA will be based. Overall, the pathologic and clinical features of AIHA relates to the autoantibody isotype (IgG or IgM), the thermal amplitude of reactivity with RBCs, and the ability to cause intravascular hemolysis upon complement binding and activation.

If a warm-type AIHA is suspected, IgG autoantibodies may be present as they are usually optimally reactive at 37°C. However, further workup to identify an underlying cause such as autoimmune disease, malignancy, or lymphoma is recommended. Drug-induced causes should also be considered and possible pertinent drugs should be discontinued.

If the clinical evaluation suggests cold agglutinins inducing CAD, IgM autoantibodies may be present as these are usually cold reactive (optimal binding at 4°C). Further testing should include cold agglutinin titer, thermal amplitude of the cold agglutinin, and Donath Landsteiner test to exclude PCH. Low titer (<1:10) cold agglutinins are common and are not clinically significant as they do not cause RBC destruction in vivo. However, some IgM autoantibodies may present with high titers (>1:000), exhibit wider thermal amplitude, activate complement, and cause intravascular hemolysis. Underlying infections should be ruled out by ordering antibody titers for viruses (i.e., EBV, parvovirus) and mycoplasma. Lastly, lymphoproliferative disorders should be ruled out by examining the patient for abnormal lymph nodes and abnormally large spleen.

Atypical AIHA with Negative Serologic Workup

About 10% of patients with warm reactive AIHA will have a negative DAT result. DAT-negative AIHA is often due to technical limitations of diagnostic tools. Indeed, DAT-negative AIHA can be due to non-IgG antibodies such as IgA and IgM, which will not be detected by the routinely used polyspecific anti-IgG or C3d Coombs reagent.[31] IgA-mediated hemolysis is difficult to detect, as the dimeric structure of the IgA is incapable of directly agglutinating red cells such as the pentameric IgM can. Flow cytometry or a specific anti-IgA antiglobulin test may be used to detect the presence of these alternative antibodies. Additionally some IgG subtypes such as IgG3 can cause hemolysis below the detection level of the Coombs reagent. Indeed, IgG3 autoantibodies induce hemolysis to a greater extent than IgG1 and IgG2, as these can bind and activate complement (Fig. 3.3). Importantly, macrophages can detect a low density of IgG3 on RBC surface and induce phagocytosis and hemolysis below the limit of detection of the DAT, resulting in a negative DAT. When antibody characteristics (i.e., quantity, specificity, subclass) are not enough to explain AIHA clinical outcomes, it is beneficial to use in vitro assays that probe how antibodies interact with immune cells: ADCC, the chemiluminescence test, and the monocyte monolayer assay (MMA). These techniques may be useful for patients with DAT-negative results, where AIHA is suspected, as strong outcomes in the MMA and ADCC have been correlated with hemolysis in DAT-negative patients.[32] Lastly, autoantibodies with low affinity to RBC surfaces may be susceptible to the washing steps performed during the Coombs test or DAT. Chassis et al. demonstrated that even transient binding of antibodies against GPA, an erythrocyte transmembrane protein, induced an irreversible increase in membrane rigidity that may leave cells more susceptible to hemolysis,[29] thus low affinity autoantibodies may induce damage that is not supported by DAT results.

TREATMENTS

The therapeutic management of AIHA will vary with the properties of the autoantibody (i.e., cold reactive or warm reactive), ability to bind complement, and whether the AIHA is associated with an underlying disease, such as malignancy, infection, or autoimmunity.

Warm-Type AIHA

In warm-type AIHA, lymphoid malignancies should be ruled out first and once ruled out steroids should be used as the first line of treatment.[33] Steroids-based therapy inhibits auto-antibody production and decreases extravascular hemolysis through downregulation of Fc-γ receptor expression on splenic macrophages. Splenectomy is only recommended as a second-line treatment for patients with no underlying autoimmune disease or hematologic malignancy.[3,34]

In warm-type AIHA secondary to an underlying disorder, efforts should be made to treat the underlying condition without exacerbating the patient's anemia because secondary AIHA resolves concurrently with the correction of the associated disease. For patients with warm-type AIHA secondary to cancer, chemotherapy drugs that do not induce hemolysis as a side effect, such as ibrutinib or nonpurine nucleoside analogs idelalisib, obinutuzumab, ofatumumab, and venetoclax, should be preferred. Similarly, drugs that may cause hemolysis such as purine analogs should be withheld, as these carry a higher risk of AIHA compared to patients receiving nonpurine nucleoside analog treatment (6% vs. 2%, respectively).[2,35]

Cold-Reactive AIHA: Cold Agglutinin Disorder—Idiopathic Cold-Type AIHA

As in all cases of cold-reactive AIHA, patients are recommended to wear warm clothing and avoid low ambient

temperatures. RBC transfusions can be safely administered when indicated using an in-line blood warmer, as long as the patient is kept warm.[36] Similarly, patients with CAD should be evaluated before surgery for the activity of the cold agglutinin at warmer temperature.

Rituximab, a monoclonal antibody against B-cell CD20 antigen inducing B-cell destruction by cytotoxicity, is the most widely used pharmacological agent for CAD treatment, but prospective studies have also shown that rituximab in combination with chemotherapy agents such as fludarabine or bendamustine may be more efficacious.[37] In addition, bortezomib, a proteasome inhibitor on myeloma plasma cells, may be an alternative therapy for patients with AIHA who do not respond to rituximab.[38]

Besides mainstay antineoplastic agents, researchers are also investigating other targeted therapies to treat CAD, including complement inhibitors and vaccines. To date, there is only one complement inhibitor used to treat CAD, C5 inhibitor eculizumab, although more beneficial results may be seen in targeted inhibitors of the classical complement pathway (i.e., inhibitors against C1 esterase or C3 convertase), as this is the pathway that leads to the hemolysis of most erythrocytes in CAD. Moreover, because the light chain genotypes seen in CAD are highly restricted, antiimmunoglobulin light chain vaccination are being investigated, similar to experimental therapies under investigation to manage treatments used in B-cell non-Hodgkin lymphomas.[14,16]

Splenectomy is not indicated in CAD because most cold agglutinin-mediated erythrocyte destruction occurs either intravascularly or in the liver, not the spleen.[3] Furthermore, Barcellini et al. advise to defer splenectomy after rituximab treatment, citing increased risk of thromboembolism, infections, and fatality in splenectomized patients.[33] Similarly, corticosteroids, azathioprine, interferon-α, or monotherapy with alkylating agents should not be used to treat CAD, as high dosages are required to induce an effect.[39]

Cold Agglutinin Syndrome—Secondary to Infections or Malignancies

Patients with secondary CAD due to lymphoproliferative disorders or infection, including PCH, should be treated for these pathologies and subsequently the CAD should resolve. If patients present with hemolysis but no infection, patient should be evaluated for non-Hodgkin's lymphoma and other possible underlying B-cell disorders.

Transfusion Recommendations—All AIHA Cases

Lastly, when RBC transfusion is required, advances in RBC genotyping technology have allowed successful RBC unit selection and crossmatch for patients with severe AIHA. In a 2002 study, Shirey and colleagues demonstrated that providing antigen-matched donor blood decreases 4.5 adsorption procedures per patient with warm-type autoantibody, leading to a simplification in pretransfusion adsorption studies and overall increase in transfusion safety.[40] In all, genotypically matched RBC transfusion serves as a valuable alternative to overcome the limitations and resource strain of serological phenotyping and crossmatches for patients with AIHA who require regular RBC transfusions.[34]

CONCLUSION AND FUTURE CONSIDERATIONS

Overall, current findings support the use of both laboratory tests and clinical presentations to diagnose the different types of AIHA. Even though the clinical diagnosis of AIHA can be puzzling and delay treatment, every effort should be made to diagnose and treat patients early, as earlier onset of therapy is associated with a lower probability of relapse.[33] As AIHA is a relatively rare disorder, the treatment recommendations are not well defined, and prospective studies are still needed to establish firm recommendations for physician providers. Specifically, the temporal sequence of second-line therapy options in AIHA is undecided and no predictors of outcome are available based on the timeline of treatment. Besides AIHA drug therapy shortcomings in general, specific attention is warranted in improving cold-reactive autoantibody outcomes, as response rates for CAD treatment are lower than equivalent treatment in warm-type AIHA patients.[3] Prospective studies would be invaluable in testing the efficacy of new therapies, notably targeted therapies against B-cell receptor pathways including ibrutinib, idelalisib, and venetoclax, as well as inhibitors of the complement pathway: C3 inhibitor compstatin and complement C1s inhibitor BIVV009. Although robust clinical trials have investigated the utility of these drugs to treat chronic lymphocytic lymphoma and other lymphoproliferative conditions, the clinical transition for these treatments in ameliorating AIHA is only beginning to be realized.[22,38]

REFERENCES

1. Mauro FR, Trastulli F, Alessandri C, et al. Clinical relevance of silent red blood cell autoantibodies. *Haematologica*. 2017;102:e473–e475.
2. Petz LD, Garratty G. *Immune Hemolytic Anemias*. 2nd ed. Philadelphia, Pa: Churchill Livingstone/Elsevier Science; 2004.
3. Go RS, Winters JL, Kay NE. How I treat autoimmune hemolytic anemia. *Blood*. 2017;129:2971–2979.
4. Salama A, Berghöfer H, Mueller-Eckhardt C. Red blood cell transfusion in warm-type autoimmune haemolytic anaemia. *Lancet*. 1992;340:1515–1517.
5. Ahrens N, Pruss A, Kähne A, Kiesewetter H, Salama A. Coexistence of autoantibodies and alloantibodies to red blood cells due to blood transfusion. *Transfusion*. 2007; 47:813–816.
6. Young PP, Uzieblo A, Trulock E, Lublin DM, Goodnough LT. Autoantibody formation after alloimmunization: are blood transfusions a risk factor for autoimmune hemolytic anemia? *Transfusion*. 2004;44:67–72.
7. Garratty G. Autoantibodies induced by blood transfusion. *Transfusion*. 2004;44:5–9.
8. Kaminski ER, Hows JM, Goldman JM, Batchelor JR. Lymphocytes from multi-transfused patients exhibit cytotoxicity against autologous cells. *Br J Haematol*. 1992;81: 23–26.
9. Molica S, Polliack A. Autoimmune hemolytic anemia (AIHA) associated with chronic lymphocytic leukemia in the current era of targeted therapy. *Leuk Res*. 2016;50: 31–36.
10. Zhao Y-B, Li J-M, Wei B-W, Xu Z-Z. BAFF level increased in patients with autoimmune hemolytic anemia. *Int J Clin Exp Med*. 2015;8:3876–3882.
11. Ravindran A, Sankaran J, Jacob EK, et al. High prevalence of monoclonal gammopathy among patients with warm autoimmune hemolytic anemia. *Am J Hematol*. 2017;92: E164–E166.
12. Randen U, Trøen G, Tierens A, et al. Primary cold agglutinin-associated lymphoproliferative disease: a B-cell lymphoma of the bone marrow distinct from lymphoplasmacytic lymphoma. *Haematologica*. 2014;99: 497–504.
13. Małecka A, Trøen G, Tierens A, et al. Frequent somatic mutations of KMT2D (MLL2) and CARD11 genes in primary cold agglutinin disease. *Br J Haematol*. 2018;183:838–842.
14. Martorelli D, Guidoboni M, De Re V, et al. IGKV3 proteins as candidate "off-the-shelf" vaccines for kappa-light chain-restricted B-cell non-Hodgkin lymphomas. *Clin Cancer Res*. 2012;18:4080–4091.
15. Henry Dunand CJ, Wilson PC. Restricted, canonical, stereotyped and convergent immunoglobulin responses. *Philos Trans R Soc Lond B Biol Sci*. 2015;370.
16. Małecka A, Trøen G, Tierens A, et al. Immunoglobulin heavy and light chain gene features are correlated with primary cold agglutinin disease onset and activity. *Haematologica*. 2016;101:e361–364.
17. Barzilai O, Ram M, Shoenfeld Y. Viral infection can induce the production of autoantibodies. *Curr Opin Rheumatol*. 2007;19:636–643.
18. Kivity S, Agmon-Levin N, Blank M, Shoenfeld Y. Infections and autoimmunity–friends or foes? *Trends Immunol*. 2009; 30:409–414.

19. Rivera-Correa J, Guthmiller JJ, Vijay R, et al. Plasmodium DNA-mediated TLR9 activation of T-bet+ B cells contributes to autoimmune anaemia during malaria. *Nat Commun.* 2017;8:1282.

20. Chambers LA, Rauck AM. Acute transient hemolytic anemia with a positive Donath-Landsteiner test following parvovirus B19 infection. *J Pediatr Hematol Oncol.* 1996; 18:178–181.

21. Wong W, Merker JD, Nguyen C, et al. Cold agglutinin syndrome in pediatric liver transplant recipients. *Pediatr Transplant.* 2007;11:931–936.

22. Meulenbroek EM, Wouters D, Zeerleder SS. Lyse or not to lyse: clinical significance of red blood cell autoantibodies. *Blood Rev.* 2015;29:369–376.

23. Alberts B, Johnson A, Lewis J, Raff M, Roberts K, Walter P. B cells and antibodies. In: *Molecular Biology of the Cell.* New York: Garland Science; 2002.

24. Jandl JH, Kaplan ME. The destruction of red cells by antibodies in man. III. Quantitative factors influencing the patterns of hemolysis in vivo. *J Clin Investig.* 1960;39: 1145–1156.

25. Holm G. Lysis of antibody-treated human erythrocytes by human leukocytes and macrophages in tissue culture. *Int Arch Allergy Appl Immunol.* 1972;43:671–682.

26. Shaw GM, Levy PC, LoBuglio AF. Human lymphocyte antibody-dependent cell-mediated cytotoxicity (ADCC) toward human red blood cells. *Blood.* 1978;52:696–705.

27. Braun A, Gessner JE, Varga-Szabo D, et al. STIM1 is essential for Fcgamma receptor activation and autoimmune inflammation. *Blood.* 2009;113:1097–1104.

28. Schreiber AD, Frank MM. Role of antibody and complement in the immune clearance and destruction of erythrocytes. I. In vivo effects of IgG and IgM complement-fixing sites. *J Clin Investig.* 1972;51:575–582.

29. Chasis JA, Reid ME, Jensen RH, Mohandas N. Signal transduction by glycophorin A: role of extracellular and cytoplasmic domains in a modulatable process. *J Cell Biol.* 1988;107:1351–1357.

30. Brain MC, Prevost JM, Pihl CE, Brown CB. Glycophorin A-mediated haemolysis of normal human erythrocytes: evidence for antigen aggregation in the pathogenesis of immune haemolysis. *Br J Haematol.* 2002;118:899–908.

31. Garratty G. Immune hemolytic anemia associated with negative routine serology. *Semin Hematol.* 2005;42: 156–164.

32. Biondi CS, Cotorruelo CM, Ensinck A, Racca LL, Racca AL. Use of the erythrophagocytosis assay for predicting the clinical consequences of immune blood cell destruction. *Clin Lab.* 2004;50:265–270.

33. Barcellini W, Fattizzo B, Zaninoni A, et al. Clinical heterogeneity and predictors of outcome in primary autoimmune hemolytic anemia: a GIMEMA study of 308 patients. *Blood.* 2014;124:2930–2936.

34. Ziman A, Cohn C, Carey PM, et al. Warm-reactive (immunoglobulin G) autoantibodies and laboratory testing best practices: review of the literature and survey of current practice. *Transfusion.* 2017;57:463–477.

35. Berentsen S. Diagnosis and treatment of cold agglutinin mediated autoimmune hemolytic anemia. *Blood Rev.* 2012;26:107–115.

36. Hill QA. Autoimmune hemolytic anemia. *Hematology.* 2015;20:553–554.

37. Berentsen S, Randen U, Vågan AM, et al. High response rate and durable remissions following fludarabine and rituximab combination therapy for chronic cold agglutinin disease. *Blood.* 2010;116:3180–3184.

38. Berentsen S. Complement activation and inhibition in autoimmune hemolytic anemia: focus on cold agglutinin disease. *Semin Hematol.* 2018;55:141–149.

39. Berentsen S, Ulvestad E, Langholm R, et al. Primary chronic cold agglutinin disease: a population based clinical study of 86 patients. *Haematologica.* 2006;91: 460–466.

40. Shirey RS, Boyd JS, Parwani AV, Tanz WS, Ness PM, King KE. Prophylactic antigen-matched donor blood for patients with warm autoantibodies: an algorithm for transfusion management. *Transfusion.* 2002;42:1435–1441.

CHAPTER 4

Allergic Transfusion Reactions

KATHLEEN M. MADDEN, MD • JAY S. RAVAL, MD

INTRODUCTION

Allergic transfusion reactions (ATRs) are type I hypersensitivity reactions and are some of the most common adverse reactions that occur with blood component infusion. Reaction rates vary depending on the particular blood component and range from 1% to 4%.[1,2] ATRs correlate with the amount of plasma proteins in the blood component and thus occur more commonly with plasma and platelet transfusions.[3–5] Most ATRs are clinically mild and typically only have cutaneous manifestations, such as urticarial rash and pruritus. However, more serious findings, such as bronchospasm, angioedema, respiratory distress, hypotension, and shock, can occur.

Treatments of ATRs involve use of antihistamines, along with possibly glucocorticoids and epinephrine in more severe cases. Premedication with antihistamines and glucocorticoids before transfusion to prevent ATRs is common, although there is limited data to support such practices.[6] However, manipulations of blood components that result in lower volumes of plasma, and concomitantly the amount of allergenic stimuli, have been shown to decrease occurrence of ATRs. Additionally, in those with known deficiencies of immunoglobulin (Ig) A or haptoglobin, blood components from donors with similar deficiencies can be obtained to decrease the risk of ATRs. In this chapter, ATR mechanisms, occurrences with various blood component transfusions, diagnostics, treatments, and prevention strategies will be reviewed.

MECHANISMS OF ALLERGY

Both IgE-dependent and -independent mechanisms can cause allergic reactions.[7–9] In the first mechanistic pathway, allergen-specific IgE is produced from B cells stimulated by T helper cells exposed to the allergen.[10] These IgE molecules bind to high-affinity Fc receptors on the allergy effector cells, i.e., basophils and mast cells. Upon reexposure to the specific allergen and subsequent binding to the previously formed cell-anchored IgE molecules, basophil and mast cell activation occurs with the release of a variety of substances that promote smooth muscle relaxation, vasodilation, and increased vascular permeability.[8,11] Some of these substances, such as histamine, are preformed and ready to be released immediately from granules within allergy effector cells. Other substances are not stored but rather generated on-demand, such as leukotrienes, prostaglandins, platelet activating factor, and other lipid mediators of inflammation.[7] This culminates in the various findings observed in allergic reaction findings.

IgE-independent mechanisms of allergic reactions include direct stimulation or IgG-dependent anaphylatoxin generation.[7,9] Histamine release from allergy effector cells has been shown to occur by direct exposure to bradykinins, leukotrienes, platelet activating factor, CCL5, and a variety of diagnostic and therapeutic drugs routinely used in patient care.[8,11] In IgG-dependent allergic pathways, binding of allergens to IgG molecules and subsequent low-affinity IgG receptors has been shown to result in allergy effector cell activation via the anaphylatoxins C3a and C5a.

MECHANISMS OF ALLERGIC TRANSFUSION REACTIONS

ATRs have similarity to allergic reactions from other causes; thus, it is believed that the underlying mechanisms of ATRs are related. Most of these reactions occur starting during the transfusion and up to 4 hours after completion.[2] The fact that ATRs occur in such temporal proximity to the blood component infusion suggests that upstream allergy effectors are either preformed or rapidly generated via mechanisms that are both IgE-dependent and -independent.[8,12] It should be noted, however, that there is a paucity of definitive proof regarding the contributions of IgE and allergy effector cells in the pathologic mechanisms of ATRs.[1,8] Investigations in those that experienced ATRs have demonstrated elevated serum tryptase levels suggestive of

Immunologic Concepts in Transfusion Medicine. https://doi.org/10.1016/B978-0-323-67509-3.00004-4

mast cell degranulation and increased spontaneous histamine release from allergy effector cells compared with those without ATRs.[13,14] Substances that initiate allergy are thought to be present in blood components. These compounds could be allergens that induce antibody formation in atopic individuals, intrinsic components of the blood component, or substances formed ex vivo within the component bag (Table 4.1). Reported allergens in blood components include normal endogenous plasma proteins (e.g., IgA and haptoglobin) that are absent in a recipient as well as exogenous compounds in the plasma of healthy donor to which a recipient is allergic (e.g., peanut or shellfish proteins).[15,16] The passive infusion of donor atopic antibodies to recipients having circulating cognate allergens has also been described as a mechanism for ATRs.[8] Several reports have identified blood component recipients without previous allergies to have severe ATRs when transfused with components from donors with demonstrable atopic antibodies and then exposure to the cognate allergens.[17,18] Indeed, blood donors have reported severe allergies and been found to have IgE directed against various allergens,[19–23] and allergy effector cell sensitization and degranulation have been reported in recipients of passively acquired atopic antibodies from transfusion.[14,24] However, for the vast majority of transfusions, the relationship between infused atopic antibodies and ATRs is likely not a significant one as investigations of donor allergy status and infusion of atopic antibodies do not reliably correlate with development of ATRs.[19,20,25–29] Intrinsic elements of blood components or substances formed within a blood component bag may be allergic agonists and cause ATRs; these include β-thromboglobulin, brain-derived neurotrophic factor, C5a, CCL5 (RANTES), CD40 ligand, histamine, platelet factor 4, serotonin, soluble CD40 ligand, thromboxane, transforming growth factor-β1, and vascular endothelial growth factor.[27,28,30] While histamine is an appealing suspect for ATRs, as its concentration should be related to leukocyte content and storage duration, passive infusion of histamine likely has a minor role in these reactions as leukoreduction does not cause a significant reduction in ATR rates.[31,32] Investigations in transfusion recipients that experienced ATRs have demonstrated elevated serum tryptase levels suggestive of mast cell degranulation,[14,33] as well as increased spontaneous histamine release from allergy effector cells in these subjects compared to those who did not have ATRs.[13] Notably, ATRs have even been reported to occur with transfusion of autologous red blood cells.[34] Our understanding of donor and recipient factors, as well as other elements of allergy pathophysiology associated with transfusion, is incomplete; further investigations to more fully characterize the relevant mechanisms in ATRs are necessary.

SPECIFIC DEFICIENCIES ASSOCIATED WITH ATRS

IgA Deficiency

IgA is found in circulation and secretions throughout the body. It plays an important role in immunity, assisting in cell-dependent processes as well as being present in secretions to prevent penetration by mucosal bacteria.[35,36] Selective IgA deficiency is recognized as the most common primary antibody deficiency; the incidence ranges from 1:18,000 Japanese patients to 1:600 Caucasian patients.[37] Within the United States, the frequency has been estimated at 1:300 to 1:3000 healthy donors.[38] Total IgA deficiency is defined by the American Rare Donor Program as serum IgA level < 5 mg/dL,[39] though the lower limit of detection in most laboratories is 7 mg/dL. Although these individuals may be labeled as having relative IgA deficiency and have increased risk of severe ATRs, IgA concentrations at significantly lower levels (<0.05 mg/dL) are typically used to characterize severe deficiency and has a prevalence of 1:1000.[38,40,41]

ATRs and anaphylaxis have been reported to occur in selective IgA-deficient patients.[42–44] These reactions are thought to be secondary to IgG, IgE, or IgM anti-IgA that have been identified in up to 40% of IgA-deficient patients.[45] Transfusion of a blood component containing even trace amounts IgA to an IgA-deficient recipient with anti-IgA antibodies could cause severe ATRs and anaphylaxis. However, it should be noted that deficiency of IgA does not imply the presence of IgA antibodies, many IgA-deficient patients receiving transfusions do not have severe ATRs or anaphylactic reactions, and ATRs can occur in those with IgA deficiency without measurable anti-IgA.[37,46,47] Hypersensitivity transfusion reactions due to IgA deficiency are rare according to French hemovigilance data.[48]

Haptoglobin Deficiency

Haptoglobin irreversibly binds oxygenated cell-free hemoglobin, thus preventing the accumulation of free radicals and resultant oxidative tissue damage.[49] The haptoglobin-hemoglobin complex then is removed from circulation by binding the CD163 receptor on monocytes and macrophages.[50] Clinically, this is used as an important laboratory marker in hemolytic anemia.[51] Inherited haptoglobin deficiency is found in East Asian populations.[52] Compared to rates of IgA deficiency in these populations (1:18,000), primary haptoglobin deficiency appears to occur more frequently (1:4,000 Japanese, 1:1,500 Koreans, and 1:1,000 Chinese).[53] Secondary haptoglobin deficiency occurs at a much higher frequency. This is likely a consequence of congenital and acquired hemolytic disorders, such as sickle cell anemia, thalassemia, hereditary red blood cell membrane or enzyme defects, and malaria.[54] Patients with primary or secondary haptoglobin deficiency may develop IgG or IgE antihaptoglobin. Case reports have described patients who experience severe ATRs or anaphylactic reactions and have undetectable haptoglobin levels upon investigation.[55–57] Severe deficiencies of other normal proteins, such as components of the complement system,[58–60] may also result in severe ATRs.

DONOR AND PATIENT CHARACTERISTICS

ATRs can occur repeatedly in some patients, suggesting that hypersensitivity or susceptibility may play an important part in the development of these reactions.[26] As ATRs occur more frequently with platelet and plasma transfusions compared to red blood cell transfusions, it has been hypothesized that the donor antibody and allergen attributes at the time of donation may have a role in mediating ATRs. In one analysis comparing overall institutional ATR rate to the concordance rate of ATRs for split apheresis platelet components transfused to at least two different recipients, no difference was observed and suggested that donor factors were not a significant influence on ATRs.[26] However, when donors of split components associated with concordant ATRs in two or more recipients were queried for development of ATRs in other recipients of other components from these same donors, a significantly higher ATR rate was observed compared to the overall ATR rate (5.8% vs. 1.7%, respectively), leaving open the possibility that donor factors may influence the ATR rate.

Recipients experiencing ATRs tend to be more atopic than those who do not experience ATRs[29]; given that the prevalence of atopy is as high as 35% of recipients,[61] this may have an impact on occurrence of ATRs. In an analysis comparing patients who experienced ATRs with apheresis platelet transfusions to those who did not, the ATR cohort had approximately sevenfold greater IgE levels.[29] Additionally, aeroallergen-specific IgE testing of the two cohorts demonstrated significantly higher concentrations in those that had an ATR compared to those who did not. Notably, there were no significant differences in total or antigen-specific IgE in the supernatants of these single-donor components. Similarly, recipients of blood components with subsequent ATR in a longitudinal cohort study were also significantly more likely to report a hay fever or food allergy history and aeroallergen sensitization compared to those that did not have ATRs.[62,63] Blood component and transfusion characteristics, including infusion rate and volume, ABO mismatch, unit age, and premedication before infusion, were not found to be significantly associated with ATRs.[63] Therefore, the cumulative body of evidence to date appears to indicate that patient but not donor characteristics are most strongly associated with ATRs.

PRESENTATION

ATRs to blood components are very common, occurring in 0.4% of red blood cell transfusions and up to 4.1% of platelet transfusions.[2,5,64] ATRs occur when patients are exposed to an agent that causes activation of allergy effector cells. Findings can be observed within seconds of beginning the transfusion, may develop at any point during the transfusion, or not begin until the transfusion has finished; in general, more severe reactions occur sooner after initiation of transfusion. ATRs can occur across a spectrum of severity (Table 4.2). Mild ATRs are the most common and are characterized by isolated cutaneous involvement (e.g., pruritus, urticarial rash, flushing). Moderate ATRs progress to localized angioedema of the head and neck and can have respiratory involvement including bronchospasm characterized by wheezing, stridor, desaturations requiring supplemental oxygen, and dyspnea. Angioedema of the gastrointestinal system can also occur and cause findings including abdominal pain or cramps, nausea, vomiting, and diarrhea. The sine qua non of a severe ATR is hypotension; this can occur in conjunction with previously mentioned findings or in isolation. Progression to the most severe ATR—anaphylaxis—occurs rarely and is characterized by hypotension, shock, respiratory compromise, and complete cardiovascular collapse. Anaphylactic transfusion reactions can develop extremely rapidly, with transfusion of only a few milliliters of whole blood or plasma.[65] Fewer than 10% of all ATRs are considered severe ATRs or anaphylactic reactions, with the latter, most severe reactions occurring at a frequency of approximately 8 per 100,000 blood components.[2,8]

DIAGNOSIS AND DIFFERENTIAL DIAGNOSIS

The National Healthcare Safety Network Biovigilance Component of the Centers for Disease Control and Prevention guidelines classifies ATR as a "definitive" adverse reaction when ≥ 2 of the following findings are present during or within 4 hours of cessation of transfusion: conjunctival edema; edema of lips, tongue, and uvula; erythema and edema of the periorbital area; generalized flushing; hypotension; localized angioedema; maculopapular rash; pruritus; respiratory distress; bronchospasm; and urticaria.[66] The diagnosis of ATR is only "probable" with any one of the following present either during or within 4 hours of cessation of transfusion: conjunctival edema; edema of lips, tongue, and uvula; erythema and edema of the periorbital area; localized angioedema; maculopapular rash; pruritus; or urticaria. The imputability of the ATR is determined by the likelihood that other underlying factors could be contributing to the findings. Although no laboratory tests or radiologic findings specifically characterize ATRs, tryptase testing, when available and ordered promptly, can be used in conjunction with clinical findings to support a diagnosis of anaphylactic reaction.[33] Importantly, in patients with no prior transfusions or no available transfusion histories that have severe ATRs and anaphylactic reactions, assessments for IgA deficiency, haptoglobin deficiency, and anti-Ch or anti-Rg can be performed on a pretransfusion specimen.

As can be seen from the list of possible findings in ATRs, a wide range of signs and symptoms impacting multiple organ systems can be observed. When cutaneous manifestations of ATRs are identified, they can assist in differentiating this reaction from other transfusion reactions in the differential; however, this does not always occur. Severe ATRs and anaphylactic transfusion reactions may present with findings similar to other transfusion-related adverse reactions, including acute hemolytic transfusion reactions, hypotensive transfusion reactions, septic transfusion reactions, transfusion-associated circulatory overload, and transfusion-related acute lung injury.[2] Thorough administrative, immunohematologic, and clinical investigations should be conducted to distinguish ATRs from these other reactions.

TREATMENT

When a patient develops signs or symptoms suggestive of an ATR, the first step in treatment is to stop the transfusion. After this, supportive care for any issues must be provided, particularly from the cardiovascular and pulmonary perspectives.[67] When an ATR is suspected, therapeutic interventions can vary depending on reaction severity (Table 4.3). Antihistamines (H1 and H2 blockers), glucocorticoids, bronchodilators, and epinephrine are all possible treatments in addition to supportive care.[2,68,69] Selective H1 receptor antagonists including diphenhydramine, doxylamine, chlorpheniramine, hydroxyzine, and cyproheptadine can be used to counter the effects of histamine on the smooth muscle and vasculature,[68] as can H2 receptor antagonists such as cimetidine, famotidine, nizatidine, and ranitidine to lesser extent. A variety of glucocorticoids and bronchodilators are also available to treat ATRs. Premedication with antihistamines has not been clearly demonstrated to prevent reoccurrence of mild ATRs,[70] yet both antihistamines and glucocorticoids are used routinely for this purpose.[6] Of all the transfusion reactions, only in cases of mild ATRs with cutaneous involvement that promptly resolve with treatment may transfusion of the same unit be resumed.

Anaphylactic reactions attributed to transfusion are managed similarly to anaphylaxis from other causes. Rapid recognition of the patient's clinical condition with initiation of treatment is necessary to prevent respiratory failure and cardiovascular collapse. Intramuscular epinephrine should be administered as soon as possible, with the epinephrine dose dependent on the patient's weight.[71] This may be repeated with additional intramuscular injections or slow intravenous infusion if the patient's signs and symptoms do not improve. Epinephrine is a nonselective adrenergic agonist, stimulating $\alpha 1$ and $\alpha 2$ receptors to cause arteriolar vasoconstriction, $\beta 1$ receptors to increase inotropy and chronotropy, and $\beta 2$ receptors to cause arteriolar vasodilation, bronchial smooth muscle relaxation, and increased glycogenolysis. This ultimately results in bronchodilation, cardiac stimulation, and, with high doses, skeletal muscle vasoconstriction.[72]

In addition to epinephrine administration, the patient should be given supplemental oxygen and volume resuscitation. Bronchodilators, such as albuterol, may be given for patients with bronchospasm not responsive to epinephrine. Additional adjunctive treatments that may be provided for the patient include H1 and H2 receptor antagonists and glucocorticoids. In patients with severe ATRs or anaphylactic reactions, concomitant assessments for IgA deficiency, haptoglobin deficiency, or other allergy issues should be performed.

PREVENTION

There are several maneuvers commonly employed to decrease the risk of ATRs (Table 4.4). Although the data to support some practices are lacking, many institutions still treat these patients with standard protocols using such interventions. However, blood component manipulations appear to have the best evidence to support decreasing the risk of ATRs. Additionally, consistent application of evidence-based thresholds to avoid unnecessary transfusions is essential.[73–75]

Premedication

A variety of medications are being used for pretransfusion prophylaxis to decrease the incidence of ATR despite a lack of convincing evidence demonstrating efficacy.[2,6,8,76,77] Selective H1 and H2 receptor antagonists are frequently used for treating ATRs, most commonly diphenhydramine, but data supporting its application for preventing ATRs are limited.[68,69] Studies performed in the 1950s formed the initial basis for the use of pretransfusion medication, with this later becoming standard practice.[68,77] Several studies found no difference in ATR rates when pretransfusion antihistamines were ordered. A systemic review of randomized controlled trials evaluating the use of antihistamine premedication to prevent ATRs concluded that there was no difference in ATR rates with or without premedication.[70,78–80] However, continued recommendation and administration of antihistamines to prevent mild ATRs, especially for patients with a history of ATRs or who will be transfused a large volume of plasma product, persists.[67,77,81,82]

Patients who have frequent or severe ATRs may also be administered pretransfusion medication with glucocorticoids 1–3 hours before future transfusion, in addition to other premedications. Through their leukocyte inhibitory functions, glucocorticoids have antiinflammatory and immunosuppressive qualities.[83] They also have β2 adrenergic receptor agonist functions. Glucocorticoids can be used to treat severe ATRs and anaphylactic reactions; however, their use has not been specifically studied for the prevention or treatment of severe ATRs.[84] Given our knowledge of other ATRs and the mechanism of action of glucocorticoids, this has potential application as premedication for patients with a history of severe ATRs or anaphylaxis but requires further investigations.

Plasma Reduction Strategies

Washing cellular blood components removes cell-free fluid and associated plasma proteins or other substances that may trigger severe ATRs and anaphylaxis.[82,85] Notably, washing is a manipulation that can only be performed on cellular blood components, i.e., red blood cells and platelets. The washing process may be done manually or by automated methods and typically using 0.9% normal saline.[86] The amount of plasma and plasma components removed depends on the volume of saline used during washing. However, this process

also produces a quantitatively and qualitatively inferior component as red blood cells are hemolyzed and endure sublethal injury, and platelets are activated and lost.[82,87–90] The use of larger saline volumes for washing will remove more plasma and plasma proteins; however, this may also increase red blood cell or platelet loss. It has been reported that washing with Plasma-Lyte A in lieu of normal saline decreases hemolysis and improves platelet function.[91] By removing plasma, and thus the allergenic stimuli responsible for ATRs, washed blood components have been demonstrated to decrease ATRs.[92] A retrospective analysis of the incidence of ATRs in patients who received unmanipulated and subsequently washed transfusions demonstrated that washing apheresis platelets significantly decreased the incidence of ATRs from 5.5% to 0.7%[4]; washing red blood cells also significantly decreased the incidence of ATRs from 2.7% to 0.3%. Another study evaluated the use of washed platelet concentrates for patients with recurrent or severe transfusion reactions, including ATRs and anaphylaxis, and found that washed platelets reduced the incidence of ATRs to <1%.[93] Cellular components can also be washed to prevent severe ATRs and anaphylactic transfusion reactions in IgA- or haptoglobin-deficient recipients.[37,53] For IgA-deficient patients, washing protocols should aim to reduce the IgA concentration to <0.05 mg/dL, or as low as possible while maintaining function and viability of the red blood cells or platelets.[39] These individuals can also receive blood components from IgA- or haptoglobin-deficient donors.

Volume reduction refers to the removal of excess cell-free fluid via centrifugation in an open or closed system for patients at high risk of repeat severe ATRs or who are sensitive to the added volume.[82,86] This process is typically utilized for platelets. Small quantities of cells in the blood component may be lost in the centrifugation process. Postvolume reduction cell recoveries have been reported to range from 79% to 95% with variable impacts on corrected count increment after transfusion.[3,89] Similar to washing, manipulation of the blood component via volume reduction may cause platelet activation and some platelet function may be decreased; however, studies have shown comparable functional outcomes of these manipulated blood products with nonvolume reduced platelet units.[94–96] Regarding ATR risk reduction, a retrospective study examining the incidence of ATRs in patients who received unmanipulated and subsequently volume-reduced apheresis platelet transfusions found that volume reduction was effective at significantly reducing the incidence of ATRs from 5.0% to 1.7%.[4]

Platelet Additive Solutions and Other Strategies

Platelet additive solutions are balanced electrolyte solutions that have been developed to suspend platelets and decrease the quantity of residual donor plasma.[82] Multiple platelet additive solutions exist, each with a different composition of specific electrolytes in solution.[97] Similar to washing and volume reduction that also decrease plasma in the blood component, use of platelet additive solutions can reduce the incidence of ATRs. Indeed, several studies have shown a significant decrease in ATRs with the use of platelet additive solution-suspended platelets compared to plasma-suspended platelets.[98–101] Although corrected count increments have been found to be generally lower in platelet additive solution-suspended platelets compared to platelets stored in plasma, particularly at 1-h posttransfusion, hemostatic efficacy of these products has not been found to be altered.[99–102]

For cases of severe ATRs or anaphylactic reactions in patients with IgA- or haptoglobin deficiency, blood components from donors negative for the specific allergen can be requested.[82] In individuals with IgA deficiency and transfusion-associated anaphylactic reactions, desensitization strategies that successfully permitted transfusion of components containing IgA have been reported.[103] Novel approaches to facilitate desensitization and immune tolerance in allergic conditions are currently underway in clinical trials and may have applications in transfusion recipients with repeated ATRs.[104]

CONCLUSION

ATRs are among the most commonly observed adverse reactions to blood components. Early recognition of such a reaction, followed by cessation of transfusion, providing supportive care, and administering treatment to alleviate findings of ATR, is vital. Although agents such as H1 receptor antagonists and glucocorticoids are commonly utilized as premedication before transfusion to decrease risks of ATRs, this practice is not supported by clinical trials to date. Blood component manipulations, such as washing, volume reduction, and use of platelet additive solutions, have been demonstrated to decrease occurrence of ATRs. There is still much to learn about the mechanisms and treatments of ATRs, as well as donor and recipient attributes that can contribute to these reactions. Additional investigations are required to optimize the management and prevention of ATRs.

TABLE 4.1
Causes of Allergic Transfusion Reactions.

- Normal endogenous plasma proteins (e.g., IgA, haptoglobin, complement)
- Exogenous compounds in donor plasma (e.g., peanut or shellfish allergens)
- Donor atopic antibodies
- Intrinsic components of blood products or substances formed within blood component units during storage (e.g., RANTES)

TABLE 4.2
Clinical Findings of Allergic Transfusion Reactions.

MILD SEVERITY

- Conjunctival edema
- Erythema and edema of the periorbital area
- Generalized flushing
- Localized angioedema
- Maculopapular rash
- Pruritus
- Urticaria

MODERATE−SEVERE SEVERITY

- Edema of lips, tongue, and uvula
- Respiratory distress
- Bronchospasm
- Abdominal pain and cramping
- Nausea
- Vomiting
- Diarrhea
- Hypotension

ANAPHYLACTIC

- Shock
- Respiratory compromise
- Complete cardiovascular collapse

TABLE 4.3
Therapeutic Interventions for Patients Having Allergic Transfusion Reactions.

- Stop the transfusion
- Provide supportive care (i.e., cardiopulmonary support)
- Antihistamines (e.g., H1 or H2 receptor antagonists)
- Glucocorticoids
- Bronchodilators
- Epinephrine
- Intravenous fluids
- Supplemental oxygen

TABLE 4.4
Strategies to Prevent Allergic Transfusion Reactions.

- Application of evidence-based transfusion thresholds
- Premedication (e.g., antihistamines, glucocorticoids)[a]
- Plasma reduction (e.g., washing, volume reduction)
- Use of platelet products suspended in platelet additive solutions
- Use of components from allergen-deficient donors (e.g., IgA-deficient donors)
- Desensitization

[a] Insufficient evidence to strongly support this practice.

REFERENCES

1. Savage WJ. Transfusion reactions. *Hematol Oncol Clin N Am.* 2016;30:619–634.
2. Delaney M, Wendel S, Bercovitz RS, et al. Transfusion reactions: prevention, diagnosis, and treatment. *Lancet.* 2016;388:2825–2836.
3. Heddle NM, Blajchman MA, Meyer RM, et al. A randomized controlled trial comparing the frequency of acute reactions to plasma-removed platelets and prestorage WBC-reduced platelets. *Transfusion.* 2002;42:556–566.
4. Tobian AA, Savage WJ, Tisch DJ, Thoman S, King KE, Ness PM. Prevention of allergic transfusion reactions to platelets and red blood cells through plasma reduction. *Transfusion.* 2011;51:1676–1683.
5. Carson JL, Triulzi DJ, Ness PM. Indications for and adverse effects of red-cell transfusion. *N Engl J Med.* 2017;377:1261–1272.
6. Tobian AA, King KE, Ness PM. Prevention of febrile nonhemolytic and allergic transfusion reactions with pretransfusion medication: is this evidence-based medicine? *Transfusion.* 2008;48:2274–2276.
7. Galli SJ, Tsai M, Piliponsky AM. The development of allergic inflammation. *Nature.* 2008;454:445–454.
8. Savage WJ, Tobian AA, Savage JH, Wood RA, Schroeder JT, Ness PM. Scratching the surface of allergic transfusion reactions. *Transfusion.* 2013;53:1361–1371.
9. Justiz Vaillant AA, Zito PM. *Immediate Hypersensitivity Reactions.* Treasure Island (FL): StatPearls; 2019.
10. Oliphant CJ, Barlow JL, McKenzie AN. Insights into the initiation of type 2 immune responses. *Immunology.* 2011;134:378–385.
11. Lieberman P, Garvey LH. Mast cells and anaphylaxis. *Curr Allergy Asthma Rep.* 2016;16:20.
12. Matsuyama N, Yasui K, Amakishi E, et al. The IgE-dependent pathway in allergic transfusion reactions: involvement of donor blood allergens other than plasma proteins. *Int J Hematol.* 2015;102:93–100.
13. Azuma H, Yamaguchi M, Takahashi D, et al. Elevated Ca(2)+ influx-inducing activity toward mast cells in pretransfusion sera from patients who developed transfusion-related adverse reactions. *Transfusion.* 2009;49:1754–1761.
14. Abe T, Shimada E, Takanashi M, et al. Antibody against immunoglobulin E contained in blood components as causative factor for anaphylactic transfusion reactions. *Transfusion.* 2014;54:1953–1960.
15. Jacobs JF, Baumert JL, Brons PP, Joosten I, Koppelman SJ, van Pampus EC. Anaphylaxis from passive transfer of peanut allergen in a blood product. *N Engl J Med.* 2011; 364:1981–1982.
16. Gao L, Sha Y, Yuan K, et al. Allergic transfusion reaction caused by the shrimp allergen of donor blood: a case report. *Transfus Apher Sci.* 2014;50:68–70.
17. Arnold DM, Blajchman MA, Ditomasso J, Kulczycki M, Keith PK. Passive transfer of peanut hypersensitivity by fresh frozen plasma. *Arch Intern Med.* 2007;167: 853–854.
18. Ching JC, Lau W, Hannach B, Upton JE. Peanut and fish allergy due to platelet transfusion in a child. *CMAJ.* 2015; 187:905–907.
19. Stern A, van Hage-Hamsten M, Sondell K, Johansson SG. Is allergy screening of blood donors necessary? A comparison between questionnaire answers and the presence of circulating IgE antibodies. *Vox Sang.* 1995;69:114–119.
20. Wilhelm D, Kluter H, Klouche M, Kirchner H. Impact of allergy screening for blood donors: relationship to nonhemolytic transfusion reactions. *Vox Sang.* 1995;69: 217–221.
21. Goldman M, O'Brien SF. Frequency of severe allergies in blood donors. *Transfusion.* 2011;51:2520–2521.
22. Apelseth TO, Kvalheim VL, Kristoffersen EK. Detection of specific immunoglobulin E antibodies toward common airborne allergens, peanut, wheat, and latex in solvent/detergent-treated pooled plasma. *Transfusion.* 2016;56: 1185–1191.
23. Johansson SG, Nopp A, Florvaag E, et al. High prevalence of IgE antibodies among blood donors in Sweden and Norway. *Allergy.* 2005;60:1312–1315.
24. Johansson SG, Nopp A, van Hage M, et al. Passive IgE-sensitization by blood transfusion. *Allergy.* 2005;60: 1192–1199.
25. Winters JL, Moore SB, Sandness C, Miller DV. Transfusion of apheresis PLTs from IgA-deficient donors with anti-IgA is not associated with an increase in transfusion reactions. *Transfusion.* 2004;44:382–385.
26. Savage WJ, Tobian AA, Fuller AK, Wood RA, King KE, Ness PM. Allergic transfusion reactions to platelets are associated more with recipient and donor factors than with product attributes. *Transfusion.* 2011;51: 1716–1722.
27. Savage WJ, Savage JH, Tobian AA, et al. Allergic agonists in apheresis platelet products are associated with allergic transfusion reactions. *Transfusion.* 2012;52:575–581.
28. Idzko M, Pitchford S, Page C. Role of platelets in allergic airway inflammation. *J Allergy Clin Immunol.* 2015;135: 1416–1423.
29. Savage WJ, Tobian AA, Savage JH, Hamilton RG, Ness PM. Atopic predisposition of recipients in allergic transfusion reactions to apheresis platelets. *Transfusion.* 2011;51:2337–2342.

30. Hirayama F. Current understanding of allergic transfusion reactions: incidence, pathogenesis, laboratory tests, prevention and treatment. *Br J Haematol*. 2013;160:434–444.

31. Muylle L, Beert JF, Mertens G, Bult H. Histamine synthesis by white cells during storage of platelet concentrates. *Vox Sang*. 1998;74:193–197.

32. Yazer MH, Podlosky L, Clarke G, Nahirniak SM. The effect of prestorage WBC reduction on the rates of febrile nonhemolytic transfusion reactions to platelet concentrates and RBC. *Transfusion*. 2004;44:10–15.

33. Schwartz LB, Yunginger JW, Miller J, Bokhari R, Dull D. Time course of appearance and disappearance of human mast cell tryptase in the circulation after anaphylaxis. *J Clin Investig*. 1989;83:1551–1555.

34. Domen RE, Hoeltge GA. Allergic transfusion reactions: an evaluation of 273 consecutive reactions. *Arch Pathol Lab Med*. 2003;127:316–320.

35. Conley ME, Delacroix DL. Intravascular and mucosal immunoglobulin A: two separate but related systems of immune defense? *Ann Intern Med*. 1987;106:892–899.

36. Woof JM, Kerr MA. The function of immunoglobulin A in immunity. *J Pathol*. 2006;208:270–282.

37. Anani W, Triulzi D, Yazer MH, Qu L. Relative IgA-deficient recipients have an increased risk of severe allergic transfusion reactions. *Vox Sang*. 2014;107:389–392.

38. Yel L. Selective IgA deficiency. *J Clin Immunol*. 2010;30:10–16.

39. Meny GM, Flickinger C, Marcucci C. The American rare donor plrogram. *J Crit Care*. 2013;28:110 e9–e18.

40. Sandler SG, Eckrich R, Malamut D, Mallory D. Hemagglutination assays for the diagnosis and prevention of IgA anaphylactic transfusion reactions. *Blood*. 1994;84:2031–2035.

41. Yazdani R, Azizi G, Abolhassani H, Aghamohammadi A. Selective IgA deficiency: epidemiology, pathogenesis, clinical phenotype, diagnosis, prognosis and management. *Scand J Immunol*. 2017;85:3–12.

42. Vyas GN, Perkins HA, Fudenberg HH. Anaphylactoid transfusion reactions associated with anti-IgA. *Lancet*. 1968;2:312–315.

43. Nadorp JH, Voss M, Buys WC, et al. The significance of the presence of anti-IgA antibodies in individuals with an IgA deficiency. *Eur J Clin Investig*. 1973;3:317–323.

44. Schmidt AP, Taswell HF, Gleich GJ. Anaphylactic transfusion reactions associated with anti-IgA antibody. *N Engl J Med*. 1969;280:188–193.

45. Lilic D, Sewell WA. IgA deficiency: what we should-or should not-be doing. *J Clin Pathol*. 2001;54:337–338.

46. Robitaille N, Delage G, Long A, Thibault L, Robillard P. Allergic transfusion reactions from blood components donated by IgA-deficient donors with and without anti-IgA: a comparative retrospective study. *Vox Sang*. 2010;99:136–141.

47. Sandler SG, Eder AF, Goldman M, Winters JL. The entity of immunoglobulin A-related anaphylactic transfusion reactions is not evidence based. *Transfusion*. 2015;55:199–204.

48. Tacquard C, Boudjedir K, Carlier M, Muller JY, Gomis P, Mertes PM. Hypersensitivity transfusion reactions due to IgA deficiency are rare according to French hemovigilance data. *J Allergy Clin Immunol*. 2017;140:884–885.

49. Carter K, Worwood M. Haptoglobin: a review of the major allele frequencies worldwide and their association with diseases. *Int J Lab Hematol*. 2007;29:92–110.

50. Kristiansen M, Graversen JH, Jacobsen C, et al. Identification of the haemoglobin scavenger receptor. *Nature*. 2001;409:198–201.

51. Ko DH, Chang HE, Kim TS, et al. A review of haptoglobin typing methods for disease association study and preventing anaphylactic transfusion reaction. *BioMed Res Int*. 2013;2013:390630.

52. Soejima M, Koda Y, Fujihara J, Takeshita H. The distribution of haptoglobin-gene deletion (Hp del) is restricted to East Asians. *Transfusion*. 2007;47:1948–1950.

53. Nishiki S, Hino M, Kumura T, et al. Effectiveness of washed platelet concentrate and red cell transfusions for a patient with anhaptoglobinemia with antihaptoglobin antibody. *Transfus Med*. 2002;12:71–73.

54. Delanghe J, Langlois M, De Buyzere M. Congenital anhaptoglobinemia versus acquired hypohaptoglobinemia. *Blood*. 1998;91:3524.

55. Morishita K, Shimada E, Watanabe Y, Kimura H. Anaphylactic transfusion reactions associated with antihaptoglobin in a patient with ahaptoglobinemia. *Transfusion*. 2000;40:120–121.

56. Shimada E, Tadokoro K, Watanabe Y, et al. Anaphylactic transfusion reactions in haptoglobin-deficient patients with IgE and IgG haptoglobin antibodies. *Transfusion*. 2002;42:766–773.

57. Kim H, Choi J, Park KU, et al. Anaphylactic transfusion reaction in a patient with anhaptoglobinemia: the first case in Korea. *Ann Lab Med*. 2012;32:304–306.

58. Lambin P, Le Pennec PY, Hauptmann G, Desaint O, Habibi B, Salmon C. Adverse transfusion reactions associated with a precipitating anti-C4 antibody of anti-Rodgers specificity. *Vox Sang*. 1984;47:242–249.

59. Westhoff CM, Sipherd BD, Wylie DE, Toalson LD. Severe anaphylactic reactions following transfusions of platelets to a patient with anti-Ch. *Transfusion*. 1992;32:576–579.

60. Wibaut B, Mannessier L, Horbez C, et al. Anaphylactic reactions associated with anti-Chido Antibody following platelet transfusions. *Vox Sang*. 1995;69:150–151.

61. Law M, Morris JK, Wald N, Luczynska C, Burney P. Changes in atopy over a quarter of a century, based on cross sectional data at three time periods. *BMJ*. 2005;330:1187–1188.

62. Savage WJ, Hamilton RG, Tobian AA, et al. Defining risk factors and presentations of allergic reactions to platelet transfusion. *J Allergy Clin Immunol*. 2014;133, 1772-5 e9.

63. Savage WJ, Tobian AA, Savage JH, et al. Transfusion and component characteristics are not associated with allergic transfusion reactions to apheresis platelets. *Transfusion*. 2015;55:296–300.

64. Savage WJ, Hod EA. Noninfectious complications of blood transfusion. In: Fung MK, Eder AF, Spitalnik SL, Westhoff CM, eds. *Technical Manual*. 19th ed. Bethesda, MD: AABB Press; 2017:569−598.

65. Gilstad CW. Anaphylactic transfusion reactions. *Curr Opin Hematol*. 2003;10:419−423.

66. *National Healthcare Safety Network Biovigilance Component Hemovigilance Module Surveillance Protocol*. National Healthcare Safety Network; 2018. https://www.cdc.gov/nhsn/pdfs/biovigilance/bv-hv-protocol-current.pdf.

67. Davenport RD. Management of transfusion reactions. In: Mintz PD, ed. *Transfusion Therapy: Clinical Principles and Practice*. Bethesda, MD: AABB Press; 2011:757−784.

68. Banerji A, Long AA, Camargo Jr CA. Diphenhydramine versus nonsedating antihistamines for acute allergic reactions: a literature review. *Allergy Asthma Proc*. 2007;28:418−426.

69. Geiger TL, Howard SC. Acetaminophen and diphenhydramine premedication for allergic and febrile nonhemolytic transfusion reactions: good prophylaxis or bad practice? *Transfus Med Rev*. 2007;21:1−12.

70. Marti-Carvajal AJ, Sola I, Gonzalez LE, Leon de Gonzalez G, Rodriguez-Malagon N. Pharmacological interventions for the prevention of allergic and febrile non-haemolytic transfusion reactions. *Cochrane Database Syst Rev*. 2010:CD007539.

71. Sicherer SH, Simons FER, Section On A, Immunology. Epinephrine for first-aid management of anaphylaxis. *Pediatrics*. 2017;139.

72. Epinephrine. *Drug Summary*. ConnectiveRx; 2019. https://www.pdr.net/drug-summary/EpiPen-epinephrine-134.6164.

73. Carson JL, Guyatt G, Heddle NM, et al. Clinical practice guidelines from the AABB: red blood cell transfusion thresholds and storage. *J Am Med Assoc*. 2016;316:2025−2035.

74. Roback JD, Caldwell S, Carson J, et al. Evidence-based practice guidelines for plasma transfusion. *Transfusion*. 2010;50:1227−1239.

75. Kaufman RM, Djulbegovic B, Gernsheimer T, et al. Platelet transfusion: a clinical practice guideline from the AABB. *Ann Intern Med*. 2015;162:205−213.

76. Fry JL, Arnold DM, Clase CM, et al. Transfusion premedication to prevent acute transfusion reactions: a retrospective observational study to assess current practices. *Transfusion*. 2010;50:1722−1730.

77. Tobian AA, King KE, Ness PM. Transfusion premedications: a growing practice not based on evidence. *Transfusion*. 2007;47:1089−1096.

78. Wang JS, Sackett DJ, Yuan YM. Randomized clinical controlled cross-over trial (RCT) in the prevention of blood transfusion febrile reactions with small dose hydrocortisone versus anti-histamines. *Zhonghua Nei Ke Za Zhi*. 1992;31(536−8):85−86.

79. Wang SE, Lara Jr PN, Lee-Ow A, et al. Acetaminophen and diphenhydramine as premedication for platelet transfusions: a prospective randomized double-blind placebo-controlled trial. *Am J Hematol*. 2002;70:191−194.

80. Kennedy LD, Case LD, Hurd DD, Cruz JM, Pomper GJ. A prospective, randomized, double-blind controlled trial of acetaminophen and diphenhydramine pretransfusion medication versus placebo for the prevention of transfusion reactions. *Transfusion*. 2008;48:2285−2291.

81. Jorgenson M. Administration of blood components. In: Fung MK, Eder AF, Spitalnik SL, Westhoff CM, eds. *Technical Manual*. Bethesda, MD: AABB Press; 2017:489−504.

82. Campbell-Lee SA, Cooling LW, Cushing MM, et al. *Blood Transfusion Therapy: A Physician's Handbook*. 12th ed. Bethesda, MD: AABB Press; 2017.

83. Williams DM. Clinical pharmacology of corticosteroids. *Respir Care*. 2018;63:655−670.

84. Choo KJ, Simons FE, Sheikh A. Glucocorticoids for the treatment of anaphylaxis. *Cochrane Database Syst Rev*. 2012:CD007596.

85. *Proven and Potential Clinical Benefits of Washing Red Blood Cells before Transfusion: Current Perspectives*. Dovepress; 2016. https://www.dovepress.com/proven-and-potential-clinical-benefits-of-washing-red-blood-cells-befo-peer-reviewed-fulltext-article-IJCTM.

86. *Circular of Information*. AABB Press; 2017. http://www.aabb.org/tm/coi/Documents/coi1017.pdf.

87. Pineda AA, Zylstra VW, Clare DE, Dewanjee MK, Forstrom LA. Viability and functional integrity of washed platelets. *Transfusion*. 1989;29:524−527.

88. Vo TD, Cowles J, Heal JM, Blumberg N. Platelet washing to prevent recurrent febrile reactions to leucocyte-reduced transfusions. *Transfus Med*. 2001;11:45−47.

89. Karafin M, Fuller AK, Savage WJ, King KE, Ness PM, Tobian AA. The impact of apheresis platelet manipulation on corrected count increment. *Transfusion*. 2012;52:1221−1227.

90. Harm SK, Raval JS, Cramer J, Waters JH, Yazer MH. Haemolysis and sublethal injury of RBCs after routine blood bank manipulations. *Transfus Med*. 2012;22:181−185.

91. Refaai MA, Conley GW, Henrichs KF, et al. Decreased hemolysis and improved platelet function in blood components washed with plasma-lyte a compared to 0.9% sodium chloride. *Am J Clin Pathol*. 2018;150:146−153.

92. Buck SA, Kickler TS, McGuire M, Braine HG, Ness PM. The utility of platelet washing using an automated procedure for severe platelet allergic reactions. *Transfusion*. 1987;27:391−393.

93. Fujiwara SI, Fujishima N, Kanamori H, et al. Released washed platelet concentrates are effective and safe in patients with a history of transfusion reactions. *Transfus Apher Sci*. 2018;57:746−751.

94. Holme S, Heaton WA, Moroff G. Evaluation of platelet concentrates stored for 5 days with reduced plasma volume. *Transfusion*. 1994;34:39−43.

95. Ali AM, Warkentin TE, Bardossy L, Goldsmith CH, Blajchman MA. Platelet concentrates stored for 5 days in a reduced volume of plasma maintain hemostatic function and viability. *Transfusion*. 1994;34:44−47.

96. Schoenfeld H, Muhm M, Doepfmer UR, Kox WJ, Spies C, Radtke H. The functional integrity of platelets in volume-

reduced platelet concentrates. *Anesth Analg.* 2005;100: 78–81.

97. Ashford P, Gulliksson H, Georgsen J, Distler P. Standard terminology for platelet additive solutions. *Vox Sang.* 2010;98:577–578.

98. de Wildt-Eggen J, Nauta S, Schrijver JG, van Marwijk Kooy M, Bins M, van Prooijen HC. Reactions and platelet increments after transfusion of platelet concentrates in plasma or an additive solution: a prospective, randomized study. *Transfusion.* 2000;40:398–403.

99. Kerkhoffs JL, Eikenboom JC, Schipperus MS, et al. A multicenter randomized study of the efficacy of transfusions with platelets stored in platelet additive solution II versus plasma. *Blood.* 2006;108:3210–3215.

100. Cohn CS, Stubbs J, Schwartz J, et al. A comparison of adverse reaction rates for PAS C versus plasma platelet units. *Transfusion.* 2014;54:1927–1934.

101. Tobian AA, Fuller AK, Uglik K, et al. The impact of platelet additive solution apheresis platelets on allergic transfusion reactions and corrected count increment (CME). *Transfusion.* 2014;54:1523–1529. quiz 2.

102. Drawz SM, Marschner S, Yanez M, et al. Observational study of corrected count increments after transfusion of platelets treated with riboflavin pathogen reduction technology in additive solutions. *Transfusion.* 2015;55: 1745–1751.

103. Kiani-Alikhan S, Yong PF, Grosse-Kreul D, et al. Successful desensitization to immunoglobulin A in a case of transfusion-related anaphylaxis. *Transfusion.* 2010;50: 1897–1901.

104. *Immune Tolerance in Allergy & Asthma.* National Institute of Allergy and Infectious Diseases; 2019. https://www. immunetolerance.org/researchers/clinical-trials/allergy-asthma.

CHAPTER 5

Changing Landscaping in Transfusion-Transmitted Infections

HONG HONG, MD, PHD • MELISSA PESSIN, MD, PHD •
ESTHER BABADY, PHD, D(ABMM)

INTRODUCTION

Treatment of patients with human blood components has improved significantly in the last century. However, complications, such as transmission of pathogens, remain a known risk of transfusion. Although the U.S. blood supply is safer than it has ever been, some bacteria, viruses, prions, and parasites can still be transmitted by blood transfusions. Additionally, emerging pathogens continue to present a considerable threat to the safety of the blood supply.

Most morbidity and mortality related to blood transfusion is caused by the transmission of infectious agents.[1] To attain the desired lowest risk blood supply, actions to enhance safety at multiple levels are needed (Fig. 5.1).[2] Donor evaluation, donor laboratory screening tests, and pathogen inactivation procedures are considered crucial tools to help reduce the risk of transfusion-transmitted infections (TTI), although these methods do not completely eliminate all potential risks.

APPROACHES TO REDUCING TTI

Most blood components (e.g., red blood cells [RBCs], platelets, plasma, and cryoprecipitate) are infused without pasteurization, sterilization, or other treatments used to inactivate infectious agents. Any blood-borne pathogen has the potential to be transmitted directly to recipients by blood transfusion. Several strategies exist to reduce the risk of TTI.

Donor Screening Approach

Blood donation is a multiple-sequential step process. Blood donors are asked a set of standard questions

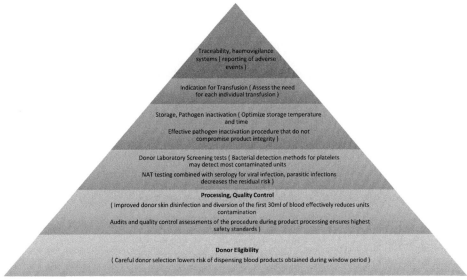

FIG. 5.1 Strategies to reduce risk of transfusion-transmitted infections.

Immunologic Concepts in Transfusion Medicine. https://doi.org/10.1016/B978-0-323-67509-3.00005-6

before the donation to assist in determining whether they are in good health and free of any diseases that could be transmitted by blood transfusion. If the donor's answers indicate that they are not well or are at risk for having a disease transmissible by blood transfusion, they are excluded from blood donation. If the donor is eligible to donate, the donated blood is then tested to rule out the presence of pathogens, such as syphilis, hepatitis B virus (HBV), hepatitis C viruses (HCV), and human immunodeficiency virus (HIV).[3]

Donor screening methods to prevent TTI include, but are not limited to donor education material, donor selection criteria, donor medical history interview, donor deferral registries, donor laboratory screening tests, donor telephone call backs after blood donation, and modification of the donated blood component (Table 5.1).[3] The current paradigm for increasing the safety of the blood supply is the development and implementation of laboratory screening methods and restrictive donor criteria. Exclusion of potential donors with an increased likelihood of exposure is the most straightforward way of protecting the safety of the blood supply. To test blood for all pathogens that are prevalent in a given population and can cause serious disease is not practical. For many diseases such as malaria and babesiosis, no licensed laboratory donor screening tests are available to increase transfusion safety. In contrast, for infectious diseases in which routine donor screening tests are performed (e.g., HIV, human T-lymphotropic virus [HTLV], HBV, HCV), there is a window period that could pose a potential risk on transfusion safety. Table 5.1 lists the types of screening

approaches used for different infectious agents.[4] Donor evaluation and donor laboratory screening tests are the key components in this process.

Donor Evaluation and Donor History Questionnaire

As biologics, blood components fall under the Food and Drug Administration (FDA)'s Center for Biologics Evaluation and Research (CBER), which is responsible for overseeing and regulating all aspects of the U.S. blood supply including enforcing standards for blood collection and blood component distribution. The agency also inspects blood collection centers and monitors reports of errors, accidents, and adverse events related to blood collection and transfusion. In recent years, the FDA has significantly increased its oversight of blood centers, with mandatory, annual inspection of all blood transfusion facilities.

The FDA has progressively strengthened the overlapping safeguards that protect patients from unsuitable blood and blood components. Blood donors are asked specific questions concerning risk factors associated with exposure to or clinical evidence of a relevant TTI at time of donation. Blood donors are deferred from donation if risk factors are acknowledged. Prospective donors must meet specific eligibility criteria required by the FDA 21 *Code of Federal Regulation* (CFR) Section 630.10 on the day of donation and before collection to ensure the safety of the blood supply. Besides donor evaluation, the FDA also requires blood centers to maintain lists of unsuitable donors to prevent further donations from these individuals.

TABLE 5.1
Approaches to Donor Screening.

Approach	Context for Use	Examples
Questioning only	Pathogens with defined risk factors and no sensitive and/or specific test	Plasmodium species, prions
Testing only	Pathogens with sensitive and/or specific test available, but no way to identify individuals at risk	West Nile virus, Zika virus
Questioning and testing	Pathogens for which there are both identified risk factors and effective tests	HIV, HBV, HCV, babesiosis
Use of blood components that test negative for specific recipients	Pathogens with a high prevalence in donors but for which an identifiable subset of recipients can benefit from blood components that test negative	Cytomegalovirus
Testing of blood components	Pathogens not detected in donor samples	Bacteria

Blood banks and their communities such as AABB (American Association of Blood Banks) have also aggressively pursued strategies to increase blood safety in all steps of the transfusion chain. AABB standards are often considered throughout the United States (U.S.) as defining a standard of practice in the blood banking community and therefore are widely implemented. The AABB task force produced a streamlined system for evaluating blood donors that satisfied U.S. requirements, and developed the "Donor History Questionnaire," commonly abbreviated DHQ, a standardized set of questions to screen volunteer blood donors at time of donation.

An FDA guidance document published in May 2016 recognized the AABB standardized full-length and abbreviated donor history questionnaires (FL-DHQ and aDHQ, respectively) and accompanying materials, version 2.0 dated February 2016. These documents are consistent with the FDA requirements and recommendations for collecting donor history information from donors of blood and blood components. AABB's DHQ is used by most blood centers in the U.S. for donor screening. Implementation of new eligibility criteria would require changes to the DHQ documents.

Donor Screening Tests

Since the 1970s, remarkable advances have been made to improve blood safety, particularly through the detection and identification of blood-borne viruses. Donor screening tests remain a reactive approach to blood safety. After donation, blood banks test a sample of the blood from each donation to identify donors and their donated components that might harbor infectious agents. The donor infectious disease tests should meet the FDA requirement as specified in Title 21, Section 610.40, of the CFR. All tests must be negative before the blood is deemed suitable for transfusion.

Various types of assays have been developed for use in blood screening over the past 3 decades. The assays most commonly in use are designed to detect antibodies against or the antigens and/or nucleic acids of the infectious agent. However, not all assays are suitable in all situations, and each assay has its limitations, which needs to be understood and taken into consideration when selecting the most appropriate for this use. Furthermore, the assays must be approved by the FDA with the intended use of donor screening.

The main types of assays used for blood screening are as follows:
- Immunoassays (IAs) including
  Enzyme Immunoassay (EIA) or Enzyme-linked Immunoassay (ELISA)

Chemiluminescent Immunoassay (ChLIA)
hemagglutination/particle agglutination assay
lateral flow immunoassay, Western Blot (WB), Enzyme Strip Assay (ESA)
- Nucleic acid amplification tests (NAT) including Polymerase Chain Reaction (PCR), Transcription-Mediated Amplification (TMA) and Nucleic Acid Sequence Based Amplification (NASBA).

The primary cause of present day transfusion-transmissible viral infections is thought to be related to donations made by individuals in the window period, the interval between the time of infection and the appearance of clinical symptoms or detectable disease markers, such as specific antibodies or viral nucleic acid sequences. Implementation of NAT with lower limits of detection (LOD) for donor screening has significantly improved the frequency of detection of donors in the window period compared to IA targeting viral antibodies or antigens.[5,6] Although the window period has considerably been reduced, rare cases of TTIs may still occur and have been reported including a case of HIV transmission from an RBC component, reinforcing the need for continued donor screening.[4]

The selection of assays to detect potential TTI is based on several criteria including assay characteristics (e.g., sensitivity and specificity), the loss of potential donors, the risk of testing errors, as well as cost and ease of use.[7] A screening algorithm may be developed for each TTI depending on pathogen characteristics. The design of an algorithm will be determined by the specific infection marker to be screened for, the expertise of the users, the infrastructure, testing conditions, and quality systems of individual screening facilities. Once an algorithm has been defined, this guides the procurement of the specific test kits, reagents, and laboratory-testing systems required.

Tests suitable for screening of blood donations are available for many of the infectious agents capable of causing significant morbidity in recipients. All the tests that can be used to screen donated blood approved by FDA as of Feb 2019 are listed in Table 5.2.

Screening of all blood donations is mandatory for HIV-1/2, HBV, HCV, HTLV I/II, ZIKV, and *T. pallidum* (syphilis). Additional testing that is not required but often performed based on special circumstances (e.g., special patient population) include testing for *T. cruzi* and Cytomegalovirus (CMV). The local epidemiology may dictate further testing for endemic infections (e.g., *Plasmodium* and *Babesia* species). Where feasible, blood screening should be consolidated in strategically located facilities at national and/or regional levels to

TABLE 5.2
Summary of Complete List of Donor Screening Assays for Infectious Agents.[4]

Pathogen	Laboratory Test Format	Marker Detected
Bacteria	Bacterial culture	Bacterial growth
Hepatitis B virus (HBV)	ChLIA/ELISA	HBV surface antigen
	ChLIA/ELISA	HBV core antibodies
	PCR	HBV DNA
Hepatitis C virus (HCV)	ChLIA/ELISA	HCV antibodies
	Reverse Transcriptase RCR	HCV RNA
Human immunodeficiency virus types 1 and 2 (HIV)	WB	HIV-1 antibodies
	PCR/TMA	HIV-1 RNA
	ELISA	HIV-2 antibodies
	ChLIA/ELISA	HIV-1/2 antibodies
Human T-Lymphotropic virus types I and II (HTLV I/II)	ChLIA/ELISA/WB	HTLV I/II antibodies
Treponema pallidum (*T. pallidum*)	ELISA/Hemagglutination	*T. pallidum* antibodies
ZIKA virus (ZIKV)	PCR/TMA	ZIKV RNA
West Nile virus (WNV)	PCR/TMA	WNV RNA
Trypanosoma cruzi (*T. cruzi*)	ChLIA/ELISA/ESA	*T. cruzi* antibodies
Cytomegalovirus (CMV)	Solid phase red cell adherence assay/ Passive particle agglutination assay	CMV antibodies
Babesia species	TMA	*Babesia RNA*

achieve uniformity of standards, increased safety, and economies of scale.

TRANSFUSION-TRANSMITTED INFECTIONS

At present, with the implementation of efficient donor screening and testing, the risk of pathogen transmission from transfusion has significantly decreased, particularly for HIV, HCV, and HBV (Table 5.3). Bacterial contamination of platelet components continues to be an issue despite all the efforts to improve platelet sterility. Emerging pathogens, such as Zika virus and Ebola virus, may potentially cause TTI and therefore are targeted for removal by testing and/or inactivation. *Plasmodium* species are still major parasites in endemic countries and potentially infected components in those countries are monitored for removal. Syphilis is still a significant bacterial blood-borne target in developing countries, though less so in developed countries.

Bacteria

Transmission of bacteria to recipients through transfusion of contaminated blood components was first documented more than 60 years ago[9] and remains one of the leading causes of morbidity and mortality in modern transfusion medicine. In combined fatalities reported to FDA from 2012 through 2016, of a total of 186 transfusion-related fatalities, 19 cases were attributed to microbial infections, 14 of which were bacterial, accounting for 73% of fatalities. Platelet components were implicated in 78% of all cases.[1]

Platelet bacterial contamination

Most platelet component contaminants are commensal skin flora introduced by venipuncture at the time of blood collection. Gram-negative bacteria such as *Escherichia coli* (*E. coli*), *Acinetobacter*, and *Klebsiella* species can also be present in blood donations from asymptomatic donors and cause infections such as pneumonia, meningitis, or other severe illnesses in blood recipients.[10,11]

Bacteria associated with the skin microflora are traditionally considered nonpathogenic; however, the ability of certain strains to form biofilms (i.e., surface-associated populations of cells encased in an extracellular polymeric matrix) increases their virulence by enhancing their capacity to adhere to and colonize surfaces, evade the immune response, and resist antimicrobial chemotherapy.[12] Several strains of Gram-positive (*Staphylococcus epidermidis*, *Staphylococcus capitis*) and

TABLE 5.3
Risk per Unit of Selected Transfusion-Transmitted Pathogens.[8]

Pathogen	Component	United States	Canada	Europe
HIV	All	1:2,000,000	1:7,800,000	1:900,000–5,500,000
HCV	All	1:2,000,000	1:2,300,000	1:2,000,000–4,400,000
HBV	All	1:277,000	1 in 153,000	1:77,000–1,100,000
WNV	All	1:350,000	Rare	No reported cases
HTLV-I and/or -II	RBCs and/or PLTs	1:3,000,000	1:4,300,000	Not tested
Bacterial transmission	RBCs	1:40,000–1: 5,000,000		
Bacterial sepsis	PLTs	1:59,000 single donor	1:41,000 single donor	1:11,000 (pooled)
Malaria	RBCs	1:1,000,000–1: 5,000,000	Three cases in 10 years	11 cases in 10 years

Gram-negative (*Serratia marcescens*) bacteria that have been recovered from contaminated platelet units can form biofilms in the platelet storage environment.[13,14] Studies also indicate that the platelet storage environment may actually stimulate biofilm formation.[14] Biofilm-forming strains can rapidly attach to the surface of the platelet bag in just 20 minutes and this reduces the number of organisms available for automated culture systems to detect. Those biofilm-forming strains are three times more likely to be undetected by the BacT/ALERT system compared to nonbiofilm formers, leading to missed detection of contaminated platelet components.[13]

Although Gram-negative organisms (e.g., *Serratia*, *Enterobacter*, *Salmonella* spp.) are typically implicated in the most severe adverse transfusion reactions, Gram-positive bacteria (e.g., *Staphylococcus epidermidis*) constitute most organisms responsible for platelet component contamination.[15] Several factors can influence platelet component contamination rates, including platelet collection and preparation methods, donor arm disinfection, diversion systems, volume cultured, aerobic and/or anaerobic culture, time to inoculation, and interpretation of results.[16] These methods have been shown to reduce bacterial contamination of the unit substantially, from 44% to 77%, but do not completely eliminate them.[17–19]

Platelet components are especially susceptible to contamination as their storage conditions of 20–24°C with agitation is particularly amenable to bacterial growth.[20] In 1984, to improve the supply and availability of platelets, the storage of platelet components was extended from 5 to 7 days. This extension was based strictly on the functional quality of the platelets. However, soon thereafter, due to the concern from an increase in platelet transfusion-related fatalities, the FDA mandated a reduction of the storage duration of platelet component back from 7 to 5 days in an effort to limit the extent of bacterial contamination.[21] It was not until 2004 that blood centers started to introduce screening of all platelet components for bacteria postdonation as a further risk reduction measure. Currently, only two automatic bacterial screening systems have been cleared and approved by FDA for detecting platelet bacterial contamination: the BacT/ALERT (bioMérieux) and the eBDS (Pall Medical). The BacT/ALERT is an automated microbial detection system, which checks bacterial growth by detecting increased CO_2 production while the eBDS system is based on detecting bacterial growth from O_2 consumption.

In practice, platelet components are held for at least 24 hours postdonation before sampling to allow bacteria to grow to sufficient numbers for detection in the testing systems.[22] The sample volume screened is a compromise between sensitivity of detection and loss of product to the patient. Souza and colleagues compared bacterial screening data for 4- and 8-mL samples and showed a relative improvement in culture sensitivity of 31% with 8-mL samples.[23] This increased volume also reduced the time to detection of positive cultures by 23% in the automated culture system.[23] Eder and colleagues also noted an improvement in sensitivity after an increase in sample volume from 4 to 8 mL.[16]

Sampled platelet components are held in collection facilities for another 12 hours while waiting for bacterial culture results. If bacterial culture initial reading is negative, the platelet components can be distributed for transfusion, but the bacterial culture will continue to be monitored for up to 7 days. A positive initial reactive signal results in the hold, or recall, of all associated components, including RBCs with pooled platelet components. If there is a delayed positive bacterial culture result, the collection center contacts the transfusion facility immediately to stop the transfusion. Additional investigations are undertaken if a component was already transfused, including informing the hospital that they may have transfused a potentially contaminated unit so that the patient can be monitored accordingly and treatment initiated if required.[3]

Implementation of the routine use of microbial detection systems as a prerelease test for platelet collections has resulted in significant safety improvements. As reviewed by Benjamin and McDonald, automated bacterial screening systems detect about 1 in 539−10,606 (0.054%−1.061%) apheresis platelet donations that are contaminated and confirmed positive or about 1/127 to 1/1035 per million (0.013%−0.104%) donations.[24] Before the implementation of bacterial culture-based testing systems, an average of 6−8 fatalities/year from contaminated platelets were reported to the FDA. Today, on average, only 1 death/year is reported to FDA.[1]

Although multiple measures have been implemented to reduce the risk, platelet contamination continues to occur.[25] Low-load bacterial contamination might evade the bacterial screening testing system. Some bacterial pathogens such as *C. perfringens* do not grow in the BacT/ALERT system. One study showed that *C. perfringens* was not consistently detected by a rapid test even when high levels of contamination were present causing a septic transfusion reaction.[11] A study from the University Hospitals of Cleveland suggested that contamination of platelet components was still undetected following implementation of a bacterial culture testing system. In this study, all platelet units were cultured 24 hours after collection and initially released as negative from the collection center. All platelet units were further cultured at time of release for transfusion at their medical center. A total of 20 out of 51,440 platelet units transfused (0.004%; 389 per million) were bacterially contaminated as

determined by active surveillance, resulting in five septic transfusion reactions occurring 9−24 hours posttransfusion.[20]

As of January 2019, no final guidelines have been issued regarding risk mitigation of bacterial platelet contamination. Per the newly issued draft guidelines in December 2018,[26] the FDA agreed that no further measures were needed to limit bacterial contamination of 5-day storage platelets that have been treated by pathogen reduction. However, regular platelets with 5-day storage need either primary culture followed by secondary culture performed no earlier than day 3, or primary culture, followed by secondary rapid testing approved by the FDA. To date, the Verax PGD test is the only FDA-cleared rapid test for this use. These guidelines also provide options to extend platelet shelf life from 5 to 7 days. For storage of platelets beyond 5 days, to 7 days, the component needs either primary culture followed by a secondary culture with a device labeled as a "safety measure" performed no earlier than day 4, or primary culture followed by a secondary rapid test labeled as a "safety measure." Large volume delayed sampling is also an acceptable method to extend platelet storage from 5 to 7 days.

Traditionally, a septic transfusion reaction would be expected to occur during or within 4 hours posttransfusion.[27] However, the study from University Hospitals of Cleveland mentioned earlier showed that in all five septic transfusion reactions after implementation of the bacterial screening testing system, patient symptoms were not immediate as had been previously described, but rather their onset was significantly delayed. In practice, with the changing clinical picture of a septic transfusion reaction, the transfusion medicine service should always maintain a high index of suspicion for platelet bacterial contamination and septic transfusion reactions. One should always stop the transfusion and start an investigation if there is concern for a septic transfusion reaction. Clinical services should be educated to immediately report any suspected septic transfusion reactions to both the transfusion service and to the blood supplier, even if they remain uncertain as to the cause.

RBC bacterial contamination

Although platelet components are the most likely blood components at risk for bacterial contamination, mainly with Gram-positive skin flora, contamination of RBCs has also been reported, primarily with endogenous enteric Gram-negative organisms. Storage of RBCs at 4°C for longer than 24 hours will inactivate some bacterial species (e.g., *T. pallidum*), but other species (e.g., *Listeria monocytogenes*, *Yersinia enterocolitica*) are still capable of growth at this temperature and may induce septic shock when such contaminated RBCs are transfused.[28]

Y. enterocolitica usually causes relatively mild gastro-intestinal disease but may cause severe infection post-transfusion.[29] Transfusion of preformed endotoxin from *Y. enterocolitica* contaminated RBCs can elicit a systemic inflammatory response that is often dramatic and rapidly fatal. A systematic review of 55 published cases showed that those septic shocks were sometimes heralded by atypical symptoms such as vomiting, explosive diarrhea, and abdominal pain. The mortality rate exceeded 50%.[29] Studies have shown that *Y. enterocolitica* is particularly apt at contaminating RBCs. This is due to its cryophilic nature, its ability to utilize glucose and adenine present in red cell anticoagulant and additive solutions as energy sources, and the RBCs' pH of 7.3, which is optimal for its growth. The longer RBCs are in storage, the greater the amount of iron released following RBC hemolysis, and thus a corresponding increase is seen in the growth of *Y. enterocolitica* following 3–5 weeks of storage.[30]

Viruses

To minimize the risk of potential blood donors transmitting transmissible viruses to patients, all donations are subjected to stringent screening procedures. As mentioned earlier, mandatory testing includes screening of donations for several transfusion-transmissible viruses including HIV, HBV, HCV, HTLVs, and ZIKV. Additional viruses that may be transmitted by blood transfusions but not routinely tested in blood donors include Hepatitis E viruses, Dengue virus, West Nile virus, Chikungunya virus, and Parvovirus B19.

HIV

HIV, including HIV-1 and HIV-2, are two species of *Lentivirus* (a subgroup of retrovirus) that cause HIV infection and if left untreated, over time result in the acquired immunodeficiency syndrome (AIDS). HIV infection is primarily a sexually transmitted infection and occurs through contact with contaminated blood, pree-jaculate, semen, and vaginal fluids.

The risk of HIV through infected blood components transfusion exceeds that of any other risk exposure. Moreover, 90% of transfused recipients would acquire HIV infection when given an HIV seropositive blood component.[31] Transmission rates of HIV are equivalent for red cells, platelets, or plasma. However, red cells stored for more than 21 days or red cells that are saline washed (and therefore have lower leukocyte concentrations) may transmit HIV infection at a lower rate than other stored components.[32]

Since the early 1980s, tremendous progress has been made in understanding, as well as decreasing, the risk of HIV transmission from blood transfusions.[33] The major interventions that are used to minimize this risk include questioning of donors concerning HIV risk behaviors and laboratory testing of each donated unit of blood for antibodies to HIV-1 and HIV-2 and for HIV-1 RNA.

Before the implementation of HIV antibody (HIV Ab) testing, it was estimated that 12,000 to 25,000 cases of transfusion-associated AIDS cases may have resulted from HIV untested blood components transfused in the U.S.[34] By 1995, the risk of HIV-1 transmission per unit transfused in the U.S. was estimated to be between 1 in 450,000 and 1 in 660,000.[35] By 2003, this estimated risk had further decreased to between 1 in 1.4 million and 1 in 1.8 million units with the implementation of NAT.[36] In the U.S., donor HIV NAT testing is done by pooling of 6−16 specimens (mini-pool NAT, or MP-NAT), whereas in some other HIV endemic countries such as South Africa, this is done as individual donation NAT (ID-NAT).[37]

Although ID-NAT (with or without antibody testing) shows the highest sensitivity for identifying infected donors, studies suggest that HIV Ab testing remains useful, particularly in first-time donations, unless other blood safety measures can be put in place.[6,38−40] From a regulatory standpoint, testing by ID-NAT without serologic screening is not yet approved nor recommended by any national or international regulatory authority. HIV Ab testing further provides another safeguard against possible failure of HIV NAT, due to either primer or probe mismatches with circulating HIV genetic variants, or due to testing error.[38]

Despite all efforts, HIV transmission may still occur for the following reasons: donations collected during the window period of infection; infection with variant strains of HIV that may escape detection by current screening assays; testing or clerical errors.[39−44] Pathogen reduction technology has proven to be a potential alternative to further improve blood safety for HIV.[45]

HBV

Over the last 4 decades, the risk of transfusion-transmitted HBV has steadily decreased, yet HBV transmission remains the most frequent transfusion-transmitted viral infection.[46] Before 1970, approximately 6% of multitransfused recipients acquired a transfusion-transmitted HBV (TT HBV) infection.[46] The risk of TT HBV infection started to fall following the introduction of the HBV surface antigen (HBsAg) testing in the early 1970s. In the mid-1980s, hepatitis B core antibody (HBcAb) testing was introduced to screen blood donors in HBV nonendemic countries to detect chronic virus carriers with low-level viremia who may not have detectable HBsAg levels. Studies of anti-HBc-positive donors have revealed an HBV DNA positivity rate of 0%–15%.[47] Since 2012, with the introduction of HBV NAT in blood donor screening, the residual risk of HBV infection by transfusion further decreased.[48,49]

Implementation of NAT further revealed the occurrence of HBsAg-negative occult HBV infection (OBI) in blood donors. OBI is defined as the presence of HBV DNA in the liver (with very low amount or undetectable HBV DNA in the serum) of individuals who tested negative for HBsAg.[50] OBIs are mainly found in older donors; nearly 100% are positive for anti-HBc, and approximately 50% are positive for anti-HBsAg. On the basis of the HBV antibody profile, OBI may be stratified into seropositive OBI (anti-HBc and/or anti-HBsAg positive) and seronegative OBI (anti-HBc and anti-HBsAg-negative).[50] Potential biological explanations for OBI include the chronic carrier state in which HBsAg has declined over the years to a subdetectable level, individuals having recovered from infection but are unable to develop a totally effective immune control, and mutations in the HBV genome affecting viral replication, S antigen production, or detection.[51]

Blood components from donors with OBI carry a high risk of HBV transmission by transfusion. The clinical outcome of occult HBV transmission primarily depends on recipient immune status and the viral load of HBV DNA copies present in the blood components. The presence of donor anti-HBsAg reduces the risk of HBV infection by approximately fivefold.[52] Notably, the risk of HBV transmission may be lower in endemic areas than in nonendemic areas, because most recipients have already been exposed to HBV.[47] OBI transmission by plasma containing components has been reported, but not by RBCs, possibly due to only small amounts of plasma present in RBC units hence with much lower levels of viral particles.[53,54]

The potential for OBI transmission remains despite the implementation of HBsAg, anti-HBc, and HBV NAT screening. Similar to HIV, pathogen inactivation technologies using chemical agents and ultraviolet illumination may provide an alternative method to further improve blood safety for HBV.

HCV

HCV infections result primarily from parenteral exposure, with high rates of infections in intravenous (IV) drug users and recipients of contaminated blood components.[55] Approximately 70%–75% of HCV infections become chronic, whereas 25%–30% of exposed individuals have self-limited infection and succeed in clearing the virus.[56]

In early HCV infection, the viremia levels rapidly ramp up to a plateau concentration and remain very high for approximately 2 months before antibody seroconversion. Intermittent low-level HCV viremia can occur as much as 2 months before the period of exponential increase in viral load and the high-titer plateau-phase viremia that usually precedes seroconversion.[57] Blood transfusions from donors in the early stage of acute HCV infection can be infectious before RNA detection by NAT screening.[58] Furthermore, NAT cannot completely exclude the risk of TT HCV given the high-level infectivity of acute HCV.[33]

The discovery of HCV as the causative agent of non-A/non-B hepatitis in 1989 and the following development of first-generation EIAs for the detection of antibodies to HCV (anti-HCV) in 1990 represents the major breakthrough in the prevention of transfusion-transmitted HCV.[59,60] Retrospective studies of blood donors and recipients repositories from the mid 1960s and early 1970s demonstrated that almost 25% of transfusion recipients in the U.S. were infected with HCV.[61,62] Several key events in the 1970s, such as moving to a 100% volunteer blood donation as opposed to paid donors, as well as implementation of screening and exclusion of HBsAg-positive blood, allowed for a reduction in TT HCV to about 7% of recipients.[63,64]

The sensitivity of anti-HCV immunoassays (IAs) improved, as second-, third-, and fourth-generation (antigen-antibody "combo") IAs were developed.[55,65,66] The fourth-generation HCV IA, which targets both antigen and antibody, has increased its sensitivity as two infectious markers of HCV are detected in the same assay, but it is limited by the infectious window period of approximately 66 days. Initiation of molecular testing for HCV-RNA by NAT further shortened the window period to only 3–5 days.[65] Stringent blood bank practices as well as serological assays and NAT have successfully minimized the residual risk from TT HCV in the U.S. to less than 1 in a million (0.0001%) per unit transfused.[55]

The American Red Cross analyzed HCV prevalence and NAT yield rates from 66 million donations in the U.S. tested during the period of 1999–2008. The NAT yield rate among first-time donors was 0.872 (1 per 115,000) and for repeat donors was 0.038 (1 per 2,660,000). Males and females were equally represented among the HCV NAT yield donors, and the highest yield occurred in donors between the ages of 16–29 years and those who lived in the Southern portion of the U.S.[67,68]

HCV infection can be classified into three categories: HCV window period infection (anti-HCV Ab negative and HCV RNA reactive), anti-HCV Ab and HCV RNA concordantly positive chronic infection, and probably resolved HCV infection (anti-HCV Ab positive and HCV NAT nonreactive).[69] In rare cases such as large in-frame deletions in structural genes of HCV, high viral load HCV carriers may never develop detectable anti-HCV Ab.[5,70]

Among anti-HCV repeatedly reactive donations, about 40% were reactive by HCV ID-NAT demonstrating acute or chronic HCV infection in these donors.[71] In contrast, about 25%−30% of donors with confirmed anti-HCV did not have detectable HCV RNA.[71,72] Those donors may have had (1) a false-reactive screening test and be uninfected, (2) a resolved HCV infection, (3) an occult HCV infection, or (4) a chronic persistent infection characterized by the presence of detectable HCV RNA in liver or peripheral blood mononuclear cells but transient or intermittent low-level viremia.[69] The risk of TT occult HCV infection is uncertain. In September 2018, the FDA issued a new draft guidance to provide additional information about the status of a donor infection for those with repeatedly reactive anti-HCV screening results using currently available licensed HCV NAT and licensed anti-HCV donor screening tests.[73]

El Ekiaby M et al. studied HCV-RNA levels in Egyptian blood donors in the preseroconversion window period and in later anti-HCV-positive stages of infection. Almost 99% of anti-HCV-reactive donations without detectable HCV-RNA on initial ID-NAT screening had eradicated circulating virus, while the other 1% had extremely low viral loads and were likely not infectious. The incremental safety offered by serologic testing of ID-NAT-screened blood seems minimal.[69] Another retrospective study in 15 countries across seven international regions also showed minimal incremental efficacy of anti-HCV testing when ID-NAT screening is performed, particularly for screening lapsed and repeat donations.[74] The small difference in TT HCV risk between the anti-HCV Ab with HCV ID-NAT strategy versus the HCV ID-NAT alone strategies is widely applicable across regions and only becomes significant in HCV endemic areas such as Egypt.[74,75] Although anti-HCV Ab screening is currently of doubtful benefit, it still remains part of the testing algorithm. With the implementation of pathogen reduction technology for RBC and whole blood, the cost-effectiveness of current HCV testing strategy might need reevaluation.

HTLV

HTLV-I and HTLV-II were the first human retroviruses discovered.[76,77] They both belong to the oncovirus subfamily of retroviruses and can transform human lymphocytes so that they are self-sustaining in vitro.[78] HTLV-I has been associated with adult T-cell leukemia, HTLV-associated myelopathy/tropical spastic paraparesis, and HTLV-associated uveitis. HTLV-II has been associated with T-hairy cell leukemia, benign lymphocytosis, and chronic neurodegenerative disease; however, different from HTLV-I, its causal role in disease has not been established.[78]

HTLV-I is endemic to the Caribbean, parts of Japan, and parts of Africa and South America. HTLV-II, on the other hand, is increasingly seen in developed countries among IV drug users.[79] Transmission of HTLV-I occurs from mother to child, by sexual contact, by blood transfusion, and by sharing contaminated needles.[80,81] Transmission of HTLV-I by blood transfusion occurs with transfusion of white cell-containing cellular blood components (whole blood, RBCs, and platelets) but not with the frozen/thawed plasma components from HTLV-I-infected blood.[82−85]

Seroconversion rates of 44%−63% have been reported in recipients of HTLV-I-infected by cellular components in HTLV-I endemic areas. Lower rates (approximately 20%) have been reported in recipients of contaminated cellular components in the U.S.[79,85] The probability of transmission by whole blood or RBCs appears to diminish with greater duration of component storage; this finding has been ascribed to depletion of infected cells, presumably T-lymphocytes.[85,86]

To date, safety measures for HTLV transmission are primarily based on donor suitability assessment and leukoreduction (LR) of cellular blood components. Pathogen reduction technologies could potentially offer an additional step toward the safety of recipients.

Because HTLV-I and HTLV-II are highly white blood cell (WBC)-associated, LR is thought to reduce the risk of virus transmission by transfusion. Hewitt and co-workers performed an HTLV lookback investigation within the NHS Blood and Transplant programs. LR was associated with a 93% reduction in HTLV transmission compared to non-LR units (transfused before 1998). The maximum HTLV transmission rate with LR units was estimated at 3.7%.[87]

FDA has required blood donation screening for antibodies to HTLV-I since 1988 and to HTLV-II since 1998. The serologic diagnosis of HTLV infections is based on an EIA screen followed by confirmation with an immunoblot (IB) assay (Western blot or line immunoassay).

In the U.S., blood donors whose serum specimens are repeatedly reactive by the HTLV-I EIA and confirmed by IB are permanently deferred from blood donation. Since 1988, more than 200,000 HTLV false-positive donors tested with licensed HTLV assays but without any evidence of infection have been deferred and none have been eligible for reentry, thus impacting blood component self-sufficiency.[88] In September 2018, the FDA issued a draft guidance that proposed a requalification method for those previously deferred donors based on "a determination that their previous reactive test results for antibodies to HTLV-I/II were falsely positive."[89]

CMV

CMV is an ubiquitous β-herpesvirus, usually transmitted by direct person-to-person contact, causing mostly asymptomatic or mild mononucleosis-like infections in immunocompetent subjects.[90] Infection of immunocompromised patients with CMV is a significant cause of morbidity and mortality. Symptoms of CMV infection in these patients cover a broad range of syndromes from direct manifestations of viral replication such as fever, leukopenia, thrombocytopenia, hepatitis, enteritis, and pneumonia to indirect sequelae such as an elevated risk for renal allograft rejection or an impaired cellular immune response.[91]

CMV DNA has repeatedly been found in peripheral WBCs of healthy, CMV-seropositive individuals, especially in cells of the myeloid lineage.[92,93] One of the main reservoirs of CMV are monocytes in peripheral blood.[94] If the donated blood contains CMV-infected monocytes, theoretically the virus can reactivate in transfused monocytes and infect the recipient. An important route of infection, therefore, for high-risk groups such as seronegative recipients of marrow transplants or newborn babies is assumed to be transmission of CMV by blood components from latently infected blood donors (so-called transfusion-transmitted CMV infection [TT-CMV]).[92,93]

Patients with significant deficits in cell-mediated immunity, such as AIDS patients, hematopoietic stem cell (HSCT) and solid-organ transplantation (SOT) recipients, very low-birth weight infants, as well as in utero transfusion cases are at high risk with CMV infection.[95–97] Studies have shown prior CMV infections have been associated with an increased risk of other disorders, such as cardiovascular disease and Alzheimer's disease, so the prevention of CMV infection in the immunocompetent individual is important as well. A look back study estimated the occurrence of TT-CMV in immunocompetent recipient to be 7.4%.[98]

Similar to other herpesviruses, CMV can establish lifelong latency in the host with possible reactivations. Around 40%–70% of donors are CMV-seropositive, which suggests that a large population of adult recipients could be naive to CMV and vulnerable to TT-CMV.[91,99,100] After infection, and shortly before seroconversion, CMV DNA is detectable in plasma and WBCs. CMV DNA usually remains detectable up to 90–120 days after seroconversion.[101] CMV DNA is detected in plasma samples of 44% of newly seropositive donors (12%–62%, depending on the interval to the last seronegative donation).[102] Plasma CMV DNA was found most often at highest levels in donors who had very recently seroconverted.[103]

A "seronegative window phase" exists in which CMV DNA is present in both peripheral WBCs and plasma. This window period lasts between a few days to several weeks. Donors with short intervals between donations (e.g., apheresis platelet donors) have an increased risk of donations during such a window period.[104]

Currently, blood donors are tested for the presence of antibodies against CMV. For CMV-seronegative donors, two possibilities exist, either they truly have never been exposed to the virus, or they are within the seronegative window. NATs for CMV DNA are primarily used for viral load monitoring in HSCT and SOT recipients, and have not been applied widely to screening of blood donors.[105] Although not in routine use, CMV NAT could also be used to prepare CMV-safe units. Patients at risk for TT-CMV, including premature babies, HSCT and SOT recipients, and other oncology patients, require special attention to prevent transmission and subsequent activation of CMV. However, to date there is no consensus agreement on the best approach to prevent TT-CMV transmission.

The standard approaches to prevent TT-CMV include (1) the use of seronegative donors, which carry the risk of TT-CMV from donors in the "window period" or (2) transfusion of LR units from unscreened donors that carry the risks of TT-CMV from filter failure, donors with high CMV viral load, and cell-free CMV in plasma. Bowden and colleagues published a landmark study in 1995 that showed no significant difference between the probability of CMV infection (1.3% vs 2.4%, $P = 1.00$) or disease (0% vs 2.4%, $P = 1.00$) between recipients of seronegative and LR units. The authors concluded that the two main options, "CMV-seronegative" and "LR" blood components were essentially equivalent.[106]

TT-CMV of immunocompromised patients still occurs despite the use of CMV-seronegative or LR units.[102] Ziemann and colleagues proposed a novel third strategy for providing CMV-safe transfusions: provision of LR units from donors who seroconverted at least 1 year earlier. This approach could potentially avoid the use of recently infected (seroconverting) donors who are known to have the highest viral loads (including plasma cell-free CMV).[103]

Another option, described as the "belt and suspenders approach", uses both CMV-seronegative and LR units that theoretically carries less TT-CMV risk. Studies from the John Roback's group showed that the combined strategy is in fact very safe, at least in at-risk very-low-birth weight neonates. A total of 2061 transfusion were administered among 57.5% ($n = 310$) of infants studied. None of the neonatal CMV infections were linked to transfusion, resulting in a CMV infection incidence of 0.0% (0.0%−0.3%) per unit of CMV-seronegative and LR blood.[107]

It is still unclear whether LR of cellular blood components is sufficient to reduce TT-CMV or whether CMV serological testing adds additional benefit to LR. Nevertheless, there are wide variations in practices of using LR components alone or in combination with CMV seronegative units to prevent TT-CMV for at-risk patients.[108−110] Other approaches may also be feasible to prevent TT-CMV, including NAT of plasma samples, pathogen inactivation, and patient blood management programs that reduce the frequency of inappropriate transfusions.[111]

Zika virus

Zika virus (ZIKV) is an arthropod-borne virus (arbovirus) in the genus Flavivirus and the family Flaviviridae.[112] ZIKV is transmitted by the bite of infected mosquitoes, most commonly by *A. aegypti*, which can also transmit dengue virus (another flavivirus) and chikungunya virus (an alphavirus). Other modes of Zika virus transmission include intrauterine, perinatal, and sexual routes.[112]

The first reported outbreak of Zika fever occurred in 2007 on the Western Pacific island of Yap in the Federated States of Micronesia; this was followed by a larger epidemic in French Polynesia in the South Pacific in 2013 and 2014, with an estimated 30,000 symptomatic infections. In 2015, ZIKV emerged for the first time in the Americas and, by the end of January 2016, autochthonous circulation of ZIKV was reported in many countries or territories in South, Central, and North America and the Caribbean.[112]

ZIKV infections in the U.S. have primarily been acquired through traveler to countries where ZIKV is endemic. However, on July 29, 2016, the Florida Department of Health and the Centers for Disease Control essentially confirmed local transmission in a small area of South Florida.[113]

Most ZIKV infected people, an estimated four out of five people, are asymptomatic. When symptoms do occur, the clinical presentation of Zika fever is nonspecific and can be misdiagnosed as other infectious diseases, especially those due to other arboviruses such as dengue and chikungunya. The most common symptoms are fever, rash, joint pain, and conjunctivitis. Even in those who develop symptoms, the illness is usually mild, with symptoms lasting from several days to a week.[114] However, severe neurological complications including Guillain−Barré syndrome were reported in adults in the French Polynesia outbreak, as well as a dramatic increase in severe congenital malformations (microcephaly) in the outbreak of ZIKV in Brazil.[112]

It is believed that ZIKV RNA can be detected in plasma for 1−2 weeks following infection, consistent with infections with WNV, dengue, and chikungunya viruses.[115] A systematic review and pooled analysis of 25 ZIKV infection cases projected that median incubation period for the infection was estimated to be 5.9 days (95% credible interval (CrI): 4.4−7.6), with 95% of people who developed symptoms doing so within 11.2 days (95% CrI: 7.6−18.0) after infection. On average, seroconversion occurred 9.1 days (95% CrI: 7.0−11.6) after infection while RNA was detectable in blood for 9.9 days (95% CrI: 6.9−21.4) on average. Without screening, the estimated risk that a blood donation would come from an infected individual increased by approximately 1 in 10, 000 for every 1 per 100, 000 person-days. Symptom-based screening may reduce this rate by 7%.[116] Longer persistence of ZIKV RNA has also been observed in whole blood compared to serum, ranging from 5 to 58 days after symptom onset despite RNA-negative findings in corresponding serum samples.[117,118]

The potential for transfusion-transmitted Zika virus (TT-ZIKV) was shown in French Polynesia where 2·8% of asymptomatic blood donors tested positive for ZIKV RNA using an in-house NAT, although no symptomatic TT-ZIKV were reported during the outbreak.[112,119] Several cases of TT-ZIKV were reported in Brazil in December 20, 15[120] and later in 2016 from platelets transfusion,[121,122] confirming ZIKV as a high-risk agent that threatens blood safety and a new challenge to the blood supply.[123,124]

Measures to prevent TT-ZIKV include temporary deferral of blood donors in epidemic locations, donor self-reporting of ZIKV symptoms after donation with or without quarantine of blood components, use of blood collected from nonendemic areas, NAT of blood donations, and pathogen inactivation of blood components. However, the sensitivity of donor deferral and postdonation information reporting will be limited by the high rate of asymptomatic infections.

On February 16, 2016, the FDA issued a new guidance recommending the deferral of individuals from donating blood if they traveled to areas with active ZIKV transmission, were potentially exposed to the virus, or have had laboratory-confirmed ZIKV infection. On August 26, 2016, the FDA released further guidance that "recommends" that all U.S. blood donors be tested for ZIKV using the Cobas Zika test (Roche Molecular), which was first used under Investigational New Drug (IND) but eventually received FDA approval for screening ZIKV in blood donations on October 5, 2017.[125] Another assay, the Procleix Zika Virus Assay (Grifols Diagnostic Solutions, Inc.) was FDA-approved for donor screening on July 5, 2018. Both tests are qualitative NAT for the detection of ZIKV RNA in plasma specimens obtained from blood and organ donors. These two tests are both intended for use by blood collection establishments to detect ZIKV in blood donations, but not for the individual diagnosis of ZIKV infection.

With the significant decrease of ZIKV cases in the U.S. and its territories, the FDA issued a revised final guidance on July 6, 2018: "Revised Recommendations for Reducing the Risk of Zika Virus Transmission by Blood and Blood Components."[126] In this guidance, the FDA recommends testing of pooled donations (minipool) rather than ID, an approach that is usually more cost-effective and less burdensome for testing centers. All donations collected in the U.S. and its territories must be tested for ZIKV with a licensed NAT, using either minipool NAT or ID NAT.

An alternative method to prevent TTI-ZIKV includes the use of an FDA-approved pathogen reduction device. Based on current approvals for pathogen reduction technology, this option is limited to use with platelets and plasma.[126] Pathogen inactivation of blood components is a proactive strategy to mitigate the risk of TT-ZIKV. Inactivation of ZIKV was demonstrated by photochemical treatment with amotosalen and ultraviolet A illumination in fresh frozen plasma ($6.57\ \log_{10}$ by infectivity assay and $10.25\ \log_{10}$ by RT-PCR assay).[127,128] Complete ZIKV inactivation of more than $5.99\ \log\text{TCID}_{50}/\text{mL}$ in RBCs was also achieved using amustaline and glutathione at levels higher than those found in asymptomatic ZIKV-infected blood donors.[129]

Ebola virus

Ebola virus (EBOV), a member of the Filoviridae family, is a lipid-enveloped pathogen containing negative-sense single-stranded RNA as its genetic material. It is a zoonotic pathogen that causes severe hemorrhagic fever with morbidity and mortality rates of up to 90%.[130] The Centers for Disease Control and Prevention (CDC) has classified EBOV as a "Category A" bioterrorism agent/disease and manipulation of the virus requires the highest level of biosafety containment (BSL-4). Recent outbreaks of EBOV in Central and West Africa have highlighted the need for an improved international approach to responding to public health emergencies.[131] Currently, Ebola does not pose a significant risk to the U.S. public.[132]

EBOV infections usually present with symptoms of fever, severe headache, muscle pain, and weakness, followed by diarrhea, vomiting, abdominal pain, and sometimes diffuse hemorrhage. Symptoms most often appear within 4–10 days following infection, although onset later than 21 days has been reported.[133] There are currently no FDA-approved vaccines or drugs to prevent or treat EBOV disease (EVD).[132] Supportive therapy, including fluids replacement and managing oxygen status and blood pressure, is the primary treatment for Ebola patients.

Transmission of EBOV occurs through direct contact with blood, organs, and other body fluids and secretions from an infected host.[132,134] EBOV RNA has been detected in semen, vaginal fluids, and other body fluids long after symptoms have resolved. The virus has also been isolated by cell culture from blood, saliva, urine, aqueous humor, semen, and breast milk from infected or convalescent patients.[133] Therefore, the risk of transfusion-transmitted Ebola exists even from an asymptomatic donor.

In January 2017, the FDA issued a guidance document—*Recommendations for Assessment of Blood Donor Eligibility, Donor Deferral and Blood Product Management in Response to Ebola Virus*. In this guidance, the FDA confirmed the risk of TT-EBOV and required implementation of protocols to assess blood donor eligibility, donor deferral, and blood product management in the event of a widespread EBOV outbreak. The recommendations apply to routine collection of blood and blood components for transfusion or further manufacturing, including source plasma.

Following the FDA recommendations, the AABB Regulatory Affairs posted an analysis of the FDA Guidance for Industry, which included additional questions to be asked in the event of widespread EBOV transmission.[135] Under the existing donor eligibility regulations, a donor is deferred if found to have symptoms of a recent or current illness, as well as travel to, or residence in, an area endemic for a possible TTI. For EBOV, the FDA recommends an 8-week deferral from the date of last exposure for any of the following instances:

- Travel to or residence in an area classified by the CDC as having widespread transmission of EBOV or with cases in urban areas with uncertain control measures unless a longer deferral applies based on malarial risk.
- Close contact, as defined in the guidance, with a person under investigation, for EVD.
- Close contact with a person confirmed to have EVD.
- Sexual contact with a person known to have recovered from EVD, regardless of the time since recovery.
- Close contact with a person who was notified by a public health authority regarding possible exposure to EVD.

Lipid-enveloped viruses, such as Ebola, are known to be inactivated by solvent-detergent treatment.[136] Intercept pathogen inactivation technologies have been proven effective in Ebola virus and have received FDA approval to treat Ebola convalescent plasma (containing neutralizing EBOV antibodies, for treatment of EBOV-infected patients) in collaboration with Emory University Hospital and University of Nebraska Medical Center.[137,138] Both THERAFLEX UV-Platelets (UVC) and THERAFLEX MB-Plasma (MB/light) also have shown to be effective in reducing Ebola virus infectivity in platelets and plasma respectively.[139]

Parasites

Babesia

Babesia spp. are intraerythrocytic protozoan parasites of animals and humans that cause babesiosis, a zoonotic disease transmitted primarily by black ticks Ixodes scapularis, which also transmits Borrelia burgdorferi, the cause of Lyme disease, and Anaplasma phagocytophilum, the cause of human granulocytic anaplasmosis. From its initial case reported from California in 1966,[140] the geographic range of infections with Babesia spp. has expanded to coastal communities in Connecticut, Massachusetts, New York, Rhode Island, New Jersey and the Upper Midwest, specifically Minnesota and Wisconsin.[141,142] Babesia spp. have emerged as a growing public health concern in the U.S.

Babesiosis is caused predominantly by B. microti and B. divergens with B. microti being more common in the U.S. The vast majority of people infected with B. microti do not have symptoms and are never diagnosed. Others develop flu-like symptoms, such as fever, headache, and body aches. In immunocompromised hosts, Babesiosis can be a severe, life-threatening disease.

Beginning in the early 1980s, reports of TT B. microti (TTB) cases appeared, and over the years, cases have steadily increased in the U.S., especially in the Northeast.[143,144] In one study, 165 of 256 (64.4%) patients developed TTB following transfusion from donors positive for B. microti. TTB involved hematologic (19%), neonate (10%), cardiovascular (8%), and gastrointestinal (6%) patients. Moreover, 19% infected patients died with death attributed to babesiosis.[145] TTB cases were predominantly due to receipt of red cells (133 of 140 specified units), with RBC units processed in a variety of ways and a range of storage duration. Approximately, 5% of cases were linked to whole blood–derived platelets. TTB with complicated babesiosis and/or death occurred in patients of all age groups and with a variety of underlying medical conditions.[145] In addition, 6 of 25 deaths (24%) due to blood component contamination reported to FDA from 2010 through 2016 were TTB. The upsurge in TTB cases as well as increased fatalities in transfusion recipients has elevated TTB to be a key policy issue in transfusion medicine.[141,146]

The only interventions implemented to prevent TTB in the past were a donor screening question regarding a "history of babesiosis" and selective avoidance of blood collections in some areas of relatively high Babesia endemicity. However, the high numbers of TTB cases continuing to occur after the implementation of the babesiosis history question in DHQ suggest that the use of this question is largely ineffective.

Researchers at the Red Cross have used investigational use only (IUO) tests, arrayed fluorescence immunoassays (AFIAs), and real-time PCR assays, to screen for Babesia positive donors in selected Babesia endemic areas (Minnesota, Wisconsin, Massachusetts, and Connecticut) since June 2012. By September 2014, 335 (0.38%) of 89,153 donations screened positive for B. microti, and at least one third of these samples were considered infectious based on animal studies. However, no cases of babesiosis were transmitted via transfusion from screened samples to patients in this study. During the 2-year study period, 29 cases of TTB were reported from unscreened samples. The estimated risk of transfusion-transmission in endemic states was 1 case per 101,000 donations.[147] This study suggested that screening for both antibodies to B. microti and parasite DNA may help to reduce the risk of transfusion-transmitted B. microti infections. In 2015, the FDA's

Blood Products Advisory Committee recommended nationwide, year-round, antibody screening for *Babesia* species in addition to nucleic acid testing in endemic states.

In March 2018, the FDA approved two tests to screen whole blood and plasma samples for the detection of *B. microti*: the Imugen *Babesia microti* AFIA and NAT tests (Oxford Immunotec, Inc.). However, the manufacturer permanently discontinued both donor screening tests in November 2018.[148,149] On January 24 2019, FDA licensed the Grifols Procleix Babesia Assay for the detection of RNA from *Babesia* species (B. *microti*, B. *duncani*, B. *divergens*, and B. *venatorum*) in whole blood specimens for use in screening donors of whole blood and blood components.[150]

In July 2018, the FDA issued their updated draft guidance for reducing TTB, followed in August 2018 by the AABB recommendations for the prevention of TTB utilizing risk-based decision-making that includes collaboration between the FDA and blood collection centers. Both the FDA and AABB recommend testing of donations year-round by universal antibody testing and NAT in states with the highest *Babesia* risk. In May 2019, the FDA issued the final guidance for reducing the risk of TTB. Since a licensed *Babesia* antibody test is not currently available for blood donor screening, the FDA is recommending regional, year-round testing using a licensed NAT for *Babesia*, or using of an FDA approved pathogen reduction device, in the states at highest risk. In states that do not test donations for *Babesia* or do not pathogen reduce blood components, the FDA recommend to revise the DHQ to ask prospective donors if they have ever had a positive test result for *Babesia*, either from a medical diagnosis or a reactive donor screening test. Donors with a positive history should be indefinitely deferred or deferred for at least 2 years from the date of positive test and evaluated for requalification.[151−153]

Pathogen inactivation methods have shown complete inactivation effect of B. *microti* as well as B. *divergens* in RBCs prepared in Optisol (AS-5) using amustaline and glutathione (GSH), and in platelet components.[154,155] Mirasol pathogen reduction technology has also been shown to be effective at inactivating/reducing B. *microti* parasites in platelet and plasma components inoculated with infected hamster erythrocytes.[156] Recent studies have demonstrated the efficacy of pathogen reduction in whole blood (including RBC units), but at lower levels compared to platelet and plasma components.

Malaria

Malaria is a serious and sometimes fatal disease that can be caused by any of the following five *Plasmodium* species: *P. falciparum*, *P. malariae*, *P. ovale*, *P. vivax*, and *P. knowlesi*. About 1700 cases of malaria are diagnosed in the U.S. each year, the vast majority of which are found among travelers and immigrants returning from countries where malaria transmission occurs. The most recent FDA guidance on malaria was published in August 2014, followed by some updates for malaria endemic areas from the CDC. The guidance provides recommendations for questioning and deferring donors, reentry criteria, and component management to reduce the risk of transfusion-transmitted malaria.[157]

MEN WHO HAVE SEX WITH MEN

During the HIV/AIDS epidemic of the 1980s, most of the developed world instituted a permanent ban on blood donations from men who have sex with men (MSM). With the technological advances in HIV testing, only a very small transmission risk remains from potentially infectious units.[158] In addition, new computer systems to manage release from quarantine have made erroneously releasing HIV-positive units all but impossible. This low risk, as well as lesbian, gay, bisexual, transgender, and student activist concerns of discrimination, have prompted revision of MSM deferral policies to shorten time deferrals.[159]

In Australia, a 12-month deferral has been in place since 2000. In Canada, the deferral period was reduced to 5 years in 2013, and then to 12 months in 2016.[159] In the U.S., the FDA guideline was amended in 2016 such that men who had sexual contact with other men within the previous 12 months could not donate blood.[160] The United Kingdom and France also implemented 12-month deferrals. In late 2017, most of the United Kingdom (England and Scotland) further reduced the deferral to 3 months. Individuals who were indefinitely deferred and otherwise eligible were reinstated as potential donors. In addition, deferred donors could request reinstatement. With current evolution in changing the MSM deferral policy, the impact of these changes remains unclear.

MSM still represents the highest risk group for HIV infection in the U.S. MSM is still a frequent risk factor for HIV-positive donors. In 2016, 67% of diagnosed HIV infections in the U.S. were attributable to MSM. During 2008−16, the annual number of diagnoses of HIV infection increased 3% per year among MSM aged 13–29 years, decreased 4% per year among those aged 30–49 years, and was stable for MSM aged ≥50 years. Racial/ethnic disparities in HIV infection persisted, particularly among younger black/African American MSM who accounted for 49% of all diagnoses among MSM aged 13–29 years during 2008–16.[161]

Data about HIV in blood donors and MSM in the UK were analyzed to estimate the risk of infectious donations entering the blood supply under different scenarios of donor selection criteria (and donor compliance) for MSM and a heterosexual group with increased risk of HIV. Between 2005 and 2007, a change from lifetime exclusion of MSM to 5-year deferral or no deferral increased the point estimate of HIV risk by between 0.4% and 7.4% depending on compliance with the deferral (range −4%–15%) and 26.5% (range 18%–43%), respectively. A change from a 12-month deferral of the high-risk heterosexual group to lifetime exclusion reduced the estimated risk by about 7.2% (range 6%–9%). They conclude if prevalence is the only factor affected by a reduced deferral, then the increased risk of HIV is probably negligible. However, the impact of a change depends on compliance; if compliance stays the same or worsens, the risk is expected to increase due to increased incidence of infections in MSM who donates blood. The risk of TT-HIV could probably be reduced further by improving compliance with any exclusion criteria, particularly after recent at-risk behaviors.[162]

Noncompliance is an important factor in the overall risk of HIV transmission but does not appear to be affected by the length of the deferral period. A major U.S. study found a 2.6% noncompliance rate with the current indefinite deferral for MSM; similar or lower rates were found in other jurisdictions with shorter deferral periods.[163]

In Canada, the deferral period for MSM was reduced from a permanent deferral since 1977 to 5 years in 2013, then to 1 year in 2016. Three anonymous online compliance surveys of male whole blood donors were carried out during those three different deferral policy periods. The data showed that participation rates did not change during those three different deferral policy periods (0.21%, 0.19%, 0.24%; $P = .70$). Notably, the percentage of eligible MSM donors increased (0.13%, 0.66%, 1.21%; $P < .0001$), resulting in approximately 2500 eligible MSM donors with the 1-year deferral in place. HIV rates were unchanged after each policy change. Overall, progressively shorter time deferrals had no impact on noncompliance of MSM with a male partner in the past year, also there was no impact

on HIV rates or incidence. There was a modest increase in eligible MSM in the donor pool after each shorter time deferral.[164]

The American Red Cross began collecting blood from MSM in line with the FDA's newly changed deferral policy in December 2016. Among the 22,482 reinstated donors with prior MSM activity, 520 (2.3%) donated blood; seven of these donors were deferred for having an infectious disease (two men had syphilis; five men had HBV antibodies (one of which was also positive for HIV)). Overall, 0.4% (21,676/4,329,679) of donors were deferred for having an infectious disease compared to 1.3% (7/520) of donors with prior MSM activity ($P < .01$). However, infectious disease prevalence rates from donors with prior MSM activity were comparable to first-time male donors from the general donor pool ($P = .9$). Their study showed that the rate of infectious disease (ID) markers such as those for HIV, HBV, and HCV in donated blood is higher for MSM relative to other blood donors. However, the ID marker rates for reinstated and newly eligible. MSM donors were like those of first-time male donors (1.52%). The researchers concluded that despite the ID reactivity among MSM donors, the number of donations from reinstated MSM donors is too small to assess any meaningful impact on national blood collections.[165]

PATHOGEN REDUCTION TECHNOLOGY

Testing donations for pathogens and deferring selected blood donors has reduced the risk of transfusion-mediated transmission of known pathogens to extremely low levels. However, some risk remains, including the residual risk of bacterial contamination of platelets and emerging pathogens such as Dengue virus, Chikungunya virus, and hepatitis E virus.[8,166,167]

One potential solution to these issues is called "pathogen inactivation" (or pathogen *reduction*). Pathogen inactivation refers to a technology that applies a physical, chemical, or photochemical process to proactively inactivate or kill blood-borne pathogens. These can include methods based on solvent and detergent techniques or photochemical inactivation techniques. Some techniques focus on either plasma or other specific blood components, while others target whole blood for pathogen reduction.

Manufacturers of purified plasma protein fractions have shown that pathogen inactivation technologies can be successfully implemented and have resulted in little or no transmission of HIV, HCV, or HBV since the late 1980s. These technologies, however, cannot be applied to cellular blood components. Thus, new technologies were developed over the past decade to treat cellular blood components as well as plasma.

Pathogen reduction technologies mainly target nucleic acids by using chemicals and ultraviolet/visible light to inactivate pathogens within the blood component, thus providing the potential to reduce TTI. These systems include Mirasol Pathogen Reduction Technology, INTERCEPT, and THERAFLEX. These new proactive technologies significantly reduce the risk of transmission of viruses, protozoa, and bacteria present in plasma or plasma-derived components, but all have limitations. They are licensed for use in Europe and are used in several other countries. For now, only the INTERCEPT Blood System has been approved by FDA for the manufacturing of certain pathogen-reduced platelet and plasma components in the U.S.[168]

RBCs constitute the most commonly transfused blood components. Current interest in the blood industry is focused on the development of pathogen reduction technologies that can treat whole blood and RBCs. The Mirasol system has undergone phase III clinical trials for treating whole blood in Ghana and has demonstrated some efficacy toward Plasmodium species inactivation and low risk of adverse effects.[169,170] A second generation of the INTERCEPT S-303 system for RBCs is currently undergoing a phase III clinical trial in the U.S.[171,172]

Amotosalen/UVA Light for Platelet and Plasma

INTERCEPT (Cerus, Corporation U.S.) employs the combination of a photosensitive agent (amotosalen) and UVA light and can be safely and effectively used for both plasma and platelets.[173–175] Amotosalen intercalates into the double-helical structure of DNA or RNA. After illumination with low-energy UVA light, the intercalated amotosalen undergoes photoaddition with a pyrimidine base to form a covalent monoadduct. The psoralen then undergoes another photoaddition with a pyrimidine base on the opposite strand, forming an adduct or interstrand cross-link. The interaction between amotosalen and pyrimidine inhibits replication, transcription, and translation. After the inactivation process, the amotosalen must be completely removed, due to its genotoxicity once exposed to UVA light.

This technology has been shown to inactivate meaningful titers of key viruses including HIV, chikungunya, Dengue, and ZIKV, bacteria known to contaminate platelets, and parasites including Plasmodium species, Babesia species, and Toxoplasma gondii. Enveloped viruses were uniformly sensitive to inactivation by this technology while nonenveloped viruses demonstrated variable inactivation.[127,128,176,177] Cases of passive transmission of Parvovirus B19 and Hepatitis E Virus following the transfusion of platelet/FFP treated by the Intercept blood pathogen reduction system have been reported.[178,179] It is best to think of these methods as means of pathogen load reduction or pathogen reduction, and to be aware that use of such methods may be insufficient to completely sterilize a blood component.

Transfusion-associated graft-versus-host disease (TA-GVHD) is a serious complication of blood component transfusion therapy, caused by donor T lymphocytes. γ-irradiation or pathogen inactivation methods, capable of inactivating proliferating T cells in blood components, should be selected to prevent TA-GVHD. The use of amotosalen/UVA light treatment is expected to eliminate the need for irradiation to prevent TA-GVHD as it inactivates leukocytes.[177] A literature review on all the observational studies, animal models, in vitro studies, and mechanistic studies of pathogen-reduced platelets with amotosalen/UVA light treatment showed that inactivation of T cells is equal or even superior to γ-irradiation. Pathogen-reduced platelets with amotosalen/UVA light treatment can be used as a measure to prevent TA-GVHD.[180]

Plasma treated with amotosalen/UVA light maintained adequate coagulation function while inactivating high levels of a wide range of pathogens. Retention was 72%–73% of baseline fibrinogen and Factor (F)VIII activity and 78%–98% for FII, FV, FVII, F IX, FX, FXI, FXIII, protein C, protein S, antithrombin, and α2-antiplasmin.[138]

Results from prospective randomized studies have raised questions about the ability of amotosalen/UVA light treatment to reduce pathogen transmission, as well as concerns about its impact on platelet function, as the life span and clot formation of platelets might be impaired.[181] A Cochrane review showed that corrected count increments (CCIs) at 1 hour and 24 hours were statistically significantly lower after INTERCEPT platelet transfusions as compared to standard platelets. The relative risk of platelet refractoriness (defined either as low CCIs in two successive transfusions with or without the presence of platelet antibodies depending on the study) was 2.74-fold higher with INTERCEPT platelets compared to standard platelets. Patients receiving INTERCEPT platelets required 7% more platelet transfusions, and the transfusion interval between multiple INTERCEPT platelet transfusions was shorter than with standard platelets. However, there was no difference between pathogen-reduced platelets and standard platelets in the incidence of clinically significant bleeding complications.[182]

For now, per FDA draft guideline, all blood establishments that implement a pathogen reduction device for the manufacturing of pathogen-reduced blood components (only INTERCEPT in the U.S.) should continue to use the DHQ for donor recruitment and perform the donor infectious disease testing required in 21 CFR 610.40. The FDA does consider the use of the INTERCEPT Blood System to be acceptable to control the risk of bacterial contamination in platelets, and it can be used as a substitute for bacterial detection testing to reduce bacterial contamination in platelets. The FDA acknowledges that the treatment of platelets with the INTERCEPT Blood System potentially lowers the risk of TA-GVHD. However, transfusion medicine physicians along with treating physicians should make the determination as to whether irradiation should be replaced with pathogen reduction to prevent TA-GVHD.[168]

Amustaline (S-303)/Glutathione for RBCs

The INTERCEPT Blood System for RBCs uses a chemical treatment with the small molecule amustaline (S-303) that forms covalent cross-links and adducts with nucleic acids, resulting in inactivation of a broad range of pathogens (Fig. 5.2).

S-303 has been shown to inactivate a variety of enveloped and nonenveloped viruses, Gram-positive and -negative bacteria, parasites,[183] and WBCs.[184]

S-303 has been shown to be effective against bovine viral diarrhea virus, a member of the Flaviviridae family and a model for HCV, as well as Chikungunya virus, Dengue virus, and ZIKV.[129,176,185]

All RBC components treated with amustaline (S-303)/glutathione meet specification for volume and hemoglobin content. Hemolysis, microvesicle formation, supernatant potassium, and deformability were lower, and ATP levels were higher in treated units when compared with control units. The amustaline (S-303)/glutathione treatment process did not increase red cell hemolysis or decrease ATP levels over storage.[184,186,187] No patients exhibited an immune response specific to amustaline-treated RBCs.[188]

Riboflavin/UVB For Whole Blood

The Mirasol Pathogen Reduction Technology is based on the application of riboflavin, followed by illumination with UVB light energy in the range of 265–370 nm for approximately 5 minutes[189] UVB can activate riboflavin resulting in the formation of free oxygen radicals and selective destruction of bacterial DNA and RNA, viruses, and other potential blood-borne pathogens. It can also inactivate leukocytes with minimal damage to blood components.[189,190] The system has been shown to be effective against clinically relevant

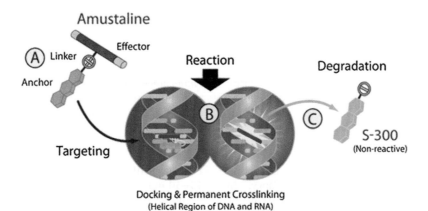

FIG. 5.2 INTERCEPT Blood System for RBCs—mechanisms of action.[129] **(A)** S-303 is a small compound with three components: an acridine anchor (an intercalator that noncovalently targets nucleic acids), an effector (a bis-alkylator group that reacts with nucleophiles such as DNA and RNA bases), and a linker (a small flexible carbon chain containing a labile ester bond that hydrolyzes at neutral pH to yield the nonreactive, negatively charged breakdown product, S-300).[129,171,176] **(B)** When S-303 is added to RBCs, the compound rapidly passes through cellular membranes and viral envelopes due to its amphipathic character. The anchor selectively targets nucleic acids where it intercalates and reversibly binds to the helical regions of the nucleic acids of pathogens and cells. The effector then irreversibly reacts with DNA and RNA guanine bases creating monoadducts and cross-links, thereby blocking nucleic acid replication, transcription, or translation. **(C)** The linker is hydrolyzed to release S-300, a nonreactive degradant resulting from the reaction. It is formulated in the presence of the natural tripeptide GSH to quench unreacted side reactions.[176,183]

pathogens, and it inactivates leukocytes without significantly compromising the efficacy of the component or resulting in component loss. It efficiently inactivates dengue virus in platelet concentrates, EBOV in vitro[191] and *P. falciparum* in whole blood.[169] It can be used to treat blood-derived cellular components as well as plasma and plasma-derived components. This technology is currently under development for the treatment of whole blood, making pathogen reduction of all blood components using one system potentially achievable.[170]

After the inactivation process, riboflavin does not need to be removed from the treated component. Riboflavin is a naturally occurring vitamin with a well-known and well-characterized safety profile. Patients receiving riboflavin/UVB-treated platelet concentrates did not demonstrate antibodies to neoantigens.[192] The procedure is safe and not toxic or carcinogenic.[192,193]

Studies have shown that the riboflavin/UVB treatment leads to a significant increase of anaerobic glycolysis rate despite functional mitochondria. The expression of active GPIIb/IIIa (PAC-1) and the adhesion to fibrinogen was significantly increased from Day 2 of storage in riboflavin/UVB-treated platelet components. It is not clear if these observations would lead to undesirable side effects. Those findings were caused by the UVB radiation alone, independently of the presence of riboflavin.[194]

Since 2009, this technology has been approved for use in more than 20 countries in Europe, the Middle East, Latin America, and Asia Pacific for plasma and platelets. No serious adverse events have been reported after more than 750,000 Mirasol disposable kits sold and about 190,000 recorded transfusions of Mirasol-treated components.[195] However, it has not yet been approved in the U.S. and has not been licensed anywhere for use in whole blood or RBCs.

UVC Light for Platelets

THERAFLEX UV-Platelets (Maco Pharma) is a novel UVC-based pathogen inactivation technology. In contrast to other PI technologies such as INTERCEPT (Cerus Corp.) and Mirasol (TerumoBCT), THERAFLEX UV-platelets work without exogenously added photoactive substances.

The pathogen reduction process is based on application of UVC light of a specific wavelength (254 nm) combined with intense agitation of the blood units to ensure a uniform treatment of all blood compartments. Shortwave UVC light directly interacts with nucleic acids, resulting in the formation of cyclobutane pyrimidine and pyrimidine-pyrimidone dimers that prevent the elongation of nucleic acid transcripts.[173,196] The illumination step takes less than 1 minute. Afterward, the pathogen-reduced platelet component can be used for transfusion.[173,196]

Due to the different absorption characteristics of nucleic acids and proteins, UVC irradiation mainly affects the nucleic acids of pathogens and leukocytes while proteins are largely preserved. UVC treatment significantly reduces the infectivity of platelet units contaminated by disease-causing bacteria, viruses, and protozoa.[139,196–200] In addition, it inactivates residual WBCs in the blood components while preserving platelet function and coagulation factors.[201]

As no photoactive compounds need to be added to the blood units, photoreagent-related adverse events are excluded. Because of its simple and rapid procedure that does not require a change to established blood component preparation procedures, UVC-based pathogen inactivation could easily be integrated into existing blood banking procedures.[196,201]

Preclinical evaluations demonstrated tolerability and immunological safety of THERAFLEX UV-Platelets using an animal model.[197] Additionally, the system has successfully completed two autologous Phase I trials on recovery and survival. Preliminary results suggest that the recovery and survival rates are consistent with other pathogen-reduced platelet components that are licensed and in use around the world. Macopharma is currently preparing a Phase III clinical trial to evaluate THERAFLEX UV-treated platelets in patients.[201]

Other Chemical Treatment for Plasma or Plasma-Derived Purified Components

Filtration/nanofiltration: Viruses may be removed from clotting factor concentrates via filtration (or nanofiltration) employing retentive filters with pores smaller than the virus diameter. These methods are used exclusively for plasma-derived purified components such as smaller molecular-weight coagulation factors (e.g., FIX or FVIII). After filtration with a 220-nm or 15–50-nm filter (filtration/nanofiltration, respectively), these components are considered free from bacteria and protozoans such as *Plasmodium*, *Trypanosoma*, or *Leishmania*. However, contamination with small viruses and prions remains a primary safety concern.[202,203]

Pasteurization: Pasteurization is done by heating proteins in an aqueous stabilized solution at 60°C for 10–11 hours, and it inactivates both lipid membrane–enveloped viruses and a range of nonenveloped viruses.[203] Coagulation factors are heat sensitive; therefore, stabilizers (usually sugars, amino acids, or acetate) are added to preserve protein integrity and are removed after pathogen inactivation. Studies have demonstrated that pasteurization inactivates a wide range of enveloped and nonenveloped viruses, including bovine viral diarrhea virus (a specific model virus for HCV), pseudorabies virus (a nonspecific model virus for HBV), herpes simplex virus-1, WNV, and poliovirus.[204]

Solvent-detergent (SD) treatment: Lipid membranes of enveloped viruses are disrupted by SD mixtures, thereby preventing binding to and infection of cells by these viruses.[205] During the SD process, prefiltered plasma is treated with an organic solvent (e.g., tri-[N-butyl]-phosphate) and a detergent (e.g., 1% polyoxyethylene-p-t-octylphenol; Triton X-100 or Tween 80); the solvent removes lipids from viral and bacterial membranes and the detergent disrupts lipid bilayers.[206–209] SD compounds are removed by chromatography or oil extraction.[207,209] Product solutions are filtered to remove viruses entrapped in particles and thus protected from exposure to SD. To further reduce the risk of blood-borne transmission of nonenveloped viruses in plasma that has undergone SD treatment, components are often subjected to a second inactivation step such as heat treatment.[210,211] SD treatment is ineffective against nonenveloped viruses such as parvovirus B19 or hepatitis A virus. SD treatment can only be used to treat plasma, but is not suitable for use with cellular components as the chemicals used would destroy RBCs or platelets cell membrane.[211] Compared with fresh frozen plasma, SD-treated plasma displayed reduced activity levels for von Willebrand factor and Protein S (67%–76% and 35% reduction, respectively).[206] FVIII treated with SD (Octaplas, Octapharma) has an FVIII activity level 10%–20% lower than that observed in fresh frozen plasma. Furthermore, SD treatment has been shown to compromise some of the in vitro coagulation function of plasma and is contraindicated by the FDA for patients undergoing liver transplant.

Dry heat treatment of lyophilized components: Most plasma-derived concentrates are lyophilized and subsequently treated with dry heat to inactivate nonenveloped viruses that resist SD treatment. Lyophilization confers a certain degree of virus inactivation; the moisture content of lyophilized components undergoing dry heat treatment should be kept low (typically <2%), as residual moisture may affect component stability. Dry heat treatment of lyophilized components has demonstrated favorable results for inactivation of relevant or model viruses of HAV, HBV, HCV, and HIV.[212–215] However, Parvovirus B19 transmission by heat-treated clotting factor concentrates has been reported.[216]

Methylene-Blue (MB): The THERAFLEX-MB Plasma system is a photodynamic pathogen inactivation procedure using methylene blue (MB) and visible light and is applied to single donor units of plasma. It employs a 0.65 μm membrane filter (Plasmaflex PLAS4, Macopharma), which removes residual leukocytes, RBCs, platelets, and aggregates. A dry pill integrated in the disposable of 85 μg anhydrous MB chloride is dissolved into the filtered plasma, which provides a final concentration of 0.8–1.2 μM MB in a volume of plasma between 235 and 330 mL. The illumination is achieved by a microprocessor-controlled device (Maco-Tronic B2, Macopharma). After treatment, residual MB combined with its photo components is removed by a Blueflex filter.[217,218]

SUMMARY

Testing blood donations for pathogens, as well as deferring selected blood donors, have together reduced the risk of transmission by transfusion of known pathogens to extremely low levels. Protecting the blood supply from emerging infectious threats remains a concern in the transfusion medicine community. To mitigate the risk of transfusion-transmitted infections, transfusion services can employ either indirect measures such as surveillance, hemovigilance, and donor questionnaires, or direct measures such as protein and/or nucleic acid-based testing or pathogen inactivation of blood components. Pathogen inactivation systems are increasing in use here and around the globe. As a result, improving the safety of the blood supply from infectious disease risk is ongoing and will continue to require a combination of innovative proactive surveillance, detection, and pathogen avoidance or inactivation.

REFERENCES

1. FDA. *Fatalities Reported to FDA Following Blood Collection and Transfusion.* 2017.
2. Bihl F, Castelli D, Marincola F, Dodd RY, Brander C. Transfusion-transmitted infections. *J Transl Med.* 2007; 5, 25-25.
3. AABB. *Standards for Blood Banks and Transfusion Services.* 2018.
4. Fung MK. *Technical Manual AABB.* 19th ed. Bethesda: AABB; 2018.
5. Stramer SL, Glynn SA, Kleinman SH, et al. Detection of HIV-1 and HCV infections among antibody-negative blood donors by nucleic acid-amplification testing. *N Engl J Med.* 2004;351(8):760–768.

6. Jarvis LM, Dow BC, Cleland A, et al. Detection of HCV and HIV-1 antibody negative infections in Scottish and Northern Ireland blood donations by nucleic acid amplification testing. *Vox Sang.* 2005;89(3):128–134.

7. WHO. *Screening Donated Blood for Transfusion Transmitted Infections.* 2009.

8. Klein HG, Anderson D, Bernardi MJ, et al. Pathogen inactivation: making decisions about new technologies. Report of a consensus conference. *Transfusion.* 2007; 47(12):2338–2347.

9. Borden CW, Hall WH. Fatal transfusion reactions from massive bacterial contamination of blood. *N Engl J Med.* 1951;245(20):760–765.

10. Eder AF, Kennedy JM, Dy BA, et al. Bacterial screening of apheresis platelets and the residual risk of septic transfusion reactions: the American Red Cross experience (2004–2006). *Transfusion.* 2007;47(7):1134–1142.

11. Eder AF, Meena-Leist CE, Hapip CA, Dy BA, Benjamin RJ, Wagner SJ. *Clostridium perfringens* in apheresis platelets: an unusual contaminant underscores the importance of clinical vigilance for septic transfusion reactions (CME). *Transfusion.* 2014;54(3 Pt 2):857–862. quiz 856.

12. Flemming HC, Wingender J. The biofilm matrix. *Nat Rev Microbiol.* 2010;8(9):623–633.

13. Greco-Stewart VS, Brown EE, Parr C, et al. *Serratia marcescens* strains implicated in adverse transfusion reactions form biofilms in platelet concentrates and demonstrate reduced detection by automated culture. *Vox Sang.* 2012;102(3):212–220.

14. Greco-Stewart VS, Ali H, Kumaran D, et al. Biofilm formation by Staphylococcus capitis strains isolated from contaminated platelet concentrates. *J Med Microbiol.* 2013;62(Pt 7):1051–1059.

15. CDC. *Bacterial Contamination of Platelets;* 2019. https://www.cdc.gov/bloodsafety/bbp/bacterial-contamination-of-platelets.html.

16. Eder AF, Kennedy JM, Dy BA, et al. Limiting and detecting bacterial contamination of apheresis platelets: inlet-line diversion and increased culture volume improve component safety. *Transfusion.* 2009;49(8):1554–1563.

17. McDonald C, McGuane S, Thomas J, et al. A novel rapid and effective donor arm disinfection method. *Transfusion.* 2010;50(1):53–58.

18. Satake M, Mitani T, Oikawa S, et al. Frequency of bacterial contamination of platelet concentrates before and after introduction of diversion method in Japan. *Transfusion.* 2009;49(10):2152–2157.

19. McDonald CP, Roy A, Mahajan P, Smith R, Charlett A, Barbara JA. Relative values of the interventions of diversion and improved donor-arm disinfection to reduce the bacterial risk from blood transfusion. *Vox Sang.* 2004;86(3):178–182.

20. Hong H, Xiao W, Lazarus HM, Good CE, Maitta RW, Jacobs MR. Detection of septic transfusion reactions to platelet transfusions by active and passive surveillance. *Blood.* 2016;127(4):496–502.

21. FDA. *Reduction of the Maximum Platelet Storage Period to 5 Days in an Approved Container. Memo to All Registered Blood Establishments;* 1986. https://www.fda.gov/downloads/BiologicsBloodVaccines/GuidanceComplianceRegulatoryInformation/OtherRecommendationsforManufacturers/MemorandumtoBloodEstablishments/UCM063013.pdf.

22. McDonald CP, Rogers A, Cox M, et al. Evaluation of the 3D BacT/ALERT automated culture system for the detection of microbial contamination of platelet concentrates. *Transfus Med.* 2002;12(5):303–309.

23. Souza S, Bravo M, Poulin T, et al. Improving the performance of culture-based bacterial screening by increasing the sample volume from 4 mL to 8 mL in aerobic culture bottles. *Transfusion.* 2012;52(7):1576–1582.

24. Benjamin RJ, McDonald CP. The international experience of bacterial screen testing of platelet components with an automated microbial detection system: a need for consensus testing and reporting guidelines. *Transfus Med Rev.* 2014;28(2):61–71.

25. Corash L. Bacterial contamination of platelet components: potential solutions to prevent transfusion-related sepsis. *Expert Rev Hematol.* 2011;4(5):509–525.

26. FDA. *Bacterial Risk Control Strategies for Blood Collection Establishments and Transfusion Services to Enhance the Safety and Availability of Platelets for Transfusion.* Draft Guidance for Industry; 2018.

27. Eder AF, Goldman M. How do I investigate septic transfusion reactions and blood donors with culture-positive platelet donations? *Transfusion.* 2011;51(8): 1662–1668.

28. Tolomelli G, Tazzari PL, Paolucci M, Arpinati M, Landini MP, Pagliaro P. Transfusion-related *Listeria monocytogenes* infection in a patient with acute myeloid leukaemia. *Blood Transfus.* 2014;12(4):611–614.

29. Guinet F, Carniel E, Leclercq A. Transfusion-transmitted *Yersinia enterocolitica* sepsis. *Clin Infect Dis.* 2011;53(6): 583–591.

30. Gibb AP, Martin KM, Davidson GA, Walker B, Murphy WG. Modeling the growth of *Yersinia enterocolitica* in donated blood. *Transfusion.* 1994;34(4):304–310.

31. Donegan E, Stuart M, Niland JC, et al. Infection with human immunodeficiency virus type 1 (HIV-1) among recipients of antibody-positive blood donations. *Ann Intern Med.* 1990;113(10):733–739.

32. Donegan E, Lenes BA, Tomasulo PA, Mosley JW. Transmission of HIV-1 by component type and duration of shelf storage before transfusion. *Transfusion.* 1990; 30(9):851–852.

33. Kleinman SH, Lelie N, Busch MP. Infectivity of human immunodeficiency virus-1, hepatitis C virus, and hepatitis B virus and risk of transmission by transfusion. *Transfusion.* 2009;49(11):2454–2489.

34. Kalbfleisch JD, Lawless JF. Estimating the incubation time distribution and expected number of cases of transfusion-associated acquired immune deficiency syndrome. *Transfusion.* 1989;29(8):672–676.

35. Schreiber GB, Busch MP, Kleinman SH, Korelitz JJ. The risk of transfusion-transmitted viral infections. The Retrovirus Epidemiology Donor Study. *N Engl J Med.* 1996; 334(26):1685–1690.

36. Goodnough LT, Shander A, Brecher ME. Transfusion medicine: looking to the future. *Lancet.* 2003; 361(9352):161–169.

37. Vermeulen M, Lelie N, Coleman C, et al. Assessment of HIV transfusion transmission risk in South Africa: a 10-year analysis following implementation of individual donation nucleic acid amplification technology testing and donor demographics eligibility changes. *Transfusion.* 2019;59(1):267–276.

38. Bruhn R, Lelie N, Custer B, Busch M, Kleinman S. Prevalence of human immunodeficiency virus RNA and antibody in first-time, lapsed, and repeat blood donations across five international regions and relative efficacy of alternative screening scenarios. *Transfusion.* 2013;53(10 Pt 2):2399–2412.

39. Melve GK, Myrmel H, Eide GE, Hervig T. Evaluation of the persistence and characteristics of indeterminate reactivity against hepatitis C virus in blood donors. *Transfusion.* 2009;49(11):2359–2365.

40. Cappy P, Barlet V, Lucas Q, et al. Transfusion of HIV-infected blood components despite highly sensitive nucleic acid testing. *Transfusion.* 2019;59(6):2046–2053.

41. Hitziger T, Schmidt M, Schottstedt V, et al. Cellular immune response to hepatitis C virus (HCV) in nonviremic blood donors with indeterminate anti-HCV reactivity. *Transfusion.* 2009;49(7):1306–1313.

42. Bes M, Esteban JI, Casamitjana N, et al. Hepatitis C virus (HCV)-specific T-cell responses among recombinant immunoblot assay-3-indeterminate blood donors: a confirmatory evidence of HCV exposure. *Transfusion.* 2009;49(7):1296–1305.

43. Delwart EL, Kalmin ND, Jones TS, et al. First report of human immunodeficiency virus transmission via an RNA-screened blood donation. *Vox Sang.* 2004;86(3):171–177.

44. Phelps R, Robbins K, Liberti T, et al. Window-period human immunodeficiency virus transmission to two recipients by an adolescent blood donor. *Transfusion.* 2004; 44(6):929–933.

45. Kwon SY, Kim IS, Bae JE, et al. Pathogen inactivation efficacy of Mirasol PRT system and Intercept Blood System for non-leucoreduced platelet-rich plasma-derived platelets suspended in plasma. *Vox Sang.* 2014;107(3):254–260.

46. Niederhauser C. Reducing the risk of hepatitis B virus transfusion-transmitted infection. *J Blood Med.* 2011;2: 91–102.

47. Seo DH, Whang DH, Song EY, Han KS. Occult hepatitis B virus infection and blood transfusion. *World J Hepatol.* 2015;7(3):600–606.

48. Roth WK, Weber M, Petersen D, et al. NAT for HBV and anti-HBc testing increase blood safety. *Transfusion.* 2002;42(7):869–875.

49. Cable R, Lelie N, Bird A. Reduction of the risk of transfusion-transmitted viral infection by nucleic acid amplification testing in the Western Cape of South Africa: a 5-year review. *Vox Sang.* 2013;104(2):93–99.

50. Raimondo G, Allain JP, Brunetto MR, et al. Statements from the Taormina expert meeting on occult hepatitis B virus infection. *J Hepatol.* 2008;49(4):652–657.

51. Candotti D, Allain J-P. Transfusion-transmitted hepatitis B virus infection. *J Hepatol.* 2009;51(4):798–809.

52. Allain JP, Mihaljevic I, Gonzalez-Fraile MI, et al. Infectivity of blood components from donors with occult hepatitis B virus infection. *Transfusion.* 2013;53(7):1405–1415.

53. Coppola N, Loquercio G, Tonziello G, et al. HBV transmission from an occult carrier with five mutations in the major hydrophilic region of HBsAg to an immunosuppressed plasma recipient. *J Clin Virol.* 2013;58(1): 315–317.

54. Furuta RA, Kondo Y, Saito T, et al. Transfusions of red blood cells from an occult hepatitis B virus carrier without apparent signs of transfusion-transmitted hepatitis B infection. *Transfus Med.* 2008;18(6):379–381.

55. Selvarajah S, Busch MP. Transfusion transmission of HCV, a long but successful road map to safety. *Antivir Ther.* 2012;17(7 Pt B):1423–1429.

56. CDC. 2015; https://www.cdc.gov/hepatitis/hcv/index.htm, 2018.

57. Glynn SA, Wright DJ, Kleinman SH, et al. Dynamics of viremia in early hepatitis C virus infection. *Transfusion.* 2005;45(6):994–1002.

58. Busch MP, Murthy KK, Kleinman SH, et al. Infectivity in chimpanzees (*Pan troglodytes*) of plasma collected before HCV RNA detectability by FDA-licensed assays: implications for transfusion safety and HCV infection outcomes. *Blood.* 2012;119(26):6326–6334.

59. Choo QL, Kuo G, Weiner AJ, Overby LR, Bradley DW, Houghton M. Isolation of a cDNA clone derived from a blood-borne non-A, non-B viral hepatitis genome. *Science.* 1989;244(4902):359–362.

60. Alter HJ, Purcell RH, Shih JW, et al. Detection of antibody to hepatitis C virus in prospectively followed transfusion recipients with acute and chronic non-A, non-B hepatitis. *N Engl J Med.* 1989;321(22):1494–1500.

61. Grady GF, Chalmers TC. Risk of post-transfusion viral hepatitis. *N Engl J Med.* 1964;271:337–342.

62. Tobler LH, Busch MP. History of post-transfusion hepatitis. *Clin Chem.* 1997;43(8 Pt 2):1487–1493.

63. Walsh JH, Purcell RH, Morrow AG, Chanock RM, Schmidt PJ. Posttransfusion hepatitis after open-heart operations. Incidence after the administration of blood from commercial and volunteer donor populations. *Jama.* 1970;211(2):261–265.

64. Alter HJ, Holland PV, Purcell RH, et al. Posttransfusion hepatitis after exclusion of commercial and hepatitis-B antigen-positive donors. *Ann Intern Med.* 1972;77(5): 691–699.

65. Marwaha N, Sachdev S. Current testing strategies for hepatitis C virus infection in blood donors and the way forward. *World J Gastroenterol.* 2014;20(11):2948–2954.

66. Courouce AM, Le Marrec N, Girault A, Ducamp S, Simon N. Anti-hepatitis C virus (anti-HCV) seroconversion in patients undergoing hemodialysis: comparison of second- and third-generation anti-HCV assays. *Transfusion.* 1994;34(9):790–795.

67. Zou S, Stramer SL, Dodd RY. Donor testing and risk: current prevalence, incidence, and residual risk of

transfusion-transmissible agents in US allogeneic donations. *Transfus Med Rev.* 2012;26(2):119–128.

68. Zou S, Dorsey KA, Notari EP, et al. Prevalence, incidence, and residual risk of human immunodeficiency virus and hepatitis C virus infections among United States blood donors since the introduction of nucleic acid testing. *Transfusion.* 2010;50(7):1495–1504.

69. El Ekiaby M, Moftah F, Goubran H, et al. Viremia levels in hepatitis C infection among Egyptian blood donors and implications for transmission risk with different screening scenarios. *Transfusion.* 2015;55(6):1186–1194.

70. Bernardin F, Stramer SL, Rehermann B, et al. High levels of subgenomic HCV plasma RNA in immunosilent infections. *Virology.* 2007;365(2):446–456.

71. Kleinman SH, Stramer SL, Brodsky JP, Caglioti S, Busch MP. Integration of nucleic acid amplification test results into hepatitis C virus supplemental serologic testing algorithms: implications for donor counseling and revision of existing algorithms. *Transfusion.* 2006; 46(5):695–702.

72. Busch MP, Glynn SA, Stramer SL, et al. Correlates of hepatitis C virus (HCV) RNA negativity among HCV-seropositive blood donors. *Transfusion.* 2006;46(3): 469–475.

73. FDA. *Further Testing of Donations that Are Reactive on a Licensed Donor Screening Test for Antibodies to Hepatitis C Virus;* 2018. https://www.fda.gov/downloads/Biologics BloodVaccines/GuidanceComplianceRegulatoryInformation/Guidances/Blood/UCM621294.pdf.

74. Bruhn R, Lelie N, Busch M, Kleinman S. Relative efficacy of nucleic acid amplification testing and serologic screening in preventing hepatitis C virus transmission risk in seven international regions. *Transfusion.* 2015; 55(6):1195–1205.

75. Kiely P. Screening blood donors for hepatitis C virus: the challenge to consider cost-effectiveness. *Transfusion.* 2015;55(6):1143–1146.

76. Poiesz BJ, Ruscetti FW, Gazdar AF, Bunn PA, Minna JD, Gallo RC. Detection and isolation of type C retrovirus particles from fresh and cultured lymphocytes of a patient with cutaneous T-cell lymphoma. *Proc Natl Acad Sci U S A.* 1980;77(12):7415–7419.

77. Kalyanaraman VS, Sarngadharan MG, Robert-Guroff M, Miyoshi I, Golde D, Gallo RC. A new subtype of human T-cell leukemia virus (HTLV-II) associated with a T-cell variant of hairy cell leukemia. *Science.* 1982;218(4572): 571–573.

78. Gonçalves DU, Proietti FA, Ribas JGR, et al. Epidemiology, treatment, and prevention of human T-cell leukemia virus type 1-associated diseases. *Clin Microbiol Rev.* 2010;23(3):577–589.

79. Recommendations for counseling persons infected with human T-lymphotrophic virus, types I and II. Centers for disease control and prevention and U.S. Public health service working group. *MMWR Recomm Rep (Morb Mortal Wkly Rep).* 1993;42(Rr-9):1–13.

80. Hakre S, Manak MM, Murray CK, et al. Transfusion-transmitted human T-lymphotropic virus Type I infection in a United States military emergency whole blood transfusion recipient in Afghanistan, 2010. *Transfusion.* 2013; 53(10):2176–2182.

81. Verdonck K, Gonzalez E, Van Dooren S, Vandamme AM, Vanham G, Gotuzzo E. Human T-lymphotropic virus 1: recent knowledge about an ancient infection. *Lancet Infect Dis.* 2007;7(4):266–281.

82. Vrielink H, Zaaijer HL, Reesink HW. The clinical relevance of HTLV type I and II in transfusion medicine. *Transfus Med Rev.* 1997;11(3):173–179.

83. Centers For Disease C, Prevention, the USPHSWG. Guidelines for counseling persons infected with human t-lymphotropic virus type I (HTLV-I) and type II (HTLV-II). *Ann Intern Med.* 1993;118(6):448–454.

84. San Martin H, Balanda M, Vergara N, et al. Human T-Lymphotropic Virus Type 1 and 2 Seroprevalence among first-time blood donors in Chile, 2011–2013. *J Med Virol.* 2016;88(6):1067–1075.

85. Marano G, Vaglio S, Pupella S, et al. Human T-lymphotropic virus and transfusion safety: does one size fit all? *Transfusion.* 2016;56(1):249–260.

86. Chang YB, Kaidarova Z, Hindes D, et al. Seroprevalence and demographic determinants of human T-lymphotropic virus type 1 and 2 infections among first-time blood donors–United States, 2000–2009. *J Infect Dis.* 2014;209(4):523–531.

87. Hewitt PE, Davison K, Howell DR, Taylor GP. Human T-lymphotropic virus lookback in NHS Blood and Transplant (England) reveals the efficacy of leukoreduction. *Transfusion.* 2013;53(10):2168–2175.

88. AABB. *A Statement Presented before the Food and Drug Administration's Blood Components Advisory Committee;* 2013. http://www.aabb.org/advocacy/statements/Pages/statement110113.aspx.

89. FDA. *Recommendations for Requalification of Blood Donors Deferred Because of Reactive Test Results for Antibodies to Human T-Lymphotropic Virus Types I and II (anti-HTLV-I/II);* 2018. https://www.fda.gov/downloads/BiologicsBlood Vaccines/GuidanceComplianceRegulatoryInformation/Guidances/Blood/UCM621245.pdf.

90. Klemola E, Kaariainen L. Cytomegalovirus as a possible cause of a disease resembling infectious mononucleosis. *Br Med J.* 1965;2(5470):1099–1102.

91. de Jong MD, Galasso GJ, Gazzard B, et al. Summary of the II international symposium on cytomegalovirus. *Antivir Res.* 1998;39(3):141–162.

92. Sinclair J, Sissons P. Latency and reactivation of human cytomegalovirus. *J Gen Virol.* 2006;87(Pt 7): 1763–1779.

93. Sinclair J. Human cytomegalovirus: latency and reactivation in the myeloid lineage. *J Clin Virol.* 2008;41(3): 180–185.

94. Larsson S, Soderberg-Naucler C, Moller E. Productive cytomegalovirus (CMV) infection exclusively in CD13-positive peripheral blood mononuclear cells from CMV-infected individuals: implications for prevention of CMV transmission. *Transplantation.* 1998;65(3): 411–415.

95. Gilbert GL, Hayes K, Hudson IL, James J. Prevention of transfusion-acquired cytomegalovirus infection in infants by blood filtration to remove leucocytes. Neonatal Cytomegalovirus Infection Study Group. *Lancet.* 1989; 1(8649):1228–1231.

96. Einsele H, Ehninger G, Hebart H, et al. Polymerase chain reaction monitoring reduces the incidence of cytomegalovirus disease and the duration and side effects of antiviral therapy after bone marrow transplantation. *Blood.* 1995;86(7):2815–2820.

97. Spector SA, Merrill R, Wolf D, Dankner WM. Detection of human cytomegalovirus in plasma of AIDS patients during acute visceral disease by DNA amplification. *J Clin Microbiol.* 1992;30(9):2359–2365.

98. Ziemann M, Juhl D, Brockmann C, Gorg S, Hennig H. Infectivity of blood components containing cytomegalovirus DNA: results of a lookback study in nonimmunocompromised patients. *Transfusion.* 2017;57(7):1691–1698.

99. Adler SP. Transfusion-associated cytomegalovirus infections. *Rev Infect Dis.* 1983;5(6):977–993.

100. Furui Y, Satake M, Hoshi Y, Uchida S, Suzuki K, Tadokoro K. Cytomegalovirus (CMV) seroprevalence in Japanese blood donors and high detection frequency of CMV DNA in elderly donors. *Transfusion.* 2013;53(10): 2190–2197.

101. Ziemann M, Unmack A, Steppat D, Juhl D, Gorg S, Hennig H. The natural course of primary cytomegalovirus infection in blood donors. *Vox Sang.* 2010;99(1):24–33.

102. Ziemann M, Krueger S, Maier AB, Unmack A, Goerg S, Hennig H. High prevalence of cytomegalovirus DNA in plasma samples of blood donors in connection with seroconversion. *Transfusion.* 2007;47(11):1972–1983.

103. Ziemann M, Juhl D, Gorg S, Hennig H. The impact of donor cytomegalovirus DNA on transfusion strategies for at-risk patients. *Transfusion.* 2013;53(10):2183–2189.

104. Ziemann M, Heuft HG, Frank K, Kraas S, Gorg S, Hennig H. Window period donations during primary cytomegalovirus infection and risk of transfusion-transmitted infections. *Transfusion.* 2013;53(5):1088–1094.

105. Roback JD, Josephson CD. New insights for preventing transfusion-transmitted cytomegalovirus and other white blood cell-associated viral infections. *Transfusion.* 2013; 53(10):2112–2116.

106. Bowden RA, Slichter SJ, Sayers M, et al. A comparison of filtered leukocyte-reduced and cytomegalovirus (CMV) seronegative blood components for the prevention of transfusion-associated CMV infection after marrow transplant. *Blood.* 1995;86(9):3598–3603.

107. Josephson CD, Caliendo AM, Easley KA, et al. Blood transfusion and breast milk transmission of cytomegalovirus in very low-birth-weight infants : a prospective cohort study. *JAMA Pediatrics.* 2014;168(11):1054–1062.

108. Thiele T, Kruger W, Zimmermann K, et al. Transmission of cytomegalovirus (CMV) infection by leukoreduced blood components not tested for CMV antibodies: a single-center prospective study in high-risk patients undergoing allogeneic hematopoietic stem cell transplantation (CME). *Transfusion.* 2011;51(12):2620–2626.

109. Finlay L, Nippak P, Tiessen J, Isaac W, Callum J, Cserti-Gazdewich C. Survey of institutional policies for provision of "CMV-Safe" blood in Ontario. *Am J Clin Pathol.* 2016;146(5):578–584.

110. Weisberg SP, Staley EM, Williams 3rd LA, et al. Survey on transfusion-transmitted cytomegalovirus and cytomegalovirus disease mitigation. *Arch Pathol Lab Med.* 2017; 141(12):1705–1711.

111. Heddle NM, Boeckh M, Grossman B, et al. AABB Committee Report: reducing transfusion-transmitted cytomegalovirus infections. *Transfusion.* 2016;56(6 Pt 2):1581–1587.

112. Musso D, Gubler DJ. Zika virus. *Clin Microbiol Rev.* 2016; 29(3):487–524.

113. *Florida Health Announcement of Local Transmission;* 2016. http://www.floridahealth.gov/newsroom/2016/07/072916-local-zika.html.

114. *Zika Virus Response Updates From FDA;* 2019. https://www.fda.gov/EmergencyPreparedness/Counterterrorism/Medical Countermeasures/MCMIssues/ucm485199.htm.

115. AABB. *AABB Association Bulletin #16-07.* 2016.

116. Lessler J, Ott CT, Carcelen AC, et al. Times to key events in Zika virus infection and implications for blood donation: a systematic review. *Bull World Health Organ.* 2016; 94(11):841–849.

117. Lustig Y, Mendelson E, Paran N, Melamed S, Schwartz E. Detection of Zika virus RNA in whole blood of imported Zika virus disease cases up to 2 months after symptom onset, Israel, December 2015 to April 2016. *Euro Surveill.* 2016;21(26).

118. Rossini G, Gaibani P, Vocale C, Cagarelli R, Landini MP. Comparison of Zika virus (ZIKV) RNA detection in plasma, whole blood and urine - case series of travel-associated ZIKV infection imported to Italy, 2016. *J Infect.* 2017;75(3):242–245.

119. Musso D, Nhan T, Robin E, et al. Potential for Zika virus transmission through blood transfusion demonstrated during an outbreak in French Polynesia, November 2013 to February 2014. *Euro Surveill.* 2014;19(14).

120. Promed. *International Society for Infectious Diseases;* 2015. http://www.promedmail.org/.

121. Barjas-Castro ML, Angerami RN, Cunha MS, et al. Probable transfusion-transmitted Zika virus in Brazil. *Transfusion.* 2016;56(7):1684–1688.

122. Motta IJ, Spencer BR, Cordeiro da Silva SG, et al. Evidence for transmission of Zika virus by platelet transfusion. *N Engl J Med.* 2016;375(11):1101–1103.

123. Lanteri MC, Kleinman SH, Glynn SA, et al. Zika virus: a new threat to the safety of the blood supply with worldwide impact and implications. *Transfusion.* 2016;56(7): 1907–1914.

124. Musso D, Stramer SL, Busch MP. Zika virus: a new challenge for blood transfusion. *Lancet.* 2016;387(10032): 1993–1994.

125. FDA. *FDA Approves First Test for Screening Zika Virus in Blood Donations;* 2017. https://www.fda.gov/News Events/Newsroom/PressAnnouncements/ucm579313.htm.

126. FDA. *Revised Recommendations for Reducing the Risk of Zika Virus Transmission by Blood and Blood Components.* 2018.

127. Aubry M, Richard V, Green J, Broult J, Musso D. Inactivation of Zika virus in plasma with amotosalen and ultraviolet A illumination. *Transfusion.* 2016;56(1):33–40.

128. Musso D, Richard V, Broult J, Cao-Lormeau VM. Inactivation of dengue virus in plasma with amotosalen and ultraviolet A illumination. *Transfusion.* 2014;54(11):2924–2930.

129. Laughhunn A, Santa Maria F, Broult J, et al. Amustaline (S-303) treatment inactivates high levels of Zika virus in red blood cell components. *Transfusion.* 2017;57(3pt.2):779–789.

130. WHO. *Ebola Virus Disease*; 2018. https://www.who.int/en/news-room/fact-sheets/detail/ebola-virus-disease.

131. Delgado R, Simon F. Transmission, human population, and pathogenicity: the Ebola case in point. *Microbiol Spectr.* 2018;6(2).

132. FDA. *Ebola Preparedness and Response Updates from FDA*; 2019. https://www.fda.gov/EmergencyPreparedness/Counterterrorism/MedicalCountermeasures/MCMIssues/ucm608358.htm.

133. Vetter P, Fischer 2nd WA, Schibler M, Jacobs M, Bausch DG, Kaiser L. Ebola virus shedding and transmission: review of current evidence. *J Infect Dis.* 2016;214(suppl 3):S177–S184.

134. Katz LM, Tobian AA. Ebola virus disease, transmission risk to laboratory personnel, and pretransfusion testing. *Transfusion.* 2014;54(12):3247–3251.

135. AABB, Analysis of FDA Guidance for Industry. *Recommendations for Assessment of Blood Donor Eligibility, Donor Deferral and Blood Product Management in Response to Ebola Virus – January 2017*; 2018. http://www.aabb.org/advocacy/regulatorygovernment/Pages/analysis013117.aspx.

136. El-Ekiaby M, Sayed MA, Caron C, et al. Solvent-detergent filtered (S/D-F) fresh frozen plasma and cryoprecipitate minipools prepared in a newly designed integral disposable processing bag system. *Transfus Med.* 2010;20(1):48–61.

137. Tedder RS, Samuel D, Dicks S, et al. Detection, characterization, and enrollment of donors of Ebola convalescent plasma in Sierra Leone. *Transfusion.* 2018;58(5):1289–1298.

138. Singh Y, Sawyer LS, Pinkoski LS, et al. Photochemical treatment of plasma with amotosalen and long-wavelength ultraviolet light inactivates pathogens while retaining coagulation function. *Transfusion.* 2006;46(7):1168–1177.

139. Eickmann M, Gravemann U, Handke W, et al. Inactivation of Ebola virus and Middle East respiratory syndrome coronavirus in platelet concentrates and plasma by ultraviolet C light and methylene blue plus visible light, respectively. *Transfusion.* 2018;58(9):2202–2207.

140. Scholtens RG, Braff EH, Healey GA, Gleason N. A case of babesiosis in man in the United States. *Am J Trop Med Hyg.* 1968;17(6):810–813.

141. Leiby DA. Transfusion-transmitted Babesia spp.: bull's-eye on *Babesia microti*. *Clin Microbiol Rev.* 2011;24(1):14–28.

142. Goss C, Giardina P, Simon M, Kessler DA, Shaz B, Cushing M. *Increasing Rate of Babesiosis in Transfused Patients at a New York City Hospital*. 2012.

143. Cable RG, Leiby DA. Risk and prevention of transfusion-transmitted babesiosis and other tick-borne diseases. *Curr Opin Hematol.* 2003;10(6):405–411.

144. Linden JV, Prusinski MA, Crowder LA, et al. Transfusion-transmitted and community-acquired babesiosis in New York, 2004 to 2015. *Transfusion.* 2018;58(3):660–668.

145. Fang DC, McCullough J. Transfusion-transmitted *Babesia microti*. *Transfus Med Rev.* 2016;30(3):132–138.

146. AABB. *Association Bulletin 14-05*; 2014. https://www.aabb.org/programs/publications/bulletins/documents/ab14-05.pdf.

147. Moritz ED, Winton CS, Tonnetti L, et al. Screening for *Babesia microti* in the U.S. Blood supply. *N Engl J Med.* 2016;375(23):2236–2245.

148. FDA. *FDA Approves First Tests to Screen for Tickborne Parasite in Whole Blood and Plasma to Protect the U.S. Blood Supply*; 2018. https://www.fda.gov/newsevents/newsroom/pressannouncements/ucm599782.htm.

149. FDA. *Complete List of Donor Screening Assays for Infectious Agents and HIV Diagnostic Assays*; 2019. www.fda.gov/BiologicsBloodVaccines/BloodBloodComponents/ApprovedComponents/LicensedComponentsBLAs/BloodDonorScreening/InfectiousDisease/ucm080466.htm.

150. FDA. *Recommendations for Reducing the Risk of Transfusion-Transmitted Babesiosis*; May 2019. https://www.fda.gov/media/114847/download.

151. Shaz BH. Risk-based decision making: a good start to aiding US blood policy decisions? *Transfusion.* 2018;58(8):1827–1830.

152. Ward SJ, Stramer SL, Szczepiorkowski ZM. Assessing the risk of Babesia to the United States blood supply using a risk-based decision-making approach: report of AABB's Ad Hoc Babesia Policy Working Group (original report). *Transfusion.* 2018;58(8):1916–1923.

153. FDA. *Recommendations for Reducing the Risk of Transfusion-Transmitted Babesiosis*. 2018.

154. Castro E, Gonzalez LM, Rubio JM, Ramiro R, Girones N, Montero E. The efficacy of the ultraviolet C pathogen inactivation system in the reduction of *Babesia divergens* in pooled buffy coat platelets. *Transfusion.* 2014;54(9):2207–2216.

155. Tonnetti L, Laughhunn A, Thorp AM, et al. Inactivation of *Babesia microti* in red blood cells and platelet concentrates. *Transfusion.* 2017;57(10):2404–2412.

156. Tonnetti L, Proctor MC, Reddy HL, Goodrich RP, Leiby DA. Evaluation of the *Mirasol pathogen* [corrected] reduction technology system against *Babesia microti* in apheresis platelets and plasma. *Transfusion.* 2010;50(5):1019–1027.

157. FDA. *Recommendations for Donor Questioning, Deferral, Reentry and Product Management to Reduce the Risk of Transfusion- Transmitted Malaria*. 2014.

158. Germain M. The risk of allowing blood donation from men having sex with men after a temporary deferral: predictions versus reality. *Transfusion.* 2016;56(6 Pt 2):1603–1607.

159. Jubran B, Billick M, Devlin G, Cygler J, Lebouche B. Reevaluating Canada's policy for blood donations from men who have sex with men (MSM). *J Public Health Policy.* 2016;37(4):428–439.

160. FDA. *Revised Recommendations for Reducing the Risk of Human Immunodeficiency Virus Transmission by Blood and Blood Components.* 2015.

161. Mitsch A, Singh S, Li J, Balaji A, Linley L, Selik R. Age-associated trends in diagnosis and prevalence of infection with HIV among men who have sex with men - United States, 2008–2016. *MMWR Morb Mortal Wkly Rep.* 2018;67(37):1025–1031.

162. Davison KL, Brant LJ, Presanis AM, Soldan K. A re-evaluation of the risk of transfusion-transmitted HIV prevented by the exclusion of men who have sex with men from blood donation in England and Wales, 2005–2007. *Vox Sang.* 2011;101(4):291–302.

163. Goldman M, O'Brien SF. Donor deferral policies for men who have sex with men: where are we today? *Curr Opin Hematol.* 2016;23(6):568–572.

164. O'Brien SF, Osmond L, Fan W, Yi QL, Goldman M. Compliance with time based deferrals for men who have sex with men. *Transfusion.* 2019;59(3):916–920.

165. Miller YM, GK, Apostoli A, et al. Infectious disease (ID) rates among donors reinstated after changes to the men who have sex with other men (MSM) deferral policy. *Transfusion.* 2018;58(s2):8A–9A.

166. Jacobs MR, Lazarus HM, Maitta RW. The safety of the blood supply–time to raise the bar. *N Engl J Med.* 2015;373(9):882.

167. Snyder EL, Stramer SL, Benjamin RJ. The safety of the blood supply–time to raise the bar. *N Engl J Med.* 2015;372(20):1882–1885.

168. FDA. *Implementation of Pathogen Reduction Technology in the Manufacture of Blood Components in Blood Establishments: Questions and Answers;* 2017. https://www.fda.gov/downloads/BiologicsBloodVaccines/GuidanceCompliance RegulatoryInformation/Guidances/Blood/UCM590405.pdf.

169. Allain JP, Owusu-Ofori AK, Assennato SM, Marschner S, Goodrich RP, Owusu-Ofori S. Effect of Plasmodium inactivation in whole blood on the incidence of blood transfusion-transmitted malaria in endemic regions: the African Investigation of the Mirasol System (AIMS) randomised controlled trial. *Lancet.* 2016;387(10029):1753–1761.

170. Marschner S, Goodrich R. Pathogen reduction technology treatment of platelets, plasma and whole blood using riboflavin and UV light. *Transfus Med Hemotherapy.* 2011;38(1):8–18.

171. Henschler R, Seifried E, Mufti N. Development of the S-303 pathogen inactivation technology for red blood cell concentrates. *Transfus Med Hemotherapy.* 2011;38(1):33–42.

172. Drew VJ, Barro L, Seghatchian J, Burnouf T. Towards pathogen inactivation of red blood cells and whole blood targeting viral DNA/RNA: design, technologies, and future prospects for developing countries. *Blood Transfus.* 2017;15(6):512–521.

173. Seltsam A, Muller TH. Update on the use of pathogen-reduced human plasma and platelet concentrates. *Br J Haematol.* 2013;162(4):442–454.

174. Knutson F, Osselaer J, Pierelli L, et al. A prospective, active haemovigilance study with combined cohort analysis of 19,175 transfusions of platelet components prepared with amotosalen-UVA photochemical treatment. *Vox Sang.* 2015;109(4):343–352.

175. Lozano M, Cid J. Pathogen inactivation: coming of age. *Curr Opin Hematol.* 2013;20(6):540–545.

176. Laughhunn A, Huang YS, Vanlandingham DL, Lanteri MC, Stassinopoulos A. Inactivation of chikungunya virus in blood components treated with amotosalen/ultraviolet a light or amustaline/glutathione. *Transfusion.* 2018;58(3):748–757.

177. Group Apitrw. *Questions and Answers about Pathogen-Reduced Apheresis Platelet Components;* 2017. https://www.aabb.org/programs/clinical/Documents/Q-and-A-about-Pathogen-Reduced-Apheresis-Platelet-Components.pdf.

178. Gowland P, Fontana S, Stolz M, Andina N, Niederhauser C. Parvovirus B19 passive transmission by transfusion of intercept(R) blood system-treated platelet concentrate. *Transfus Med Hemother.* 2016;43(3):198–202.

179. Hauser L, Roque-Afonso AM, Beyloune A, et al. Hepatitis E transmission by transfusion of intercept blood system-treated plasma. *Blood.* 2014;123(5):796–797.

180. Cid J. Prevention of transfusion-associated graft-versus-host disease with pathogen-reduced platelets with amotosalen and ultraviolet A light: a review. *Vox Sang.* 2017;112(7):607–613.

181. Snyder E, McCullough J, Slichter SJ, et al. Clinical safety of platelets photochemically treated with amotosalen HCl and ultraviolet A light for pathogen inactivation: the SPRINT trial. *Transfusion.* 2005;45(12):1864–1875.

182. Estcourt LJ, Malouf R, Hopewell S, et al. Pathogen-reduced platelets for the prevention of bleeding. *Cochrane Database Syst Rev.* 2017;(7).

183. Mufti NA, Erickson AC, North AK, et al. Treatment of whole blood (WB) and red blood cells (RBC) with S-303 inactivates pathogens and retains in vitro quality of stored RBC. *Biologicals.* 2010;38(1):14–19.

184. Wiltshire M, Meli A, Schott MA, et al. Quality of red cells after combination of prion reduction and treatment with the intercept system for pathogen inactivation. *Transfus Med.* 2016;26(3):208–214.

185. Aubry M, Laughhunn A, Santa Maria F, Lanteri MC, Stassinopoulos A, Musso D. Pathogen inactivation of Dengue virus in red blood cells using amustaline and glutathione. *Transfusion.* 2017;57(12):2888–2896.

186. Winter KM, Johnson L, Kwok M, et al. Red blood cell in vitro quality and function is maintained after S-303 pathogen inactivation treatment. *Transfusion.* 2014;54(7):1798–1807.

187. Cancelas JA, Gottschall JL, Rugg N, et al. Red blood cell concentrates treated with the amustaline (S-303) pathogen reduction system and stored for 35 days retain post-transfusion viability: results of a two-centre study. *Vox Sang.* 2017;112(3):210–218.

188. Brixner V, Kiessling AH, Madlener K, et al. Red blood cells treated with the amustaline (S-303) pathogen reduction system: a transfusion study in cardiac surgery. *Transfusion.* 2018;58(4):905–916.

189. Tormey CA, Santhanakrishnan M, Smith NH, et al. Riboflavin-ultraviolet light pathogen reduction treatment does not impact the immunogenicity of murine red blood cells. *Transfusion.* 2016;56(4):863–872.

190. Marschner S, Fast LD, Baldwin 3rd WM, Slichter SJ, Goodrich RP. White blood cell inactivation after treatment with riboflavin and ultraviolet light. *Transfusion.* 2010;50(11):2489–2498.

191. Cap AP, Pidcoke HF, Keil SD, et al. Treatment of blood with a pathogen reduction technology using ultraviolet light and riboflavin inactivates Ebola virus in vitro. *Transfusion.* 2016;56(Suppl 1):S6–S15.

192. Ambruso DR, Thurman G, Marschner S, Goodrich RP. Lack of antibody formation to platelet neoantigens after transfusion of riboflavin and ultraviolet light-treated platelet concentrates. *Transfusion.* 2009;49(12):2631–2636.

193. Reddy HL, Dayan AD, Cavagnaro J, Gad S, Li J, Goodrich RP. Toxicity testing of a novel riboflavin-based technology for pathogen reduction and white blood cell inactivation. *Transfus Med Rev.* 2008;22(2):133–153.

194. Abonnenc M, Sonego G, Crettaz D, et al. In vitro study of platelet function confirms the contribution of the ultraviolet B (UVB) radiation in the lesions observed in riboflavin/UVB-treated platelet concentrates. *Transfusion.* 2015;55(9):2219–2230.

195. Mirasol® Pathogen Reduction Technology (Prt) System. https://www.terumobct.com/Public/306690407.pdf. Accessed Feb 4th, 2019.

196. Seltsam A, Muller TH. UVC irradiation for pathogen reduction of platelet concentrates and plasma. *Transfus Med Hemother.* 2011;38(1):43–54.

197. Gravemann U, Handke W, Muller TH, Seltsam A. Bacterial inactivation of platelet concentrates with the THERA-FLEX UV-Platelets pathogen inactivation system. *Transfusion.* 2018;59(4):1324–1332.

198. Faddy HM, Fryk JJ, Prow NA, et al. Inactivation of dengue, chikungunya, and Ross River viruses in platelet concentrates after treatment with ultraviolet C light. *Transfusion.* 2016;56(6 Pt 2):1548–1555.

199. Fryk JJ, Marks DC, Hobson-Peters J, et al. Reduction of Zika virus infectivity in platelet concentrates after treatment with ultraviolet C light and in plasma after treatment with methylene blue and visible light. *Transfusion.* 2017;57(11):2677–2682.

200. Steinmann E, Gravemann U, Friesland M, et al. Two pathogen reduction technologies–methylene blue plus light and shortwave ultraviolet light–effectively inactivate hepatitis C virus in blood components. *Transfusion.* 2013;53(5):1010–1018.

201. Seghatchian J, Tolksdorf F. Characteristics of the THERA-FLEX UV-Platelets pathogen inactivation system – an update. *Transfus Apher Sci.* 2012;46(2):221–229.

202. Burnouf T, Radosevich M. Nanofiltration of plasma-derived biopharmaceutical components. *Haemophilia.* 2003;9(1):24–37.

203. WHO. *Guidelines on Viral Inactivation and Removal Procedures Intended to Assure the Viral Safety of Human Blood Plasma Components;* 2004. www.who.int/bloodcomponents/publications/WHO_TRS_924_A4.pdf.

204. Groner A. Pathogen safety of plasma-derived components - Haemate P/Humate-P. *Haemophilia.* 2008;14(Suppl 5):54–71.

205. Horowitz B. Inactivation of viruses found with plasma proteins. *Biotechnology.* 1991;19:417–430.

206. Horowitz B, Bonomo R, Prince AM, Chin SN, Brotman B, Shulman RW. Solvent/detergent-treated plasma: a virus-inactivated substitute for fresh frozen plasma. *Blood.* 1992;79(3):826–831.

207. Hellstern P, Solheim BG. The use of solvent/detergent treatment in pathogen reduction of plasma. *Transfus Med Hemother.* 2011;38(1):65–70.

208. Hellstern P, Sachse H, Schwinn H, Oberfrank K. Manufacture and in vitro characterization of a solvent/detergent-treated human plasma. *Vox Sang.* 1992;63(3):178–185.

209. Prince AM, Horowitz B, Brotman B. Sterilisation of hepatitis and HTLV-III viruses by exposure to tri(n-butyl)phosphate and sodium cholate. *Lancet.* 1986;1(8483):706–710.

210. Lindholm PF, Annen K, Ramsey G. Approaches to minimize infection risk in blood banking and transfusion practice. *Infect Disord Drug Targets.* 2011;11(1):45–56.

211. Klamroth R, Groner A, Simon TL. Pathogen inactivation and removal methods for plasma-derived clotting factor concentrates. *Transfusion.* 2014;54(5):1406–1417.

212. Kim IS, Choi YW, Kang Y, Sung HM, Shin JS. Dry-heat treatment process for enhancing viral safety of an antihemophilic factor VIII concentrate prepared from human plasma. *J Microbiol Biotechnol.* 2008;18(5):997–1003.

213. Stadler M, Gruber G, Kannicht C, et al. Characterisation of a novel high-purity, double virus inactivated von Willebrand Factor and Factor VIII concentrate (Wilate). *Biologicals.* 2006;34(4):281–288.

214. Effect of dry-heating of coagulation factor concentrates at 80 degrees C for 72 hours on transmission of non-A, non-B hepatitis. Study group of the UK Haemophilia centre directors on surveillance of virus transmission by concentrates. *Lancet.* 1988;2(8615):814–816.

215. Roberts PL, Dunkerley C, McAuley A, Winkelman L. Effect of manufacturing process parameters on virus inactivation by dry heat treatment at 80 degrees C in factor VIII. *Vox Sang.* 2007;92(1):56–63.

216. Blumel J, Schmidt I, Effenberger W, et al. Parvovirus B19 transmission by heat-treated clotting factor concentrates. *Transfusion.* 2002;42(11):1473–1481.

217. Seghatchian J, Struff WG, Reichenberg S. Main properties of the THERAFLEX MB-plasma system for pathogen reduction. *Transfus Med Hemother.* 2011;38(1):55–64.

218. Williamson LM, Cardigan R, Prowse CV. Methylene blue-treated fresh-frozen plasma: what is its contribution to blood safety? *Transfusion.* 2003;43(9):1322–1329.

CHAPTER 6

Transfusion-Related Immunomodulation

ROBERT W. MAITTA, MD, PHD

INTRODUCTION

Blood transfusions represent to date one of the most common clinical approaches to treat patients with a myriad of etiologies that lead to anemia, thrombocytopenia, or deficient coagulation requiring factor supplementation. With a growing aging population, the demands on transfusion medicine facilities and donation centers are likely to continue to increase in the coming years. However, use of blood either whole or its components in the treatment of patients is not without risks. One such entity that has been the reason of heightened concern over the last 40 years is known as transfusion-related immunomodulation (TRIM). Importantly, the question we continue to ask is if this should still be a matter of concern today when blood components are safer than they have ever been. Considering that in the United States there is a red blood cell (RBC) transfusion every 2 seconds that translates into approximately 16 million units transfused in the country on an annual basis,[1] immunomodulatory adverse events if common could represent a major public health issue that would need to be addressed by the medical community.

RBC transfusions in particular have been the focus of years of research to understand the potential effects that they may have once transfused in the recipient. Specifically, transfusion of RBC units results in immune exposure to cell-bound and cell-free antigens or metabolites that lead to changes in a recipient's immune response.[2] These effects can also potentially occur when transfused with either pooled or single-donor derived platelet units. Therefore, in this chapter, data will be presented to guide the reader to take into consideration those changes that blood component preparation have undergone since the initial studies were published decades ago. With this in mind, studies will be presented in the context of how components were prepared at the

time for transfusion so that there is a better understanding of the effects that these components may have had and to facilitate comparison of findings from older studies to more recent ones.

HISTORICAL PERSPECTIVE

As mentioned earlier, it has been known for quite some time that RBC units can contain immunomodulatory mediators that lead to changes in the way the immune system of a recipient responds posttransfusion. However, this potentially complex response to blood transfusions needs to be properly defined to grasp its true effects especially in those critically ill who may be particularly susceptible to potentially deleterious effects of transfusions in either the adult or the pediatric settings.[3,4] In its simplest form, TRIM can be seen as those potentially proinflammatory or immunosuppressive effects that can occur because of a transfusion due to mediators that are preformed and present in the unit or that are produced by the recipient as a response to the transfusion.

First, we should step back in time and look at the early reports that first described these potential effects of blood. It is agreed upon in the literature that it was the report in the 1970s by Opelz and colleagues of lower rejection rates of patients who underwent renal transplantation and received allogeneic transfusions, which the authors argued was secondary to lower concentrations of antihuman leukocyte antigen (HLA) antibodies post-RBC transfusion, that provided the foundation for TRIM.[5] This observation resulted in deliberate transfusions of transplant patients regardless of need to have better posttransplantation outcomes; this is something that would be more difficult to do today.[6] Nevertheless, this important finding would define the next 40 years in how blood transfusions were seen and utilized in clinical settings.

Immunologic Concepts in Transfusion Medicine. https://doi.org/10.1016/B978-0-323-67509-3.00006-8

Early data from animal models appeared to indicate that transfusion of blood made more likely metastasis of solid organ malignancies.[7,8] However, this association since then has been disputed by others who have not seen such an association; as a result, this still remains a matter of debate.[4] Nevertheless, it can be said that any degree of immunosuppression by blood transfusions as that defined as TRIM would have detrimental effects in other clinical settings such as patients dealing with malignancies, either in remission or not, and those patients fighting infections.[9–12] Undoubtedly, early studies indicating that the post-transfusion risk of infection was greater also inferred that this correlated with the number of units transfused, especially, when compared to infectious rates of patients who did not receive transfusions.[13,14] Therefore, this risk had to be taken into consideration when the decision to transfuse was made. However, specific variables such as patients' complex and significant health impairments, and lack of risk-stratification when determining the effects of transfusion in relation to a patient's condition may have had immediate bearing on the effects seen in these early studies.

NEWER PERSPECTIVES

Despite increased awareness, this has not stopped the controversy of how to best define TRIM and attempts have been made to limit its definition to those secondary to length of storage of RBC units (Fig. 6.1).[15] In this redefinition, the focus shifts almost exclusively to the changes that RBC units undergo while in storage and the deleterious effects of using these older RBC units.[15] This distinction, however, allows to differentiate TRIM from those processes that lead to alloimmunization to RBC antigens and/or iron overload secondary to iron present in RBC units; similarly, it also sets forth that this and any other definition should be limited to the effects of blood components over the function of the recipient's immune system. In support of this definition, it has been reported that the length of storage causes physiological and metabolic changes that can result in deleterious effects as shown in an in vivo model of transfusion comparing stored versus fresh RBCs. In this model, mortality and tumor progression were not mediated either by the leukocytes still present in the transfused blood or by the RBC supernatant but instead by the aged RBC themselves.[16] Additionally, depending upon the timing of the patient's response,

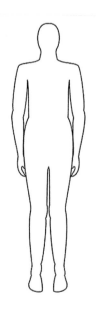

Pre-leukoreduction
WBC:
Cytokines, chemokines, soluble mediators
Apoptosis derivatives, Cell activation/suppression signals

RBC:
Heme, iron, metabolic/physiologic changes (storage lesion)
Phosphatidylserine
Ubiquitin
Vesicles
Endothelial adherence

Platelets:
Microparticles,
Cytokines, chemokines,
WBC/platelet aggregates,
Immune activity

Bioactive lipids

Post-leukoreduction
RBC:
Heme, Iron, metabolic/physiologic changes (storage lesion)
Phosphatidylserine
Ubiquitin
Vesicles
Endothelial adherence

Platelets
Microparticles,
Cytokines, chemokines,
WBC/platelet aggregates,
Immune activity

Bioactive lipids

WBC:
Cytokines, chemokines, soluble mediators
Apoptosis derivatives, Cell activation/suppression signals

FIG. 6.1 Diagram of role of each blood cell or soluble mediator potentially involved in TRIM before and after prestorage leukoreduction. Smaller font postleukoreduction signifies decreased role of WBC-mediated factors leading to TRIM.

RBC transfusion effects could be seen as part of a continuum that are either immediate or delayed, and in some cases elicit memory responses that result in reactions to other RBC units at a later time point.[15]

Existing clinical evidence has also described at least temporal association between RBC transfusions and higher incidence of organ dysfunction, nosocomial infections in addition to possible cancer recurrence.[17] Reports have also indicated that the remaining plasma supernatant of stored RBCs may increase the metastatic (immunosuppressive) effects of transfusion,[18,19] which in animal models could be worse when cells/plasma are derived from female mice.[20] However, opinions of this potential association have changed over the years as it became clearer that remaining white blood cell (WBC) in RBC units, or factors released by them, mediated at least some of the negative effects secondary to RBC transfusions (Fig. 6.1). Over time, this drove home the argument for wide use of leukoreduced RBC units.[21–23] Nevertheless, despite greater awareness immunomodulatory effects are still seen, though less frequently, in the postleukoreduction era.

BIOLOGICAL MECHANISMS
The cumulative weight of the data indicates that these mechanisms are likely multifactorial. RBC transfusions appear to activate a recipients' WBC resulting in decreased neutrophil chemotaxis, phagocyte activation, exacerbation of a patient's limited immune response, and cytokine dysregulation.[4,17,24,25] Of these, neutrophil

chemotaxis has been shown to be mediated by RBC supernatants containing transforming growth factor (TGF)-β, and these inhibitory effects can be replicated either by using plasma from RBC recipients (containing endogenous TGF-β among other mediators) or by using exogenous TGF-β (Fig. 6.2).[26]

An interesting hypothesis that is supported by increasing literature is that blood represents a "second immunological hit" that brings about those physiological changes characteristic of TRIM.[25] This is similar to what has been suggested in severe transfusion reactions such as transfusion-related acute lung injury,[27] which is the focus of discussion elsewhere in this book. This implies that there must be a primary insult to the immune system that predisposes the transfusion recipient to TRIM. Therefore, even though the focus of research has been to some extent limited to the composition/content of a unit, the condition of the recipient is equally relevant when one analyzes data reporting these adverse events to transfusion.[28] Unfortunately, this may be the one unintended bias introduced by studies reporting TRIM that will prove difficult to eliminate. This would explain why a meta-analysis of available randomized trials and of the literature found the data inconsistent to establish if RBC storage influences TRIM; however, data from this analysis did point out that when these adverse events do occur they may be limited to specific patient subpopulations such as those in cardiac settings and/or trauma.[29] This is one area that will be discussed later in this chapter.

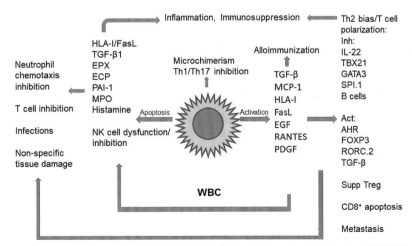

FIG. 6.2 Representation of white blood cell–driven mediators and mechanisms leading to TRIM. To the right, representation of processes dependent upon WBC activation and to the left those processes driven by cell apoptosis. Arrows represent the flow of mediators and the potential role in a particular immunomodulatory process. *Inh*, inhibition; *Act*, Activation; *Supp*, Suppressor.

Regarding immunosuppressive effects, a number of cellular and tissue targets can be affected in a recipient because of transfusions, which explains the profound systemic effects that have been reported. For example, it has been shown that RBC transfusions inhibit natural killer (NK)-cell activity and that this is mediated by decreases in soluble HLA-I, soluble Fas ligand (L), and changes in production of TGF-β.[30] Similarly, in a time-dependent manner, nonleukoreduced RBC units showed a bias toward greater number of T helper (h)2 cells versus Th1 (Fig. 6.2). This occurs in the setting of decreases in transcription factors TBX21, GATA3, SPI.1, and cytokine IL-22 with concomitant increases in AHR, FOXP3, RORC.2, and TGF-β.[31] Of note, regardless of leukoreduction, RBC units appear to induce proliferation of suppressive regulatory T cells suggesting that, at least regarding this effect, leukoreduction may have limited effectiveness.[32]

Over the years, studies looking at the effect of leukocytes in transfused units focused on patients undergoing cardiac surgery who needed transfusions. These studies indicated that patients who received nonleukoreduced units were more likely to have complications during their hospitalization and increased mortality,[33] and in surgical patients have a higher propensity for infections.[13,34] Authors of these studies, therefore, favored leukoreduction of RBC units to avoid such complications. Larger studies and meta-analyses have also pointed out that leukoreduction results in significant reduction in complications and mortality in adults.[23,35] However, a similar benefit of leukoreduction in mortality was not observed in transfused low-birth-weight premature patients, but use of leukoreduced units did reduce the incidence of bacteremia, bronchopulmonary dysplasia, retinopathy, intravascular hemorrhage and necrotizing enterocolitis.[36] Taken together, these reports indicated that the effects over the immune system in critical patient settings appeared dependent upon the leukocyte load in units that were not leukoreduced.[37]

One important element that earlier studies alluded to is that the patient population receiving blood is an important variable in TRIM occurrence as likely recipient factors play a major role in the responses to blood components regardless of leukoreduction. If an analogy could be made, this is similar to what has been seen in the infectious diseases literature in which microorganisms normally innocuous to the general population as a whole become pathogenic in immunocompromised patients. As a result, as patients who receive blood tend to be more severely ill at the time of transfusions this inevitably adds factors that may be exacerbated and "prime" the recipient to react negatively to a blood transfusion. This possibility could provide a physiological explanation to the early discrepant results observed in randomized clinical trials looking at the effect of transfusion in blood recipients.[2]

Leukocytes in the blood unit are also involved in processes leading to alloimmunization (Fig. 6.2). Evidence indicating that leukocytes in transfused blood also play a role in RBC alloimmunization have come from mouse studies indicating that apoptotic WBCs in transfused blood release factors that regulate RBC alloimmunization such as TGF-β, and by among other mechanisms causing polarization of naïve $CD4^+CD25^+$ T cells.[38] This is not at all unexpected, because it has been known for some time that RBC units have increases in inflammatory cytokines in a time-dependent manner during storage.[39,40] Leukoreduction does result in marked decreases in these soluble mediators.[39] However, data of the immunosuppressive effects of increasing TGF-β levels secondary to apoptotic WBCs in the unit does not exclude endogenous production of this cytokine by recipients' macrophages as shown post-transfusion of RBCs expressing phosphatidylserine that results in immunosuppression.[41]

T-cell activation and deactivation are likely to mediate either the reported proinflammatory or the immunosuppressive effects of RBCs. This has been suggested by data indicating that transfusion of both fresh and RBCs stored for longer periods leads to suppression of cytokine production by isolated T cells in vitro.[42] Nevertheless, of the two, older RBCs result in greater decreases in cytokine production including interleukin (IL)-10, IL-17a, interferon (IFN)-γ, tumor necrosis factor (TNF)-α, and granulocyte macrophage colony-stimulating factor compared to fresh RBCs.[42] However, RBCs may not need to be stored for long time periods to exert an immune effect. RBCs stored for as little as 2–3 weeks can inhibit both $CD4^+$ and $CD8^+$ T cells stimulated with anti-CD3/CD28, inhibit B cells stimulated with lipopolysaccharide, and both of these effects could be reversed by transfusing fresh RBCs.[43] Similarly, comparisons of transfusions of fresh versus older RBCs in a mouse model have indicated that the latter results in increased IL-6, keratinocyte-derived chemokine/CXCL1 and monocyte chemoattractant protein-1.[24]

OLD VERSUS FRESH UNITS

Based on what was described in the prior paragraph, older RBCs seem to result in higher incidence of TRIM compared to fresh cells. Yet, the data indicating this remain controversial. As mentioned earlier, responses to RBCs may not be totally dependent upon storage times as a trend toward less mortality has been described using stored RBCs.[29] Later on, authors of this earlier study reanalyzed observational data and came to a markedly different conclusion that though RBC units stored greater than 30 days did not correlate with greater incidence of nosocomial infections, mortality did appear to correlate with longer RBC storage.[44] These conflicting results exemplify the difficulties in determining the true effect of RBC storage.

This debate between fresh versus not fresh units leading to different patient outcomes has been reason for concern in the mind of clinicians for decades. Indeed, there is data describing that decreased deformability of erythrocyte membranes may occur because of storage duration but more importantly that this change can continue even after cells are transfused.[45] This later point is an important one as it would imply that older units would not provide full therapeutic benefit due to their storage age. However, results from randomized clinical trials may shed more light into this issue and their results will be discussed next.

Randomized clinical trials provide the best evidence regarding the role that the age of the unit and changes related to the storage lesion can cause in patients. A recent large multinational trial, the Age of Blood Evaluation (ABLE), which included European and Canadian medical centers found that use of fresh RBC units (7 day or less) provided no survival advantage and did not lead to significant economic benefit compared to standard issue RBC units.[46] Even though the focus of this large trial of over 1200 patients in each investigational arm was not pediatric patients, among those included in the study were teenagers, and results were similar to those described for the whole study population. Similarly, the Age of Red Blood Cells in Premature Infants trial indicated that the age of RBC units did not have a noticeable effect on outcomes among neonatal patients.[47] Similarly, the Red-Cell Storage Duration Study that looked at outcomes in cardiac patients undergoing surgery and required transfusions did not show that outcomes of patients receiving units >21 days were worse than those patients receiving fresh units.[48] Finally, the findings reported by the ABLE trial were also similar in critically ill adults requiring transfusion.[49] One major randomized clinical trial in pediatric patients that at the time of writing this chapter is still underway is The Age of Blood in Children in Pediatric Intensive Care Unit and its results hopefully in the near future will provide further insight into the potential differences between older versus fresher units in

this patient population.[50] As a result, based on the information conveyed by these large trials, the age of the unit may not necessarily be a determinant of poor outcomes in diverse patient populations.

Despite results obtained by these trials, differing opinions of the role of older versus fresh RBC units in pediatric settings have not ended with the previously mentioned data. Contrary to what has been described by others, in the pediatric setting transfusion of older (>21 days) RBC units has been reported to lead to persistence of systemic inflammation and innate immunity suppression (measured by ex vivo lipopolysaccharide stimulation leading to TNF-α production) when compared to patients receiving fresher units or fewer number of units.[51] In this same study, IL-6 production was decreased by use of fresher RBC units. The differences in this study's observations could be due in part to being observational in nature, have a relatively small patient cohort while the ones listed earlier were well-controlled randomized clinical trials. This inevitably adds variables to each study that are likely to add confounders leading to markedly different conclusions. Along these lines, additional reports have found an association between the age of RBC units and high incidence of complications including mortality in both adult and pediatric cardiac patients in intensive care units.[52–54] Similarly, there is literature indicating that older RBC units lead to innate immunity (cytokines) suppression.[55–58] This immune suppression would result in higher infectious rates and mortality as shown in trauma patients receiving transfusions that could be made worse by transfusing a greater number of units.[59,60] Something that will require closer investigation in future studies is what role higher levels of IL-10 play in TRIM responses. This is because in patients who have had repeated reactions to blood components, they are found to have increased concentrations of IL-10 upon transfusion suggesting that in this cohort this may represent one of the mechanisms leading to immunomodulation (Fig. 6.3).[61] Likely, this contentious topic will continue and future studies will need to be carried out to provide further insight and resolve the role that metabolic and cellular changes that occur while in storage play in TRIM.

WBCS IN UNITS AND LEUKOREDUCTION

As eluded earlier, WBC in the unit can produce mediators that lead to the unforseen reactions that qualify as TRIM. It should be of interest to the reader that in some instances these negative effects have been described as lasting long after transfusion exposure. For example, it was reported that 2 weeks posttransfusion, plasma samples from blood recipients had high levels of TGF-β1

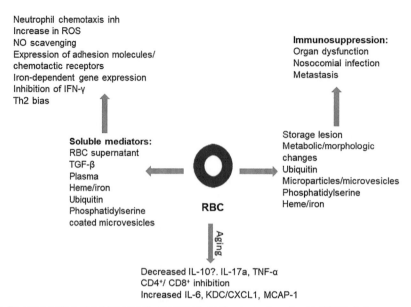

FIG. 6.3 Representation of red blood cell—mediated mechanisms described in TRIM. Aging represents data referring to age of unit. To the right, potential effects secondary to storage lesion are indicated. To the left, mechanisms possibly mediated by soluble mediators are indicated.

synthesized by recipients' neutrophils that were the result of direct interaction with soluble FasL and HLA-I molecules present in nonleukoreduced transfused units (Fig. 6.2).[62] This in turn inhibits neutrophil chemotaxis leading to increased susceptibility to infections. Similarly, blood units derived from placentas have high TGF-β1 produced by apoptotic or necrotic WBC that increases over time, and this may be associated with erythrocyte lysis in a time-dependent manner.[63] This mechanism also appears to mediate the response to intravenous immunoglobulin through induction of TGF-β1 that is also mediated by soluble FasL and HLA-I,[64] suggesting that these mediators are involved in multiple immunomodulatory responses. Interestingly, soluble HLA-I free chains increase in both RBC and platelet units during storage, are produced by remaining WBC in the units in a time-dependent manner, and at some threshold cause apoptosis of CD8$^+$ T cells suggesting that this could be an additional immunosuppressive effect that has been described in both allogeneic and autologous blood transfusions.[65]

RBC units also increase perioperative inflammatory responses as described in patients receiving transfusions during cardiopulmonary bypass surgery,[66] and these effects can be lessened if leukoreduced RBC units are utilized.[67] These findings represented an additional reason to push for leukoreduction of units that has

resulted in an overall decrease in the number of reports of potential immunomodulatory effects of blood, including associated mortality, organ dysfunction, and infectious rates.[22,23,68] Likewise, leukoreduction has translated into improved postsurgery survival of cardiac patients thanks to potentially lower proinflammatory rates.[69] However, despite benefits seen post leukoreduction, survival of patients transfused with leukoreduced units is still lower than patients who are not transfused, and regarding cancer recurrence rates it has shown not to have made a difference.[70] Nevertheless, reports from animal models indicate that use of leukoreduced blood results in fewer recipient splenic T cells undergoing apoptosis that is mediated by Fas/FasL,[71] and decreased rates of solid tumor metastasis.[72] As a result, reported results of positive benefits of restrictive transfusion strategies that minimize blood usage whenever possible can be understood, as this approach results in fewer nosocomial infections compared to patients liberally transfused.[73]

One point that needs to be reemphasized is that despite almost universal prestorage leukoreduction of units across the United States, up to 5×10^6 WBCs/unit still remain in the bag and these cells can still cause some of the reactions described thus far.[74-76] Despite initial data indicating the role that HLA-I played in some of the immunomodulatory processes mediated by WBCs in the unit, there is evidence that class II may also mediate some of these effects. MHC class II molecules on antigen presenting cells (APCs) such as monocytes and dendritic cells in the donated unit are also capable of initiating a cascade of events that activate T cells and result in either immunosuppression or alloimmunization.[77,78] Immune responses can be further complicated by differences between a recipient's and donor's HLA antigens, and depending on the recipient's clinical condition lead to alloimmunization, or when costimulation is incomplete result in immune tolerance and T-cell anergy.[17] This latter effect provides for an explanation when microchimerism occurs after allogeneic blood transfusions, due to lack of an immune response, allowing allogeneic cells to survive in a recipient's circulation.[79] Survival of allogeneic cells could last for years posttransfusion due to engraftment of donor leukocytes as seen in multilineage microchimerism of trauma patients who received intense transfusion support (Fig. 6.2).[79,80] Mechanistically, the extent of this microchimerism is secondary to Th2 activation and TGF-β increases resulting in immunosuppression posttransfusion,[81,82] reduction in both Th1 and Th17 responses,[83] and even changes to patterns of gene expression needed for a healthy immune response.[84]

ROLE OF APOPTOSIS AND SOLUBLE MEDIATORS

Cell death and/or apoptosis can cause release of mediators that can be immunomodulatory in nature. One of these molecules released during cell death is phosphatidylserine that is expressed on RBC-derived microparticles and cellular debris produced postapoptosis.[85] Upon exposure to phosphatidylserine, synthesis of cytokines such as IL-10 and TGF-β increases, and inhibition of NFκB and p38 MAPK occur as early as 72 hours poststorage downregulating dendritic cells and activating T regulatory cells (Fig. 6.3).[86,87] These apoptotic effects, however, are not unique to RBC units, as they have also been reported to occur in platelet units as well.[88]

Apoptosis leads not only to cell fragmentation but also to the release of cell content including bioactive substances from cytoplasmic granules. Among such contents are histamine, eosinophil protein X (EPX), myeloperoxidase, eosinophil cationic protein (ECP), and plasminogen activator inhibitor 1 that are released by both leukocytes and platelets in a time-dependent manner during storage.[89] Importantly, these mediators are significantly decreased by prestorage leukoreduction.[90] Of these, histamine, EPX, and ECP have been shown to inhibit neutrophil chemotaxis and T lymphocyte proliferation in vitro,[91,92] and in some instances result in diffuse nonspecific tissue damage (Fig. 6.3).[93]

It has also been reported that supernatant of stored RBC units can suppress monocytes, and washing of units can remove soluble mediators responsible for this inhibition.[51,94] Since mediators that can cause TRIM symptomatology are found in solution and are released by remaining WBCs still present in RBC units, leukoreduction would not fully remove the potential risk represented by these mediators to cause unforseen adverse events in the recipient. Mediators such as soluble FasL and TGF-β that as mentioned earlier lead to TRIM,[26,38] and to a lesser extent soluble HLA-I molecules work through direct inhibition of a recipient's immune responses even when autologous RBC units are transfused.[64,95] These mediators can activate apoptotic signals, or result in dysfunctional neutrophil chemotaxis and NK cell activity.[1] This is one point that needs to be emphasized that use of autologous units does not exempt the recipient from reacting adversely to these soluble mediators which may have significant effects over a recipient's immune responses.

Additional soluble immune mediators in the form of cytokines can also be released by WBC present in the unit, although these are likely to be less of a factor in the era of leukoreduction. Data indicate that procarcinogenic cytokines such as monocyte chemotactic protein-1 (MCP-1), RANTES, epidermal growth factor, and platelet-derived growth factor increase over time during storage; however, all of these cytokines are markedly reduced but not eliminated through leukoreduction.[19] Therefore, it should be no surprise that in patients with impaired immunity such as young infants reports that MCP-1, IL-1β, IL-8, IL-17, TNF-α, IFN-γ, IFN-γ-induced protein 10, soluble intracellular adhesion molecule, and plasma macrophage inhibitory factor are increased in recipients posttransfusion. These mediators in some instances lead to TRIM-associated symptomatology in this patient population.[96,97]

HEME, IRON, AND RBC MEDIATORS

It is clear that prolonged storage results in RBCs, which as they complete their life cycle, release their contents into suspension and this may be increasingly more significant toward the end of the unit's shelf life. However, this is a constant process that starts at time of collection since donated RBCs when drawn from the recipient span in age from young to older RBCs as they enter the bag. As mentioned earlier, storage itself may cause changes to RBCs partly driving some of the deleterious changes associated with TRIM and increased mortality as shown in in vivo models.[98,99] These storage-length changes define the storage lesion. These negative effects can be minimized by washing older units resulting in better animal survival, less lung injury, better cardiac and liver functional responses, and above all reduced levels of nontransferrin-bound iron and plasma labile iron.[100] Despite these findings, available data from randomized clinical trials does not support that storage significantly affects outcomes after transfusion that are likely dependent upon a recipient's clinical condition or a given patient subpopulation rather than to the age of units used.[101]

We therefore need to look at biochemical changes caused by storage to understand the potential mechanisms mediating the reported deleterious effects. Among changes that RBCs undergo in the bag are oxygen affinity, decreased pH, cell morphological changes, and increased membrane permeability[102]; fortunately, some of these can be reversed using RBC rejuvenation techniques that improve energy metabolism (Fig. 6.3).[103,104] However, these techniques cannot reverse the senescence of cells that continues as cells reach their expected lifespan. Nevertheless, despite these storage-dependent changes, reviews of the literature have failed to find evidence that fresh units are necessarily superior to older units[105,106]; and in some instances the opposite could be true.[107] Undoubtedly, the lack of uniformity in defining what an old unit is for a given population (adult vs. pediatric, trauma, surgery, numerous comorbidities among others) may prove a difficult obstacle to overcome and find consistency among reports showing that exposure to older units correlates with poorer outcomes.

However, two mediators are constantly released in a unit while in storage, and they are heme and iron. Presence of either one of these bioactive substances in solution at the time of transfusion could immediately influence the recipient's response to transfusion. Yet, the question that needs to be asked is if iron and/or heme can sufficiently affect the recipient's immune system to result in changes associated with TRIM. Furthermore, RBC units need not to be old to generate free hemoglobin and iron as phagocytes in the spleen among other organs can remove aging cells in fresher units via extravascular hemolysis.[108] Once free, iron deposition can occur in a variety of organs or by itself lead to inflammatory responses.[109] Both heme and iron can also cause tissue damage directly due to formation of reactive oxygen species (ROS), or indirectly through activation and increased migration of leukocytes via enhanced expression of adhesion molecules and chemotactic receptors.[110–112]

Iron released during storage can be found as transferrin-bound, nontransferrin-bound, or in plasma form.[1] Of these, nontransferrin-bound iron causes release of inflammatory cytokines in mice,[109] but such effects thus far have failed to be shown to occur in either adults,[113] or in pediatric patients.[114] In this latter patient group, however, transfusion itself and not iron specifically may be behind transfusion-associated neonatal enterocolitis,[97] and evidence points that MCP-1 mediates these immunomodulatory responses in neonates.[115] Different from iron, upon cell lysis free hemoglobin can be removed from circulation by the action of haptoglobin but this capability can be overwhelmed when the concentration of hemoglobin exceeds compensatory mechanisms. Free hemoglobin can also undergo biochemical changes that result in the formation of methemoglobin and release of heme that can further catalyze iron release.[116]

Uptake and degradation of RBCs by macrophages drives heme and iron levels to increase in the cell's cytoplasm working as a signal for cytokine release and iron-mediated generation of reactive oxygen forms that father enhance proinflammatory signals.[1] Intracytoplasmic iron in phagocytes can also result in changes to the cell's gene expression profile so that alternative phagocyte phenotypes that are characteristic of immunosuppression are elicited.[117] This immunosuppressive phenotype would be characterized by higher inducible nitric oxide synthetase expression and therefore couple nitric oxide (NO) regulation to iron homeostasis.[118] In this manner, iron could trigger a cascade of immunosuppressive events that results in inhibition of activating cytokines such as IFN-γ and therefore, inhibit pathways that depend on these active mediators for competent immunological responses.[117] Inhibition of IFN-γ-dependent pathways can also hinder other immune cell types leading to a broader immunosuppressive effect.

MICROPARTICLES AND ADDITIONAL MEDIATORS

Microparticles derived from RBCs are elements that could also play a role in TRIM. RBC-derived microparticles contain hemoglobin and cell-free-hemoglobin that when in the ferrous state can deplete and result in vasoconstriction and inability to vasoregulate (Fig. 6.3).[119] Interestingly, this ability to scavenge NO appears to be more evident when older RBC units are used.[120] Leukoreduction also has limited effect when RBC unit changes are due to storage. This is because reduction in red cell size due to cell membrane losses and increase in rates of nitrite oxidation to nitrate when using leukoreduced RBC units stored for greater than 25 days may also represent an important element in the storage lesion.[121] Release of ROS by RBCs can also bind NO and potentiate those processes outlined previously.[122] This mechanism may have high relevance, as ROS release by RBC units may be greater in older units.[116,123] Additionally, previously discussed phosphatidylserine is also found on RBC microvesicles that form during storage, resulting in thrombin-dependent complement activation that worsens lipopolysaccharide-induced proinflammatory cytokine production in a mouse model.[124]

Reports have also pointed out that release of ubiquitin by RBCs during storage may also be involved in TRIM. Among cells, ubiquitin is highly expressed in RBCs and just as other mediators its concentration is quantitatively higher in units in a time-dependent manner.[125] Ubiquitin can induce changes in gene expression so that the net result is a Th2 bias in cytokine expression and gene expression.[126] This Th2 activation bias has been the focus of earlier discussion in this chapter. Specifically, exposure to ubiquitin in supernatant from RBC units toward the end of their shelf lives resulted in significant increases in IL-4 and IL-8, while lowering IFN-γ and TNF-α postmitogen stimulation.[126,127]

Biologically active lipids also present in RBC units can also mediate immunoregulation. These lipids such as lysophosphatidylcholine appear to be derived from the remaining plasma in units rather than cells as plasma substitution with buffers significantly reduced their concentration.[128] These lipids can activate neutrophils and this may be one of the factors (first hit) leading to the constellation of symptoms known as transfusion-related acute lung injury (TRALI).[129] Importantly, being plasma-derived would explain why leukoreduction has had limited effect in the reduction of these lipids. Furthermore, as shown in an in vivo transfusion model, the higher the plasma content the greater the concentration of these lipids as seen in immunomodulatory effects of platelet units that have high plasma content.[130] The effect of these lipids will be further covered elsewhere in this book under TRALI.

CELL-DERIVED VESICLES

Cells in the unit release vesicles such as microparticles and ectosomes during storage that increase over time and have been implicated in TRIM. These vesicles are released by aging RBCs,[131] by leukocytes,[132] and by platelets[133,134] with higher concentrations later in a unit's storage life resulting in significant immunomodulatory effects[135]; and in some cases higher mortality in critically

ill patients.[136] As most blood cells have been found to release these vesicles, their functions are likely complex with distinct physiology depending on the originating cell lineage. Case in point, platelets have two types of these vesicles, microparticles, and exosomes that have distinct functions not limited to procoagulant activity.[137] On the other hand, those vesicles derived from RBCs and leukocytes may be physiologically immunosuppressive decreasing inflammatory responses.[131,138] They potentially exert some of these functions by direct cell binding or through uptake by leukocytes.[139] Consequently, these vesicular functions reach beyond those in the immune system and include roles in coagulation, vascular homeostasis, and cell development to name a few, and when in excess may increase incidence of adverse outcomes.[140]

ENDOTHELIUM ADHERENCE

One observation that may be of interest is that when RBCs are transfused in an animal model after prolonged storage, leukocytes in the transfused unit lead to higher levels of RBC adherence to capillaries and endothelium as a whole that can be reduced with prestorage leukoreduction.[141] In particular, time-dependent increases in RBC adherence to endothelial cell layers are almost abrogated by prestorage leukoreduction.[142,143] Of interest, poststorage rejuvenation of RBC units, which was covered earlier in the text, also reverses the observed adhesion to endothelial cells.[144] These observations suggest that adherence is secondary to RBC aging while the former places WBCs as the cell group mediating this process. This apparent contradiction will require future research but regardless of the initiating trigger, this adherence is clinically important in the inflammatory dysregulation and binding of RBC to endothelial cells seen in sickle cell disease.[145]

ROLE OF PLATELETS IN TRIM

An increasing number of patients require platelet transfusions, and this number is likely to increase as more patients qualify for hematopoietic stem cell transplantation. Platelet units have in addition to thrombocytes, plasma, leukocytes (remaining postleukoreduction), and RBCs all of which could cause potential complications posttransfusion. Similarly, RBC units also contain platelets that in the preleukoreduction era could cause complex aggregate formation with WBCs leading to a more procoagulable effect and increase the potential for adverse events even with units early in storage.[146,147] Therefore, at this point in the narrative we shift the focus to platelets and their derivatives as possible mediators of TRIM.

Platelets are not just hemostatic mediators but are essential members of the immune system through their ability to release immunomodulatory cytokines and chemokines, activate neutrophils and form neutrophil extracellular traps, increase expression of endothelial adhesion markers, mediate lymphocyte modulation, leukocyte recruitment, direct killing of infected cells, pathogen sequestration, and direct phagocytosis of invading microorganisms (Fig. 6.1).[148] As a result, platelet transfusions should be seen as an infusion of innate immune hemocytes that will mediate hemostasis, are potentially involved in all arms of the immune response, and in some circumstances be mediators of autoimmunity.[149] Just as in the case of other blood cells, platelets also actively generate microparticles, which are smaller versions of mature platelets that can mediate both activation and suppression of immune responses, and regulate immune cell differentiation.[133,134,150] This immune nature of platelets will likely make them an important participant in responses associated with TRIM and should be the focus of future investigation.

CONCLUSION

Blood component utilization is not without risk, and this can be seen with the 40 years of reports describing TRIM. One think that it is clear that the incidence of TRIM appears to have decreased with the advent of pre-storage leukoreduction; nevertheless, as units still have remaining leukocytes, the possibility of TRIM has not fully disappeared. Evidence that TRIM can also be caused by RBCs themselves as they age may signify that these adverse outcomes will prove difficult to avoid. This is further complicated by data showing that soluble mediators found in plasma can also cause TRIM. Furthermore, links of microvesicles, microparticles, and platelets to TRIM implies that a sense of proactive vigilance is needed when using blood. As a result, increased awareness of these responses to transfusion will lead to rapid recognition of these reactions, and implies that a more judicious use of blood components will result in fewer potential cases of TRIM being reported.

REFERENCES

1. Remy KE, Hall MW, Cholette J, et al. Mechanisms of red blood cell transfusion-related immunomodulation. *Transfusion.* 2018;58(3):804–815.
2. Blajchman MA. Transfusion immunomodulation or TRIM: what does it mean clinically? *Hematology.* 2005;10(Suppl 1):208–214.
3. Muszynski JA, Spinella PC, Cholette JM, et al. Transfusion-related immunomodulation: review of the literature and implications for pediatric critical illness. *Transfusion.* 2017;57(1):195–206.
4. Vamvakas EC, Blajchman MA. Deleterious clinical effects of transfusion-associated immunomodulation: fact or fiction? *Blood.* 2001;97(5):1180–1195.
5. Opelz G, Sengar DP, Mickey MR, Terasaki PI. Effect of blood transfusions on subsequent kidney transplants. *Transplant Proc.* 1973;5(1):253–259.
6. Opelz G, Graver B, Terasaki PI. Induction of high kidney graft survival rate by multiple transfusion. *Lancet.* 1981;1(8232):1223–1225.
7. Shirwadkar S, Blajchman MA, Frame B, Orr FW, Singal DP. Effect of blood transfusions on experimental pulmonary metastases in mice. *Transfusion.* 1990;30(2):188–190.
8. Shirwadkar S, Blajchman MA, Frame B, Singal DP. Effect of allogeneic blood transfusion on solid tumor growth and pulmonary metastases in mice. *J Cancer Res Clin Oncol.* 1992;118(3):176–180.
9. Mezrow CK, Bergstein I, Tartter PI. Postoperative infections following autologous and homologous blood transfusions. *Transfusion.* 1992;32(1):27–30.
10. Tartter PI. The association of perioperative blood transfusion with colorectal cancer recurrence. *Ann Surg.* 1992;216(6):633–638.
11. Tartter PI. Transfusion-induced immunosuppression and perioperative infections. *Beitr Infusionsther.* 1993;31:52–63.
12. Amato A, Pescatori M. Perioperative blood transfusions for the recurrence of colorectal cancer. *Cochrane Database Syst Rev.* 2006;(1):CD005033.
13. Carson JL, Altman DG, Duff A, et al. Risk of bacterial infection associated with allogeneic blood transfusion among patients undergoing hip fracture repair. *Transfusion.* 1999;39(7):694–700.
14. Vamvakas EC, Carven JH. Transfusion and postoperative pneumonia in coronary artery bypass graft surgery: effect of the length of storage of transfused red cells. *Transfusion.* 1999;39(7):701–710.
15. Youssef LA, Spitalnik SL. Transfusion-related immunomodulation: a reappraisal. *Curr Opin Hematol.* 2017;24(6):551–557.
16. Atzil S, Arad M, Glasner A, et al. Blood transfusion promotes cancer progression: a critical role for aged erythrocytes. *Anesthesiology.* 2008;109(6):989–997.
17. Vamvakas EC, Blajchman MA. Transfusion-related immunomodulation (TRIM): an update. *Blood Rev.* 2007;21(6):327–348.
18. Barnett Jr CC, Beck AW, Holloway SE, et al. Intravenous delivery of the plasma fraction of stored packed erythrocytes promotes pancreatic cancer growth in immunocompetent mice. *Cancer.* 2010;116(16):3862–3874.
19. Benson DD, Beck AW, Burdine MS, Brekken R, Silliman CC, Barnett Jr CC. Accumulation of pro-cancer cytokines in the plasma fraction of stored packed red cells. *J Gastrointest Surg.* 2012;16(3):460–468.

20. Moore PK, Benson D, Kehler M, et al. The plasma fraction of stored erythrocytes augments pancreatic cancer metastasis in male versus female mice. *J Surg Res.* 2010;164(1): 23−27.

21. Blumberg N, Fine L, Gettings KF, Heal JM. Decreased sepsis related to indwelling venous access devices coincident with implementation of universal leukoreduction of blood transfusions. *Transfusion.* 2005;45(10): 1632−1639.

22. Bassuni WY, Blajchman MA, Al-Moshary MA. Why implement universal leukoreduction? *Hematol Oncol Stem Cell Ther.* 2008;1(2):106−123.

23. Hebert PC, Fergusson D, Blajchman MA, et al. Clinical outcomes following institution of the Canadian universal leukoreduction program for red blood cell transfusions. *J Am Med Assoc.* 2003;289(15):1941−1949.

24. Hendrickson JE, Hod EA, Hudson KE, Spitalnik SL, Zimring JC. Transfusion of fresh murine red blood cells reverses adverse effects of older stored red blood cells. *Transfusion.* 2011;51(12):2695−2702.

25. Bilgin YM, Brand A. Transfusion-related immunomodulation: a second hit in an inflammatory cascade? *Vox Sang.* 2008;95(4):261−271.

26. Ghio M, Ottonello L, Contini P, et al. Transforming growth factor-beta1 in supernatants from stored red blood cells inhibits neutrophil locomotion. *Blood.* 2003;102(3):1100−1107.

27. Vlaar AP, Hofstra JJ, Levi M, et al. Supernatant of aged erythrocytes causes lung inflammation and coagulopathy in a "two-hit" in vivo syngeneic transfusion model. *Anesthesiology.* 2010;113(1):92−103.

28. Vamvakas EC. White-blood-cell-containing allogeneic blood transfusion and postoperative infection or mortality: an updated meta-analysis. *Vox Sang.* 2007;92(3): 224−232.

29. Ng MS, Ng AS, Chan J, Tung JP, Fraser JF. Effects of packed red blood cell storage duration on post-transfusion clinical outcomes: a meta-analysis and systematic review. *Intensive Care Med.* 2015;41(12): 2087−2097.

30. Ghio M, Contini P, Negrini S, Mazzei C, Zocchi MR, Poggi A. Down regulation of human natural killer cell-mediated cytolysis induced by blood transfusion: role of transforming growth factor-beta(1), soluble Fas ligand, and soluble Class I human leukocyte antigen. *Transfusion.* 2011;51(7):1567−1573.

31. Bal SH, Heper Y, Kumas LT, et al. Effect of storage period of red blood cell suspensions on helper T-cell subpopulations. *Blood Transfus.* 2018;16(3):262−272.

32. Baumgartner JM, Silliman CC, Moore EE, Banerjee A, McCarter MD. Stored red blood cell transfusion induces regulatory T cells. *J Am Coll Surg.* 2009;208(1):110−119.

33. Bilgin YM, van de Watering LM, Eijsman L, et al. Double-blind, randomized controlled trial on the effect of leukocyte-depleted erythrocyte transfusions in cardiac valve surgery. *Circulation.* 2004;109(22): 2755−2760.

34. Bilgin YM, van de Watering LM, Eijsman L, Versteegh MI, van Oers MH, Brand A. Is increased mortality associated with post-operative infections after leukocytes containing red blood cell transfusions in cardiac surgery? An extended analysis. *Transfus Med.* 2007;17(4):304−311.

35. Blumberg N, Zhao H, Wang H, Messing S, Heal JM, Lyman GH. The intention-to-treat principle in clinical trials and meta-analyses of leukoreduced blood transfusions in surgical patients. *Transfusion.* 2007;47(4): 573−581.

36. Fergusson D, Hebert PC, Lee SK, et al. Clinical outcomes following institution of universal leukoreduction of blood transfusions for premature infants. *J Am Med Assoc.* 2003;289(15):1950−1956.

37. Vamvakas EC. WBC-containing allogeneic blood transfusion and mortality: a meta-analysis of randomized controlled trials. *Transfusion.* 2003;43(7):963−973.

38. Vallion R, Bonnefoy F, Daoui A, et al. Transforming growth factor-beta released by apoptotic white blood cells during red blood cell storage promotes transfusion-induced alloimmunomodulation. *Transfusion.* 2015;55(7):1721−1735.

39. Sparrow RL, Patton KA. Supernatant from stored red blood cell primes inflammatory cells: influence of pre-storage white cell reduction. *Transfusion.* 2004;44(5): 722−730.

40. Shanwell A, Kristiansson M, Remberger M, Ringden O. Generation of cytokines in red cell concentrates during storage is prevented by prestorage white cell reduction. *Transfusion.* 1997;37(7):678−684.

41. Dzik S, Mincheff M, Puppo F. Apoptosis, transforming growth factor-beta, and the immunosuppressive effect of transfusion. *Transfusion.* 2002;42(9):1221−1223.

42. Long K, Woodward J, Procter L, et al. In vitro transfusion of red blood cells results in decreased cytokine production by human T cells. *J Trauma Acute Care Surg.* 2014; 77(2):198−201.

43. Long K, Meier C, Ward M, Williams D, Woodward J, Bernard A. Immunologic profiles of red blood cells using in vitro models of transfusion. *J Surg Res.* 2013;184(1): 567−571.

44. Ng MSY, David M, Middelburg RA, et al. Transfusion of packed red blood cells at the end of shelf life is associated with increased risk of mortality − a pooled patient data analysis of 16 observational trials. *Haematologica.* 2018; 103(9):1542−1548.

45. Frank SM, Abazyan B, Ono M, et al. Decreased erythrocyte deformability after transfusion and the effects of erythrocyte storage duration. *Anesth Analg.* 2013;116(5): 975−981.

46. Walsh TS, Stanworth S, Boyd J, et al. The Age of BLood Evaluation (ABLE) randomised controlled trial: description of the UK-funded arm of the international trial, the UK cost-utility analysis and secondary analyses exploring factors associated with health-related quality of life and health-care costs during the 12-month follow-up. *Health Technol Assess.* 2017;21(62):1−118.

47. Fergusson DA, Hebert P, Hogan DL, et al. Effect of fresh red blood cell transfusions on clinical outcomes in premature, very low-birth-weight infants: the ARIPI randomized trial. *J Am Med Assoc.* 2012;308(14):1443–1451.

48. Steiner ME, Ness PM, Assmann SF, et al. Effects of red-cell storage duration on patients undergoing cardiac surgery. *N Engl J Med.* 2015;372(15):1419–1429.

49. Lacroix J, Hebert PC, Fergusson DA, et al. Age of transfused blood in critically ill adults. *N Engl J Med.* 2015; 372(15):1410–1418.

50. Tucci M, Lacroix J, Fergusson D, et al. The age of blood in pediatric intensive care units (ABC PICU): study protocol for a randomized controlled trial. *Trials.* 2018;19(1):404.

51. Muszynski JA, Frazier E, Nofziger R, et al. Red blood cell transfusion and immune function in critically ill children: a prospective observational study. *Transfusion.* 2015;55(4):766–774.

52. Koch CG, Li L, Sessler DI, et al. Duration of red-cell storage and complications after cardiac surgery. *N Engl J Med.* 2008;358(12):1229–1239.

53. Manlhiot C, McCrindle BW, Menjak IB, et al. Longer blood storage is associated with suboptimal outcomes in high-risk pediatric cardiac surgery. *Ann Thorac Surg.* 2012;93(5):1563–1569.

54. Ranucci M, Carlucci C, Isgro G, et al. Duration of red blood cell storage and outcomes in pediatric cardiac surgery: an association found for pump prime blood. *Crit Care.* 2009;13(6):R207.

55. Biedler AE, Schneider SO, Seyfert U, et al. Impact of alloantigens and storage-associated factors on stimulated cytokine response in an in vitro model of blood transfusion. *Anesthesiology.* 2002;97(5):1102–1109.

56. Karam O, Tucci M, Toledano BJ, et al. Length of storage and in vitro immunomodulation induced by prestorage leukoreduced red blood cells. *Transfusion.* 2009;49(11): 2326–2334.

57. Mynster T. Effects of red cell storage and lysis on in vitro cytokine release. *Transfus Apher Sci.* 2001;25(1):17–23.

58. Muszynski J, Nateri J, Nicol K, Greathouse K, Hanson L, Hall M. Immunosuppressive effects of red blood cells on monocytes are related to both storage time and storage solution. *Transfusion.* 2012;52(4):794–802.

59. Offner PJ, Moore EE, Biffl WL, Johnson JL, Silliman CC. Increased rate of infection associated with transfusion of old blood after severe injury. *Arch Surg.* 2002;137(6): 711–716. discussion 716-717.

60. Weinberg JA, McGwin Jr G, Vandromme MJ, et al. Duration of red cell storage influences mortality after trauma. *J Trauma.* 2010;69(6):1427–1431. discussion 1431-1422.

61. Fontaine MJ, Shih H, Schubert R, et al. Leukocyte and plasma activation profiles in chronically transfused patients with a history of allergic reactions. *Transfusion.* 2017;57(11):2639–2648.

62. Ottonello L, Ghio M, Contini P, et al. Nonleukoreduced red blood cell transfusion induces a sustained inhibition of neutrophil chemotaxis by stimulating in vivo production of transforming growth factor-beta1 by neutrophils:

role of the immunoglobulinlike transcript 1, sFasL, and sHLA-I. *Transfusion.* 2007;47(8):1395–1404.

63. Widing L, Bechensteen AG, Mirlashari MR, Vetlesen A, Kjeldsen-Kragh J. Evaluation of nonleukoreduced red blood cell transfusion units collected at delivery from the placenta. *Transfusion.* 2007;47(8):1481–1487.

64. Ghio M, Contini P, Negrini S, et al. sHLA-I contaminating molecules as novel mechanism of ex vivo/in vitro transcriptional and posttranscriptional modulation of transforming growth factor-beta in CD8+ T lymphocytes and neutrophils after intravenous immunoglobulin treatment. *Transfusion.* 2010;50(3):547–555.

65. Ghio M, Contini P, Ubezio G, Mazzei C, Puppo F, Indiveri F. Immunomodulatory effects of blood transfusions: the synergic role of soluble HLA Class I free heavy-chain molecules detectable in blood components. *Transfusion.* 2008;48(8):1591–1597.

66. Miyaji K, Miyamoto T, Kohira S, et al. The influences of red blood cell transfusion on perioperative inflammatory responses using a miniaturized biocompatible bypass with an asanguineous prime. *Int Heart J.* 2009;50(5): 581–589.

67. Miyaji K, Miyamoto T, Kohira S, et al. The effectiveness of prestorage leukocyte-reduced red blood cell transfusion on perioperative inflammatory response with a miniaturized biocompatible bypass system. *J Thorac Cardiovasc Surg.* 2010;139(6):1561–1567.

68. Lannan KL, Sahler J, Spinelli SL, Phipps RP, Blumberg N. Transfusion immunomodulation–the case for leukoreduced and (perhaps) washed transfusions. *Blood Cells Mol Dis.* 2013;50(1):61–68.

69. van de Watering LM, Hermans J, Houbiers JG, et al. Beneficial effects of leukocyte depletion of transfused blood on postoperative complications in patients undergoing cardiac surgery: a randomized clinical trial. *Circulation.* 1998;97(6):562–568.

70. van de Watering LM, Brand A, Houbiers JG, et al. Perioperative blood transfusions, with or without allogeneic leucocytes, relate to survival, not to cancer recurrence. *Br J Surg.* 2001;88(2):267–272.

71. Hashimoto MN, Kimura EY, Yamamoto M, Bordin JO. Expression of Fas and Fas ligand on spleen T cells of experimental animals after unmodified or leukoreduced allogeneic blood transfusions. *Transfusion.* 2004;44(2): 158–163.

72. Blajchman MA, Bardossy L, Carmen R, Sastry A, Singal DP. Allogeneic blood transfusion-induced enhancement of tumor growth: two animal models showing amelioration by leukodepletion and passive transfer using spleen cells. *Blood.* 1993;81(7):1880–1882.

73. Rohde JM, Dimcheff DE, Blumberg N, et al. Health care-associated infection after red blood cell transfusion: a systematic review and meta-analysis. *J Am Med Assoc.* 2014; 311(13):1317–1326.

74. Sut C, Tariket S, Chou ML, et al. Duration of red blood cell storage and inflammatory marker generation. *Blood Transfus.* 2017;15(2):145–152.

75. Shapiro MJ. To filter blood or universal leukoreduction: what is the answer? *Crit Care.* 2004;8(Suppl 2):S27—S30.

76. Blajchman MA. The clinical benefits of the leukoreduction of blood products. *J Trauma.* 2006;60(6 Suppl): S83—S90.

77. Desmarets M, Cadwell CM, Peterson KR, Neades R, Zimring JC. Minor histocompatibility antigens on transfused leukoreduced units of red blood cells induce bone marrow transplant rejection in a mouse model. *Blood.* 2009;114(11):2315—2322.

78. Patel SR, Zimring JC. Transfusion-induced bone marrow transplant rejection due to minor histocompatibility antigens. *Transfus Med Rev.* 2013;27(4):241—248.

79. Reed W, Lee TH, Norris PJ, Utter GH, Busch MP. Transfusion-associated microchimerism: a new complication of blood transfusions in severely injured patients. *Semin Hematol.* 2007;44(1):24—31.

80. Lee TH, Paglieroni T, Ohto H, Holland PV, Busch MP. Survival of donor leukocyte subpopulations in immunocompetent transfusion recipients: frequent long-term microchimerism in severe trauma patients. *Blood.* 1999; 93(9):3127—3139.

81. Gafter U, Kalechman Y, Sredni B. Blood transfusion enhances production of T-helper-2 cytokines and transforming growth factor beta in humans. *Clin Sci (Lond).* 1996;91(4):519—523.

82. Leal-Noval SR, Munoz-Gomez M, Arellano V, et al. Influence of red blood cell transfusion on CD_4^+ T-helper cells immune response in patients undergoing cardiac surgery. *J Surg Res.* 2010;164(1):43—49.

83. Fragkou PC, Torrance HD, Pearse RM, et al. Perioperative blood transfusion is associated with a gene transcription profile characteristic of immunosuppression: a prospective cohort study. *Crit Care.* 2014;18(5):541.

84. Torrance HD, Brohi K, Pearse RM, et al. Association between gene expression biomarkers of immunosuppression and blood transfusion in severely injured polytrauma patients. *Ann Surg.* 2015;261(4): 751—759.

85. Saas P, Angelot F, Bardiaux L, Seilles E, Garnache-Ottou F, Perruche S. Phosphatidylserine-expressing cell by-products in transfusion: a pro-inflammatory or an anti-inflammatory effect? *Transfus Clin Biol.* 2012;19(3): 90—97.

86. Doffek K, Chen X, Sugg SL, Shilyansky J. Phosphatidylserine inhibits NFkappaB and p38 MAPK activation in human monocyte derived dendritic cells. *Mol Immunol.* 2011;48(15—16):1771—1777.

87. Frabetti F, Musiani D, Marini M, et al. White cell apoptosis in packed red cells. *Transfusion.* 1998; 38(11—12):1082—1089.

88. Frabetti F, Tazzari PL, Musiani D, et al. White cell apoptosis in platelet concentrates. *Transfusion.* 2000; 40(2):160—168.

89. Nielsen HJ, Reimert CM, Pedersen AN, et al. Time-dependent, spontaneous release of white cell- and platelet-derived bioactive substances from stored human blood. *Transfusion.* 1996;36(11—12):960—965.

90. Nielsen HJ, Skov F, Dybkjaer E, et al. Leucocyte and platelet-derived bioactive substances in stored blood: effect of prestorage leucocyte filtration. *Eur J Haematol.* 1997;58(4):273—278.

91. Bury TB, Corhay JL, Radermecker MF. Histamine-induced inhibition of neutrophil chemotaxis and T-lymphocyte proliferation in man. *Allergy.* 1992;47(6):624—629.

92. Peterson CG, Skoog V, Venge P. Human eosinophil cationic proteins (ECP and EPX) and their suppressive effects on lymphocyte proliferation. *Immunobiology.* 1986; 171(1—2):1—13.

93. Fredens K, Dybdahl H, Dahl R, Baandrup U. Extracellular deposit of the cationic proteins ECP and EPX in tissue infiltrations of eosinophils related to tissue damage. *APMIS.* 1988;96(8):711—719.

94. Cholette JM, Henrichs KF, Alfieris GM, et al. Washing red blood cells and platelets transfused in cardiac surgery reduces postoperative inflammation and number of transfusions: results of a prospective, randomized, controlled clinical trial. *Pediatr Crit Care Med.* 2012;13(3):290—299.

95. Ghio M, Contini P, Mazzei C, et al. In vitro immunosuppressive activity of soluble HLA class I and Fas ligand molecules: do they play a role in autologous blood transfusion? *Transfusion.* 2001;41(8):988—996.

96. Keir AK, McPhee AJ, Andersen CC, Stark MJ. Plasma cytokines and markers of endothelial activation increase after packed red cell transfusion in the preterm infant. *Pediatr Res.* 2013;73(1):75—79.

97. Dani C, Poggi C, Gozzini E, et al. Red blood cell transfusions can induce proinflammatory cytokines in preterm infants. *Transfusion.* 2017;57(5):1304—1310.

98. Solomon SB, Wang D, Sun J, et al. Mortality increases after massive exchange transfusion with older stored blood in canines with experimental pneumonia. *Blood.* 2013; 121(9):1663—1672.

99. Wang D, Cortes-Puch I, Sun J, et al. Transfusion of older stored blood worsens outcomes in canines depending on the presence and severity of pneumonia. *Transfusion.* 2014;54(7):1712—1724.

100. Cortes-Puch I, Wang D, Sun J, et al. Washing older blood units before transfusion reduces plasma iron and improves outcomes in experimental canine pneumonia. *Blood.* 2014;123(9):1403—1411.

101. Qu L, Triulzi DJ. Clinical effects of red blood cell storage. *Cancer Control.* 2015;22(1):26—37.

102. Alshalani A, Acker JP. Red blood cell membrane water permeability increases with length of ex vivo storage. *Cryobiology.* 2017;76:51—58.

103. D'Alessandro A, Gray AD, Szczepiorkowski ZM, Hansen K, Herschel LH, Dumont LJ. Red blood cell metabolic responses to refrigerated storage, rejuvenation, and frozen storage. *Transfusion.* 2017;57(4):1019—1030.

104. Gehrke S, Srinivasan AJ, Culp-Hill R, et al. Metabolomics evaluation of early-storage red blood cell rejuvenation at 4 degrees C and 37 degrees C. *Transfusion.* 2018;58(8): 1980—1991.

105. Lelubre C, Vincent JL. Relationship between red cell storage duration and outcomes in adults receiving red cell

transfusions: a systematic review. *Crit Care.* 2013;17(2): R66.

106. Vamvakas EC. Purported deleterious effects of "old" versus "fresh" red blood cells: an updated meta-analysis. *Transfusion.* 2011;51(5):1122–1123.

107. Wang D, Sun J, Solomon SB, Klein HG, Natanson C. Transfusion of older stored blood and risk of death: a meta-analysis. *Transfusion.* 2012;52(6):1184–1195.

108. Spitalnik SL. Stored red blood cell transfusions: iron, inflammation, immunity, and infection. *Transfusion.* 2014;54(10):2365–2371.

109. Hod EA, Zhang N, Sokol SA, et al. Transfusion of red blood cells after prolonged storage produces harmful effects that are mediated by iron and inflammation. *Blood.* 2010;115(21):4284–4292.

110. Ganz T, Nemeth E. Iron homeostasis in host defence and inflammation. *Nat Rev Immunol.* 2015;15(8): 500–510.

111. Maccio A, Madeddu C, Gramignano G, et al. The role of inflammation, iron, and nutritional status in cancer-related anemia: results of a large, prospective, observational study. *Haematologica.* 2015;100(1):124–132.

112. Porto BN, Alves LS, Fernandez PL, et al. Heme induces neutrophil migration and reactive oxygen species generation through signaling pathways characteristic of chemotactic receptors. *J Biol Chem.* 2007;282(33): 24430–24436.

113. Berra L, Coppadoro A, Yu B, et al. Transfusion of stored autologous blood does not alter reactive hyperemia index in healthy volunteers. *Anesthesiology.* 2012;117(1): 56–63.

114. Stark MJ, Keir AK, Andersen CC. Does non-transferrin bound iron contribute to transfusion related immune-modulation in preterms? *Arch Dis Child Fetal Neonatal Ed.* 2013;98(5):F424–F429.

115. Kalhan TG, Bateman DA, Bowker RM, Hod EA, Kashyap S. Effect of red blood cell storage time on markers of hemolysis and inflammation in transfused very low birth weight infants. *Pediatr Res.* 2017;82(6): 964–969.

116. Spinella PC, Sparrow RL, Hess JR, Norris PJ. Properties of stored red blood cells: understanding immune and vascular reactivity. *Transfusion.* 2011;51(4):894–900.

117. Theurl I, Fritsche G, Ludwiczek S, Garimorth K, Bellmann-Weiler R, Weiss G. The macrophage: a cellular factory at the interphase between iron and immunity for the control of infections. *Biometals.* 2005;18(4): 359–367.

118. Fritsche G, Nairz M, Theurl I, et al. Modulation of macrophage iron transport by Nramp1 (Slc11a1). *Immunobiology.* 2007;212(9–10):751–757.

119. Donadee C, Raat NJ, Kanias T, et al. Nitric oxide scavenging by red blood cell microparticles and cell-free hemoglobin as a mechanism for the red cell storage lesion. *Circulation.* 2011;124(4):465–476.

120. Liu C, Liu X, Janes J, et al. Mechanism of faster NO scavenging by older stored red blood cells. *Redox Biol.* 2014;2: 211–219.

121. Stapley R, Owusu BY, Brandon A, et al. Erythrocyte storage increases rates of NO and nitrite scavenging: implications for transfusion-related toxicity. *Biochem J.* 2012; 446(3):499–508.

122. Rifkind JM, Mohanty JG, Nagababu E, Salgado MT, Cao Z. Potential modulation of vascular function by nitric oxide and reactive oxygen species released from erythrocytes. *Front Physiol.* 2018;9:690.

123. Tinmouth A, Fergusson D, Yee IC, Hebert PC, Investigators A, Canadian Critical Care Trials G. Clinical consequences of red cell storage in the critically ill. *Transfusion.* 2006;46(11):2014–2027.

124. Zecher D, Cumpelik A, Schifferli JA. Erythrocyte-derived microvesicles amplify systemic inflammation by thrombin-dependent activation of complement. *Arterioscler Thromb Vasc Biol.* 2014;34(2):313–320.

125. Patel MB, Proctor KG, Majetschak M. Extracellular ubiquitin increases in packed red blood cell units during storage. *J Surg Res.* 2006;135(2):226–232.

126. Zhu X, Yu B, You P, et al. Ubiquitin released in the plasma of whole blood during storage promotes mRNA expression of Th2 cytokines and Th2-inducing transcription factors. *Transfus Apher Sci.* 2012;47(3):305–311.

127. Majetschak M, Krehmeier U, Bardenheuer M, et al. Extracellular ubiquitin inhibits the TNF-alpha response to endotoxin in peripheral blood mononuclear cells and regulates endotoxin hyporesponsiveness in critical illness. *Blood.* 2003;101(5):1882–1890.

128. Vlaar AP, Kulik W, Nieuwland R, et al. Accumulation of bioactive lipids during storage of blood products is not cell but plasma derived and temperature dependent. *Transfusion.* 2011;51(11):2358–2366.

129. Maslanka K, Smolenska-Sym G, Michur H, Wrobel A, Lachert E, Brojer E. Lysophosphatidylcholines: bioactive lipids generated during storage of blood components. *Arch Immunol Ther Exp.* 2012;60(1):55–60.

130. Vlaar AP, Hofstra JJ, Kulik W, et al. Supernatant of stored platelets causes lung inflammation and coagulopathy in a novel in vivo transfusion model. *Blood.* 2010;116(8): 1360–1368.

131. Sadallah S, Eken C, Schifferli JA. Erythrocyte-derived ectosomes have immunosuppressive properties. *J Leukoc Biol.* 2008;84(5):1316–1325.

132. Eken C, Sadallah S, Martin PJ, Treves S, Schifferli JA. Ectosomes of polymorphonuclear neutrophils activate multiple signaling pathways in macrophages. *Immunobiology.* 2013;218(3):382–392.

133. Sadallah S, Eken C, Martin PJ, Schifferli JA. Microparticles (ectosomes) shed by stored human platelets downregulate macrophages and modify the development of dendritic cells. *J Immunol.* 2011;186(11):6543–6552.

134. Sadallah S, Schmied L, Eken C, Charoudeh HN, Amicarella F, Schifferli JA. Platelet-derived ectosomes reduce NK cell function. *J Immunol.* 2016;197(5): 1663–1671.

135. Cocucci E, Racchetti G, Meldolesi J. Shedding microvesicles: artefacts no more. *Trends Cell Biol.* 2009;19(2): 43–51.

136. Danesh A, Inglis HC, Abdel-Mohsen M, et al. Granulocyte-derived extracellular vesicles activate monocytes and are associated with mortality in intensive care unit patients. *Front Immunol.* 2018;9:956.

137. Heijnen HF, Schiel AE, Fijnheer R, Geuze HJ, Sixma JJ. Activated platelets release two types of membrane vesicles: microvesicles by surface shedding and exosomes derived from exocytosis of multivesicular bodies and alpha-granules. *Blood.* 1999;94(11):3791–3799.

138. Gasser O, Schifferli JA. Activated polymorphonuclear neutrophils disseminate anti-inflammatory microparticles by ectocytosis. *Blood.* 2004;104(8):2543–2548.

139. Danesh A, Inglis HC, Jackman RP, et al. Exosomes from red blood cell units bind to monocytes and induce proinflammatory cytokines, boosting T-cell responses in vitro. *Blood.* 2014;123(5):687–696.

140. Pilzer D, Gasser O, Moskovich O, Schifferli JA, Fishelson Z. Emission of membrane vesicles: roles in complement resistance, immunity and cancer. *Springer Semin Immunopathol.* 2005;27(3):375–387.

141. Chin-Yee IH, Gray-Statchuk L, Milkovich S, Ellis CG. Transfusion of stored red blood cells adhere in the rat microvasculature. *Transfusion.* 2009;49(11):2304–2310.

142. Anniss AM, Sparrow RL. Storage duration and white blood cell content of red blood cell (RBC) products increases adhesion of stored RBCs to endothelium under flow conditions. *Transfusion.* 2006;46(9):1561–1567.

143. Luk CS, Gray-Statchuk LA, Cepinkas G, Chin-Yee IH. WBC reduction reduces storage-associated RBC adhesion to human vascular endothelial cells under conditions of continuous flow in vitro. *Transfusion.* 2003;43(2):151–156.

144. Koshkaryev A, Zelig O, Manny N, Yedgar S, Barshtein G. Rejuvenation treatment of stored red blood cells reverses storage-induced adhesion to vascular endothelial cells. *Transfusion.* 2009;49(10):2136–2143.

145. Kaul DK, Finnegan E, Barabino GA. Sickle red cell-endothelium interactions. *Microcirculation.* 2009;16(1):97–111.

146. Keating FK, Butenas S, Fung MK, Schneider DJ. Platelet-white blood cell (WBC) interaction, WBC apoptosis, and procoagulant activity in stored red blood cells. *Transfusion.* 2011;51(5):1086–1095.

147. Keating FK, Fung MK, Schneider DJ. Induction of platelet white blood cell (WBC) aggregate formation by platelets and WBCs in red blood cell units. *Transfusion.* 2008;48(6):1099–1105.

148. Jenne CN, Urrutia R, Kubes P. Platelets: bridging hemostasis, inflammation, and immunity. *Int J Lab Hematol.* 2013;35(3):254–261.

149. Jenne CN, Kubes P. Platelets in inflammation and infection. *Platelets.* 2015;26(4):286–292.

150. Nguyen XD, Muller-Berghaus J, Kalsch T, Schadendorf D, Borggrefe M, Kluter H. Differentiation of monocyte-derived dendritic cells under the influence of platelets. *Cytotherapy.* 2008;10(7):720–729.

CHAPTER 7

Transfusion-Related Acute Lung Injury

IAN M. HARROLD, MD • MELISSA R. GEORGE, DO, FCAP, FASCP

HISTORY

By the 1950s, transfusions were known to be a cause of acute lung injury. Brittingham demonstrated that transfusing plasma from a patient with a known leukoagglutinin to a previously healthy volunteer caused immediate faintness, fever, hypotension, tachypnea, dyspnea, and persistent cyanosis. Leukoagglutinin was the phrase used at the time to describe substances in donor sera that caused white cells to agglutinate; these were later understood to be antibodies.[1] Additionally, the volunteer developed marked bilateral pulmonary edema and small pleural effusions. From then until the 1980s, very little was published or defined about how severe this reaction could be or what was causing the edema. Through the 1970s, multiple case studies were published describing some instances of lung injury with symptoms described as hypersensitivity reactions,[2] allergic pulmonary edema,[3] leukoagglutinin transfusion reactions,[4] and noncardiogenic pulmonary edema.[5] Most of these early studies refer to a leukoagglutinin reaction similar to the one Brittingham described in 1957. These authors were starting to circle around the idea that this reaction was clinically significant and had an immunologic basis. The consistent finding in these early cases was the leukoagglutinins, pulmonary overload due to a noncardiogenic cause and bilateral widespread patchy opacities in the lungs.

By 1985, only 31 cases had been reported and the lack of any unifying terminology kept this reaction from becoming a major concern within the transfusion community.[6] This changed when Popovsky and Moore reported a case series of 36 patients with acute respiratory distress, hypoxemia, and fulminant pulmonary edema.[7] This was a follow-up from a previous study of five patients that they had reported who had developed lung injury after transfusion.[8] All of the patients in both studies developed severe lung injury and pulmonary edema within 4 hours of transfusion, and all required respiratory support. Most patients in their study (81%) had rapid recovery within 48 hours, but

fatalities were also noted (5%). Granulocyte and lymphocytotoxic antibodies were found in 89% of the cases. Popovsky and Moore were the first authors to use the phrase transfusion-related acute lung injury and coined the acronym TRALI for this entity.[7]

Through the 1990s, TRALI was greatly underdiagnosed due to the fact that many clinicians did not understand this entity. The underlying immunologic basis for TRALI was still being defined at this time.[6,9] Brittingham believed even back in 1957 that a leukoagglutinin in the donor unit was responsible for the reaction that he was seeing. It was later determined that these leukoagglutinins were most frequently directed against human leukocyte antigens (HLA)[10–13] and human neutrophil antigens (HNA).[14] Although not every case of TRALI has identifiable antibodies (reports ranging from 61% to 89%),[7,10] this does appear to be the prevailing mechanism in most cases.

DEFINITION

The national healthcare safety network hemovigilance module surveillance protocol from the Center for Disease Control (CDC) and the National Heart, Lung, and Blood Institute (NHLBI) Working Group on TRALI define it as acute lung injury (ALI) occurring within 6 h of cessation of transfusion in the presence of hypoxemia. Hypoxemia is defined by any of the following methods: the ratio of arterial oxygen partial pressure to fractional inspired oxygen (PaO_2/FiO_2) less than or equal to 300 mm Hg, oxygen saturation less than 90% on room air, or other clinical evidence. Additionally, radiographic evidence of bilateral infiltrates needs to be identified with no previous evidence of ALI before the transfusion and no evidence for left atrial hypertension leading to circulatory overload[15–18] (Table 7.1). Using this definition, cases of ALI that are worsened after a transfusion are not included. Although these cases perhaps should be considered in the same category as TRALI, differentiating them can be very difficult.[16]

Immunologic Concepts in Transfusion Medicine. https://doi.org/10.1016/B978-0-323-67509-3.00007-X

TABLE 7.1
Criteria for the Diagnosing of TRALI.

Criteria for TRALI

- ALI developing within 6 hours of cessation of transfusion
- Radiographic evidence of new bilateral infiltrates
- Hypoxemia defined by ≥1 of the following:
  - PaO_2/FiO_2 ≤300 mg Hg
  - O_2 saturation <90% on room air
  - Other clinical evidence of hypoxemia
- No previous evidence of ALI

ALI, acute lung injury; *FiO2*, fractional inspired oxygen; *PaO2*, arterial oxygen partial pressure.
Adapted from the Center for Disease Control and Prevention. National healthcare safety network biovigilance component hemovigilance module durveillance protocol. https://www.cdc.gov/nhsn/pdfs/biovigilance/bv-hv-protocol-current.pdf; Toy P, Popovsky MA, Abraham E, et al. Transfusion-related acute lung injury: definition and review. Crit Care Med 2005;33(4):721−726[15,16].

Despite the plethora of evidence that TRALI is strongly related to antibodies from donor units,[1−5,7,10−14] finding HLA, HNA, or other donor-derived antibodies is not required to define TRALI by accepted CDC and other consensus guidelines.

PRESENTATION

The initial presentation of TRALI is indistinguishable from ALI with the one major difference being that TRALI is typically transient. Patients usually present with *hypotension*, cyanosis, fever, tachycardia, and hypoxemia. The pulmonary edema starts in the dependent parts of the lung and then develops into whiteout patterns of interstitial and alveolar infiltrates as seen by X-ray.[6] Occasionally, cases of TRALI can present with hypertension, but these cases are in the minority.[7] Patients with TRALI most often recover on their own with just supportive care and respiratory support after 48−72 hours as Popovsky and Moore first described in 1985,[7] though morality rates of 45% and 43% have also been seen in recent reports.[19,20] The differences in mortality rates likely has to do with the underlying disease states of the patients included in those studies. Specifically, studies with higher mortality rates focused on patients in the intensive-care units (ICUs) and those with cardiac disease. It is possible that those hospitals had cases of TRALI in lower acuity patients that were not identified and these cases would have increased the denominator when calculating the mortality rate. Additionally, Li et al. showed that TRALI is associated with lower long-term survival especially when compared with the other major pulmonary transfusion reaction, transfusion-associated circulatory overload (TACO).[20]

RISK FACTORS

Recipient

TRALI presents evenly between males and females with no ethnic or age predispositions.[6,10] Studies by Silliman et al. demonstrated through a nested case-control study of 46 patients with TRALI compared to 225 controls that there was a higher predilection for TRALI in patients with underlying hematologic malignancies ($P < .0004$) and those with cardiac disease ($P < .0006$).[21] Toy et al. outlined other specific patient-centric risk factors to include shock, liver surgery (especially transplantation), chronic alcohol abuse, positive fluid balance, peak airway pressure greater than 30 cm H_2O if mechanically ventilated before transfusion, smoking and increased plasma interleukin (IL)-8 levels if measured before transfusion.[22]

BLOOD FRACTION

Perhaps more important than the recipients' underlying physiological status is the blood fraction itself. TRALI has been seen to occur much more commonly with plasma-rich units such as fresh frozen plasma (FFP) and platelets,[13,19,23] but it has been associated with all types of blood components including red blood cells (RBCs),[24] granulocytes,[25] intravenous immune globulin (IVIG),[26] stem cell infusions,[27] and cryoprecipitate.[21] Additionally, a study from 2007 showed that plasma from female donors had a higher likelihood of causing TRALI in their patients (odds ratio of 5.09 for female plasma vs. 1.60 for male plasma).[28] This finding of female plasma being more commonly implicated would become one of the most important concepts to help with TRALI mitigation in recent years. These findings helped to confirm that the immunologic status of the donor units is a vitally important topic in understanding the pathophysiology and cause of TRALI. Even with the strong correlations to preexisting illnesses, TRALI can still occur after transfusions in patients who were perfectly healthy beforehand.[1,29] It appears that both the underlying patient characteristics as well as the type of blood component and demographics of the donor make a difference in TRALI incidence.

An additional risk factor for the development of TRALI is the use of directed donations from a mother to a child. If a mother is sensitized to paternally derived HLA antigens during a previous pregnancy, she may develop HLA antibodies against those antigens. A directed donation from mother to child would then have a higher risk of leading to TRALI. This risk would also be present if that same mother gave a directed donation to the father of her child after sensitization. The foreign antigens that she was potentially exposed to would have been the antigens present in the father.[30] For these, and many other reasons, directed donations should be avoided in routine transfusion services.

Incidence

Identifying the exact incidence of TRALI can be difficult. The blood bank is dependent on the clinical team's recognition and reporting of a transfusion reaction. A study from 2016 showed that in a lookback of 5,000 transfusion episodes, among the 43 cases that were determined to be likely TRALI or TACO, only 27 (63%) were documented in the clinical notes and only 3 (7%) were actually reported to the transfusion service.[31] Another study showed that only around 14% of suspected TRALI cases were reported to the transfusion service.[32] Kopko et al. conducted a clinical lookback study of 50 patients who all received blood components from a donor who was linked to a fatal transfusion reaction. Seven of the patients in the study had moderate reactions recorded in the chart and eight had severe reactions reported. Of all of those cases, 5/7 of the moderate and only 2/8 of the severe were reported to the transfusion service. To protect against TRALI, cases need to be reported back to the regional blood supplier, but in only 2 of the 15 cases did that occur.[33]

With these studies in mind, the current reported incidence ranges from 1 in 1,300 transfusions to 1 in 7,900 transfusions. The most common reported number is typically around 1 in 5,000 transfusions,[7,19] although a recent study out of the University of Texas reports a rate of 1 reaction in every 47,000 blood components or 1 in 20,000 plasma units after a retrospective lookback over 10 years at a large urban tertiary care center.[34] An additional reason for the diversity of reported numbers was discussed by Kleinman et al. They theorized that the wide variation in how TRALI is defined and measured leads to vast differences in how often TRALI is reported.[18] Some studies require the presence of HLA antibodies while others focus more solely on the clinical history. As previously mentioned, TRALI also seems to present in different frequencies depending on what, if any, underlying conditions a patient may have.[35] In a study of patients in the ICU, TRALI was found to develop at a rate of up to 8% and was seen more commonly in patients who had a history of alcohol abuse and a current diagnosis of sepsis.[28] Similarly patients who presented for cardiac surgery were found to develop TRALI at a rate of 2.4%.[36]

Fatalities

From 2001 to 2015, TRALI was the leading cause of mortality among transfusion-related reactions according to the US Food and Drug Administration (FDA). In 2016 (the most recent reported year from the FDA at the time of this writing), TRALI dropped to number two leading cause behind TACO.[37,38] The number of TRALI fatalities drastically dropped from 2007 to 2008 after the use of primarily male-only plasma was implemented in the United States of America (USA). The incidence has been steadily dropping since that time as well.[38] This drop is mirrored in the United Kingdom (UK) through their serious hazards of transfusion (SHOT) hemovigilance scheme with TACO accounting for 44.1% of the transfusion-related deaths and TRALI only accounting for 3.7% of the deaths from transfusion.[39] Similarly, hemolytic transfusion reactions and allergic/febrile reactions also accounted for a larger number of the reported deaths from transfusions in the UK than did TRALI. A report by the International Haemovigilance Network Database stated that from 2006 to 2012, 132.8 million blood components were issued with an adverse reaction reported at a rate of 77.5 per 100,000 components. Three hundred forty-nine deaths were reported with 58% of them due to pulmonary complications. TACO had the highest rate at 27% with TRALI at 19% and transfusion-associated dyspnea (TAD) at 12%.[40]

Although the rate of fatal reactions to TRALI have been decreasing, it may appear that the number of diagnoses are increasing. Countless papers and reports have been published over the past 20 years while only 31 cases were reported from 1957 to 1985. This likely has nothing to do with an increase in the actual incidence but more to do with a better understanding of the pathophysiology of this reaction and how to recognize it.

PATHOPHYSIOLOGY

The pathophysiology of TRALI remains somewhat controversial. Similar to many illnesses, one proposed model for TRALI is a two hit hypothesis (Fig. 7.1). The first hit usually involves the patient's underlying condition. Particular risk factors for this first hit include hematologic malignancy,[21] higher IL-8 levels, recent surgery (particularly liver transplant), chronic alcohol abuse, shock, mechanical ventilation, and positive fluid balance.[22]

The second hit, which is generally attributed to the transfused blood component, activates the neutrophils within the pulmonary vasculature, which in turn causes endothelial damage. HLA/HNA antibodies are believed to be one of the most common factors involved in the second hit of the theory.

MULTICAUSAL MODEL

Greater interest has developed in recent years into multicausal theories of TRALI, so as to not exclude other factors that may warrant further research. Such models include the threshold and the sufficient cause models.[41]

THE THRESHOLD MODEL

Threshold models must define a final common pathway of disease. The model starts with a single system with modifiable activity level, beyond which disease develops. The TRALI threshold model is no exception, and is based on the two hit hypothesis. It postulates that a certain threshold must be overcome to induce TRALI. In mild TRALI, the threshold in which oxygen supply is sufficient is overcome, and is lower than that

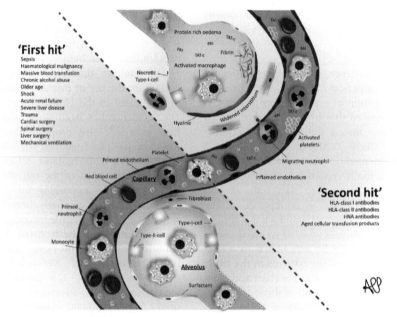

FIG. 7.1 **Two-hit model of TRALI.** A "first hit," an underlying clinical condition of the patient, results in priming of neutrophils and their attraction to the lung capillary by release of cytokines and chemokines by lining endothelium as evidenced in histological sections of patients who succumbed to TRALI. L-selectin loosely binds the neutrophils after which E-selectin, platelet-derived P-selectin, and intracellular adhesion molecules (ICAM1) facilitate firm adhesion. The "second hit," the transfusion of a blood component, causes activation of neutrophils and coagulation pathways resulting in TRALI. Neutrophil activation results in margination of neutrophils through the interstitium into the alveoli, which are filled with protein-rich edema. Here, cytokines, interleukin-1β, -6, -8 (IL-1β, IL-6, IL-8), that further stimulate neutrophil chemotaxis and neutrophil formation of elastase-α1-antitrypsin (EA) complex are secreted. Increase in thrombin-anti-thrombin complexes (TATc) and reduction of plasminogen activator activity indicate activation of coagulation. The "second hit," the transfused component, may contain accumulated solubles, aged cells, human leukocyte antigen (HLA)-antibodies, or human neutrophil antigen (HNA)-antibodies. PAI: plasminogen activator inhibitor. (Used with permission from John Wiley & Sons, Inc. Wiley Publishing: Peters AL, Van Stein D, Vlaar APJ. Antibody mediated transfusion-related acute lung injury; from discovery to prevention. Br *J Hameatol* 2015; 170: 597–614.[41] Bux J, Sachs, UJ. The pathogenesis of transfusion-related acute lung injury (TRALI). Br J Haematol 2007;136:788–799[42].)

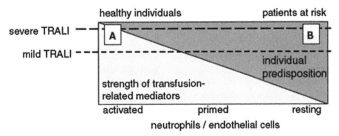

FIG. 7.2 The Bux and Sachs threshold model. A threshold for TRALI is established by the degree of neutrophil priming, and ability of substances in the transfused blood component to further activate primed pulmonary neutrophils. (Used with permission from John Wiley & Sons, Inc. Wiley Publishing: Bux J, Sachs, UJ. The pathogenesis of transfusion-related acute lung injury (TRALI). *Br J Haematol* 2007;136:788−799[42]; Peters AL, Van Stein D, Vlaar APJ. Antibody-mediated transfusion-related acute lung injury; from discovery to prevention. *Br J Haematol* 2015;170:597−614.[41])

seen in severe TRALI where mechanical ventilation is required. To overcome these thresholds, a number of factors act together. This model was summarized by Bux and Sachs in Fig. 7.2, showing the balanced relationship between the strength of transfusion-related mediators and patient predisposition. The model demonstrates graphically how a transfusion must have more influence on the activation of pulmonary neutrophils and endothelium if patient predisposition is weaker and shows how high patient predisposition may require less activating factors from transfusion.[42]

SUFFICIENT CAUSE MODEL

In the sufficient cause model, individual contributing factors called component causes add up in any possible combination sufficient to cause disease. This model described in early epidemiological literature can often be presented as a pie chart with component pieces adding up to complete the pie.[43] Regardless of the model, the underlying pathophysiological principles outlined below apply.

SPECIFIC EVIDENCE OF ANTIBODY-RELATED CAUSE

The link between leukocyte antibodies and TRALI was first posited by Brittingham, who demonstrated that antibodies (called leukoagglutinins at the time) caused an acute pulmonary reaction when transfused to a healthy volunteer.[1] These findings were reproducible in healthy volunteers receiving a gamma globulin concentrate rich in antileukocyte antibodies, especially antimonocyte antibodies, later suggesting a role for HLA class II antibodies.[44] Numerous animal models have supported the antibody-mediated mechanism of TRALI, including

murine models with true or functional neutropenia or monocytopenia, and therefore decreased reaction to anti-HLA or anti-HNA antibodies, demonstrating protection against TRALI.[45,46] However, a case of TRALI in a neutropenic patient has been reported, suggesting that activated neutrophils are not the only cause.[47]

ANTIBODY MEDIATED

The majority (approximately 80%) of TRALI cases are believed to be caused by passive transfer of HLA or HNA antibodies from donor blood to a transfusion recipient.[48] HLA is a class of genes encoding the most highly polymorphic molecules in the human body. The HLA-complex is also known as the major histocompatibility complex. HLA has three classes: HLA class I molecules consist of the A, B, and C antigens carried on nucleated cells (including both leukocytes and endothelial cells) and platelets, while HLA class II molecules consist of DP, DR, and DQ antigens found mainly on dendritic, macrophage and B cells,[48] and class III encodes portions of the complement system.[49] Recent studies have begun to evaluate genome-wide sequence association of HLA alloimmunization, particularly in previously pregnant women. Much is still to be learned about factors that may predispose an individual to alloimmunization.[50]

HNA are structures predominantly expressed on neutrophils, but are also found on monocytes, lymphocytes, and platelets.[51] Exposure to foreign HLA or HNA molecules through transfusion, transplantation, or pregnancy can cause alloimmunization or production of antibodies against the foreign antigens. These antibodies produce a robust immune response with near immediate destruction of cells expressing cognate antigens. Such an antibody-antigen reaction is associated with TRALI.[52] The presence of HLA antibodies is not always a given in causing TRALI as some reports based on lookbacks of TRALI-implicated donors have demonstrated numerous transfusions of antibodies against common HLA antigens without causing TRALI.[33,53]

SPECIFICITIES OF INVOLVED ANTIBODIES

Antibodies against HLA antibodies are rather common in the general donor population. Studies evaluating previously pregnant female apheresis platelet donors, previously transfused male donors, and a control group of nulliparous female donors found an overall alloimmunization rate of 20.2%. Moreover, 31% of parous women versus 4.2% of nulliparous women demonstrated anti-HLA antibodies. Rates of alloimmunization, not surprisingly, increased with parity. In transfused male donors, up to 1.3% demonstrated HLA-alloimmunization.[49] The incidence of associated antibodies in TRALI cases, based on retrospective review, is as follows: HLA class I antibodies in 14.3% −26.7%; HLA class II antibodies in 0.0%−46.7%; and HNA antibodies in 16.7%−28.6%.[11,54−59]

HLA Class I

Cognate HLA class I antigens are found on neutrophils and endothelial cells, which are the primary cell types playing a pathophysiological role in TRALI. HLA class I antibodies when bound to neutrophils initiate priming, which in turn initiate a cascade of effects to include mechanical plugging of capillary beds and overt endothelial damage. Numerous cases and models of TRALI featuring antibodies against HLA-A2, a frequent antigen, have been reported.[60] A recent study has suggested that this particular antibody may induce endothelial permeability that plays a major role in the alveolar edema seen in TRALI.[61]

HLA Class II

There is growing evidence for the association between anti-HLA class II antibodies and TRALI. Although class II antigens are not generally found on resting neutrophils, their expression may be induced through neutrophil stimulation.[62] Antibodies directed against class II antigens may bind to monocytes and subsequently cause release of cytokines and neutrophil activation through an alternate TRALI pathway as proposed by Kopko et al.[11]

HUMAN NEUTROPHIL ANTIGENS

Human neutrophil antigens are also expressed on neutrophils, but different from HLA, they are not expressed on the endothelium. Anti-HNA antibodies have been isolated in many patients during the serological work-up of TRALI.[63,64] Antibodies against HNA-3a have been singled out as a potent initiating factor for TRALI with or without modulation from other substances in plasma.[65] An elegant ex vivo animal lung model demonstrated severe vascular leakage induced by HNA-3a antibodies. The same did not occur in the absence of HNA-3a antibodies, or HNA-3a positive neutrophils. This lent further evidence for the antibody-mediated mechanism.[64,65]

Heterogeneous expression of certain HNA such as HNA-2a on either a majority or minority subpopulation of circulating human neutrophils also appears to have an impact on the pathogenesis. In an ex vivo rodent lung model, TRALI was only induced when HNA-2a was present on most neutrophils in the presence of the cognate antibody.[66]

NEUTROPHIL PASSAGE THROUGH MICROVASCULATURE

Neutrophil migration from the blood stream into peripheral tissues at sites of inflammation has been extensively modeled. This process is believed to follow a series of adhesive steps starting with tethering on endothelium in a shear stress environment. This process is normally highly dependent on adhesion molecules, particularly E-selectin and P-selectin found on endothelium, and L-selectin found on neutrophils, as well as a variety of ligands found on both cell types. In the lungs, the alveolar capillary bed is the primary site of neutrophil emigration during an inflammatory response, as opposed to postcapillary venules in other organs.[67−69] This region has unique anatomy in that it constitutes a complex network of short capillary segments in which the path from arteriole to venule crosses alveolar walls and contains many capillary segments. These complex vascular structures contain many fold more neutrophils, lymphocytes, and monocytes than other anatomic vascular beds.[69]

Neutrophils are normally relatively spherical in shape with a diameter of 6−8 μm. This is larger than the diameter of many capillaries, which range from 2 to 15 μm, which forces the neutrophils to change shape, essentially flattening out into an oval shape that allows them to pass through these tiny capillary branches en route from arteriole to venule.[42] (Fig. 7.3) Red cells with their biconcave disc shape are better able to deform through narrow blood vessels. Neutrophils with their need to deform more dramatically, therefore, have slower transit time through pulmonary capillaries. This helps to explain why the pulmonary circulation

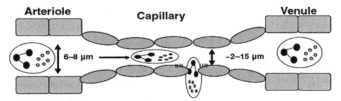

FIG. 7.3 Pulmonary microvasculature influences neutrophil passage. Normal neutrophil diameter is larger than pulmonary capillaries, causing deformation. Neutrophil response to inflammation in the lungs is uniquely targeted to the alveolar capillary bed. (Used with permission from John Wiley & Sons, Inc, Wiley Publishing: Bux J, Sachs, UJ. The pathogenesis of transfusion-related acute lung injury (TRALI). *Br J Haematol* 2007;136:788–799.[42])

normally contains about 30% of circulating neutrophils in an essentially marginated pool.[70–72] Due to the small diameter of pulmonary capillaries, neutrophils are unable to roll. Thus, the usual model of neutrophil rolling, adhesion, and arrest in response to injured endothelium does not apply here. Rather, true mechanical arrest from the plugging of capillaries by primed neutrophils with decreased deformability is likely the initial insult in TRALI.[70-72]

PRIMING AND ACTIVATION OF NEUTROPHILS

Neutrophils in resting state circulate without expressing their full microbicidal activity unless they are first primed. Priming potentiates the response of neutrophils when encountering an activating substance. Activated neutrophils, cluster surface receptors form NADPH oxidase complex, and thus synthesize reactive oxygen species (ROS). Neutrophil priming can enhance ROS release by up to 20-fold.[73] In TRALI, it is thought that neutrophils undergo both priming and activation likely by two separate substances or stimuli and that at least one of these stimuli must be derived from the transfused blood component.

Priming may occur because of underlying disease. Epidemiologic studies and hemovigilance monitoring have shown recent surgery to be an independent risk factor for TRALI, corroborating Popovsky and Moore's initial paper in 1985.[7] Additionally, infection, cardiovascular disease, and hematological malignancies are also recognized risk factors.[21,37,74] Neutrophils can be primed by infectious agents, as in viruses and lipopolysaccharides (LPS) from bacteria.[73–75] It is thought that once primed, neutrophils remain primed for at least 24 hours.[75] This correlates well with the observation that recent surgery (within 48 hours) appears to be a priming risk factor.

Priming and activation of neutrophils as in inflammation may cause failure of neutrophils to successfully pass through these small capillary beds. This is likely the result of mediators such as chemotactic factors (e.g., complement C5a) to neutrophil receptors causing resistance to cellular deformation. Additional inflammatory mediators may cause neutrophils to further concentrate at the alveolar walls physically trapping them in these vessels. Decreases in deformability may also be correlated with upregulation of adhesive factors such as β_2-integrins, which further promote trapping and adhesiveness to the endothelial cells within the alveolar capillaries. Pulmonary inflammation, as in TRALI, causes profound emigration of neutrophils from capillary beds into the alveolar spaces. Adjacent alveoli are separated by a capillary network in contact with alveolar air on both sides and a single alveolus is in contact with about 1,000 capillary segments. Noteworthy, neutrophils appear to be able to squeeze through small gaps between endothelial cells and pass into the alveolar spaces.[70]

ACTIVATION OF PULMONARY ENDOTHELIAL CELLS

Inflammatory cytokines and mediators appear to create conditions that favor endothelial cytoskeletal rearrangements that facilitate leukocyte transmigration. Activated endothelial cells use selectins, and produce more adhesive proteins and inflammatory mediators, promoting further neutrophil adherence and additionally further enhance the neutrophil, monocyte, and platelet activation that is already occurring. These processes can cause alveolar damage that allows for the secretion of fluid and migration of neutrophils into the alveolar spaces.[70] Additionally, there is some experimental evidence that activated pulmonary endothelium may be an initiating factor in TRALI and that primed neutrophils are not always the first hit. Activated endothelial cells upregulate various surface receptors that promote neutrophil adhesion, and may also produce other chemokines/cytokines such as platelet-activating factor, leukotrienes, and IL-8. These substances interact further with nearby neutrophils. Furthermore, antibodies directed against alloantigens present on the endothelium of transplanted organs have been reported to cause TRALI.[76]

PARTICIPATION OF OTHER CELLS

It is a subject of debate as to whether cells other than neutrophils contribute to TRALI. However, this mystery began to unravel with greater insights into HLA class II antibody-mediated TRALI. HLA class II is not generally expressed on neutrophils or endothelial cells; however, it is well expressed on monocytes. It appears that HLA class II antibodies bind to monocytes, and then monocytes release neutrophil-activating substances such as IL-8, which in turn trigger the cascade of events leading to neutrophil activation, emigration, and ultimately TRALI.[11,12] Additionally, monocytes may even be involved in HLA class I antibody-mediated TRALI, as murine knock-out models with severe monocytopenia appeared to be protected from HLA class I-mediated TRALI.[77]

INTERACTIONS BETWEEN WHITE BLOOD CELLS AND ENDOTHELIAL CELLS

Neutrophils that are physically trapped in small alveolar capillaries can then release their granules, which contain various substances with toxic/microbicidal activity and in turn damage the endothelium. Damaged endothelium causes capillary leak, which allows fluid and neutrophils to pass into the alveolar spaces, causing even more damage. In turn, endothelial damage unsheathes subendothelial collagen producing a surface conducive for thrombosis and even more neutrophils being sequestered in the vessels, thus keeping the process going.

NEUTROPHIL TRANSENDOTHELIAL MIGRATION

Neutrophil transendothelial migration is a complex process and is thought to be regulated by a number of substances including platelet/endothelial cell adhesion molecule-1 (PECAM-1; CD31), junctional adhesion molecules, endothelial-cadherin (E-cadherin), and CD99.[70]

Normally, tight junctions between alveolar epithelial cells protect against fluid leakage into the alveoli. In cardiogenic or volume overload scenarios, fluid moves into the alveolar interstitial space but does not directly enter the alveoli. From the interstitium, this low protein content fluid (transudate) is normally filtered by lymphatics and returned to systemic circulation.[78] However, once primed and trapped, neutrophils in pulmonary capillaries release toxic granules and start damaging endothelium; fluid and protein leakage can occur through small gaps between capillary endothelial cells. This noncardiogenic, unfiltered fluid has high protein content (exudate) and enters alveolar spaces, causing the respiratory failure seen in TRALI.[78]

INVERSE TRALI—TRANSFUSION OF WBC

As previously discussed, most cases of TRALI are due to antibodies or other neutrophil-priming substances present in a transfused blood component. However, TRALI can occur in HLA or HNA alloimmunized patients receiving blood components that contain neutrophils. Not surprisingly, granulocyte transfusion would be of particular risk, as antibodies in the recipient could interact with the plentiful cognate alloantigens on the transfused cells and initiate TRALI.[25] In vivo studies transfusing 111-indium labeled neutrophils to recipients with antineutrophil antibodies demonstrated abnormal sequestration in the lungs.[79] As leukoreduction is gaining more widespread acceptance, the incidence of inverse TRALI should decrease accordingly.

NONANTIBODY FACTORS

Adding to the debate over blood storage, various TRALI models have demonstrated that stored blood poses a greater risk than fresh blood.[80,81] Other studies have not found such an effect.[82,83] Blood components stored in a bag are never quite as physiologic as blood elements circulating in the body. During storage, blood components accumulate various metabolic breakdown products. Among these are bioactive lipids such as lysophosphatidylcholines, known to prime neutrophils. Bioactive lipids only accumulate in components containing RBCs and do not accumulate in acellular plasma. Initial studies demonstrated that transfusion of supernatant from stored packed (p) RBCs caused TRALI in a murine model, adding to the already contentious debate about the significance of the age of stored blood components.[74,80–83] Nonpolar lipids such as arachidonic acid, 5-hydroxyeicosatetraenoic acid (HETE), 12-HETE, and 15-HETE have also been investigated as potential players in the "two-hit" model of TRALI. These compounds also accumulate during blood component storage, but this accumulation appears to occur more profoundly at temperatures well above normal storage conditions of pRBC and is less pronounced in platelet components. In a model of human volunteers primed with LPS, infusion of RBCs with increased levels of nonpolar lipids did not appear to induce TRALI.[83] Overall, there is not compelling evidence for or against the potential role of bioactive lipids in TRALI. Other factors theorized to play a role in TRALI include damage-associated molecular patterns (DAMPs) that may be formed during the collection, processing, and storing of blood components. The innate immune system and, in particular, inflammatory cells are equipped with receptors that can recognize DAMPs. In this process, the immune cells are activated, which may lead to neutrophil priming and contribute to the endothelial damage and cascade of events leading to TRALI.[84] Unfortunately, it is unlikely that the fresh versus stored blood debate will reach a conclusive end in the near future.[80–83]

NEUTROPHIL EXTRACELLULAR TRAPS

Neutrophil extracellular traps (NETs) are strands of neutrophil DNA and histones impregnated with antimicrobial proteins from neutrophil granules that can be expelled from a neutrophil in response to a microbe. These NETs allow for the trapping and killing of bacteria and yeast. However, NETs when activated inappropriately or not cleared effectively may injure host tissues and play a role in autoimmune diseases. NETs may play a role in TRALI. The role of NETs was studied in an in vivo model of antibody (HNA-3a)-mediated TRALI in mice. Results from this study suggest that anti-HNA-3a antibodies trigger neutrophil activation, and NETosis, likely through an Fcγ-RIIa-mediated process. The same study identified NET biomarkers (DNA, myeloperoxidase, and nucleosomes) in the bloodstream of patients with TRALI. Disruption of NETs in the alveoli using a DNase improved oxygenation in this murine model.[85] Platelets may also play a role in inducing extracellular traps in TRALI. In an experimental TRALI model, targeting platelet activation with aspirin or other antiplatelet agent decreased NET formation and lung injury.[86]

T-REGULATORY LYMPHOCYTES AND DENDRITIC CELLS

T-regulatory cells or T-regs are CD4$^+$, CD25$^+$, FoxP3$^+$ T-lymphocytes, and CD11c$^+$ dendritic cells appear to protect against TRALI in a murine model. These cells appear to be associated with increased plasma IL-10 levels and low IL-10 appears to be a risk factor for TRALI.[87]

Radiographic Findings in TRALI Patients

The radiographic findings in TRALI patients can be seen below in figure 7.4 demonstrating unremarkable chest x-ray findings before the reaction and bilateral opacities afterwards, with resolution over time.[88]

Pathological Findings in TRALI Patients

Evaluating the histological findings in patients who died from TRALI has provided further evidence of its pathophysiology. Histological findings are consistent with acute respiratory distress syndrome (ARDS) with extensive intraalveolar edema and presence of neutrophils.[2,3,7,74,89,90] Hyaline membranes and distortion of pulmonary architecture have also been reported.[2,89,90] Capillary leukostasis is also a prominent feature. Electron microscopy has demonstrated that neutrophils were degranulated and in direct contact with injured stretches of capillary endothelium, supporting the theory of neutrophil adhesion and retention in pulmonary capillaries as a causative feature[90] (Figs. 7.4, 7.5 and 7.6).

DIAGNOSIS

TRALI can be difficult to diagnose as there are no highly pathognomonic signs and symptoms associated with it. The initial step in diagnosing TRALI would be to identify if there is respiratory distress and pulmonary edema in the patient. The edema can be evaluated by physical exam or by chest X-ray. Other causes of respiratory distress that are associated with transfusion, such as circulatory overload, bacterial infection, hemolytic transfusion reactions, and myocardial infarction, need to be ruled out before reaching a diagnosis of TRALI. Circulatory overload can present in a very similar way to TRALI and extra care needs to be taken to differentiate between the entities. TRALI will typically present with a normal central venous pressure and the patient should not have any predisposition for developing circulatory overload.

Although no laboratory tests are completely sensitive or specific, there are a few tests that can be done that would be consistent with a diagnosis of TRALI. Leukopenia often occurs within the first hour after a transfusion and can even occur before the evidence of lung injury presents. The leukopenia will normally develop into leukocytosis within 6 hours of the transfusion. Seeing this pattern in the complete blood count is a strong indication that the lung injury may be due to the transfusion.[1,19,91] The leukopenia usually manifests as a neutropenia in patients who had antibodies against HNA-2 and HNA-3a and as a monocytopenia in patients with antibodies against HLA class II.[29] Other laboratory values that may have clinical utility in this setting are a posttransfusion to pretransfusion B-type (or brain) natriuretic peptide

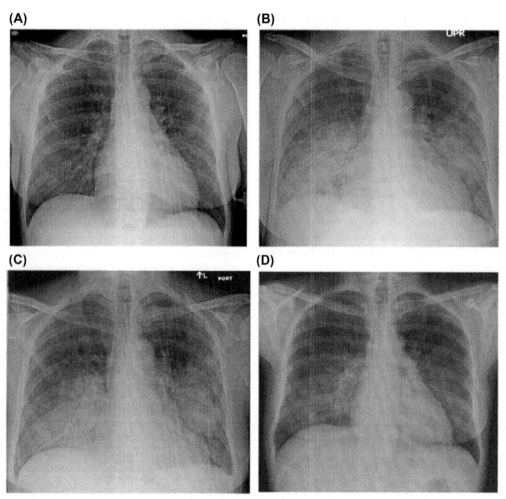

FIG. 7.4 Four anteroposterior (AP) radiographs of the chest **(A–D)** of a patient who developed TRALI. **(A)** Pretransfusion chest radiograph shows clear lungs. **(B** and **C)** Posttransfusion chest radiographs obtained approximately 5 and 40 h after transfusion show developing confluent alveolar opacities with perihilar predominance in the bilateral mid and lower lung zones. AP radiograph 72 h after transfusion **(D)** shows partial resolution of lung opacities. (Used with permission from Elsevier: Carcano C, Okafor N, Martinez F, Ramirez J, Kanne J, Kirsch J. Radiographic manifestations of transfusion-related acute lung injury. *Clinical Imaging* 2013; 37:1020–1023.[88])

(BNP) ratio of <1.5 and an edema fluid/plasma protein ratio of ≥0.75, which helps to exclude TACO and favor TRALI.[92,93] Even though finding lymphotoxic, HLA, or granulocyte antibodies in the donor unit is not part of the official criteria definition, it is a strong indication that TRALI is the appropriate diagnosis.

DIFFERENTIAL

The main diagnosis that needs to be ruled out when evaluating a case of TRALI is TACO (Table 7.2). TACO has now become the most common cause of fatality among

transfusions in the USA and UK.[38,39] Different from TRALI, the pathophysiology of TACO does not have an immunologic underpinning. TACO is caused by an increased pulmonary capillary pressure that leads to a cardiogenic edema, while TRALI is due to a noncardiogenic edema from the activated neutrophils and endothelial leak. Patients who develop TACO typically have a preexisting condition that predisposes them to volume overload. All blood components have been implicated in TACO with no particular type contributing more cases. This is due to the fact that this disease process is primarily

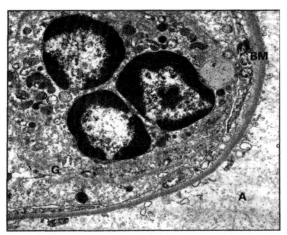

FIG. 7.5 Electron micrograph of alveolar basement membrane (BM) with intravascular, adherent granulocyte (G), desquamated alveolar epithelium and amorphous proteinaceous alveolar material (A) ($\times$10,000). (Used with permission from Oxford University Press: Dry SM, Bechard KM, Milford EL, Hallowell Churchill W, Benjamin RJ. The pathology of transfusion-related acute lung injury. *Am J Clin Pathol* 1999;112(2):216–221.[90])

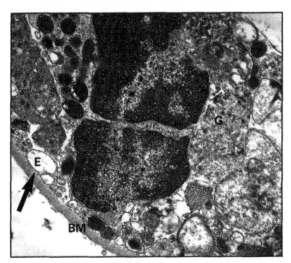

FIG. 7.6 Electron micrograph of adherent degranulated granulocyte (G) in contact with the basement membrane (BM) and with vesicular "blebbing" of an endothelial cell (E) ($\times$14,000). (Used with permission of Oxford University Press from Dry SM, Bechard KM, Milford EL, Hallowell Churchill W, Benjamin RJ. The pathology of transfusion-related acute lung injury. *Am J Clin Pathol* 1999;112(2):216–221.[90])

due purely to volume overload. The type of fluid is inconsequential (RBCs, plasma, crystalloids, and colloids), as long as the volume exceeds the patient's ability

TABLE 7.2 Key Points to Distinguish the Three Major Pulmonary-Related Transfusion Reactions.	
TRALI	• ALI due to microvascular injury • Immunologic based pathophysiology • Hypotension • Pretransfusion: post transfusion BNP ratio <1.5
TACO	• ALI due to circulatory overload • Volume-based pathophysiology • Hypertension • Pretransfusion: post transfusion BNP ratio ≥1.5
TAD	• Dyspnea after transfusion • Does not meet the criteria for TRALI and TACO

to compensate. TACO presents with *hypertension* in the setting of pulmonary edema, although it is not impossible for a patient to present with both symptoms of TRALI and volume overload. As TACO has no immunologic basis, prevention is simpler with mindfulness of fluid balance the goal, achievable by avoiding unnecessary transfusions and transfusing at a slower rate. The most effective lab test that can be used to differentiate TACO and TRALI is measuring the patient's posttransfusion to pretransfusion BNP level. BNP is a hormone secreted by myocytes in the heart ventricles in response to stretching caused by increased ventricular blood volume. BNP's name is derived from the fact that the original isolate was from extracts of pig brain. A diagnosis of TACO is more likely than TRALI if the post- to pretransfusion ratio of BNP is ≥ 1.5. This indicates that the BNP level has increased after the transfusion that would be due to the increased stretching of the ventricles due to volume overload.[92]

The other transfusion-associated respiratory disorder that needs to be ruled out in the work-up of TRALI is the catch-all definition of TAD. This is defined as acute respiratory distress that does not meet the definition of TRALI or TACO.[15] Although this is important to note from a regulatory perspective, the actual usefulness of this diagnosis is unclear. No specific underlying mechanism has been identified with no immunologic or physiologic cause seen.

MANAGEMENT

The management of TRALI patients typically is focused on supportive care. Respiratory support is needed in most cases in the form of oxygen alone, positive pressure, or intubation.[7] More severe cases of TRALI may require fluid replacement depending on the level of hypotension and hypovolemia. Although diuretics are the mainstay of therapy for TACO, they are contraindicated in TRALI. TACO, as should be remembered, is a problem of volume overload. TRALI presents initially with hypotension and hypovolemia due to microvascular injury from antibodies or other substances; diuretics will just worsen the condition.[94] Some clinical trials have tried to evaluate how effective corticosteroids are in the treatment of ARDS but not specifically in TRALI. These studies showed no benefit to using corticosteroids in the treatment of ARDS and that persistent use could in fact worsen the condition.[95,96] This finding can be extrapolated into a contraindication of using steroids to treat TRALI. Other modalities that have been tried with limited success and limited data include infusion with albumin that resulted in marked improvement,[97] extracorporeal membrane oxygenation in a child,[98] and therapeutic plasma exchange to remove the offending antibody.[99] Although each of these showed some success in anecdotal reports and case reports, the use of these treatments should be considered experimental at this time.

NOVEL FUTURE TREATMENT TARGETS
IL-10 Therapy
Low plasma IL-10 levels have been demonstrated in murine and human TRALI models. In Kapur et al.'s murine TRALI model, IL-10 injection appeared to prevent or rescue the mice from TRALI and represent a potential novel treatment for humans. Caution in using IL-10 is warranted as it may impair host defenses against infection and cost may be another prohibitive factor. However, IL-10 administration in healthy volunteers has been demonstrated to be safe with side effects mainly limited to flu-like symptoms. Additionally, only a short IL-10 effect would be needed as TRALI occurs within 6 hours of transfusion, thus minimizing the dosing needed.[87,100,101]

C-Reactive Protein Down-Modulation
As an acute phase reactant, C-reactive protein (CRP) is upregulated during infection or inflammation. Inflammation is a known risk factor for TRALI, and CRP has been demonstrated to enhance HLA class I antibody-mediated TRALI in a murine model.[102] CRP might, therefore, be a novel target for TRALI therapy. Animal models have demonstrated benefits from blocking CRP in other diseases. In addition, caution is warranted as CRP inhibition may adversely decrease bacterial clearance.[101]

Anti-ROS Therapy
ROS generated by activated neutrophils are likely to play a part in the pathogenesis of TRALI due to their damaging effects on endothelium. Therefore, the use of antioxidants in the form of high dose vitamins or other inhibitors may warrant further investigation.[101]

IL-8 Receptor Blockade
As IL-8 has been shown to promote neutrophil chemotaxis and degranulation, blocking its receptor might have an inhibitory effect on the ongoing pathological effects of these processes in TRALI. One such receptor, CXC-chemokine receptor (CXCR 2), is currently being studied in other pulmonary conditions such as asthma, cystic fibrosis, and chronic obstructive pulmonary disease. TRALI may be another potential application, especially if receptor blockade can cause a rapid effect.[101]

IV IMMUNOGLOBULIN AND BLOCKING FCγ-RECEPTORS
IVIG therapy has been attempted for many autoimmune-type processes, and in a severe combined immune deficiency mouse TRALI model. Its use after TRALI induction reduced severe lung injury. As the exact mechanism of action for IVIG remains elusive, its use in the treatment of TRALI might be limited.[101]

Neutrophil Extracellular Trap Disruption
Increased NETosis has been described in TRALI. Disruption of NETs in the alveoli using a DNase improved oxygenation in a murine model and might prove to be a useful therapeutic target in human TRALI. However, more research is needed to definitively delineate a causative effect of NETs in the pathogenesis of TRALI before therapeutic studies can proceed.[85,86,101]

Antiplatelet Agents
The role of platelets in TRALI remains unclear. Despite some murine models demonstrating an attenuating effect from aspirin and other antiplatelet agents, this finding has not been consistently reproducible, and given the risk of dyspnea and bleeding, the use of antiplatelet agents in TRALI cannot yet be recommended.[101]

Targeting Bioactive Lipid, Damage-Associated Molecular Pathogens
The role of nonimmune substances that accumulate in blood components during storage remains to be more conclusively elucidated.[80–83,101] There appears to be a fairly even balance in the literature of studies for and against "old" blood, thus negating any substantial conclusions.

Prevention

With TRALI being the leading cause of transfusion-related mortality in many countries in the early 2000s,[103] ways to mitigate the risk of TRALI became of utmost importance. As TRALI typically has an antibody-mediated etiology, prevention usually is aimed at reducing the likelihood of transfusing the causative antibodies.

The finding that plasma from female donors had a higher correlation with the development of TRALI than any blood component from male donors became the focal point of prevention strategies.[28,104] This risk mitigation strategy relied upon the antibody-mediated pathway for the development of TRALI. Women who had been pregnant would have a higher chance of developing HLA and HNA antibodies, due to sensitization from the fetus, that could be passively transferred to the recipient during the transfusion.[105,106] As antibodies circulate in the plasma, FFP and apheresis platelets were the most important products to initially evaluate. Therefore, many countries started to develop policies to limit the amount of plasma that was transfused from female donors.

With the use of male-only plasma in the UK, rates of TRALI were seen to drop from 15.5 per million to 3.2 per million units of FFP.[107] They were able to decrease the number of fatalities from TRALI to a single case by 2006 and have been able to stay at that rate over the past 12 years.[39] Other European countries have seen similar results in their efforts to decrease the rate of TRALI. Germany showed a decrease in the rate of TRALI from 12.71 per million to 6.81 per million[57] and the Netherlands saw a 33% reduction in the rate of TRALI.[108]

The Canadian Blood Service (CBS) has also endeavored to use blood from male-only donors and to defer females from donating apheresis platelets if they had a high likelihood of harboring HLA antibodies. They reported a compliance rate of 93%–96%. Initially, they saw an increase in the rate of TRALI over the first 3 years of the study, but this was theorized to be likely due to the increased awareness of the disease as opposed to an actual increase. The rates of TRALI started to stabilize and then decrease over the latter half of the 9-year study.[103,109]

The United States had a slower implementation of the accepted TRALI mitigation strategies. Initially, the problem may have been that there was no standardization in how blood banks were implementing TRALI mitigation strategies.[110,111] Starting in 2006, the American Association of Blood Banks (AABB) introduced a standard that required blood banks to evaluate donors implicated in TRALI and determine if they should be able to continue to donate blood.[112] AABB bulletins from 2006 to 2007 stated that accepting high plasma-volume components from donors with a known leukocyte antibody or any patients at a high risk for developing one should be minimized and that each institution should develop strategies to mitigate TRALI risk without compromising the blood supply.[113,114] In 2007, the American Red Cross (ARC) started to distribute plasma from male-only donors (save for group AB plasma) for transfusion and diverting female-derived plasma to pharmaceutical companies for manufacturing. By the end of 2007, 95% of the plasma that was transfused came from male donors. Subsequently, there was a large decrease in the number of reported cases of TRALI and thus a decrease in the number of transfusion-related fatalities in the USA.[38,104] (Fig. 7.7). The current work in using whole blood in massively bleeding patients is using the same

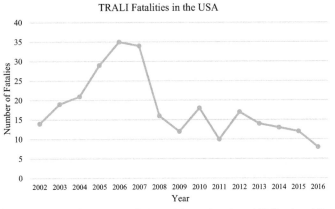

FIG. 7.7 TRALI fatalities in the USA by year. (Adapted from data from US Food and Drug Administration. Fatalities Reported to FDA Following Blood Collection and Transfusion: Annual Summary for FY2016; 2016: 15. https://www.fda.gov/BiologicsBloodVaccines/SafetyAvailability/ReportaProblem/ TransfusionDonationFatalities/default.htm.)

mitigation strategy by only using whole blood from male donors.[115] Despite the use of blood components from male donors being theoretically safer, there may still be a small percentage of male donors who harbor anti-HLA antibodies.[116]

Donor lookback and deferral is a critical part of TRALI prevention and highlights the need for reporting of suspected transfusion reactions. However, guidance for donor deferral is still quite variable. Different from other transfusion reactions, TRALI is typically due to a cognate antibody-antigen match that is present in the donor unit. If that donor's HLA or HNA antibodies caused a reaction in a random patient, it is very possible that the antibody would react against additional blood recipients. The first step in managing the donor is to contact the blood supplier and have any other units that exist from that donor quarantined. There is much variation in opinions on the handling of implicated donors.[117] Although the 19th edition of the AABB Technical Manual states that donors implicated in TRALI should be deferred for life,[118] this strategy could defer many donors who have a very rare antibody that has an extremely small chance of causing a reaction. Additionally, it follows from that strategy that every donor should be screened for HLA antibodies before any donation and those who screen positive should also be deferred for life. This would devastate the donor pool and be associated with untenable cost. The AABB released bulletins in 2005 and 2014 with summaries of their recommendations for how to handle implicated donors.[119,120] (Fig. 7.8) They recommend that if a donor is conclusively determined to have an HLA/HNA antibody that is specific for the recipients HLA/HNA type, then the donor should be deferred from donating whole blood and high plasma-volume components. Further strategies would be to only defer the donor if it was proven that they were positive for an HLA antibody for which the recipient had the corresponding antigen or to only defer donors who were implicated in TRALI from donating high plasma-volume components.[121] Although more efficient assays for HLA and HNA antibody detection are starting to be developed, they are not widely available at this time.[116,117,122] Variable scenarios in suspected TRALI cases greatly complicate the handling of potentially implicated donors. The overarching goal is to balance minimizing risk of TRALI without unnecessary donor deferral.

Currently, it is believed that a patient who has a previous history of TRALI is not at any greater risk developing TRALI again after an additional transfusion.

Most efforts in eliminating TRALI therefore, focus on the components that are being collected as opposed to the patient being transfused.

Additional strategies that have been attempted have focused on decreasing the number of unnecessary transfusions, especially of high plasma-volume components such as FFP and platelet units. FFP has been found to be ineffective in correcting minor coagulopathies and should not be used for that purpose.[123,124] The recent emphasis on patient blood management has also led to an almost universal overall decrease in blood transfusions.[125] The more that unnecessary transfusions can be avoided, the more likely that cases of TRALI will decrease.

These strategies for TRALI mitigation have been fairly simple but have demonstrated a high yield. One interesting side effect is that TRALI due to RBCs is now almost as common as TRALI from high plasma components.[24] This is likely not related to an increase in the number of cases from RBCs but from the large decrease in the number of cases from FFP. It is important to note that TRALI can be caused by very small amounts of residual plasma. The study by Weber et al. in 2014 showed that RBCs had a residual plasma content approaching 100 mL. In the setting of a high-strength antibody, severe or even fatal TRALI could occur.[24] Additionally, a study by Win in 2008 showed that residual plasma levels of as low as 10−20 mL in pooled platelet units from male donors could still induce a TRALI reaction.[23] This demonstrates that while the TRALI mitigation strategies have been very successful, there is still a risk of this severe reaction.

Cost

The importance of prevention can be seen both from the patient care perspective and also from the hospital cost perspective. A study out of the Netherlands from 2017 set out to evaluate the cost to a hospital due to transfusion reactions. They evaluated the direct costs of transfusion complications (costs of extended length of stay, hospital diagnostics, and additional care). TRALI was found to be the most expensive transfusion reaction to work up and evaluate at a median cost of €6652 (approximately $7600) for severe reactions and €2086 (approximately $2400) for nonsevere reactions.[126] The increased costs were due to extra days needed in an ICU, HLA work-ups, additional physician, nurse, and technologist time, and chest X-rays. Therefore, greater prevention of TRALI has not only significant clinical benefit, but economic as well.

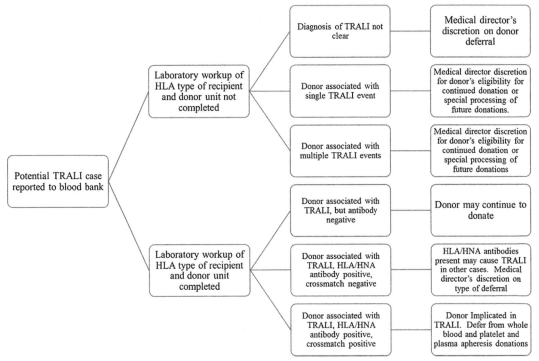

FIG. 7.8 Potential TRALI cases are divided into cases that have had a laboratory work-up to identify the recipient's HLA/HNA antigens and the donor's HLA/HNA antibodies and cases that have not. For cases without a work-up, if the diagnosis of TRALI is unclear then it is under the discretion of the medical director if that donor should be deferred from donating. If there is a clear diagnosis of TRALI but no laboratory work-up for a donor who has been implicated in one or more TRALI cases, associated blood components from that donor should be identified and removed from circulation and the donor should be evaluated for conditions that may have led to antibody development. Further donations are by the discretion of the medical director. For cases with a laboratory work-up, if the donor is HLA/HNA antibody negative, they are able to continue to donate normally. If HLA/HNA antibodies that match the recipient's type by crossmatch are identified, then the donor should be deferred from future donations. If HLA/HNA antibodies are identified, but specificity is not directed against a recipient antigen evidenced by antigen typing or crossmatching then donor management is unclear. The most appropriate course of action is not defined due to many multiparous women having numerous HLA/HNA antibodies yet never being implicated in a TRALI reaction. (Adapted from Mintz PD, Lipton KS. AABB Association Bulletin #05-09 Transfusion-Related Acute Lung Injury; 2005. http://www.aabb.org/programs/publications/bulletins/Documents/ab05-9.pdf; Sher G, Markowitz MA. AABB Association Bulletin #14-02: TRALI Risk Mitigation for Plasma and Whole Blood for Allogeneic Transfusion; 2014. https://www.aabb.org/programs/publications/bulletins/Documents/ab14-02.pdf.)

TRALI in Pediatrics

TRALI can occur at any age, but most of the current guidance and criteria focus on adults. Lieberman et al. with the CBS set out to determine how TRALI differed in presentation, outcomes, antibody profile, and demographic when comparing the adult and pediatric populations.[127] The review used a definition of less than 18 years old as pediatric. Among the 434 cases of TRALI reported to CBS between 2001 and 2011, 26 (6%) were identified in pediatric patients. Among these cases, 284 total and 17 pediatrics were determined to be definite,

probably or possible cases of TRALI. The point was that pediatric TRALI patients were primarily either under 1 year of age or over 14 years of age with only one TRALI victim between these two age points. There was no clinically significant difference between overall mortality (5.2% for adults and 5.9% for pediatrics; $P = .99$) or the likelihood of identifying an antibody-antigen pair from the donor to the recipient (13% for adults and 18% for pediatrics; $P = .6255$). Though, a study out of Pakistan did show a higher mortality rate of 10.7% in pediatric intensive-care patients.[35] The pediatric population in the Canadian study did have a high incidence of TRALI in the pediatric patients of 5.58 per 100,000 compared to 3.75 per 100,000 in adults. Other studies have shown that TRALI presents much more commonly in pediatric patients who have a history of a hematologic malignancy.[128]

Neonates are found to be extremely difficult to diagnose with TRALI and are likely underdiagnosed.[127,129,130] As most neonates are already critically ill and often intubated before needing a transfusion, it can be difficult to determine if there was a previous history of lung injury before the blood was given. This is compounded by the fact that a neonate's chest radiograph may be abnormal at baseline. With the fact that neonates have a relative immunosuppression and immature immune system, different criteria may need to be used to diagnosis TRALI in this population.

CONCLUSION

From the 1950s to the present, TRALI has been a major concern within the transfusion medicine community and the medical field as a whole. The evolution of understanding of the pathogenesis of this disease has led to major advancements in treatment and prevention strategies. Simple, yet effective methods to mitigate TRALI risk have demonstrated substantial benefit. However, these benefits have come at the cost of a decreased donor pool. More efficient and less costly means to screen out high risk donors while avoiding unnecessary donor deferral would further optimize prevention strategies while allowing for the maintenance of an adequate blood supply. The significant decline in the number of deaths from TRALI that occur in the last 2 decades demonstrates the power of an effective hemovigilance program.

REFERENCES

1. Brittingham TE. Immunologic studies on leukocytes. *Vox Sang.* 1957;2(4):242–248.
2. Wolf CFW, Canale VC. Fatal pulmonary hypersensitivity reaction to HL-A incompatible blood transfusion. *Transfusion (Paris).* 1976;16(2):135–140.
3. Kernoff PBA, Durrant IJ, Rizza CR, Wright FW. Severe allergic pulmonary oedema after plasma transfusion. *Br J Haematol.* 1972;23(6):777–781.
4. Ward HN. Pulmonary infiltrates associated with leukoagglutinin transfusion reactions. *Ann Intern Med.* 1970; 73(5):689.
5. Carilli AD, Ramanamurty MV, Chang YS, Shin D, Sethi V. Noncardiogenic pulmonary edema following blood transfusion. *Chest.* 1978;74(3):310–312.
6. Popovsky MA, Chaplin HC, Moore SB. Transfusion-related acute lung injury: a neglected, serious complication of hemotherapy. *Transfusion (Paris).* 1992;32(6): 589–592.
7. Popovsky MA, Moore SB. Diagnostic and pathogenetic considerations in transfusion-related acute lung injury. *Transfusion (Paris).* 1985;25(6):573–577.
8. Popovsky MA, Abel MD, Moore SB. Transfusion-related acute lung injury associated with passive transfer of antileukocyte antibodies. *Am Rev Respir Dis.* 1983;128(1):185–189.
9. Wallis JP. Transfusion-related lung injury. *Transfus Apher Sci Off J World Apher Assoc Off J Eur Soc Haemapheresis.* 2008;39(2):155–159.
10. Popovsky MA, Haley NR. Further characterization of transfusion-related acute lung injury: demographics, clinical and laboratory features, and morbidity. *Immunohematology.* 2000;16(4):157–159.
11. Kopko PM, Paglieroni TG, Popovsky MA, Muto KN, MacKenzie MR, Holland PV. TRALI: correlation of antigen-antibody and monocyte activation in donor-recipient pairs. *Transfusion (Paris).* 2003;43(2):177–184.
12. Kopko PM, Popovsky MA, MacKenzie MR, Paglieroni TG, Muto KN, Holland PV. HLA class II antibodies in transfusion-related acute lung injury. *Transfusion (Paris).* 2001;41(10):1244–1248.
13. Win N, Massey E, Lucas G, et al. Ninety-six suspected transfusion related acute lung injury cases: investigation findings and clinical outcome. *Hematology.* 2007;12(5): 461–469.
14. Seeger W, Schneider U, Kreusler B, et al. Reproduction of transfusion-related acute lung injury in an ex vivo lung model. *Blood.* 1990;76(7):1438–1444.
15. Center for Disease Control and Prevention. National Healthcare Safety Network Biovigilance Component Hemovigilance Module Surveillance Protocol. https://www.cdc.gov/nhsn/pdfs/biovigilance/bv-hv-protocol-current.pdf. Accessed October 16, 2018.
16. Toy P, Lowell C. TRALI - definition, mechanisms, incidence and clinical relevance. *Best Pract Res Clin Anaesthesiol.* 2007;21(2):183–193.
17. Toy P, Popovsky MA, Abraham E, et al. Transfusion-related acute lung injury: definition and review. *Crit Care Med.* 2005;33(4):721–726.
18. Kleinman S, Caulfield T, Chan P, et al. Toward an understanding of transfusion-related acute lung injury: statement of a consensus panel. *Transfusion (Paris).* 2004; 44(12):1774–1789.
19. Wallis JP, Lubenko A, Wells AW, Chapman CE. Single hospital experience of TRALI. *Transfusion (Paris).* 2003; 43(8):1053–1059.
20. Li G, Kojicic M, Reriani MK, et al. Long-term survival and quality of life after transfusion-associated pulmonary edema in critically ill medical patients. *Chest.* 2010; 137(4):783–789.
21. Silliman CC, Boshkov LK, Mehdizadehkashi Z, et al. Transfusion-related acute lung injury: epidemiology and a prospective analysis of etiologic factors. *Blood.* 2003;101(2):454–462.

22. Toy P, Gajic O, Bacchetti P, et al. Transfusion-related acute lung injury: incidence and risk factors. *Blood.* 2012;119(7):1757−1767.

23. Win N, Chapman CE, Bowles KM, et al. How much residual plasma may cause TRALI? *Transfus Med.* 2008;18(5):276−280.

24. Weber LL, Roberts LD, Sweeney JD. Residual plasma in red blood cells and transfusion-related acute lung injury. *Transfusion (Paris).* 2014;54(10):2425−2430.

25. Sachs UJ, Bux J. TRALI after the transfusion of cross-match-positive granulocytes. *Transfusion (Paris).* 2003;43(12):1683−1686.

26. Rizk A, Gorson KC, Kenney L, Weinstein R. Transfusion-related acute lung injury after the infusion of IVIG. *Transfusion (Paris).* 2001;41(2):264−268.

27. Leach V, Jones L. Transfusion-related acute lung injury (TRALI) following autologous stem cell transplant for relapsed acute myeloid leukaemia: a case report and review of the literature. *Transfus Med.* 1998;8(4):333−337.

28. Gajic O, Rana R, Winters JL, et al. Transfusion-related acute lung injury in the critically ill. *Am J Respir Crit Care Med.* 2007;176(9):886−891.

29. Flesch BK, Neppert J. Transfusion-related acute lung injury caused by human leucocyte antigen class II antibody. *Br J Haematol.* 2002;116(3):673−676.

30. Yang X, Ahmed S, Chandrasekaran V. Transfusion-related acute lung injury resulting from designated blood transfusion between mother and child: a report of two cases. *Am J Clin Pathol.* 2004;121(4):590−592.

31. Hendrickson JE, Roubinian NH, Chowdhury D, et al. Incidence of transfusion reactions: a multicenter study utilizing systematic active surveillance and expert adjudication. *Transfusion (Paris).* 2016;56(10):2587−2596.

32. Hendrickson JE, Hillyer CD. Noninfectious serious hazards of transfusion. *Anesth Analg.* 2009;108(3):759−769.

33. Kopko PM, Marshall CS, MacKenzie MR, Holland PV, Popovsky MA. Transfusion-related acute lung injury: report of a clinical look-back investigation. *J Am Med Assoc.* 2002;287(15):1968−1971.

34. Meyer DE, Reynolds JW, Hobbs R, et al. The incidence of transfusion-related acute lung injury at a large, urban tertiary medical center: a decade's experience. *Anesth Analg.* 2018;127(2):444−449.

35. Jamil MT, Dhanani ZN, Abbas Q, Jurair H, Mahar FK, Haque A. Transfusion-related acute lung injury in a pediatric intensive care unit of Pakistan. *J Ayub Med Coll Abbottabad.* 2017;29(4):702−705.

36. Vlaar APJ, Hofstra JJ, Determann RM, et al. The incidence, risk factors, and outcome of transfusion-related acute lung injury in a cohort of cardiac surgery patients: a prospective nested case-control study. *Blood.* 2011;117(16):4218−4225.

37. Holness L, Knippen MA, Simmons L, Lachenbruch PA. Fatalities caused by TRALI. *Transfus Med Rev.* 2004;18(3):184−188.

38. US Food and Drug Administration. *Fatalities Reported to FDA Following Blood Collection and Transfusion: Annual Summary for FY2016*; 2016:15. https://www.fda.gov/BiologicsBloodVaccines/SafetyAvailability/ReportaProblem/TransfusionDonationFatalities/default.htm.

39. Bellamy M, Watt A, Poles D, et al. *Annual SHOT Report 2017*; 2017:206. http://www.isbtweb.org/about-isbt/news/article/2017-annual-shot-report-published/.

40. Politis C, Wiersum JC, Richardson C, et al. The International Haemovigilance Network Database for the surveillance of adverse reactions and events in donors and Recipients of blood components: technical issues and results. *Vox Sang.* 2016;111(4):409−417.

41. Peters AL, Van Stein D, Vlaar APJ. Antibody-mediated transfusion-related acute lung injury: from discovery to prevention. *Br J Haematol.* 2015;170:597−614.

42. Bux J, Sachs U. The pathogenesis of transfusion-related acute lung injury (TRALI). *Br J Hematol.* 2007;136:788−799.

43. Middelburg RA, van der Bom JG. Transfusion-related acute lung injury not a two-hit, but a multicausal model. *Transfusion (Paris).* 2015;55(5):953−960.

44. Dooren MC, Ouwehand WH, Verhoeven AJ, von dem Borne AE, Kuijpers RW. Adult respiratory distress syndrome after experimental intravenous gamma-globulin concentrate and monocyte-reactive IgG antibodies. *Lancet Lond Engl.* 1998;352(9140):1601−1602.

45. Strait RT, Hicks W, Barasa N, et al. MHC class I-specific antibody binding to nonhematopoietic cells drives complement activation to induce transfusion-related acute lung injury in mice. *J Exp Med.* 2011;208(12):2525−2544. https://doi.org/10.1084/jem.20110159.

46. McKenzie CGJ, Kim M, Singh TK, Milev Y, Freedman J, Semple JW. Peripheral blood monocyte-derived chemokine blockade prevents murine transfusion-related acute lung injury (TRALI). *Blood.* 2014;123(22):3496−3503. https://doi.org/10.1182/blood-2013-11-536755.

47. Finlayson J, Grey D, Kavanagh L, Witt C. Transfusion-related acute lung injury in a neutropenic patient. *Intern Med J.* 2011;41(8):638−641. https://doi.org/10.1111/j.1445-5994.2010.02366.x.

48. Middelburg RA, van Stein D, Briet E, van der Bom JG. The role of donor antibodies in the pathogenesis of transfusion-related acute lung injury: a systematic review. *Transfusion (Paris).* 2008;48(10):2167−2176.

49. Horton R, Wilming L, Rand V, et al. Gene map of the extended human MHC. *Nat Rev Genet.* 2004;5:889−899.

50. Seielstad M, Page GP, Gaddis N, et al. Genomewide association study of HLA alloimmunization in previously pregnant blood donors. *Transfusion (Paris).* 2018;58(2):402−412.

51. Bux J. Human neutrophil alloantigens. *Vox Sang.* 2008;94:277−285.

52. Muschter S, Berthold T, Greinacher A. Developments in the definition and clinical impact of human neutrophil antigens. *Curr Opin Hematol.* 2011;18:452−460.

53. Toy P, Hollis-Perry KM, Jun J, Nakagawa M. Recipients of blood from a donor with multiple HLA antibodies: a

lookback study of transfusion-related acute lung injury. *Transfusion (Paris)*. 2004;44(12):1683–1688.

54. Porretti L, Cattaneo A, Coluccio E, et al. Implementation and outcomes of a transfusion-related acute lung injury surveillance programme and study of HLA/HNA alloimmunization in blood donors. *Blood Transfus*. 2012;10: 351–359.

55. Fadeyi E, Adams S, Sheldon S, et al. A preliminary comparison of the prevalence of transfusion reactions in recipients of platelet components from donors with and without human leukocyte antibodies. *Vox Sang*. 2008; 94:324–328.

56. Zupanaska B, Uhrynoowska M, Michur H, Maslanka K, Zajko M. Transfusion-related acute lung injury and leukocyte-reacting antibodies. *Vox Sang*. 2007;93:70–77.

57. Funk MB, Guenay S, Lohmann A, et al. Benefit of transfusion-related acute lung injury risk-minimization measures — German haemovigilance data (2006–2010). *Vox Sang*. 2012;102(4):317–323.

58. Sachs U, Link E, Hofmann C, Wasel W, Bein G. Screening of multiparous wommen to avoid transfusion-related acute lung injury: a single centre experience. *Transfus Med*. 2008;18:348–354.

59. Reil A, Keller-Stanislawski B, Gunay S, Bux J. Specificities of leukocyte alloantibodies in transfusion-related acute lung injury and results of leukocyte antibody screening of blood donors. *Vox Sang*. 2008;95:313–317.

60. Silliman CC, Bercovitz RS, Khan SY, et al. Antibodies to the HLA-A2 antigen prime neutrophils and serve as the second event in an in vitro model of transfusion-related acute lung injury. *Vox Sang*. 2014;107(1):76–82.

61. Khoy K, Nguyen MVC, Masson D, Bardy B, Drouet C, Paclet M-H. Transfusion-related acute lung injury: critical neutrophil activation by anti-HLA-A2 antibodies for endothelial permeability. *Transfusion (Paris)*. 2017; 57(7):1699–1708.

62. Gosselin EJ, Wardwell K, Rigby WF, Guyre PM. Induction of MHC class II on human polymorphonuclear neutrophils by granulocyte/macrophage colony-stimulating factor, IFN-gamma, and IL-3. *J Immunol Baltim Md 1950*. 1993;151(3):1482–1490.

63. Yomtovian R, Press C, Engman H, et al. Severe pulmonary hypersensitivity associated with passive transfusion of a neutrophil-specific antibody. *The Lancet*. 1984; 323(8371):244–246.

64. Nordhagen R, Conradi M, Drömtorp SM. Pulmonary reaction associated with transfusion of plasma containing anti-5b. *Vox Sang*. 1986;51(2):102–107.

65. Schubert N, Berthold T, Muschter S, et al. Human neutrophil antigen-3a antibodies induce neutrophil aggregation in a plasma-free medium. *Blood Transfus Trasfus Sangue*. 2013;11(4):541–547.

66. Sachs UJH, Hattar K, Weissmann N, et al. Antibody-induced neutrophil activation as a trigger for transfusion-related acute lung injury in an ex vivo rat lung model. *Blood*. 2006;107(3):1217–1219.

67. Loosli CG, Baker RF. Acute experimental pneumococcal (type I) pneumonia in the mouse: the migration of leucocytes from the pulmonary capillaries into the alveolar spaces as revealed by the electron microscope. *Trans Am Clin Climatol Assoc*. 1962;74:15–28.

68. Lee WL, Downey GP. Leukocyte elastase: physiological functions and role in acute lung injury. *Am J Respir Crit Care Med*. 2001;164(5):896–904.

69. Burns A, Smith C, Walker D. Unique structural features that influence neutrophil emigration into the lung. *Physiol Rev*. 2003;83:309–336.

70. Gee MH, Albertine KH. Neutrophil-endothelial cell interactions in the lung. *Annu Rev Physiol*. 1993;55(1): 227–248.

71. Drost EM, Kassabain G, Meiselman HJ, Gelmont D, Fisher TC. Increased rigidity and priming of polymorphonuclear leukocytes in sepsis. *Am J Respir Crit Care Med*. 1999;159(6):1696–1702.

72. Gebb SA, Graham JA, Hanger CC, et al. Sites of leukocyte sequestration in the pulmonary microcirculation. *J Appl Physiol Bethesda Md 1985*. 1995;79(2):493–497.

73. Guthrie LA, McPhail LC, Henson PM, Johnston RBJ. Priming of neutrophils for enhanced release of oxygen metabolites by bacterial lipopolysaccharide. Evidence for increased activity of the superoxide-producing enzyme. *J Exp Med*. 1984;160(6):1656–1671.

74. Silliman CC, Paterson AJ, Dickey WO, et al. The association of biologically active lipids with the development of transfusion-related acute lung injury: a retrospective study. *Transfusion (Paris)*. 1997;37(7):719–726.

75. Ichinose Y, Hara N, Ohta M, et al. Recombinant granulocyte colony-stimulating factor and lipopolysaccharide maintain the phenotype of and superoxide anion generation by neutrophils. *Infect Immun*. 1990;58(6):1647–1652.

76. Dykes A, Smallwood D, Kotsimbos T, Street A. Transfusion-related acute lung injury (TRALI) in a patient with a single lung transplant. *Br J Haematol*. 2000;109(3): 674–676.

77. Sachs U, Wasel W, Bayat E, et al. Mechanism of transfusion-related acute lung injury induced by HLA class II antibodies. *Blood*. 2011;117(2):669–677.

78. Ware LB, Matthay MA. Clinical practice, acute pulmonary edema. *N Engl J Med*. 2005;353(26):2788–2796.

79. McCullough J, Clay M, Hurd D, Richards K, Ludvigsen C, Forstrom L. Effect of leukocyte antibodies and HLA matching on the intravascular recovery, survival, and tissue localization of 111-indium granulocytes. *Blood*. 1986; 67(2):522–528.

80. Silliman CC, Voelkel NF, Allard JD, et al. Plasma and lipids from stored packed red blood cells cause acute lung injury in an animal model. *J Clin Investig*. 1998; 101(7):1458–1467.

81. Silliman CC, Thurman GW, Ambruso DR. Stored blood components contain agents that prime the neutrophil NADPH oxidase through the platelet-activating-factor receptor. *Vox Sang*. 1992;63(2):133–136.

82. Peters AL, van Hezel ME, Cortjens B, et al. Transfusion of 35-day stored RBCs in the presence of endotoxemia does not result in lung injury in humans. *Crit Care Med*. 2016; 44(6):e412–419.

83. Peters AL, Vervaart MAT, van Bruggen R, et al. Non-polar lipids accumulate during storage of transfusion products and do not contribute to the onset of transfusion-related acute lung injury. *Vox Sang.* 2017;112(1):25–32.

84. Land WG. Transfusion-related acute lung injury: the work of DAMPs. *Transfus Med Hemotherapy Off Organ Dtsch Ges Transfusionsmedizin Immunhamatologie.* 2013;40(1):3–13.

85. Thomas GM, Carbo C, Curtis BR, et al. Extracellular DNA traps are associated with the pathogenesis of TRALI in humans and mice. *Blood.* 2012;119(26):6335–6343.

86. Caudrillier A, Kessenbrock K, Gilliss BM, et al. Platelets induce neutrophil extracellular traps in transfusion-related acute lung injury. *J Clin Investig.* 2012;122(7):2661–2671.

87. Kapur R, Kim M, Rebetz J, Rondina MT, Porcelijn L, Semple JW. Low levels of interleukin-10 in patients with transfusion-related acute lung injury. *Ann Transl Med.* 2017;5(16). http://atm.amegroups.com/article/view/14882.

88. Carcano C, Okafor N, Martinez F, Ramirez J, Kanne J, Kirsch J. Radiographic manifestations of transfusion-related acute lung injury. *Clin Imaging.* 2013;37(6):1020–1023.

89. Felbo M, Jensen KG. Death in childbirth following transfusion of leukocyte-incompatible blood. *Acta Haematol.* 1962;27(2):113–119.

90. Dry SM, Bechard KM, Milford EL, Hallowell Churchill W, Benjamin RJ. The pathology of transfusion-related acute lung injury. *Am J Clin Pathol.* 1999;112(2):216–221.

91. Nakagawa M, Toy P. Acute and transient decrease in neutrophil count in transfusion-related acute lung injury: cases at one hospital. *Transfusion (Paris).* 2004;44(12):1689–1694.

92. Zhou L, Giacherio D, Cooling L, Davenport RD. Use of B-natriuretic peptide as a diagnostic marker in the differential diagnosis of transfusion-associated circulatory overload. *Transfusion (Paris).* 2005;45(7):1056–1063.

93. Yost CS, Matthay MA, Gropper MA. Etiology of acute pulmonary edema during liver transplantation: a series of cases with analysis of the edema fluid. *Chest Chic.* 2001;119(1):219–223.

94. Levy GJ, Shabot MM, Hart ME, Mya WW, Goldfinger D. Transfusion-associated noncardiogenic pulmonary edema. *Transfusion (Paris).* 1986;26(3):278–281.

95. Bernard GR, Luce JM, Sprung CL, et al. High-dose corticosteroids in patients with the adult respiratory distress syndrome. *N Engl J Med.* 1987;317(25):1565–1570.

96. Steinberg K, Hudson L, Goodman R. Efficacy and safety of corticosteroids for persistent acute respiratory distress syndrome. *N Engl J Med Boston.* 2006;354(16):1671–1684.

97. Djalali AG, Moore KA, Kelly E. Report of a patient with severe transfusion-related acute lung injury after multiple transfusions, resuscitated with albumin. *Resuscitation.* 2005;66(2):225–230.

98. Nouraei SM, Wallis JP, Bolton D, Hasan A. Management of transfusion-related acute lung injury with extracorporeal cardiopulmonary support in a four-year-old child. *Br J Anaesth.* 2003;91(2):292–294.

99. Kuijpers R, Dooren M, Ouwehand W, Verhoeven A, von dem Borne AK. Adult respiratory distress syndrome after experimental intravenous γ-globulin concentrate and monocyte-reactive IgG antibodies. *The Lancet.* 1998;352(9140):1601–1602.

100. Kapur R, Kim M, Aslam R, et al. T regulatory cells and dendritic cells protect against transfusion-related acute lung injury via IL-10. *Blood.* 2017;129(18):2557–2569.

101. Semple JW, McVey MJ, Kim M, Rebetz J, Kuebler WM, Kapur R. Targeting transfusion-related acute lung injury: the journey from basic science to novel therapies. *Crit Care Med.* 2018;46(5):e452.

102. Kapur R, Kim M, Rondina MT, Porcelijn L, Semple JW. Elevation of C-reactive protein levels in patients with transfusion-related acute lung injury. *Oncotarget.* 2016;7(47):78048–78054.

103. Otrock ZK, Liu C, Grossman BJ. Transfusion-related acute lung injury risk mitigation: an update. *Vox Sang.* 2017;112(8):694–703.

104. Eder AF, Herron R, Strupp A, et al. Transfusion-related acute lung injury surveillance (2003–2005) and the potential impact of the selective use of plasma from male donors in the American Red Cross. *Transfusion (Paris).* 2007;47(4):599–607.

105. Payne R, Tripp M. The development and persistence of leukoagglutinins in parous women. *Blood.* 1962;19(4):411–424.

106. Densmore TL, Goodnough LT, Ali S, Dynis M, Chaplin H. Prevalence of HLA sensitization in female apheresis donors. *Transfusion (Paris).* 1999;39(1):103–106.

107. Chapman CE, Stainsby D, Jones H, et al. Ten years of hemovigilance reports of transfusion-related acute lung injury in the United Kingdom and the impact of preferential use of male donor plasma. *Transfusion (Paris).* 2009;49(3):440–452.

108. Wiersum-Osselton JC, Middelburg RA, Beckers EAM, et al. Male-only fresh-frozen plasma for transfusion-related acute lung injury prevention: before-and-after comparative cohort study. *Transfusion (Paris).* 2011;51(6):1278–1283.

109. Lin Y, Saw C-L, Hannach B, Goldman M. Transfusion-related acute lung injury prevention measures and their impact at Canadian Blood Services. *Transfusion (Paris).* 2012;52(3):567–574.

110. Kopko P, Silva M, Shulman I, Kleinman S. AABB survey of transfusion-related acute lung injury policies and practices in the United States. *Transfusion (Paris).* 2007;47(9):1679–1685.

111. Kleinman S, Grossman B, Kopko P. A national survey of transfusion-related acute lung injury risk reduction policies for platelets and plasma in the United States. *Transfusion (Paris).* 2010;50(6):1312–1321.

112. AABB Standard 5.4.2.1. *Standards for Blood Banks and Transfusion Services.* 24th ed. Bethesda, MD: AABB; 2016.

113. Strong M, Lipton K. AABB Association Bulletin #06–07: Transfusion-Related Acute Lung Injury.; 2006. www.bpro.or.jp/publication/pdf_jptrans/us/us200611en.pdf.; http://

www.aabb.org/programs/publications/bulletins/Docs/ab0 6-07.pdf. Accessed October 18, 2018.

114. Connor J, Lipton K. *AABB Association Bulletin #07-03 Clarifications to Recommendations to Reduce the Risk of TRALI*; 2007. http://www.aabb.org/programs/publications/bulletins/Pages/ab07-03.a spx.

115. Yazer MH, Cap AP, Spinella PC, Alarcon L, Triulzi DJ. How do I implement a whole blood program for massively bleeding patients? *Transfusion (Paris)*. 2018; 58(3):622−628.

116. Nguyen XD, Dengler T, Schulz-Linkholt M, Klüter H. A novel tool for high-throughput screening of granulocyte-specific antibodies using the automated flow cytometric granulocyte immunofluorescence test (Flow-GIFT). *ScientificWorldJournal*. 2011;11:302−309.

117. Müller MC, Juffermans NP. Transfusion-related acute lung injury: a preventable syndrome? *Expert Rev Hematol*. 2012;5(1):97−106.

118. Fung M, Eder A, Spitalnik S, Westhoff C, eds. *AABB Technical Manual*. 19th ed. Bethesda, MD: AABB; 2017.

119. Mintz PD, Lipton KS. *AABB Association Bulletin #05-09 Transfusion-Related Acute Lung Injury*; 2005. http://www.aabb.org/programs/publications/bulletins/Documents/ab05-9.pdf.

120. Sher G, Markowitz MA. *AABB Association Bulletin #14-02: TRALI Risk Mitigation for Plasma and Whole Blood for Allogeneic Transfusion*; 2014. https://www.aabb.org/programs/publications/bulletins/Documents/ab14-02.pdf.

121. Goldberg AD, Kor DJ. State of the art management of transfusion-related acute lung injury (TRALI). *Curr Pharmaceut Des*. 2012;18(22):3273−3284.

122. Quillen K, Medrano C, Adams S, et al. Screening platelet-pheresis donors for HLA antibodies on two high-throughput platforms and correlation with recipient outcome. *Transfusion (Paris)*. 2011;51(3):504−510.

123. Dzik WH. The James Blundell Award Lecture 2006: transfusion and the treatment of haemorrhage: past, present and future. *Transfus Med*. 2007;17(5): 367−374.

124. Wallis JP, Dzik S. Is fresh frozen plasma overtransfused in the United States? *Transfusion (Paris)*. 2004;44(11): 1674−1675.

125. Rajbhandary S, Whitaker B, Perez G. *The 2014-2015 AABB Blood Collection and Utilization Survey Report*; 2018. http://www.aabb.org/research/hemovigilance/bloodsurvey/Docs/2014-2015-AABB-Blood-Survey-Report.pdf.

126. Janssen MP, van Tilborgh AJW, de Vooght KMK, Bokhorst AG, Wiersum-Osselton JC. Direct costs of transfusion reactions − an expert judgement approach. *Vox Sang*. 2018;113(2):143−151.

127. Lieberman L, Petraszko T, Yi Q, Hannach B, Skeate R. Transfusion-related lung injury in children: a case series and review of the literature. *Transfusion (Paris)*. 2014; 54(1):57−64.

128. Sanchez R, Toy P. Transfusion related acute lung injury: a pediatric perspective. *Pediatr Blood Canc*. 2005;45(3): 248−255.

129. Gupta S, Som T, Iyer L, Agarwal R. Transfusion related acute lung injury in a neonate. *Indian J Pediatr*. 2012; 79(10):1363−1365.

130. Kelly AM, Williamson LM. Neonatal transfusion. *Early Hum Dev*. 2013;89(11):855−860.

CHAPTER 8

Alloantibodies and Platelets

GEOFFREY D. WOOL, MD, PHD • NICHOLAS BROWN, PHD

INTRODUCTION

Platelets are small (2–4 μm) anucleate corpuscles, representing ~0.25% of the total blood volume,[1,2] which are vitally important for hemostasis. Platelets interact with subendothelial collagen in damaged vessels to form the initial platelet plug (in complex with von Willebrand factor), and are a surface for the development of the fibrin clot. The formation of the platelet plug involves a complex choreography of platelet adhesion, activation, signaling, shape change, degranulation, and aggregation. Platelets express numerous surface proteins and glycoproteins involved in adhesion and signaling.

Circulating platelet counts are maintained in a range that provides a surfeit of platelets for control of endothelial damage. In the setting of thrombocytopenia, the degree of bleeding relative to the severity of the injury worsens. Thrombocytopenia of sufficient severity (generally believed to be platelet counts below 10×10^9/L for otherwise hemostatically intact patients) can predispose to spontaneous severe bleeding.

In addition to their role in hemostasis, platelets play a role in inflammation and in immune modulation. Platelet activation induces the expression of CD40L, which can lead to the recruitment of leukocytes to the site of injury by inducing endothelial cells to secrete chemokines and to express adhesion molecules.[3,4] In a mouse model, transfused platelets stimulate IFN-γ release from NK cells, and, through a nitric oxide-dependent pathway, stimulate humoral immunity.[5] Platelets can also express additional T-cell costimulatory and adhesion molecules associated with antigen presenting cells: CD44, ICAM-2, and DC-SIGN.[6]

Platelets express proteins and glycoproteins that are involved with several antigenic systems: ABO blood group antigens, human leukocyte antigen (HLA), and human platelet antigen (HPA). The human platelet antigen (HPA) system involves a series of immunogenic polymorphisms found mostly on platelet glycoproteins. Platelets also express human leukocyte antigen (HLA) class I molecules. The HLA system is involved with presentation of self and foreign peptides for cellular immune surveillance, activation, and regulation. In the setting of infection or thrombin activation, platelets can present antigen via HLA class I and stimulate naïve T-cell responses.[6]

The HLA system includes the most polymorphic genes in humans, with several thousand alleles encoding for functional surface proteins. This high level of polymorphism and heterozygosity allow the immune system to sample and defend against a diversity of microorganisms and antigens.[7] However, extreme polymorphism increases the possibility of alloimmunization upon exposure to foreign HLA, such as in the setting of transfusion, pregnancy, or transplantation. Exposure to foreign HLA epitopes is a potent immune stimulus, with frequent development of adaptive humoral and cellular immunity to the foreign HLA.

Antibody-mediated platelet clearance involves opsonization of platelets by antibodies, recognition of opsonized platelets by macrophage Fc-receptors, and phagocytosis.[8] Autoimmune disorders involving platelets, namely immune thrombocytopenic purpura and drug-induced immune thrombocytopenia, are important bleeding disorders characterized by antibodies directed toward endogenous platelet antigens, native or drug-modified, respectively.[9,10] However, this chapter will focus on alloimmune thrombocytopenias. Alloimmune thrombocytopenia involves alloantibody-mediated platelet depletion and occurs in several settings. We will provide a general review of the following disorders while also highlighting their pathophysiology and underlying immune mechanisms:

- Alloimmune platelet transfusion refractoriness
- Transplantation-associated alloimmune thrombocytopenia
- Fetal/neonatal alloimmune thrombocytopenia (FNAIT)
- Posttransfusion purpura (PTP)
- Passive alloimmune thrombocytopenia

HLA STRUCTURE AND FUNCTION

The HLA complex is found on the short arm of chromosome 6, and is genetically dense, encoding hundreds of protein-coding genes; refer to Fig. 8.1 for illustrations of the molecules discussed in this section. Among these are loci encoding for the major histocompatibility complex (MHC), otherwise known as the "classical HLA" genes. These HLA loci encode transmembrane proteins that form extracellular heterodimers. The class I HLA molecules are encoded by the HLA-A, B, and C loci, and each protein combines with β2-microglobulin, a conserved protein encoded outside of the HLA complex, to form a functional HLA-A, B, or C heterodimer. The class II heterodimers, on the other hand, are each encoded by two loci in the HLA complex: DRA and DRB, DQA1 and DQB1, and DPB1 and DPA1, which form the HLA-DR, DQ, and DP loci, respectively.

The main function of the HLA heterodimers, hereafter called as "HLA molecules," is to present peptide antigens to T cells. Class I HLA molecules are expressed on nearly all cells, and obtain their peptide antigens from the proteasome. As such, class I HLA molecules sample intracellular proteins, and present to CD8[+] cytotoxic T cells. Class II HLA molecules are expressed on a subset of immune cells known as antigen-presenting cells, including macrophages, dendritic cells, and B cells. Class II molecules bind peptides derived from phagosomes, presenting extracellularly derived antigens to CD4[+] helper T cells. In all cases, recognition of a peptide antigen by a T-cell results in some form of T-cell response, either activating or inhibitory. Therefore, HLA acts as the channel through which antigen-dependent T-cell responses are controlled.

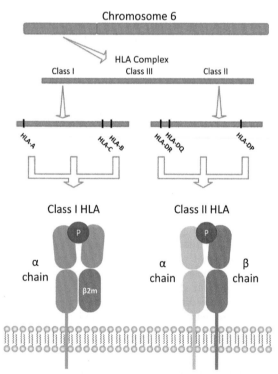

FIG. 8.1 The HLA complex and the classical HLA molecules. The HLA complex is located on the short arm of chromosome 6, and encodes for the classical HLA genes, which are found in the class I and class II regions. The class I HLA loci encode for proteins that bind to β2-microglobulin (β2m) to form a stable heterodimer, while the class II HLA loci encode for separate α- and β-chains. All HLA molecules present peptide antigens (P) in their distal, antigen-biding domain.

HLA EXPRESSION ON PLATELETS

Platelets, being derived from nonantigen presenting cells (namely megakaryocytes), express only class I HLA molecules. In addition to endogenously expressed HLA,[11] platelets also have a significant amount of HLA molecules that appear to be absorbed from circulating, soluble HLA proteins.[12,13] Each platelet expresses 1000–100,000 class I HLA molecules, with HLA-C being weakly expressed, compared to HLA-A or HLA-B.[12,14–16] Platelets express 73% of the whole blood load of class I HLA-A and HLA-B antigen.[17]

HLA DIVERSITY

During evolution, there has been selective pressure to generate immense polymorphism in the HLA loci. This is presumably due to the fact that different HLA alleles are capable of presenting different sets of peptide antigens, thereby ensuring that in a population with significant HLA diversity, HLA alleles will exist that can recognize and respond to nearly any infectious microorganism.[18] This has resulted in the HLA loci having the greatest polymorphism in the human genome, with the class I HLA locus *HLA-B* being the most polymorphic human gene.[19] Indeed, the immunogenetics community has recently coined the term "hyperpolymorphic" to describe the HLA loci's diversity, with over 20,000 alleles characterized as of September 2018, with new alleles continually being discovered.[20] This results in a very high likelihood that any two individuals in a population will express different HLA antigens.

The fact that humans express a wide range of different HLA is immunologically significant. The leading theory of the immune system posits that evolution has created a system that recognizes "self" from "nonself," with nonself being attacked. When applied to an infection with a virus, it is easy to see how it would be advantageous for the immune system to recognize viral antigens as foreign, so that an immune response can be mounted to clear the infection. However, exposure to HLA from another individual can also represent an immunizing event, and the diversity of the HLA system means that these events will often result in an immune response to the "foreign" HLA antigens. Most germane to this text, immunization with foreign HLA antigens, also known as sensitization or alloimmunization, results in production of IgG antibodies. As will be discussed later, these antibodies can bind, opsonize, and lead to the removal of platelets from the blood system. Although the frequency of HLA sensitizing events is not as great as the frequency of infection, it is not uncommon: transfusion, pregnancy, and transplantation can each expose an individual to foreign HLA antigens. Although sensitization rates differ between studied populations, a consensus is that transfusion has the lowest rate of HLA sensitization, pregnancy has a higher rate, and transplantation is the most likely to result in HLA antibodies.[21–24]

HLA ALLOIMMUNIZATION

Blood product transfusion can lead to HLA sensitization, as blood donors frequently express HLA antigens foreign to the recipient. HLA molecules are expressed poorly on erythrocytes, while platelets and lymphocytes express roughly 50,000–100,000 class I HLA molecules per cell, with the smaller size of platelets giving them the greatest density of HLA.[12] Nevertheless, the contamination of blood components by white blood cells (WBCs) is the main cause of HLA alloimmunization by transfusion, evidenced by the significant reduction in alloimmunization after transfusion with leukoreduced platelets.[25] WBCs are thought to be superior immunizers due to their expression of inflammatory and costimulatory molecules.[26]

Certain patient populations appear to be at higher risk of transfusion-related HLA alloimmunization. HLA antibodies have been identified in 30%–50% of multitransfused patients,[27] while Laundy and colleagues showed 62% of a population of aplastic anemia patients had detectable HLA antibodies.[26] However, a classic study reported no dose–response relationship existed between platelet transfusion and alloimmunization.[28] As with all immune responses, HLA antibodies take time to appear after sensitizing events, typically within 8 weeks after initial transfusion exposure.[29] A hallmark of the adaptive immune system is memory, such that an anamnestic reappearance of anti-HLA antibodies can occur as quickly as 4 days after reexposure.[30,31] Both purified RBC and platelets have the capacity to reactivate antibody production to HLA in previously sensitized recipients,[26] even though they are not efficient immunizers of a primary immune response.

Pregnancy represents a common, and the arguably only "natural," sensitizing event for HLA antigens. During pregnancy and delivery, the mother is exposed to paternally derived HLA expressed by the fetus, which can induce a maternal immune response to the foreign HLA. Not all pregnancies result in an anti-HLA immune response, however. The prevalence of HLA antibodies (class I or II) in NIH plateletpheresis donors was 17% in female donors without pregnancy or transfusion history and 47% in female donors with such history.[32] The REDS study detected HLA antibodies in 17% of all female blood donors and in 24% of female blood donors with a previous pregnancy.[33] In the Trial to Reduce Alloimmunization to Platelets (TRAP) study, the incidence of HLA alloimmunization in female patients was increased 3.5-fold by a prior history of pregnancy.[25]

HLA antibody prevalence increases with number of pregnancies: 1.7% (0 pregnancies), 11.2% (1), 22.5% (2), 27.5% (3), and 32.2% (≥4).[33] At UChicago Medicine, approximately 42% of previously pregnant females, tested to comply with AABB standards for female blood donors, have detectable HLA antibodies (unpublished results). To answer why some women develop HLA antibodies and some do not, a recent genome-wide association study probed for genetic markers associated with development of HLA antibodies and identified a few candidates with unclear involvement in the immune system.[34] Clearly, alloimmunization is a complex event, and requires further study.

Along with transfusion and pregnancy, transplantation represents the last major sensitizing event for HLA, and the most likely to result in HLA antibodies.[21–24] This is presumably due to the extended exposure of a transplant recipient to an allograft, compared to the transient nature of transfusion and pregnancy. In much the same way that HLA antibodies are a cause of platelet refractoriness, HLA sensitization is a major barrier to organ transplantation.[35] Indeed, the body of knowledge of HLA antibodies has largely come from the transplant immunology community.

TECHNIQUES OF HLA TYPING AND ANTIBODY IDENTIFICATION

The assays used to detect HLA antibodies for platelet-refractory patients were developed for, and used extensively in, the transplant immunology field. Starting in the 1960s, HLA antibodies were detected with cell-based assays, where a patient's serum was incubated with a panel of cells, complement was added, and cells were observed under a microscope for cytotoxicity.[36] These complement-dependent cytotoxicity (CDC) assays are still in use today, but have been eclipsed by so-called "solid-phase" assays, where purified HLA antigens are fixed to a solid substrate, either an ELISA microplate or fluorescent microbeads, and patient antibody binding is detected by labeled antihuman antisera[37] (see Fig. 8.2 for diagrams of the assays discussed in this section). Assays exist that can be run on an ELISA plate reader, a standard flow cytometer, or a Luminex instrument, a specialized flow cytometer that can distinguish 100 or more differentially labeled microbeads.[37] The assays also range from being able to only detect the presence or absence of HLA antibodies, to providing an estimation of the sensitization of a patient to the general population. This estimation is known as the panel-reactive antibody (PRA), and is often used synonymously with HLA antibody testing. The PRA is useful to determine the likelihood that a patient will be able to find a compatible platelet donor; a patient with a PRA of 80% would be expected to only obtain matched donor platelets from the 20% of the population to which they do not have HLA antibodies.

In addition to percent PRA, solid-phase HLA antibody assays are also able to report the specific HLA antigens to which a patient has antibodies. The assay most useful for this is the single-antigen bead (SAB) assay, of which there are two commercially available kits. As the name implies, the SAB assays are multiplexed assays of roughly 100 different bead sets, with each set of beads is coated with a single HLA antigen. This allows for results that define which specific HLA antigens are targeted by

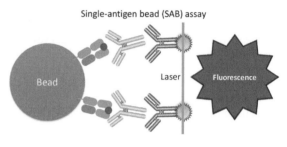

Complement-dependent cytotoxicity (CDC) assay

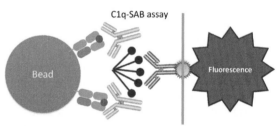

Single-antigen bead (SAB) assay

C1q-SAB assay

FIG. 8.2 HLA antibody assays. The complement-dependent cytotoxicity (CDC) assay involves incubation of patient antibodies with donor cells. Addition of complement leads to the death of any cells coated with HLA antibodies. The single-antigen bead (SAB) assay replaces donor cells with polystyrene beads coated with HLA antigens. HLA antibodies are detected with fluorochrome-labeled antihuman IgG antisera, which are detected by flow cytometry. The C1q-SAB assay replaces the anti-IgG antisera with anti-C1q antisera, so that only complement-fixing antibodies are detected.

the patient. An example result from such a test would be as follows: A2, A68, A69, B57, and B58. This would imply that the patient makes antibodies only to these HLA antigens, and so should be able to accept platelets from donors that do not express those antigens. Due to this fact, the SAB assays are the most widely used HLA antibody assays currently in use.

In addition to the fine specificity of the SAB assays, the solid-phase assays, as a group, are much more sensitive than the older CDC assays.[36] However, it is not clear that the increased sensitivity is clinically relevant.[38] Therefore, much work has been done to stratify the risk of HLA antibodies detected by the SAB assay.

One way is to use the mean fluorescence intensity (MFI) value for each detected HLA antibody. The MFI is a unitless measurement of the fluorescent signal detected by the Luminex instrument analyzing the SAB assay, and it is assumed that higher-titer antibodies result in higher MFI values.[39] However, MFI values can vary significantly between SAB assays, with one study demonstrating up to 20% variability in MFI values across labs, even when assays were rigorously standardized.[40] Very strong, or high-titer, antibodies can also appear weak or even negative on SAB assays, due to a complement-mediated interference in the assay, which is frequently called as the "prozone effect.[41]" Several methods have been reported to overcome this effect, and we and others have shown that treatment of patient serum with EDTA to inhibit complement activation is the most robust method.[42,43] There are, however, reports of rare samples for which EDTA treatment does not ameliorate the prozone effect, and in these cases, running dilutions of the patient sample is required to assess the true strength of the HLA antibodies.[44] Nevertheless, MFI is an easily available and, especially when used on EDTA-treated serum, useful value for stratifying HLA antibody risk. As such, it can be used to predict if a patient's HLA antibodies may cause platelet refractoriness, as donor specific antibody MFI negatively correlates with platelet transfusion responsiveness.[45]

To further stratify HLA antibody risk, methods to determine that antibodies are capable of fixing complement have been developed. The hypothesis here is twofold: (1) complement-fixing antibodies will be more immediately injurious to a target cell, be it a platelet or an endothelial cell and (2) complement-fixing antibodies will better correlate with the older, cell-based CDC assays. The most widely used of these assays is the C1q-SAB assay, which shows better correlation with the CDC assay than the normal SAB assay.[46] This assay was tested on platelet-refractory patients, where it was found to better predict HLA antibodies mediating platelet refractoriness.[47] This assay has subsequently been offered clinically, along with a similar test, the C3d-SAB assay (C3d is a cleavage product further down the complement cascade than C1q).[48] Many studies have been performed in the transplant setting using these assays, with the consensus that complement-fixing HLA antibodies are higher risk, compared to C1q- or C3d-negative antibodies.[49] It is important to note, however, that the C1q or C3d assays only measure the ability of an antibody to fix complement in vitro, on an HLA-coated polystyrene bead, and that results do not necessarily predict the ability of an antibody to mediate cell or platelet injury in vivo.[49] Indeed, it has been shown in several studies that the C1q and C3d assays are strongly correlated with MFI of the standard SAB assays,[50,51] suggesting that these assays simply define antibody "strength" in the SAB assay, instead of providing qualitative information on the complement-fixing ability of the antibody. Therefore, it seems that using an extra complement-fixing assay is superfluous when the same information can be gleaned from MFI values of a standard SAB assay using EDTA-treated serum.[49]

HLA TYPING AND TERMINOLOGY

As described earlier, the HLA complex contains the most polymorphic human genes. Due to this extreme variability, the nomenclature for HLA alleles is complex. Historically, HLA alleles were determined serologically, meaning that a panel of antibodies or antisera was incubated with patient cells in a CDC assay, and the resultant reaction was analyzed to determine that HLA proteins were expressed. This HLA typing was reported in "serologic" nomenclature (an example typing would be A2, A24; B8, B57), which, because it was based on detection by antibodies, directly corresponded to the terminology used for reporting HLA antibodies. This way, a patient with A68 HLA antibodies would be expected to react with platelets expressing A68. However, HLA laboratories have moved away from these serology-based typing assays, partly because regulations now require molecular typing for transplantation, and partly because the ability of the serologic assays to distinguish the alleles of the hyperpolymorphic HLA system reached its limit. Currently, therefore, nearly all HLA laboratories use molecular methods for HLA typing, with serologic HLA typing becoming increasingly rare.

Although the serologic nomenclature defines HLA proteins, the molecular nomenclature follows from methods to probe the DNA sequence of the HLA loci. As the genetic code is degenerate, and therefore different DNA sequences can encode for the same protein, a new nomenclature system was required for molecular typing.[52] The molecular nomenclature can be easily identified by the presence of an asterisk, which is not present in the serologic nomenclature. To use the example earlier, the A68 molecule can be encoded by A*68:01, A*68:02, or dozens of other A*68 alleles.[20] To complicate things further, not all molecular typing directly "translates" to serologic typing. For example, the B62 molecule is encoded by the B*15:01 allele. Therefore, when HLA is typed by molecular methods and serologic nomenclature is required, the alleles are translated to proteins using the "HLA dictionary.[53]" Whether typed directly from serologic methods or translated from molecular nomenclature, serologic HLA nomenclature is used in the matching of platelet products for sensitized patients.

APPROACH TO HLA MATCHING

Determining the need for HLA matching will be discussed in the Platelet transfusion refractoriness section. Here, we will provide background for the now somewhat historic serologic matching of platelet products.

When considering HLA antibodies binding to their cognate HLA antigens, it is important to remember that any particular antibody does not recognize the entire antigen, rather they recognize a smaller part of the protein. This site on an antigen is called an "epitope," and any given HLA antigen will have several epitopes that can potentially be bound by an antibody (refer to Fig. 8.3 for an example of epitopes expressed on HLA molecules). HLA diversity is partly generated by recombination between different alleles,[54] meaning that any given HLA molecule will likely share several epitopes with other HLA molecules. This leads to two hypotheses relevant to platelet matching: (1) any epitope that is not encoded by the patient can potentially be recognized as foreign by the patient, and may generate an antibody response, and (2) if a foreign HLA molecule shares epitope(s) with the HLA

molecules encoded by a patient, then the patient will not generate antibodies to those epitope(s), as they will be recognized as self.

These hypotheses lead to the conclusion that for HLA antibody-mediated platelet-refectory patients, to prevent further alloimmunization, the patients should not be administered any blood components that contain foreign HLA epitopes, as they could further sensitize the patient, making it increasingly difficult to find compatible donors. The ideal way to achieve this is to administer HLA-identical blood components, ensuring that the patient recognizes all donors as "self." This is, however, frequently challenging to achieve given the requirements for donor typing and platelet inventory; it is especially problematic for patients from racial/ethnic populations poorly represented in the donor pool. Another option is to administer donor components that are not HLA-matched to the individual, but rather contain HLA epitopes that are present in the patient (see Fig. 8.3 for an example). Unfortunately, different from HLA typing, which can make use of molecular methods to definitively determine a nucleic acid sequence, HLA epitopes are defined by amino acid configurations, which are generated by complex, three-dimensional protein folding patterns. As such, HLA epitopes are not yet completely defined. However, researchers have been attempting to characterize HLA epitopes for several decades. The first insight was that patient antisera

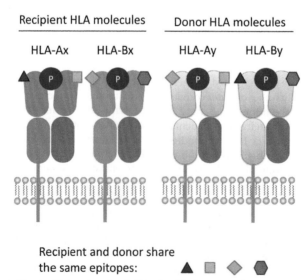

FIG. 8.3 Epitope matching for HLA molecules. In this simplified example, both recipient x and donor y encode one HLA-A and one HLA-B allele, and each molecule expresses two distinct epitopes. Although the recipient and donor do not express the same HLA molecules, they express the same epitopes. Therefore, all of the epitopes of the donor would be recognized as self by the patient.

TABLE 8.1
HLA-A and B CREGs.

CREG	Antigens Belonging to Group
1	A1, A3, A11, A29, A30, A31, A36, A80
2	A2, A9, A23, A24, A2403, A28, A68, A69, A203, A210, B17, B57, B58
5	B5, B15, B17, B18, B35, B46, B51, B5102, B5103, B52, B53, B57, B58, B53, B62, B63, B70, B71, B72, B75, B76, B77, B78
7	B7, B8, B703, B13, B22, B27, B2708, B40, B41, B42, B47, B48, B54, B55, B56, B60, B61, B73, B81
8	B8, B14, B16, B18, B38, B39, B3901, B3902, B59, B64, B65, B67
10	A11, A19, A25, A26, A28, A32, A33, A34, A66, A68, A69, A74
12	B12, B21, B37, B4005, B44, B45, B49, B50

Modified and updated from Rodey GE. HLA beyond Tears. 2nd ed. Durango, CO: De Novo; 2000.

frequently recognized multiple HLA antigens. It was inferred that these antibodies were recognizing epitopes shared by multiple HLA molecules, and these shared epitopes were termed "public" epitopes.[17,55] The HLA antigens sharing these public epitopes were called as cross-reactive epitope groups (CREGs) (see Table 8.1 for HLA-A and B CREGs). In other words, a CREG comprises antigens that all share a public epitope. Conversely, epitopes unique to a particular HLA molecule are considered "private." It was also observed that HLA antibodies were more frequently generated to public epitopes, and less frequently to private epitopes.[55,56] Therefore, in the absence of detailed HLA antibody information (as can be obtained from contemporary SAB assays), it was hypothesized that if an HLA matched donor was not available, a mismatched donor that expressed an HLA allele that was part of the same CREG as the patient would produce a superior posttransfusion response. Put another way, a foreign HLA antigen that was part of a patient's CREG group was less likely to be the target of patient antibodies, leading to better platelet responses and less chance of sensitization to the foreign HLA antigen. Indeed, Duquesnoy et al. demonstrated in 1977 that using an HLA matching schema based on CREGs (see Table 8.2 for a simplified version) resulted in postplatelet counts similar to fully HLA-matched donors, and superior to donors with a mismatch not part of the patient's CREGs. This strategy increased acceptable donors approximately 10-fold.[57]

To follow-up on this work, Rene Duquesnoy has attempted to define HLA epitopes as groups of amino acids expressed by the HLA proteins. He and his group have found that such epitopes are best described by "eplets," groups of three amino acids that are physically close together, within an approximately 3–3.5 Å radius, on the tertiary structure of HLA antigens.[59] Using software that attempts to define the eplets expressed by recipient and donors, multiple groups have shown that epitope matching can identify compatible platelet donors that would not be found with CREG-based matching[60,61] (Fig. 8.3 shows a simplified example of epitope matching). However, this matching is not yet ready for routine clinical use, as the program requires patient and donor HLA typing at a higher resolution than is often available for platelet-refractory work-ups. Nevertheless, HLA epitope definition is an active area of research, and the future will surely bring advances in platelet matching based on a better understanding of this complex subject.

THE HUMAN PLATELET ANTIGEN SYSTEM

In 1990, the Platelet Serology Working Party of the International Society of Blood Transfusion established a nomenclature for platelet antigens, defining the HPA system.[62]

The HPA system consists of a series of immunogenic polymorphisms on antigens mostly restricted to platelets. Although platelets express a wide variety of receptors and transporters on their surface, the HPA antigens are almost entirely present on platelet surface glycoproteins. These glycoproteins play crucial roles in platelet aggregation, adhesion, and clot formation.

TABLE 8.2
Serologic-Based HLA Matching.
HLA Typing That is Different in the Donor is Bolded.

Grade	Definition	Example
A	Matched at all four HLA-A and -B antigens	Recipient A2, A3; B7, B8 Donor A2, A3; B7, B8
BU	Matched at three HLA-A and -B antigens, the unmatched antigen in the recipient comes from an HLA locus that is homozygous in the donor (only three antigens detected in donor)	Recipient A2, A3; B7, B8 Donor A2, -; B7, B8
BX	Matched at three HLA-A and -B antigens, the unmatched antigen in the donor is within a CREG in the recipient	Recipient A2, A3; B7, B8 Donor A2, A3; B7, **B18**
C	Platelet product contains an HLA antigen that is not within a CREG in the recipient	Recipient A2, A3; B7, B8 Donor A2, **A25**; B7, B8
D	Platelet product contains two or more HLA antigens that are not within a CREG(s) in the recipient	Recipient A2, A3; B7, B8 Donor A2, **A25**; B7, **B37**
R	Random	

Except for R, these match grades are ideally used to describe units with no incompatible antibodies present in the recipient. Incompatible units should not be considered HLA matched.
Modified from Duquesnoy RJ, Filip DJ, Rodey GE, Rimm AA, Aster RH. Successful transfusion of platelets "mismatched" for HLA antigens to alloimmunized thrombocytopenic patients. Am J Hematol. 1977;2(3):219–226 and Forest SK, Hod EA. Management of the platelet refractory patient. Hematol Oncol Clin N Am. 2016;30(3):665–677.

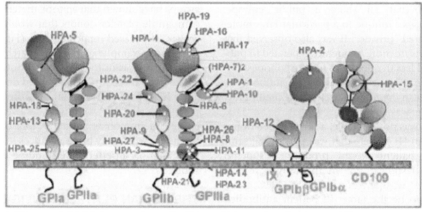

FIG. 8.4 Diagram of platelet glycoproteins and antigens with immunogenic epitopes. HPA epitopes mapped onto their sites on the platelet glycoproteins. HPA antigens are found on the extracellular surface of these glycoproteins on domains that are relatively solvent exposed. (From Brouk H, Ouelaa H. Fetal and neonatal alloimmune thrombocytopenia: advances in laboratory diagnosis and management. *Int J Blood Res Disord*. 2015;2.)

HPA epitopes are expressed on the following receptors[63] (Fig. 8.4):
- GPIIb/IIIa (αIIb/b3, CD41/CD61, fibrinogen receptor)
- GPIb-V-IX (CD42a-d, von Willebrand factor receptor)
- GPIa/IIa (a2/b1, CD49/CD29, collagen receptor)
- CD109

There are approximately 80,000 copies of gpIIbIIIa integrin and 25,000 copies of gpIbα on the surface of resting human platelets.[64] GpIbα and the IIb subunit

of the gpIIbIIIa integrin were previously believed to be expressed solely on platelets and their precursors, while the IIIa subunit of the gpIIbIIIa integrin is expressed on many other cell types such as endothelial cells and trophoblasts.[64,65] There are some reports of the IIb subunit of the gpIIbIIIa integrin being expressed on cells other than platelets.[64]

The HPA system has been numbered in order of antigen discovery. To date, 35 platelet-specific alloantigens

TABLE 8.3
Human Platelet Antigen (HPA) system.

System (If Applicable)	Antigen	Allele Frequencies (International Averages)	Glycoprotein/CD Name	Gene Name	Nucleotide Change	Mature Protein Position
HPA-1	HPA-1	a 87%, b 13%	GPIIIa (CD61)	ITGB3	176T > C	L33P
HPA-2	HPA-2	a 88%, b12%	GPIbα (CD42b)	GP1BA	482C > T	T145M
HPA-3	HPA-3	a 60%, b 40%	GPIIb (CD41)	ITGA2B	2621T > G	I843S
HPA-4	HPA-4	a >99%, b <1%	GPIIIa (CD61)	ITGB3	506G > A	R143Q
HPA-5	HPA-5	a 90%, b 10%	GPIa (CD49b)	ITGA2	1600G > A	E505K
	HPA-6w	Low frequency allele 1%	GPIIIa (CD61)	ITGB3	1544G > A	R489Q
	HPA-7w	Low frequency allele 1%	GPIIIa (CD61)	ITGB3	1297C > G	P407A
	HPA-8w	Low frequency allele <1%	GPIIIa (CD61)	ITGB3	1984C > T	R636C
	HPA-9w	Low frequency allele <1%	GPIIb (CD41)	ITGA2B	2602G > A	V837M
	HPA-10w	Low frequency allele <1%	GPIIIa (CD61)	ITGB3	263G > A	R62Q
	HPA-11w	Low frequency allele <1%	GPIIIa (CD61)	ITGB3	1976G > A	R633H
	HPA-12w	Low frequency allele <1%	GPIbb (CD42c)	GP1BB	119G > A	G15E
	HPA-13w	Low frequency allele <1%	GPIa (CD49b)	ITGA2	2483C > T	T799M
	HPA-14w	Low frequency allele 1%	GPIIIa (CD61)	ITGB3	1909_1911delAAG	K611del
HPA-15	HPA-15	a 54%, b 46%	CD109	CD109	2108C > A	S682Y
	HPA-16w	Low frequency allele <1%	GPIIIa (CD61)	ITGB3	497C > T	T140I
	HPA-17w	Low frequency allele <1%	GPIIIa (CD61)	ITGB3	662C > T	T195M
	HPA-18w	Low frequency allele <1%	GP1a (CD49b)	ITGA2	2235G > T	Q716H
	HPA-19w	Low frequency allele <1%	GPIIIa (CD61)	ITGB3	487A > C	K137Q
	HPA-20w	Low frequency allele <1%	GPIIb (CD41)	ITGA2B	1949C > T	T619M
	HPA-21w	Low frequency allele <1%	GPIIIa (CD61)	ITGB3	1960G > A	E628K
	HPA-22bw	Low frequency allele <1%[71]	GPIIb (CD41)	ITGA2B	584A > C	K164T
	HPA-23bw	Low frequency allele <1%[71]	GPIIIa (CD61)	ITGB3	1942C > T	R622W
	HPA-24bw	Low frequency allele <1%[72]	GPIIb (CD41)	ITGA2B	1508G > A	S472N
	HPA-25bw	Low frequency allele <1%[73]	GPIa (CD49b)	ITGA2	3347C > T	T1087M
	HPA-26bw	Low frequency allele <1%[74]	GPIIIa (CD61)	ITGB3	1818G > T	K580N
	HPA-27bw	Overall allelic frequency <1%. In Sub-Saharan African populations, allelic frequencies up to 8.2% are seen, as are individuals homozygous for the polymorphism[75]	GPIIb (CD41)	ITGA2B	2614C > A	L841M
	HPA-28bw	Low frequency allele <1%[76]	GPIIb (CD41)	ITGA2B	2311G > T	V740L
	HPA-29bw	Low frequency allele <1%[77]	GPIIIa (CD61)	ITGB3	98C > T	T7M

Note: For those antigens without alleles listed, no immunization against the unchanged amino acid sequence has been identified. Some FNAIT-associated glycoprotein variants have not yet been added to the EBI-IPD HPA database.[78–80]
Modified from European Bioinformatics Institute Immuno Polymorphism Database (EBI-IPD).[69] Allele frequencies based on averaged reported data to EBI-IPD as well as Refs[70–77].

have been defined by immune sera (Table 8.3). Six antithetical pairs of HPA antigens have been identified and are grouped together into six systems (HPA-1, -2, -3, -4, -5, and -15) with the higher frequency allele being designated with a lowercase "a" and the lower frequency allele being designated with a lowercase "b" (HPA-1a/1b, -2a/2b, -3a/3b, -4a/4b, -5a/5b, -15a/15b). Those 23 antigens for which alloantibodies against the thetical but not the antithetical antigen have been observed are distinguished with a "w" (workshop).[9,66] The thetical/antithetical HPA alleles differ by a single amino acid, except for HPA-14w, which is the result of a one amino acid deletion[67] (Table 8.3). An additional variant of HPA-1 (L33V) has been described as allele "c" with an allele frequency of <0.1%, but this allele variably binds anti-HPA-1a.[68]

HPA-1a and HPA-5b have been implicated in all alloimmune thrombocytopenia syndromes that will be discussed later; these two alloantigens are also implicated in most patients with FNAIT in Caucasian populations[81] (see specific discussion later). HPA-1a appears to be significantly more immunogenic than the HPA-1b antigen, as determined by the comparison of the alloimmunization rate to those antigens as compared to the expected exposure rate of susceptible individuals.[81]

HPAs are generally thought to be function-neutral and are most frequently localized to integrin gpIIbIIIa, specifically to the gpIIIa subunit (Table 8.3). Non-HPA-defining missense mutations in the β3 integrin cause Glanzmann thrombasthenia, a severe platelet function disorder. Glanzmann thrombasthenia mutations generally involve either integrin mutations that disrupt ligand binding function or integrin expression.[82,83] Why some amino acid substitutions cause glycoprotein dysfunction while others do not appear to be related to their location in the glycoprotein. The HPAs generally reside in extracellular positions on the protein surface separated from the ligand-binding site and do not play a role in the stabilization of the protein fold. These amino acid positions therefore appear to be function-neutral and lack evolutionary pressure for sequence conservation.[84] In contrast, those mutations affecting residues that are deeply buried within the fold of the protein or located near the active site, near the ligand-binding site, or at the interfaces with other protein domains are likely to alter the structure and negatively affect the protein function.

Mismatched donor/recipient or mother/fetus HPA antigens can cause alloantibody production. Up to 4.2% of previously pregnant female blood donors have detectable antiplatelet alloantibodies. Once formed, antiplatelet antibodies may persist for up to 30 years after the last pregnancy.[85] These alloantibodies can be associated with alloimmune thrombocytopenic disorders, as described later. The HPAs, though described as single amino acid substitutions, are frequently recognized by antibodies directed toward a larger epitope dependent on the intact tertiary structure of its domain.[78,84]

Different from the HPA, function-neutral platelet glycoprotein variants that do not cause an immune response exist.[84] Although HPA and these nonimmunizing variants are equally nonconserved evolutionarily, the nonimmunizing variants are less solvent-exposed. Therefore, the immunogenicity of platelet glycoprotein polymorphisms appears to be dependent mostly on the structural location of the variant residue.[84]

Finally, glycoprotein IV (CD36) deficiency occurs in 3%−7% of individuals of African or Asian ancestry. Such a deficiency is rare in Caucasians (<0.3%).[86] CD36 is a member of the class B scavenger receptor family of proteins expressed on platelets, red blood cells, endothelial cells, monocytes, and macrophages. As CD36 is expressed on multiple cells, it does not have HPA nomenclature,[64] but is included here for completeness of discussion. There are two types of CD36 deficiency: Type I, with a total absence of CD36 expression on both platelets and monocytes, and Type II, which lacks CD36 on platelets but not on monocytes. Type I CD36 loss can lead to anti-CD36 alloimmunization after transfusion of antigen-positive platelets or pregnancy.[87,88]

ANTI-HPA ANTIBODY DETECTION

Platelet serologic investigation can be challenging, with antibody identification sometimes being ambiguous, particularly in the setting of multiple antibodies. Experts in platelet serology typically recommend a multipronged investigation for platelet-specific antibodies, specifically using (1) an assay employing intact platelets, (2) a glycoprotein-specific assay (typically performed with platelet fragments or purified glycoproteins), and (3) HPA genotyping.[70]

Glycoprotein-specific assays are the most sensitive and specific for identifying the HPA specificity of alloantibodies. These assays involve capture of platelet glycoproteins by monoclonal antibodies, which exclude interference from non-HPA antibodies. Several glycoprotein-specific assays are available, with the monoclonal antibody-specific immobilization of platelet antigen (MAIPA) generally being considered the gold standard.[89] The advantage of the MAIPA is that antibody binding (both human and murine) to their respective antigen on the platelet membrane takes place while the antigen is in a native conformational state.[89] The MAIPA, described in 1987 by Kiefel et al. involves incubating intact washed platelets with patient serum, followed by addition of a mouse monoclonal antibody against the glycoprotein under investigation. Platelets are then lysed, and the supernatant is added to a microplate precoated with antimouse IgG. Any human antibodies bound to the glycoprotein are detected with an antihuman-IgG secondary antibody[67,90] (Fig. 8.5). The MAIPA relies on monoclonal antibodies, given the potential for false positivity when using polyclonal antisera for HPA that could be contaminated by antibodies to HLA class I antibodies. The MAIPA can be performed with a panel of fresh phenotyped platelets or with a panel of

cryopreserved platelets; transfected cell lines can also be used to perform the MAIPA, absent a well-characterized platelet donor cohort.[91]

An assay using intact platelets (such as flow cytometry) is useful to confirm the results of the glycoprotein-specific tests, as the process of platelet lysis with detergent used in those assays can interfere with detection of antibodies that target conformation-dependent epitopes.[70,86] Positive intact platelet assays are not specific for anti-HPA antibodies, however, as they can be indicative of HLA or HPA antibodies.[70]

Serological HPA phenotyping is limited by several factors, including the lack of available antisera to all HPA antigens as well as the inability to obtain adequate numbers of platelets from thrombocytopenic patients for typing. Therefore, while the MAIPA can be used for HPA phenotyping, patient HPA typing is often accomplished by genotyping. Accurate genotyping of patient HPA antigens provides critical confirmatory information when investigating HPA alloimmunization.[67]

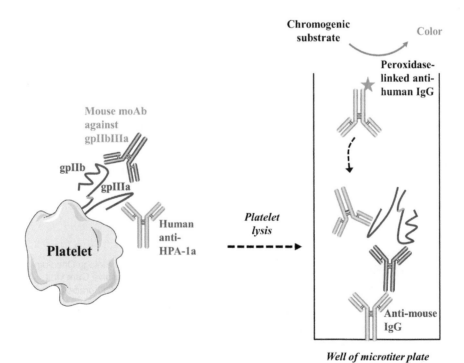

FIG. 8.5 Monoclonal antibody-specific immobilization of platelet antigen (MAIPA) technique. In this example, purified platelets are incubated with patient serum containing anti-HPA-1a and a mouse monoclonal antibody to gpIIbIIIa. After washing and detergent lysis, the glycoprotein—antibody complexes are captured in the microtiter well by an antimouse IgG antibody. The presence of anti-HPA antibodies is finally determined by the addition of a peroxidase-linked antihuman IgG secondary. (Modified from Metcalfe P. Platelet antigens and antibody detection. *Vox Sang.* 2004;87 (Suppl1):82—86.)

PLATELETS AND THE ABO ANTIGEN SYSTEM

Platelets express the ABH antigens of the ABO blood group system on their surface, on a mix of type 1 (extrinsic) and type 2 (intrinsic) chains.[92] The intrinsic ABH antigens are expressed on the platelet glycoproteins gpIb, IIa, IIb, and IIIa as well as the platelet endothelial cell adhesion molecule (PECAM-1, CD31).[16,93,94] On platelets and megakaryocytes, ABH antigen is expressed on a broad mixture of N-linked and complex O-linked structures. GPIIb/IIIa, the major carrier of N-linked glycan chains on platelets, possesses 11 N-linked glycan sites; ~5% of those glycan chains may terminate in ABH. Glycoprotein Ib, the major sialomucin on platelets, displays 3–4 N-linked and 50–60 O-linked glycans.[95]

Platelet donors show a spectrum of ABH antigen expression density and can be divided into those with low platelet ABH expression (<2000–6000 antigens/platelet, majority of population) and those with high expression (minority of population).[16,94,96,97] The presence of A and B antigens on platelets can be associated with incompatibilities due to isohemagglutinins (major incompatibility). Platelets from group A1 individuals express A antigen. However, platelets from group A2 individuals lack detectable A antigen expression in one report.[95]

Platelet products are collected in donor plasma (whole blood derived and standard plateletpheresis collection), or can be collected in a mixture of platelet additive solution (PAS) and donor plasma. Anti-A and -B isohemagglutinins are present in the donor plasma (potentially causing transfusion minor incompatibility), though clearly in lesser total amounts in platelet components collected in PAS.

PLATELET TRANSFUSION

The benefit of providing exogenous platelet support to thrombocytopenic patients was first described in 1910, with the use of fresh whole blood.[98] Platelet concentrates were developed in the late 1950s and played an important role in facilitating the development of induction chemotherapy for childhood lymphoblastic leukemia as well as other leukemias.[99,100] The goal of platelet transfusion in the setting of hypoproliferative thrombocytopenia is generally prophylactic, that is, to increase the platelet count and thereby reduce the risk of bleeding. In traumatic or operative bleeding, the goal is directly therapeutic: reduction or cessation of bleeding.[101] Modern oncologic therapies and hematopoietic stem cell transplantation are associated with severe hypoproliferative thrombocytopenia of longer durations than were historically seen,[58] and therefore require more extensive platelet transfusion support.

Platelet transfusions are now most commonly given for hypoproliferative thrombocytopenia (not acute bleeding) in the setting of chemotherapy, hematopoietic malignancy, or marrow failure (Fig. 8.6). This prophylactic usage has driven the increase in platelet transfusions over the last several decades, to reach 2.3 million platelet units transfused in the United States in 2013[102] (up from 0.92 million platelet doses transfused in the United States in 2004[103]).

Although all patients who receive red cell transfusion are screened for relevant antibodies to red cells beforehand, platelets are given without pretransfusion testing for platelet-specific incompatibility. Rather, a patient must merely have a confirmed ABO/Rh type and they can be provided with ABO/Rh compatible platelet components (or major or minor incompatible platelet

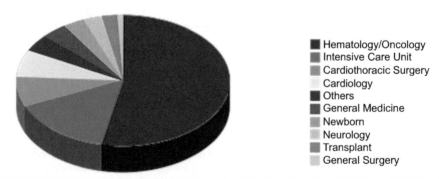

■ Hematology/Oncology
■ Intensive Care Unit
■ Cardiothoracic Surgery
  Cardiology
■ Others
■ General Medicine
■ Newborn
  Neurology
■ Transplant
  General Surgery

FIG. 8.6 Platelet transfusion at UChicago Medicine, by clinical service, from 7/2012–to 12/2015, showing most platelets going to hematology–oncology units.

components, in settings of inventory shortage). Only in the setting of inadequate response to platelet transfusion is a non-ABO platelet serologic investigation generally pursued.

PLATELET TRANSFUSION REFRACTORINESS

Reduction/cessation of bleeding is an important endpoint in hemorrhaging patients but is both rather subjective as well as polyfactorial, making it a challenging endpoint to accurately capture for platelet transfusion studies. Nevertheless, Salama et al. have used the PFA-100 device to measure the efficacy of platelet transfusion and found that those transfusions that normalized the PFA-100 closure time or caused >40 seconds shortening in closure time were associated with improved patient bleeding symptoms.[104]

Transfusion of platelets without achievement of an appropriate platelet count increment is the commonly used definition of platelet transfusion refractoriness. Platelet transfusion refractoriness represents an *inadequate* transfusion response to an *adequate* transfused dose. For that reason, platelet transfusions are often monitored using the corrected-count increment (CCI), which takes into account the recipient's size and the dose of transfused platelets

The units of CCI are 10^2 m^2 L^{-1}, but the parameter is

expected CCI is 13–16 (depending on platelet age).[108,109] Thrombocytopenic patients will always have lower CCI due to consumption of a fixed amount of transfused platelets for maintenance of endothelial integrity.[17,110] Refractoriness is often defined as CCI <7.5. Lower transfusion responses are expected in patients with significant splenomegaly or active bleeding, so a lower CCI trigger for diagnosis of transfusion refractoriness could reasonably be used for these patients.

CCI is best calculated based on 1-hour posttransfusion platelet counts, as alloimmune clearance of platelets typically occurs within 1 hour.[111–113] Clearance of platelets by other causes of transfusion refractoriness typically occur more slowly; 24-hour post-counts generally capture both immune and nonimmune clearance. 24-hour CCIs are typically approximately two-thirds of the 1-hour CCI value.[114] Patients with adequate 1-h CCI and inadequate 24-hour CCI generally have nonimmune causes of refractoriness[112] and matched platelets are typically not helpful.

A diagnosis of platelet transfusion refractoriness can be made after two inadequate platelet transfusion responses (1-hour CCI <7.5); many transfusion services require that these inadequate responses be consecutive. Of note, the TRAP study used the more stringent definition of platelet refractoriness as a 1-hour CCI of less than 5 on two sequential occasions, when using ABO

$$\text{corrected count increment (CCI)} = \frac{(\text{posttransfusion platelet count} - \text{pretransfusion platelet count}) \times \text{body surface area (BSA)}}{\text{transfused platelet dose}}$$

often treated as unitless.[17] The CCI is generally a smaller number than the absolute platelet increment. The CCI and other formulae for normalizing platelet response to recipient size and platelet dose have been criticized for being unsuitable for comparing the different platelet preparations as they are biased toward preparations with fewer platelets.[105] Therefore, CCI should not be used uncritically to compare different platelet preparations. However, for a standard modern US transfusion service that overwhelmingly provides platelet support as full plateletpheresis doses, the CCI is ideal to serially measure a patient's platelet responses.

The average CCI in a healthy subject using labeled autologous platelets is ~20.[106] In healthy volunteers transfused with radiolabeled platelets, 30%–40% of transfused platelets are sequestered by the spleen.[107] In hypoproliferative thrombocytopenia patients, the

compatible platelets.[25] Post-counts are often overlooked by busy clinical services. To increase the collection of post-counts, some have advocated the utility of a 10-minute post-count rather than a 1-hour post-count, as a 10-minute post-count is potentially more likely to be collected while clinical staff are bedside breaking down the platelet bag and tubing. However, some have found the 10-minute post-count to be inferior to the 1-hour post-count.[106]

The causes of platelet transfusion refractoriness are numerous (Table 8.4), but the mechanism is generally either increased consumption by active coagulation, increased splenic/reticuloendothelial clearance, or both. Increased splenic clearance of platelets can be caused by numerous etiologies, some of which are immune. The removal of immune incompatible platelets is mediated primarily by FcγR-mediated

TABLE 8.4
Causes of Platelet Refractoriness.[116]

		Examples
Nonimmune (>80% of cases)	Clinically significant bleeding	
	Splenomegaly	
	Medication (nonimmune)	Platelet-activating medications (heparin, amphotericin B)
	Febrile/infectious states	• Febrile neutropenia
		• Infection
		• Sepsis
	Consumptive coagulopathy	• Disseminated intravascular coagulation
		• Extracorporeal circuits (particularly when run without anticoagulant)
	Endothelial damage	• Veno-occlusive disease (VOD)
		• Stem cell transplant
		• Graft-versus-host disease (GvHD)
Immune (<20% of cases)	Medication (immune)	• Drug-dependent antibodies (quinidine, quinine, abciximab, eptifibatide, tirofiban, carbamazepine, sulfamethoxazole, vancomycin, others[117–119])
	Immune refractoriness	• Platelet autoantibodies (ITP)
		• Platelet alloantibodies (HLA, HPA)
		• Transfusion of ABO major mismatched platelets (typically only significant in the setting of other platelet-refractory risk factors)

macrophage clearance, predominantly in the spleen (Fig. 8.7). However, hepatocytes have been implicated in some particular immune thrombocytopenias.[115]

The etiology for an individual patient's transfusion refractoriness is frequently multifactorial and only a minority of cases are immune mediated. In any event, platelet transfusion refractoriness is associated with a threefold increased risk of bleeding[120] as well as doubled length of hospital admission and hospital cost.[121] Patients with platelet transfusion refractoriness also have lower survival in some studies.[120]

Alloimmune refractoriness is most commonly seen in patients with hematolymphoid malignancies,[27] with a female predominance due to prior alloimmunization by pregnancy. An analysis of transfusion data at a Canadian hospital before and after universal prestorage leukoreduction showed that the three independent factors that predicted alloimmune platelet transfusion refractoriness were the use of nonleukoreduced blood components (relative risk 2.2), a history of pregnancy and/or prior transfusion (RR 2.3), and receipt of 13 or more platelet transfusions (RR 6.0).[122] Patients with hematopoietic malignancies are more often affected by alloimmune refractoriness due to disease- and/or therapy-related severe thrombocytopenia, numerous transfusions, and frequent infectious complications.[123]

Slichter et al. showed that patients receiving numerous platelet transfusions have an incremental decrement in transfusion responsiveness, even in the absence of HLA antibodies.[111] Moreover, 25%–70% patients receiving multiple platelet transfusions will have at least one platelet transfusion with an inadequate response. Most of these patients will *not* meet criteria for alloimmune transfusion refractoriness.[120]

Splenomegaly is an important cause of thrombocytopenia and transfusion refractoriness. Although approximately one-third of a typical human's platelets are found in the spleen at any given time, in splenomegalic patients that number can increase to over 70%.[124]

ABO major incompatible platelet components are generally considered an acceptable product by most transfusion services, given the limitations of the platelet supply and expiration requirements.[125–130] In fact, ABO minor (plasma) incompatibility is often paid more attention to, given the frequent resulting positive direct antiglobulin test and possible hemolysis caused by transfusing ABO minor incompatible platelets.[131,132] ABO minor incompatible platelet transfusions have sometimes been found to cause worsened platelet transfusion response, presumably due to the formation of immune complexes that may bind onto the platelet surface and increase clearance.[133]

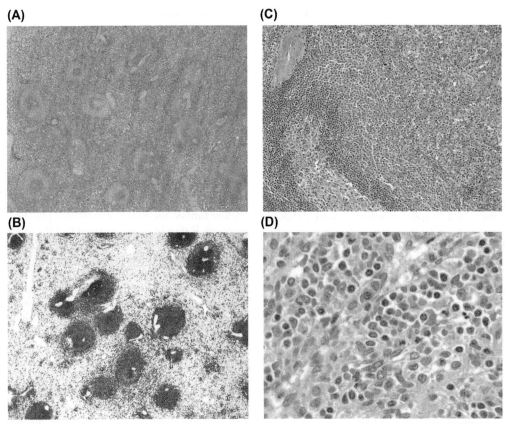

FIG. 8.7 Splenic findings in immune thrombocytopenia reflect humoral immune activation and antibody production, together with increased macrophage phagocytosis of platelets. **(A and B)** Expanded white pulp with follicular hyperplasia with increased CD20$^+$ B cells (seen in image B), **(C)** expanded marginal zones with plasmacytic differentiation, and **(D)** cords of Billroth contain increased plasma cells and debris-laden histiocytes, in addition to pigment deposition.

ABO major mismatched platelets are most commonly associated with clinical refractoriness in the setting of group A platelets transfused to group O patients, due to denser expression of the A antigen as well as higher mean recipient anti-A titers.[95] ABO major mismatched platelets show a 10%–35% decrement in platelet recovery (or CCI reduction of 6–15) compared to ABO matched platelets.[134–140] ABO major incompatible platelets can show deficits not only in CCI, but also in transfused platelet function: isohemagglutinin binding has been associated with worsened platelet response in aggregation testing.[141]The transfusion of ABO major incompatible platelets can lead to reactive subsequent increases in recipient isohemagglutinin titers, which correlates with worsened subsequent response to continued ABO major incompatible platelets.[142–144] In one randomized trial, ABO major

incompatible platelet transfusion was also associated with increased alloimmunization to HLA and HPA.[144]

For all these described reasons, an initial step in the support of platelet transfusion refractory patients is the provision of ABO matched (or at least ABO major matched) platelet components. Additionally, provision of fresher platelets (day 3 or earlier) also provides some benefit to functionally refractory patients, due to more rapid clearance of platelets activated during storage.[17,111,135] Fresher platelets cannot be provided to every patient, however, as transfusion services often first receive platelets from the supplier on day 3 and a significant proportion of platelet recipients are supported with day 4 and 5 platelets.

HLA antibodies are relatively commonly found, particularly, in previously pregnant women. Antibodies reacting with platelets (HLA and HPA) were seen in

45% of hematology-oncology patients.[145] It must be kept in mind, however, that the presence of antibodies is not diagnostic of refractoriness. In the TRAP study, 45% of the control group developed anti-HLA antibodies, but only 13% developed platelet refractoriness[25]; overall only 44% of patients with detectable HLA antibodies were truly refractory to platelet transfusion.[31] Therefore, alloimmunization is not synonymous with refractoriness; additional unknown modifying factors determine whether an alloantibody will cause refractoriness to transfusion.[58] This incomplete penetrance of immune refractoriness in the alloimmunized population means that the initial work-up of a patient with presumed platelet transfusion refractoriness by a hospital transfusion service should be to accurately document true refractoriness with platelet count increment investigation, rather than jumping straight to serologic investigation.

Once a truly refractory patient has been identified, they should be screened for relevant antibodies and, if screen positive, those antibodies should be identified. The primary alloimmune cause of platelet transfusion refractoriness is generally IgG antibodies against HLA-A and -B.[146] Such antibodies are only detected in approximately 20%–30% of transfusion refractory patients.[147,148] In refractory patients, platelet transfusion incompatibility due to HLA antibodies is associated with rapid destruction of transfused platelets.[125,125a]

Anti-HPA antibodies have also been associated with platelet transfusion refractoriness, but such antibodies are much less common. HPA antibodies are detected in 3.5%–16% of alloimmunized transfusion recipients, versus 94%–98% for HLA antibodies.[87,147,149] Overall, HPA antibodies are rare and, when present, are most often seen in combination with HLA antibodies.[145] The most commonly observed anti-HPA antibodies in transfused hematology-oncology patients have corresponding population antigen-positive frequencies of less than 30% (Table 8.3).[145] Additionally, only those anti-HPA antibodies directed against HPA epitopes on gpIIb/IIIa were found to be associated with inadequate transfusion response from incompatible platelets.[151] Therefore, anti-HPA antibodies do not generally significantly worsen difficulties finding compatible platelet units. Antibodies to a high-frequency HPA antigen are clearly a potential exception, however.

For both HLA and HPA antibodies, there is a significant amount of discordance between platelet antibody detection methods; no single methodology or clinically significant threshold has been identified as the gold standard for management of platelet transfusion refractoriness.[152] Although not generally used, a flow cytometric assay utilizing serum from transfusion refractory patients to potentiate in vitro platelet uptake by monocytes has shown the ability to predict whether patients benefit from specially matched platelets.[153]

Finally, cytotoxic T cells may play a role in platelet transfusion refractoriness, in addition to antibodies. In a mouse transfusion model, mice that were B-cell deficient and therefore unable to form alloantibodies still showed increased platelet clearance that was dependent on $CD8^+$ T cells.[154]

PROVISION OF MATCHED PLATELET PRODUCTS

Before further discussion of providing matched platelet support, it should be emphasized that the International Collaboration for Transfusion Medicine Guidelines has stated that patients with hypoproliferative thrombocytopenia who are refractory to platelet transfusions solely due to nonimmune factors should probably not receive HLA-selected or crossmatch-selected platelets.[155]

Overall, approximately 5% of hematology-oncology patients regularly transfused with leukoreduced or inactivated blood components show platelet-reactive antibodies in the serum and insufficient platelet count increments (i.e., meeting both elements of immune refractoriness).[123] Such patients generate an outsized financial and logistical burden in the clinic and the transfusion service.[123,156] Given those burdens on the transfusion service, patients with HLA PRA below 20%–30% can often be managed with random donor platelets, as more than two-thirds of all random platelet units would be expected to be compatible with such a patent.

Once the decision is made to provide compatible platelet components, three strategies of support are available (Table 8.5).[157] Platelet compatibility can be approached either by crossmatching, which is generally performed "blindly" with units at-hand, or by attempting to match donor HLA type with recipient. We have previously discussed the grades of serologic-based HLA matching (Table 8.2).

An incompatible crossmatch result predicts poor responses, but a compatible crossmatch does not exclude a poor response.[17] Historically, up to 17% of incompatible platelet–serum combinations showed false negativity in a platelet crossmatch assay.[160] Most laboratories are now using solid-phase red cell adherence (SPRCA) assays, modified antigen capture ELISA, or flow cytometric techniques for platelet crossmatching.[161] SPRCA is by far the most commonly used method.[150]

TABLE 8.5
Comparison of Methods of Platelet Matching.

	Requirements	Benefits	Pitfalls
Crossmatch compatible platelets	1. Least information required 2. Requires crossmatching reagents	1. Does not require donor or patient HLA typing or antibody identification; can use platelets on the shelf 2. Broadens available donor base[17] 3. Generally the most rapidly available option, if crossmatching can be done locally 4. Capable of detecting incompatibilities due to anti-HLA and HPA antibodies	1. By some reports, less successful than HLA matched units 2. Transfusion support with crossmatched platelets has potential to cause additional alloimmunization 3. In highly alloimmunized patients, may not find any compatible platelets 4. Must use ABO compatible platelets 5. Frequent crossmatching necessary (for ongoing platelet support, a new sample is needed every 3 days)
HLA-negative platelets (includes products meeting grade A, B, C, and D matches)	Requires identification of patient's HLA antibody specificities and donor HLA antigen typing	1. Broadens available compatible donor base by greater than 30-fold[158] compared to HLA matched platelets 2. Does not require patient HLA typing, though it is frequently performed	Has potential to cause additional alloimmunization
HLA matched platelets (includes grade A and BU matches; most transfusion services also include BX matches)	Requires patient and donor HLA antigen typing	1. Most precise match 2. Least risk of additional alloimmunization	1. May require recruitment of platelet donor, if no matched units are in supplier's inventory 2. Takes the most time to procure 3. Requires largest typed donor base (at least 3000–5000 typed donors required to ensure good potential support for 95% of recipients[159])

SPRCA can be used either as a platelet antibody screen or for platelet crossmatching. Due to the need for large numbers of apheresis platelets of a given blood group, the SPRCA platelet crossmatch is most frequently performed by blood suppliers rather than transfusion services. The SPRCA utilizes conical microwells coated with reagent platelets (platelet antibody screen) or aliquots from donor platelet units (platelet crossmatch). Patient plasma is added and incubated. The plasma is then removed, and the wells are washed. Indicator red cells coated with antihuman IgG are then added, and the microplate is centrifuged. The presence of antiplatelet antibodies will generate a red lawn, while the absence of antiplatelet antibodies will result in a red button at the bottom of the well (Fig. 8.8).

A positive SPRCA result indicates the presence of antiplatelet antibodies but does not resolve the specificity of the antibodies (HLA, HPA, and ABH if not using ABH-matched platelets). Due to variation in platelet ABH expression, Heal et al. showed that nearly 40% of group A and 80% of group B platelet donors were crossmatch compatible with group O patients.[162] Preidentification

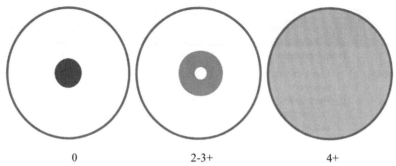

0	2-3+	4+

FIG. 8.8 Grading of the solid-phase red-cell adherence assay (SPRCA) for use in platelet antibody screening and platelet crossmatch.

of group A2 as well as group A1 low expresser platelets (seen with 10%–20% of A1 donors) could increase the available pool for performing platelet crossmatching.[95]

Crossmatch compatible platelet units show adequate 1-hour CCI 45%–65% of the time.[60,163–165] Although crossmatch compatible platelet units generally provide adequate CCI, in subgroup analysis those units that are crossmatch compatible but have lesser degrees of HLA match show inferior responses.[163] Wiita[165] and Wang[87] both describe the chronic support of patients with crossmatched platelets to be effective and without significant development of additional platelet alloantibodies.

The potential benefits of crossmatch compatible platelets over HLA-negative platelets are twofold: (1) the detection of incompatibility due to additional anti-HPA antibodies (relatively uncommon), and (2) the identification of compatible units that would not have been selected by the HLA-negative process.[17] In a platelet-refractory patient without detectable anti-HLA antibodies, the detection of significant crossmatch incompatibility should trigger an investigation for anti-HPA antibodies.[166] Patients with hypoproliferative thrombocytopenia who are refractory to platelet transfusions and have HPA antibodies should probably receive HPA-selected or crossmatch-selected platelet transfusion.[155]

A complete four-allele HLA match is clearly the ideal platelet product for an alloimmunized refractory patient, but such units are often not immediately available and represented only 16% of matched platelet units in one report.[45]

HLA-negative units were historically not a preferred option due to difficulties resolving patient antibody specificities when using cytotoxicity assays.[160] In the modern era of very accurate HLA antibody identification, the efficacy of HLA-negative units becomes similar to that of crossmatch compatible units.[158] Selecting

platelet units mismatched for recipient antigens that are nevertheless within the same CREG as the recipient provides an opportunity to expand the available platelet supply for a given patient (as previously described in detail), while maintaining a reasonable likelihood of transfusion success and not predisposing to additional alloimmunization.[17] Specifically, expanding the platelet donor pool to include grade BX matches increases the donor pool 10-fold.[57] Duquesnoy and colleagues showed that transfusing within a CREG (BX, B2UX, B2X) provided similar response as a fully matched unit (match grade A), but grade C and D matches showed slightly worse average responses.[57] Of course, patients with antibodies to so-called private HLA epitopes that are within their CREG will not be well served by CREG-based platelet selection.[116] Moroff and colleagues showed that grade BX and C platelet matches showed lower CCI efficacy (47% and 37% acceptable, respectively) than better HLA-matched units (grade A/BU, 73% acceptable CCI).[157] Some transfusions within CREGs are more successful than others. Transfusion within donor-recipient cross-reactive pairs A1/A11, A2/A28, B5/18, and B7/B22 generally resulted in good platelet increments, whereas A1/A3, A3/A11, B7/B17, B7/B21, B5/B15, B5/17, B8/B14, B5/B27, and B27/B35 did not.[167]

In one report, HLA-matched platelet support with HLA A/BU grade matches appeared to be superior to a selection method based upon cross-matching alone,[157] but such a strategy may restrict availability of platelets in some difficult to match patients. In addition, it is not uncommon for the "best" HLA-selected platelet to be an ABO-incompatible component.[146] In patients who are particularly sensitive to ABO incompatibility, HLA-matched but ABO major mismatched platelets can show poor responses.[168] In this setting, a sacrifice in the degree of HLA match may be necessary to ensure ABO match.

Overall, the platelet support strategies of HLA matched, HLA negative, and the crossmatching generally show similar effectiveness and the chosen strategy should be based on local operational convenience and cost analysis.[123,164] One workflow for work-up and management of a patient with platelet transfusion refractoriness is presented in Fig. 8.9. There are no randomized clinical trials comparing the effectiveness of different methods of matched platelet support on clinical outcomes.[58,164,169] Finally, HLA negative, HLA matched, and crossmatch compatible platelets should all be irradiated given the likelihood for a degree of HLA matching that could allow the development of transfusion-associated graft-versus-host disease.

ONGOING MANAGEMENT OF PATIENTS RECEIVING MATCHED PLATELETS

Continued collection of posttransfusion platelet counts is of considerable importance for managing patients receiving matched platelets.[170] Analyzing the CCI of matched units can highlight units with unexpectedly poor response, facilitating the identification of HPA antibodies or the emergence of additional new HLA antibodies. Monitoring of matched platelet response and periodic repeat HLA antibody identification is an important part of the transfusion service's ongoing management of platelet transfusion refractory patients. Although ~25% of patients broaden their anti-HLA PRA during treatment, HLA antibodies also disappear

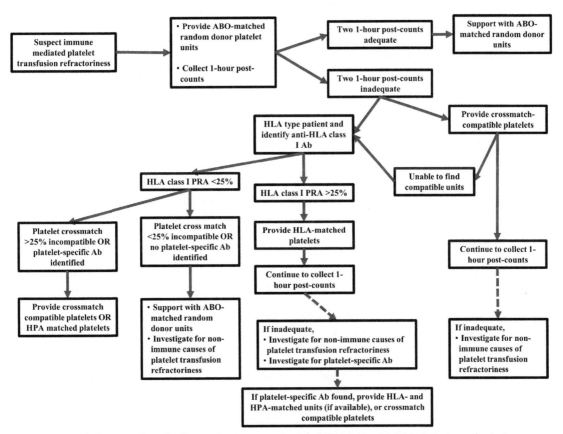

FIG. 8.9 Laboratory investigation and management of a patient with platelet transfusion refractoriness. (Modified from Brown CJ, Navarrete CV. Clinical relevance of the HLA system in blood transfusion. *Vox Sang.* 2011;101(2):93–105; Kopko PM, Warner P, Kresie L, Pancoska C. Methods for the selection of platelet products for alloimmune-refractory patients. *Transfusion.* 2015;55(2):235–244; Juskewitch JE, Norgan AP, De Goey SR, et al. How do I... manage the platelet transfusion-refractory patient? *Transfusion.* 2017;57(12): 2828–2835; Murphy ME. Manging the platelet refractory patient. *ISBT Sci Ser.* 2014;9:234–238; Hod E, Schwartz J. Platelet transfusion refractoriness. *Br J Haematol.* 2008;142(3):348–360.)

with periods of abstinence from transfusion (median HLA antibody persistence is 14 weeks).[31] Antiplatelet antibodies can also disappear during periods of active transfusion support.[171,172] Rechallenge with platelets expressing HLA for which a patient previously had a reactive antibody can sometimes be tolerated without antibody recrudescence.[173] For this reason, difficult to match patients may benefit from monthly reidentification of detectable antibodies, as this may allow greater numbers of potential compatible donors to be identified.

The increased utilization of leukoreduced (LR) cellular blood components has reduced the number of alloimmunized transfusion recipients. The TRAP study showed 62% relative reduction in class I HLA alloimmunization and 69% reduction in platelet transfusion refractoriness in those patients randomized to LR cellular blood components.[25] The randomized controlled TRAP study showed more significant reductions in alloimmunization due to LR than was seen in an observational study[122] or a randomized controlled trial in cardiothoracic surgery, however.[174] Although leukoreduction significantly reduced HLA alloimmunization, 7%–9% of previously unsensitized patients still developed antibodies to class I HLA after being treated with LR cellular blood components.[25,175] Similar to leukoreduction, pathogen reduction techniques also reduce alloimmunization caused by transfused WBC.[176,177]

Although LR filters do entrap platelets in addition to WBC, there does not seem to be any benefit of LR blood components in the incidence of anti-HPA alloimmunization.[25,58] However, as discussed earlier, anti-HPA antibodies do not seem to be as detrimental to platelet transfusion responsiveness as anti-HLA antibodies.[58,147]

In highly alloimmunized patients (PRA approaching 100%) for whom HLA-matched units cannot be found, "least incompatible" platelets can potentially be identified by utilizing additional data obtained from solid-phase HLA antibody identification, as was described earlier. First, analyzing the mean fluorescence intensity (MFI) of the patient's HLA antibodies may allow weaker antibodies to be dropped from consideration and may identify units with acceptable transfusion response.[38] Jackman and colleagues retested samples from TRAP participants who had been platelet transfusion refractory but lacked detectable HLA antibodies by CDC assay, using IgG-based flow cytometric antibody detection (not C1q-binding). Levels of HLA or HPA antibodies detected by solid phase did not correlate with refractoriness among CDC(−) recipients. These data demonstrate that weak-to-moderate HLA antibody levels detectable

by modern assays do not significantly associate with platelet refractoriness.[178] Second, a C1q-binding flow cytometric HLA detection assay may be used to identify only those HLA antibodies that fix complement. The C1q-binding flow cytometric HLA detection assay recapitulates the detection functionalities of the previous CDC, in which lymphocytes were only lysed if (1) patient antibody bound reagent WBC, and (2) the antibody fixed complement and caused the formation of the membrane attack complex. Platelet units that would be considered compatible based on a patient's C1q SAB flow assay, but incompatible based on a patient's IgG SAB flow assay had higher mean CCI (10.6) than dual incompatible units (2.5).[47] Third, some antibodies can be ignored and still provide successful platelet support.[150] Incompatible platelet transfusions are often successful, demonstrating that the presence of a donor-specific antibody is necessary but not sufficient for platelet clearance.[45] Certain HLA antigens are expressed at low density on platelets and may therefore antigen positive units may provide better responses than would be expected despite patient cognate alloantibodies.[179] Antibodies to HLA-B12 (B44 and B45) can frequently be ignored, as platelets do not express these antigens at high density.[180] Other HLA class I antigens vary in expression level. Expression varies by factors of 8–35-fold for HLA-B12, B8, Bw4, and Bw6.[17] Expression of B12 is decreased when A2, A3, or Aw28 is present.[17] Expression of Bw4 is weaker in the presence of B13. Expression of Bw6 is weaker with B8 or B14.[17]

Finally, platelet transfusion refractory patients who do not achieve platelet count goals with best matched units are extremely challenging to manage. Such patients represent about one-third of immune refractory patients.[123,181] Failure to achieve count goals can be due to extremely broad alloimmunization and failure to identify matched units, or, quite commonly, due to concurrent immune and nonimmune factors leading to refractoriness for a particular patient.[181a] Additional therapies, in addition to ongoing best platelet support, include antifibrinolytics, intravenous immune globulin (IVIG), thrombopoietin mimetics, and immunosuppressants.[58,123] It is worth acknowledging that, in patients at high risk of bleeding, even platelet transfusions that do not provide an adequate CCI still provide some detectable protection from bleeding.[182]

Patients with the severe platelet function defects Bernard–Soulier syndrome and Glanzmann thrombasthenia, which are due to marked deficiency of the relevant glycoprotein receptor on the platelet surface, are at risk of alloimmunization to glycoprotein Ib/IX/V and IIb/IIIa, respectively. Those patients who completely lack surface glycoprotein expression are at particular risk. Functional donor platelets lacking the glycoprotein receptors are clearly not available, but prophylactic HLA matching of platelet transfusions for such patients can be considered. This is a unique patient population where prophylactic HLA matching before alloimmunization may be of benefit.[2,146]

TRANSPLANTATION-ASSOCIATED ALLOIMMUNE THROMBOCYTOPENIA

Alloantibodies to HPA can rarely cause thrombocytopenia after transplantation. These alloantibodies are recipient anti-donor antibodies in the setting of affected stem cell transplants, but are donor anti-recipient antibodies in the setting of affected solid organ transplant.

Lucas and colleagues described three patients who developed prolonged alloimmune thrombocytopenia lasting up to 10 months after allogeneic stem-cell transplantation (10 out of 10 HLA allele-matched).[183] These three patients all had anti-HPA-1a antibodies that reacted against HPA-1a-positive donor megakaryocytes/platelets.[183]

Severe thrombocytopenia has also been described in three organ recipients after solid organ transplantation from the same multiparous female organ donor with normal platelet counts. Anti-HPA-la alloantibodies were detected in donor and posttransplant (but not pretransplant) recipients' sera; the recipients were homozygous HPA-la positive.[81] The transplanted organs were presumed to carry B cells and/or plasma cells that produced high-affinity anti-HPA-1a.

FETAL/NEONATAL ALLOIMMUNE THROMBOCYTOPENIA

FNAIT is caused by alloimmunization of a pregnant woman by paternal platelet antigens, leading to the production of alloantibodies against paternal antigens on fetal platelets. These IgG alloantibodies then cross the placenta (mostly IgG1 and IgG3, via the neonatal Fc receptor) and bind fetal platelets, causing increased clearance by the fetal spleen and liver, resulting in fetal immune thrombocytopenia (generally below 50×10^9/L and often below 20×10^9/L).[64] This mechanism is similar to the pathogenesis of hemolytic disease of the fetus/newborn (HDFN), where a mother is alloimmunized to paternal *red cell* antigens. Different from HDFN, FNAIT can sometimes occur in the first pregnancy.[67,184] There are two potential explanations for this disparate disease presentation:

- Fetal platelets may more rapidly mix into maternal circulation with microvascular damage to the placenta, due to their smaller size relative to red blood cells[64]

- As β3 integrin is expressed on human trophoblastic cells as part of the αVβ3 vitronectin receptor, a maternal immune response may be generated before delivery due to the expression of paternally inherited antigens on syncytiotrophoblasts[65,184]

The incidence of FNAIT is approximately 1:1000 pregnancies.[67,184] FNAIT is heavily underrecognized, however.[64,185] FNAIT is the most common cause of isolated severe thrombocytopenia in otherwise healthy term newborns.[184]

Although platelets express the three antigen groups previously described, HPA is the system consistently implicated in FNAIT. ABO and HLA discrepancy are only rarely described as a cause of FNAIT.[16,67,186] It has been hypothesized that the lack of anti-HLA mediated FNAIT is due to maternal anti-HLA antibodies being absorbed on the placenta.[16]

Despite the existence of numerous HPA, alloimmunization to only a few particular HPA is responsible for most reported cases of FNAIT. Irrespective of race, HPAs in the β3 integrin subunit of gpIIb/IIIa accounts for most reported FNAIT cases.[64] In the US and European studies, the most commonly reported causes of alloimmune thrombocytopenia are anti-HPA-1a (~75% of cases), followed by anti-HPA-5b (~10% of cases).[9] In contrast, FNAIT due to HPA-1a incompatibility is very rare in African and Asian populations,[64] due to the HPA-1b/b type being rare in nonwhite populations. Among Japanese, the most common cause of fetal alloimmune thrombocytopenia is anti-HPA-4b.[9] Although the likelihood of antigen incompatibility between mother and fetus is very high in HPA-3 and HPA-15 systems (due to their higher heterozygosity rate), they less commonly cause FNAIT compared to HPA-1 and HPA-5 systems. This implies that the HPA-1 and -5 systems are more immunogenic.[84] A small minority of FNAIT cases (~3%) show antibody specificity to multiple HPA antigens.[186]

A maternal−paternal discrepancy between HPA alleles is necessary but not sufficient for FNAIT, however. Only 10%−12% of HPA-1a-negative pregnant women become immunized.[64,187−189] Additionally, the formation of anti-HPA antibodies is not sufficient for FNAIT: while approximately 1 in 330 pregnancies are affected by the formation of anti-HPA-1a antibodies, only 1:1285 pregnancies is affected by fetal/neonatal thrombocytopenia.[187] This implies a 26%−31% disease penetrance of anti-HPA-1a antibodies for severe FNAIT.[189] This progressive narrowing from HPA-discrepant pregnancies, to HPA alloimmunized

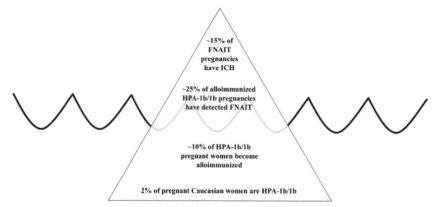

FIG. 8.10 Iceberg model of maternal HPA type, alloimmunization, and fetal/neonatal alloimmune thrombocytopenia (FNAIT). (Modified from Tiller H, Husebekk A, Ahlen MT, Stuge TB, Skogen B. Current perspectives on fetal and neonatal alloimmune thrombocytopenia - increasing clinical concerns and new treatment opportunities. *Int J Womens Health*. 2017;9:223–234.)

pregnancies, to actual FNAIT-affected pregnancies can be described as an iceberg model (Fig. 8.10).

Immunization against HPA-1a is strongly correlated with inheritance of the HLA allele HLA-DRB3*01:01,[84,184,190] and odds ratio for anti-HPA-1a immunization in women with DRB3*01:01 was 92.3.[191] However, HLA genotyping has not been shown to be predictive of the severity of anti-HPA-1a FNAIT.[192]

Not all pregnancies with a clinical diagnosis of FNAIT have a detectable anti-HPA antibody.[187] In one report, approximately 50% of pregnancies with a clinical diagnosis of FNAIT in Japan did not have detectable anti-HPA antibodies.[91] This may be due to the presence of low avidity anti-HPA antibodies that are not easily detected by the MAIPA assay.[63]

Different from HDFN due to anti-D, there is as of yet no passive immunoprophylaxis available to prevent anti-HPA-1a FNAIT.[186] Animal experiments have suggested that a passive immunization strategy (similar to RhIG for HDFN prophylaxis of RhD-negative mothers) may be beneficial for reducing FNAIT. Administration of anti-HPA-1a was able to suppress the murine antibody response to transfused human HPA-1a-positive platelets. This prophylaxis also reduced fetal loss in pregnant mice and increased the newborn pups' platelet counts.[193] An upcoming trial of passive polyclonal immune prophylaxis in pregnant women at-risk of FNAIT (HPA-1a negative, HLA DRB3*01:01 positive) is planned in Europe (http://www.profnait.eu). Eksteen and colleagues have recently developed a monoclonal antibody specific for HPA-1a derived from an immortalized B cell from an alloimmunized woman who had an infant affected by FNAIT.[194] Such monoclonal antibodies may serve as a future source

of human passive immunoprophylaxis to prevent development of FNAIT, and/or for therapeutic treatment of pregnant women who have already formed anti-HPA-1a to minimize fetal thrombocytopenia (through competitive inhibition of clearance by maternal antibodies).

Further discussion of FNAIT is available elsewhere in this textbook.

POST TRANSFUSION PURPURA

PTP is a rare immune thrombocytopenia disorder triggered by transfusion, characterized by alloantibodies to platelet-specific antigens. Moreover, 96% of PTP patients were women in one report.[195] The patient (typically a previously pregnant woman) is reexposed to HPA epitopes by the platelets in a transfused cellular blood component. Fevers and chills have been reported to occur during the implicated transfusion. The transfusion exposure causes a rapidly developing severe thrombocytopenia roughly 1 week later. Leukoreduction of blood components is associated with less PTP incidence, as whole-blood leukoreduction filters reduce contaminating platelets 100-fold.[196]

Zucker and von Loghem first described PTP in 1959. A subsequent description of two PTP cases was made by Shulman and colleagues in 1961.[197] All described cases involved previously pregnant women who developed severe purpura after transfusion of whole blood. The Zucker and von Loghem reports both demonstrated platelet alloagglutinin by the women's sera. The Shulman report showed that serum from PTP patients contained an antibody that bound and fixed complement on platelets from 12 normal donors. Shulman and colleagues described that these women both had an antibody to the Pl^{A1} antigen, the antigen now known as HPA-1a, and that both lacked that antigen on their platelets.

HPA-1a is the most common relevant antigen in PTP. Previously pregnant HPA-1a-negative women (presumably initially alloimmunized by pregnancy exposures) are the most commonly affected.[198,199] Despite the frequency of the susceptible HPA-1b/1b genotype being 2%—3% in the Caucasian population, the incidence of PTP is rare and estimated at 1 in 24,000 to 100,000 transfused components.[198,200] This implies that additional "hits"/risk factors are required for PTP. Only 250 total cases of PTP have been described in the medical literature to-date, but it is likely significantly underrecognized/underreported.

PTP typically presents 5—12 days after transfusion of a cellular blood component with severe thrombocytopenia (often $<10 \times 10^9/L$) and bleeding (including 30% with major or life-threatening bleeds).[198] Bleeding symptoms include cutaneous bruising/bleeding, epistaxis, upper and lower gastrointestinal hemorrhage, and hematuria.[201] Consensus criteria for diagnosis of PTP are included in the Centers for Disease Control Hemovigilance document.[202] A definitive PTP diagnosis requires (1) the detection of alloantibodies in the patient directed against HPA or other platelet-specific antigen, detected at the time of or after development of thrombocytopenia, and (2) otherwise unexplained thrombocytopenia (i.e., decrease in platelets to less than 20% of pretransfusion count) occurring 5—12 days after transfusion of a cellular blood component.

It is presumed that patients who develop PTP were originally alloimmunized (mostly during prior pregnancy(s)) and that reexposure to the relevant foreign epitope by transfusion triggers an anamnestic memory immune response with a dramatic rise in antibody formation. These antibodies provoke clearance of any remaining exogenous transfused platelets from the transfused blood component. This alloimmune clearance would generally be well tolerated; however, PTP causes much more severe thrombocytopenia by leading to clearance of endogenous self-platelets as well. The mechanism for this self-platelet clearance is unclear. Several mechanisms have been hypothesized:

- immune epitope spreading/peripheral loss of tolerance mechanism wherein the patient's alloimmunization broadens into an autoimmune response with resultant thrombocytopenia due to clearance of endogenous antigen-negative platelets.[203—206] This phenomenon appears limited to the early stages of PTP, as autoimmune reactivity is not often found in convalescent serum.[201,207]

- immune complexes between alloantibody and fragments of exogenous platelets deposit on the surface of self-platelets, leading to clearance[197]

- allogeneic platelets coated with alloantibodies might interact with the FcγIIa-receptor of autologous platelets to mediate the activation and ultimate destruction of autologous platelets[201]

- conversion of antigen-negative endogenous platelets to antigen-positive status by deposition of soluble free antigen (derived from the transfused component) on their surface

Watkins et al. described the existence of autoreactive circulating B cells in an acute PTP patient. The gpIIbIIIa autoantibodies that they cloned targeted an immunodominant compound epitope on the gpIIbIIIa heterodimer and showed a low level of somatic mutation.[203] Watkins et al. hypothesized that naive, autoreactive B cells receive inappropriate costimulatory signals from memory, alloreactive T cells in the setting of PTP, leading to the generation of autoantibodies.[203]

After identifying an appropriate patient with otherwise unexplained thrombocytopenia after transfusion, diagnosis of PTP is typically made by (1) identification of alloantibody to HPA and (2) genotyping the patient to confirm the lack of the target antigen. Alloantibody detection can be achieved using the MAIPA or modified antigen capture ELISA techniques. These HPA alloantibodies are high-titer IgG and fix complement.[67] Although specificity for anti-HPA-1a is the most frequently implicated alloantibody, antibodies against numerous other HPA epitopes have been implicated in PTP (HPA-1b, -2b, -3a, -3b, -5b).[200,201,208]

A diagnosis of PTP is often challenging to make due to the patient population frequently being postoperative or otherwise critically ill, and receiving multiple medications. In this setting, the thrombocytopenia often has multiple potential mechanisms other than PTP: drug-induced thrombocytopenia (including heparin-induced thrombocytopenia), immune thrombocytopenia, sepsis, and disseminated intravascular coagulopathy.[209] A frequent misdiagnosis for PTP is heparin-induced thrombocytopenia.[201] If features consistent with PTP (such as recent blood transfusion in the last 2—14 days, a more severe drop in platelet count to below $15 \times 10^9/L$, and bleeding symptoms rather than thrombosis) are present, particularly in previously pregnant women, concurrent testing for both heparin-dependent antibodies and anti-HPA antibodies should be pursued.[201]

Although PTP is usually self-limited (lasting 1–4 weeks), death from hemorrhage does occur and PTP mortality has historically been estimated at 10%–15%.[210] Platelet transfusions are frequently ineffective to raise the platelet count in acute PTP, though antigen-negative platelet products have been reported to be successful for critically bleeding patients in one report.[211] PTP is best treated by high-dose IVIG, 1 g/kg daily for 2 days, or 2 g/kg in divided doses provided over 2–5 days.[209] IVIG response rate is reported to be 85%.[198] Multiple mechanisms of action for IVIG in PTP have been hypothesized, including antiidiotype antibodies, FcR blockade, and neutralization of platelet antigens. Corticosteroids are also frequently given.[195] Therapeutic plasma exchange (TPE) can also be considered, to more rapidly decrease antiplatelet antibodies. TPE may also remove residual soluble alloantigen, given the immune complex and soluble antigen theories of PTP. TPE does seem to shorten the duration of thrombocytopenia. Therefore, if IVIG is not effective, TPE may be considered if bleeding is severe.[209] The American Society for Apheresis gives PTP a category III recommendation for TPE, meaning that the "optimum role of apheresis therapy is not established ... decision making should be individualized."[209]

Recovery from PTP (rise in platelets to greater than 50×10^9/L) is variable, occurring from after 1 day to 4 months. Antiplatelet antibody may persist for several months after clinical recovery.[212] Antiplatelet antibody titers have been followed serially in some patients, and tend to fall as the platelet count increases. Similarly, in patients treated with TPE, the antibody titer declines. Platelet count recovery occurs despite the presence of residual detectable antibody titer, though typically lower titer than at initial testing.[212]

After PTP remission, further transfusion of PTP patients with allogeneic blood components is generally discouraged, but antigen-negative products can be used if necessary.[204] Washed cellular blood components reduce the risk of PTP relapse, but do not eliminate the risk.[213]

Although PTP requires two temporally distinct "hits" (initial historic alloimmunization and subsequent reexposure to the same antigen), FNAIT results from one alloantigen exposure: a maternal alloimmunization to paternal alloantigen expressed on fetal platelets.[81] Although alloimmunization against HPA-1a is the most frequent cause of both PTP and FNAIT, only one patient with PTP has been described to have a history of an FNAIT-affected pregnancy.[214] The cause of this unexpected absence of disease correlation despite common alloantibody is unclear.

ACUTE THROMBOCYTOPENIA AFTER PASSIVE IMMUNIZATION WITH ANTI-HPA ANTIBODIES (PASSIVE ALLOIMMUNE THROMBOCYTOPENIA)

An acute thrombocytopenia syndrome has also been reported after passive immunization via plasma-rich blood components containing antiplatelet antibodies.[215] This is different from actual PTP, of course, as the donor antiplatelet antibodies cause a transient passive alloantibody-mediated platelet clearance, without any autoimmune-type clearance. A literature review by Pavenski and colleagues identified 19 cases of passive transfer of antiplatelet antibody that resulted in thrombocytopenia. The median platelet count nadir was 7×10^9/L, which was reached within a median of 6 hour after transfusion. Transfusion was accompanied by an acute transfusion reaction in 30% of recipients. Plasma-rich blood components accounted for most cases. Approximately 75% of recipients developed thrombocytopenic bleeding. The median time to platelet count recovery was 5 days. All cases involved a female donor with a history of pregnancy, and anti-HPA-1a was the most frequently implicated antibody.[216] Brunner-Bolliger and colleagues demonstrated that the passively transferred antiplatelet antibody was undetectable within 40 minutes of transfusion, likely due to rapid adsorption onto recipient platelets.[217]

As of 2008, no cases of thrombocytopenia due to passive transfer of PLT antibody involving a male donor have been described.[216] Women with previous pregnancies affected (or likely affected) by FNAIT are most frequently identified as donors positive for anti-HPA-1a antibodies and are the implicated donor population for passively acquired alloimmune thrombocytopenia reactions.[216] TRALI mitigation efforts that exclude previously pregnant women will likely reduce passively acquired alloimmune thrombocytopenia. It must be noted, however, that previously pregnant female donors cleared for plasma or platelet product manufacture by negative HLA antibody testing could still have anti-HPA antibodies.

CONCLUSION AND SUMMARY

Platelets are a vital part of the hemostatic system, providing the physical basis of primary hemostasis and the surface for formation of the secondary hemostatic fibrin clot, in addition to important roles in inflammatory and immune signaling and response. Platelets express antigens from several important antigen systems: ABO, HLA, and HPA. Antibodies to all of these systems can cause immune clearance of incompatible platelets. We have discussed the various alloimmune thrombocytopenia syndromes: posttransfusion purpura, passive alloimmune thrombocytopenia, fetal/neonatal alloimmune thrombocytopenia, transplantation-associated alloimmune thrombocytopenia, and alloimmune platelet transfusion refractoriness. Platelet transfusion refractoriness is the most commonly encountered alloimmune thrombocytopenia condition, with the others being less common (though likely underrecognized).

Antibodies to all three antigen systems (ABO, HLA, and HPA) are associated with immune platelet transfusion refractoriness, with HLA generally being the most important. In contrast, FNAIT, PTP, passive alloimmune thrombocytopenia, and transplantation-associated alloimmune thrombocytopenia are all caused by antibodies to the HPA system. PTP is unique among the alloimmune thrombocytopenia syndromes in its combined immune attack against allogeneic platelets *and* autologous platelets.

Humoral immune response appears to cause the vast majority of alloimmune thrombocytopenia in humans, although mouse models have shown a role for cytotoxic T cells for alloimmune platelet clearance. Future work investigating this possible mechanism in humans is anticipated.

REFERENCES

1. Sweeney JLM. Preface. In: SJL M, ed. *Platelet Transfusion Therapy*. Bethesda: AABB Press; 2013.
2. Bolton-Maggs PH, Chalmers EA, Collins PW, et al. A review of inherited platelet disorders with guidelines for their management on behalf of the UKHCDO. *Br J Haematol*. 2006;135(5):603–633.
3. Henn V, Slupsky JR, Grafe M, et al. CD40 ligand on activated platelets triggers an inflammatory reaction of endothelial cells. *Nature*. 1998;391(6667):591–594.
4. Henn V, Steinbach S, Buchner K, Presek P, Kroczek RA. The inflammatory action of CD40 ligand (CD154) expressed on activated human platelets is temporally limited by coexpressed CD40. *Blood*. 2001;98(4):1047–1054.
5. Bang A, Speck ER, Blanchette VS, Freedman J, Semple JW. Recipient humoral immunity against leukoreduced allogeneic platelets is suppressed by aminoguanidine, a selective inhibitor of inducible nitric oxide synthase. *Blood*. 1996;88(8):2959–2966.
6. Chapman LM, Aggrey AA, Field DJ, et al. Platelets present antigen in the context of MHC class I. *J Immunol*. 2012;189(2):916–923.
7. Crux NB, Elahi S. Human leukocyte antigen (HLA) and immune regulation: how do classical and non-classical HLA alleles modulate immune response to human immunodeficiency virus and hepatitis C virus infections? *Front Immunol*. 2017;8:832.
8. Quach ME, Chen W, Li R. Mechanisms of platelet clearance and translation to improve platelet storage. *Blood*. 2018;131(14):1512–1521.
9. Curtis BR. Genotyping for human platelet alloantigen polymorphisms: applications in the diagnosis of alloimmune platelet disorders. *Semin Thromb Hemost*. 2008;34(6):539–548.
10. Swinkels M, Rijkers M, Voorberg J, Vidarsson G, Leebeek FWG, Jansen AJG. Emerging concepts in immune thrombocytopenia. *Front Immunol*. 2018;9:880.
11. Zufferey A, Schvartz D, Nolli S, Reny JL, Sanchez JC, Fontana P. Characterization of the platelet granule proteome: evidence of the presence of MHC1 in alpha-granules. *J Proteomics*. 2014;101:130–140.
12. Kao KJ, Cook DJ, Scornik JC. Quantitative analysis of platelet surface HLA by W6/32 anti-HLA monoclonal antibody. *Blood*. 1986;68(3):627–632.
13. Lalezari P, Driscoll AM. Ability of thrombocytes to acquire HLA specificity from plasma. *Blood*. 1982;59(1):167–170.
14. Mueller-Eckhardt G, Hauck M, Kayser W, Mueller-Eckhardt C. HLA-C antigens on platelets. *Tissue Antigens*. 1980;16(1):91–94.
15. Datema G, Stein S, Eijsink C, Mulder A, Claas FH, Doxiadis II. HLA-C expression on platelets: studies with an HLA-Cw1-specific human monoclonal antibody. *Vox Sang*. 2000;79(2):108–111.
16. Bonstein L, Haddad N. Taking a wider view on fetal/neonatal alloimmune thrombocytopenia. *Thromb Res*. 2017;151(Suppl 1):S100–S102.
17. Delaflor-Weiss E, Mintz PD. The evaluation and management of platelet refractoriness and alloimmunization. *Transfus Med Rev*. 2000;14(2):180–196.
18. Trowsdale J, Knight JC. Major histocompatibility complex genomics and human disease. *Annu Rev Genom Hum Genet*. 2013;14:301–323.
19. Mungall AJ, Palmer SA, Sims SK, et al. The DNA sequence and analysis of human chromosome 6. *Nature*. 2003;425(6960):805–811.
20. Robinson J, Halliwell JA, Hayhurst JD, Flicek P, Parham P, Marsh SG. The IPD and IMGT/HLA database: allele variant databases. *Nucleic Acids Res*. 2015;43(Database issue):D423–D431.
21. Hyun J, Park KD, Yoo Y, et al. Effects of different sensitization events on HLA alloimmunization in solid organ transplantation patients. *Transplant Proc*. 2012;44(1):222–225.
22. Lopes D, Barra T, Malheiro J, et al. Effect of different sensitization events on HLA alloimmunization in kidney transplantation candidates. *Transplant Proc*. 2015;47(4):894–897.
23. Picascia A, Grimaldi V, Sabia C, Napoli C. Comprehensive assessment of sensitizing events and anti-HLA antibody development in women awaiting kidney transplantation. *Transpl Immunol*. 2016;36:14–19.

24. Akgul SU, Ciftci HS, Temurhan S, et al. Association between HLA antibodies and different sensitization events in renal transplant candidates. *Transplant Proc.* 2017;49(3):425–429.

25. Trial to Reduce Alloimmunization to Platelets Study G. Leukocyte reduction and ultraviolet B irradiation of platelets to prevent alloimmunization and refractoriness to platelet transfusions. *N Engl J Med.* 1997;337(26):1861–1869.

26. Laundy GJ, Bradley BA, Rees BM, Younie M, Hows JM. Incidence and specificity of HLA antibodies in multi-transfused patients with acquired aplastic anemia. *Transfusion.* 2004;44(6):814–825.

27. Brown CJ, Navarrete CV. Clinical relevance of the HLA system in blood transfusion. *Vox Sang.* 2011;101(2):93–105.

28. Dutcher JP, Schiffer CA, Aisner J, Wiernik PH. Alloimmunization following platelet transfusion: the absence of a dose-response relationship. *Blood.* 1981;57(3):395–398.

29. Dutcher JP, Schiffer CA, Aisner J, Wiernik PH. Long-term follow-up patients with leukemia receiving platelet transfusions: identification of a large group of patients who do not become alloimmunized. *Blood.* 1981;58(5):1007–1011.

30. Howard JE, Perkins HA. The natural history of alloimmunization to platelets. *Transfusion.* 1978;18(4):496–503.

31. Slichter SJ, Bolgiano D, Kao KJ, et al. Persistence of lymphocytotoxic antibodies in patients in the trial to reduce alloimmunization to platelets: implications for using modified blood products. *Transfus Med Rev.* 2011;25(2):102–110.

32. Quillen K, Medrano C, Adams S, et al. Screening plateletpheresis donors for HLA antibodies on two high-throughput platforms and correlation with recipient outcome. *Transfusion.* 2011;51(3):504–510.

33. Kleinman S, King MR, Busch MP, et al. The national heart, lung, and blood Institute retrovirus epidemiology donor studies (retrovirus epidemiology donor study and retrovirus epidemiology donor study-II): twenty years of research to advance blood product safety and availability. *Transfus Med Rev.* 2012;26(4):281–304, 304 e281-282.

34. Seielstad M, Page GP, Gaddis N, et al. Genomewide association study of HLA alloimmunization in previously pregnant blood donors. *Transfusion.* 2018;58(2):402–412.

35. Thomas KA, Valenzuela NM, Reed EF. The perfect storm: HLA antibodies, complement, FcgammaRs, and endothelium in transplant rejection. *Trends Mol Med.* 2015;21(5):319–329.

36. Gebel HM, Bray RA. The evolution and clinical impact of human leukocyte antigen technology. *Curr Opin Nephrol Hypertens.* 2010;19(6):598–602.

37. Tait BD, Hudson F, Cantwell L, et al. Review article: Luminex technology for HLA antibody detection in organ transplantation. *Nephrology.* 2009;14(2):247–254.

38. Schmidt AE, Refaai MA, Coppage M. HLA-mediated platelet refractoriness: an ACLPS critical review. *Am J Clin Pathol.* 2019 Mar 1;151(4):353–363. https://doi.org/10.1093/ajcp/aqy121. PubMed PMID: 30285067.

39. Sullivan HC, Gebel HM, Bray RA. Understanding solid-phase HLA antibody assays and the value of MFI. *Hum Immunol.* 2017;78(7–8):471–480.

40. Reed EF, Rao P, Zhang Z, et al. Comprehensive assessment and standardization of solid phase multiplex-bead arrays for the detection of antibodies to HLA. *Am J Transplant.* 2013;13(7):1859–1870.

41. Schwaiger E, Wahrmann M, Bond G, Eskandary F, Bohmig GA. Complement component C3 activation: the leading cause of the prozone phenomenon affecting HLA antibody detection on single-antigen beads. *Transplantation.* 2014;97(12):1279–1285.

42. Wang J, Meade JR, Brown NK, Weidner JG, Marino SR. EDTA is superior to DTT treatment for overcoming the prozone effect in HLA antibody testing. *HLA.* 2017;89(2):82–89.

43. Zhang X, Reinsmoen NL. Comprehensive assessment for serum treatment for single antigen test for detection of HLA antibodies. *Hum Immunol.* 2017;78(11–12):699–703.

44. Tambur AR, Herrera ND, Haarberg KM, et al. Assessing antibody strength: comparison of MFI, C1q, and titer information. *Am J Transplant.* 2015;15(9):2421–2430.

45. Karlström C, Linjama T, Edgren G, Lauronen J, Wikman A, Höglund P. HLA-selected platelets for platelet refractory patients with HLA antibodies: a single-center experience. *Transfusion.* 2019 Mar;59(3):945–952. https://doi.org/10.1111/trf.15108. Epub 2018 Dec 21. PubMed PMID: 30575964.

46. Chen G, Sequeira F, Tyan DB. Novel C1q assay reveals a clinically relevant subset of human leukocyte antigen antibodies independent of immunoglobulin G strength on single antigen beads. *Hum Immunol.* 2011;72(10):849–858.

47. Fontaine MJ, Kuo J, Chen G, et al. Complement (C1q) fixing solid-phase screening for HLA antibodies increases the availability of compatible platelet components for refractory patients. *Transfusion.* 2011;51(12):2611–2618.

48. Sicard A, Ducreux S, Rabeyrin M, et al. Detection of C3d-binding donor-specific anti-HLA antibodies at diagnosis of humoral rejection predicts renal graft loss. *J Am Soc Nephrol.* 2015;26(2):457–467.

49. Lan JH, Tinckam K. Clinical utility of complement dependent assays in kidney transplantation. *Transplantation.* 2018;102(1S Suppl 1):S14–S22.

50. Wiebe C, Gareau AJ, Pochinco D, et al. Evaluation of C1q status and titer of de novo donor-specific antibodies as predictors of allograft survival. *Am J Transplant.* 2017;17(3):703–711.

51. Comoli P, Cioni M, Tagliamacco A, et al. Acquisition of C3d-binding activity by de novo donor-specific HLA antibodies correlates with graft loss in nonsensitized

pediatric kidney recipients. *Am J Transplant*. 2016;16(7): 2106−2116.

52. Nunes E, Heslop H, Fernandez-Vina M, et al. Definitions of histocompatibility typing terms. *Blood*. 2011;118(23): e180−183.

53. Holdsworth R, Hurley CK, Marsh SG, et al. The HLA dictionary 2008: a summary of HLA-A, -B, -C, -DRB1/3/4/5, and -DQB1 alleles and their association with serologically defined HLA-A, -B, -C, -DR, and -DQ antigens. *Tissue Antigens*. 2009;73(2):95−170.

54. Adamek M, Klages C, Bauer M, et al. Seven novel HLA alleles reflect different mechanisms involved in the evolution of HLA diversity: description of the new alleles and review of the literature. *Hum Immunol*. 2015;76(1): 30−35.

55. Rodey GE, Neylan JF, Whelchel JD, Revels KW, Bray RA. Epitope specificity of HLA class I alloantibodies. I. Frequency analysis of antibodies to private versus public specificities in potential transplant recipients. *Hum Immunol*. 1994;39(4):272−280.

56. Rodey GE. *HLA beyond Tears*. 2nd ed. Durango, CO: De Novo; 2000.

57. Duquesnoy RJ, Filip DJ, Rodey GE, Rimm AA, Aster RH. Successful transfusion of platelets "mismatched" for HLA antigens to alloimmunized thrombocytopenic patients. *Am J Hematol*. 1977;2(3):219−226.

58. Forest SK, Hod EA. Management of the platelet refractory patient. *Hematol Oncol Clin N Am*. 2016;30(3):665−677.

59. Duquesnoy RJ. HLAMatchmaker: a molecularly based algorithm for histocompatibility determination. I. Description of the algorithm. *Hum Immunol*. 2002; 63(5):339−352.

60. Brooks EG, MacPherson BR, Fung MK. Validation of HLAMatchmaker algorithm in identifying acceptable HLA mismatches for thrombocytopenic patients refractory to platelet transfusions. *Transfusion*. 2008;48(10): 2159−2166.

61. Nambiar A, Duquesnoy RJ, Adams S, et al. HLAMatchmaker-driven analysis of responses to HLA-typed platelet transfusions in alloimmunized thrombocytopenic patients. *Blood*. 2006;107(4):1680−1687.

62. von dem Borne AE, Decary F. ICSH/ISBT Working Party on platelet serology. Nomenclature of platelet-specific antigens. *Vox Sang*. 1990;58(2):176.

63. Curtis BR. Recent progress in understanding the pathogenesis of fetal and neonatal alloimmune thrombocytopenia. *Br J Haematol*. 2015;171(5):671−682.

64. Vadasz B, Chen P, Yougbare I, et al. Platelets and platelet alloantigens: lessons from human patients and animal models of fetal and neonatal alloimmune thrombocytopenia. *Genes Dis*. 2015;2(2):173−185.

65. Giltay JC, Leeksma OC, von dem Borne AE, van Mourik JA. Alloantigenic composition of the endothelial vitronectin receptor. *Blood*. 1988;72(1):230−233.

66. Metcalfe P, Watkins NA, Ouwehand WH, et al. Nomenclature of human platelet antigens. *Vox Sang*. 2003; 85(3):240−245.

67. Metcalfe P. Platelet antigens and antibody detection. *Vox Sang*. 2004;87(Suppl1):82−86.

68. Santoso S, Kroll H, Andrei-Selmer CL, et al. A naturally occurring LeuVal mutation in beta3-integrin impairs the HPA-1a epitope: the third allele of HPA-1. *Transfusion*. 2006;46(5):790−799.

69. Database EBIIP. Human Platelet Antigen (HPA) System. Accessed 12/18/2018.

70. Lochowicz AJ, Curtis BR. Clinical applications of platelet antibody and antigen testing. *Lab Med*. 2011;42(11): 687−692.

71. Peterson JA, Pechauer SM, Gitter ML, et al. New platelet glycoprotein polymorphisms causing maternal immunization and neonatal alloimmune thrombocytopenia. *Transfusion*. 2012;52(5):1117−1124.

72. Jallu V, Dusseaux M, Kaplan C. A new Ser472Asn (Cab2(a$^+$)) polymorphism localized within the alphaIIb "thigh" domain is involved in neonatal thrombocytopenia. *Transfusion*. 2011;51(2):393−400.

73. Kroll H, Feldmann K, Zwingel C, et al. A new platelet alloantigen, Swi(a) , located on glycoprotein Ia identified in a family with fetal and neonatal alloimmune thrombocytopenia. *Transfusion*. 2011;51(8):1745−1754.

74. Sachs UJ, Bakchoul T, Eva O, et al. A point mutation in the EGF-4 domain of beta(3) integrin is responsible for the formation of the Sec(a) platelet alloantigen and affects receptor function. *Thromb Haemostasis*. 2012; 107(1):80−87.

75. Jallu V, Bertrand G, Bianchi F, Chenet C, Poulain P, Kaplan C. The alphaIIb p.Leu841Met (Cab3(a$^+$)) polymorphism results in a new human platelet alloantigen involved in neonatal alloimmune thrombocytopenia. *Transfusion*. 2013;53(3):554−563.

76. Poles A, Wozniak MJ, Walser P, et al. A V740L mutation in glycoprotein IIb defines a novel epitope (War) associated with fetomaternal alloimmune thrombocytopenia. *Transfusion*. 2013;53(9):1965−1973.

77. Sullivan MJ, Peterson J, McFarland JG, Bougie D, Aster RH, Curtis BR. A new low-frequency alloantigen (Kha(b)) located on platelet glycoprotein IIIa as a cause of maternal sensitization leading to neonatal alloimmune thrombocytopenia. *Transfusion*. 2015;55(6 Pt 2): 1584−1585.

78. Wihadmadyatami H, Heidinger K, Roder L, et al. Alloantibody against new platelet alloantigen (Lap(a)) on glycoprotein IIb is responsible for a case of fetal and neonatal alloimmune thrombocytopenia. *Transfusion*. 2015;55(12):2920−2929.

79. Jallu V, Beranger T, Bianchi F, et al. Cab4b, the first human platelet antigen carried by glycoprotein IX discovered in a context of severe neonatal thrombocytopenia. *J Thromb Haemost*. 2017;15(8):1646−1654.

80. Sullivan MJ, Kuhlmann R, Peterson JA, Curtis BR. Severe neonatal alloimmune thrombocytopenia caused by maternal sensitization against a new low-frequency alloantigen (Dom(b)) located on platelet glycoprotein IIIa. *Transfusion*. 2017;57(7):1847−1848.

81. Warkentin TE, Smith JW. The alloimmune thrombocytopenic syndromes. *Transfus Med Rev.* 1997;11(4):296–307.

82. Baker EK, Tozer EC, Pfaff M, Shattil SJ, Loftus JC, Ginsberg MH. A genetic analysis of integrin function: Glanzmann thrombasthenia in vitro. *Proc Natl Acad Sci USA.* 1997;94(5):1973–1978.

83. Nurden AT, Fiore M, Nurden P, Pillois X. Glanzmann thrombasthenia: a review of ITGA2B and ITGB3 defects with emphasis on variants, phenotypic variability, and mouse models. *Blood.* 2011;118(23):5996–6005.

84. Landau M, Rosenberg N. Molecular insight into human platelet antigens: structural and evolutionary conservation analyses offer new perspective to immunogenic disorders. *Transfusion.* 2011;51(3):558–569.

85. Schnaidt M, Wernet D. Platelet-specific antibodies in female blood donors after pregnancy. *Transfus Med.* 2000;10(1):77–80.

86. Lin M, Xu X, Lee HL, Liang DC, Santoso S. Fetal/neonatal alloimmune thrombocytopenia due to anti-CD36 antibodies: antibody evaluations by CD36-transfected cell lines. *Transfusion.* 2018;58(1):189–195.

87. Wang J, Xia W, Deng J, et al. Analysis of platelet-reactive alloantibodies and evaluation of cross-match-compatible platelets for the management of patients with transfusion refractoriness. *Transfus Med.* 2018;28(1):40–46.

88. Yamamoto N, Akamatsu N, Sakuraba H, Yamazaki H, Tanoue K. Platelet glycoprotein IV (CD36) deficiency is associated with the absence (type I) or the presence (type II) of glycoprotein IV on monocytes. *Blood.* 1994;83(2):392–397.

89. Kaplan C, Freedman J, Foxcroft Z, et al. Monoclonal platelet antigen capture assays (MAIPA) and reagents: a statement. *Vox Sang.* 2007;93(4):298–299.

90. Kiefel V, Santoso S, Weisheit M, Mueller-Eckhardt C. Monoclonal antibody–specific immobilization of platelet antigens (MAIPA): a new tool for the identification of platelet-reactive antibodies. *Blood.* 1987;70(6):1722–1726.

91. Hayashi T, Hirayama F. Advances in alloimmune thrombocytopenia: perspectives on current concepts of human platelet antigens, antibody detection strategies, and genotyping. *Blood Transfus.* 2015;13(3):380–390.

92. Dunstan RA, Simpson MB, Knowles RW, Rosse WF. The origin of ABH antigens on human platelets. *Blood.* 1985;65(3):615–619.

93. Santoso S, Kiefel V, Mueller-Eckhardt C. Blood group A and B determinants are expressed on platelet glycoproteins IIa, IIIa, and Ib. *Thromb Haemostasis.* 1991;65(2):196–201.

94. Ogasawara K, Ueki J, Takenaka M, Furihata K. Study on the expression of ABH antigens on platelets. *Blood.* 1993;82(3):993–999.

95. Cooling LL, Kelly K, Barton J, Hwang D, Koerner TA, Olson JD. Determinants of ABH expression on human blood platelets. *Blood.* 2005;105(8):3356–3364.

96. Curtis BR, Edwards JT, Hessner MJ, Klein JP, Aster RH. Blood group A and B antigens are strongly expressed on platelets of some individuals. *Blood.* 2000;96(4):1574–1581.

97. Sant'Anna Gomes BM, Estalote AC, Palatnik M, Pimenta G, Pereira Bde B, Do Nascimento EM. Prevalence, serologic and genetic studies of high expressers of the blood group A antigen on platelets*. *Transfus Med.* 2010;20(5):303–314.

98. Duke WW. The relation of blood platelets to hemorrhagic disease: description of a method for determining the bleeding time and coagulation time and report of three cases of hemorrhagic disease relieved by transfusion. *J Am Med Assoc.* 1910;55(14):1185–1192.

99. Han T, Stutzman L, Cohen E, Kim U. Effect of platelet transfusion on hemorrhage in patients with acute leukemia. An autopsy study. *Cancer.* 1966;19(12):1937–1942.

100. Hersh EM, Bodey GP, Nies BA, Freireich EJ. Causes of death in acute leukemia: a ten-year study of 414 patients from 1954-1963. *J Am Med Assoc.* 1965;193:105–109.

101. Sweeney JD, L M. Epidemiology of platelet transfusion. In: SJL M, ed. *Platelet Transfusion Therapy.* Bethesda: AABB Press; 2013.

102. Ellingson KD, Sapiano MRP, Haass KA, et al. Continued decline in blood collection and transfusion in the United States-2015. *Transfusion.* 2017;57(Suppl 2):1588–1598.

103. Whitaker B, Sullivan M. *Nationwide Blood Collection and Utilization Survey Report.* United States Department of Health and Human Services; 2005.

104. Salama ME, Raman S, Drew MJ, Abdel-Raheem M, Mahmood MN. Platelet function testing to assess effectiveness of platelet transfusion therapy. *Transfus Apher Sci.* 2004;30(2):93–100.

105. Davis KB, Slichter SJ, Corash L. Corrected count increment and percent platelet recovery as measures of posttransfusion platelet response: problems and a solution. *Transfusion.* 1999;39(6):586–592.

106. Brubaker DB, Marcus C, Holmes E. Intravascular and total body platelet equilibrium in healthy volunteers and in thrombocytopenic patients transfused with single donor platelets. *Am J Hematol.* 1998;58(3):165–176.

107. Aster RH. Pooling of platelets in the spleen: role in the pathogenesis of "hypersplenic" thrombocytopenia. *J Clin Investig.* 1966;45(5):645–657.

108. Heddle NM, Arnold DM, Boye D, Webert KE, Resz I, Dumont LJ. Comparing the efficacy and safety of apheresis and whole blood-derived platelet transfusions: a systematic review. *Transfusion.* 2008;48(7):1447–1458.

109. Schiffer CA, Lee EJ, Ness PM, Reilly J. Clinical evaluation of platelet concentrates stored for one to five days. *Blood.* 1986;67(6):1591–1594.

110. Hanson SR, Slichter SJ. Platelet kinetics in patients with bone marrow hypoplasia: evidence for a fixed platelet requirement. *Blood.* 1985;66(5):1105–1109.

111. Slichter SJ, Davis K, Enright H, et al. Factors affecting posttransfusion platelet increments, platelet refractoriness, and platelet transfusion intervals in thrombocytopenic patients. *Blood.* 2005;105(10):4106–4114.
112. Daly PA, Schiffer CA, Aisner J, Wiernik PH. Platelet transfusion therapy. One-hour posttransfusion increments are valuable in predicting the need for HLA-matched preparations. *J Am Med Assoc.* 1980;243(5):435–438.
113. Bishop JF, Matthews JP, Yuen K, McGrath K, Wolf MM, Szer J. The definition of refractoriness to platelet transfusions. *Transfus Med.* 1992;2(1):35–41.
114. Bishop JF, Matthews JP, McGrath K, Yuen K, Wolf MM, Szer J. Factors influencing 20-hour increments after platelet transfusion. *Transfusion.* 1991;31(5):392–396.
115. Li J, Callum JL, Lin Y, Zhou Y, Zhu G, Ni H. Severe platelet desialylation in a patient with glycoprotein Ib/IX antibody-mediated immune thrombocytopenia and fatal pulmonary hemorrhage. *Haematologica.* 2014;99(4):e61–63.
116. Pavenski K, Freedman J, Semple JW. HLA alloimmunization against platelet transfusions: pathophysiology, significance, prevention and management. *Tissue Antigens.* 2012;79(4):237–245.
117. George JN, Aster RH. Drug-induced thrombocytopenia: pathogenesis, evaluation, and management. *Hematology Am Soc Hematol Educ Program.* 2009:153–158.
118. Drug-Induced Thrombocytopenia. https://www.ouhsc.edu/platelets/ditp.html. Accessed 12/29/2018.
119. Aster RH, Curtis BR, McFarland JG, Bougie DW. Drug-induced immune thrombocytopenia: pathogenesis, diagnosis, and management. *J Thromb Haemost.* 2009;7(6):911–918.
120. Kerkhoffs JL, E JC, van de Watering LM, van Wordragen-Vlaswinkel RJ, Wijermans PW, Brand A. The clinical impact of platelet refractoriness: correlation with bleeding and survival. *Transfusion.* 2008;48(9):1959–1965.
121. Meehan KR, Matias CO, Rathore SS, et al. Platelet transfusions: utilization and associated costs in a tertiary care hospital. *Am J Hematol.* 2000;64(4):251–256.
122. Seftel MD, Growe GH, Petraszko T, et al. Universal prestorage leukoreduction in Canada decreases platelet alloimmunization and refractoriness. *Blood.* 2004;103(1):333–339.
123. Rebulla P. A mini-review on platelet refractoriness. *Haematologica.* 2005;90(2):247–253.
124. Wadenvik H, Kutti J. The spleen and pooling of blood cells. *Eur J Haematol.* 1988;41(1):1–5.
125. Cid J, L M. Platelet transfusion. ABO and RhD. In: SJL M, ed. *Platelet Transfusion Therapy.* Bethesda: AABB Press; 2013.
125a. Hogge DE, McConnell M, Jacobson C, Sutherland HJ, Benny WB, Massing BG. Platelet refractoriness and alloimmunization in pediatric oncology and bone marrow transplant patients. *Transfusion.* 1995 Aug;35(8):645–652. PubMed PMID: 7631404.
126. Lin Y, Callum JL, Coovadia AS, Murphy PM. Transfusion of ABO-nonidentical platelets is not associated with adverse clinical outcomes in cardiovascular surgery patients. *Transfusion.* 2002;42(2):166–172.
127. Fung MK, Downes KA, Shulman IA. Transfusion of platelets containing ABO-incompatible plasma: a survey of 3156 North American laboratories. *Arch Pathol Lab Med.* 2007;131(6):909–916.
128. Lozano M, Heddle N, Williamson LM, et al. Practices associated with ABO-incompatible platelet transfusions: a BEST Collaborative international survey. *Transfusion.* 2010;50(8):1743–1748.
129. Dunbar NM, Ornstein DL, Dumont LJ. ABO incompatible platelets: risks versus benefit. *Curr Opin Hematol.* 2012;19(6):475–479.
130. Dunbar NM, Katus MC, Freeman CM, Szczepiorkowski ZM. Easier said than done: ABO compatibility and D matching in apheresis platelet transfusions. *Transfusion.* 2015;55(8):1882–1888.
131. Harris SB, Josephson CD, Kost CB, Hillyer CD. Nonfatal intravascular hemolysis in a pediatric patient after transfusion of a platelet unit with high-titer anti-A. *Transfusion.* 2007;47(8):1412–1417.
132. Daniel-Johnson J, Leitman S, Klein H, et al. Probiotic-associated high-titer anti-B in a group A platelet donor as a cause of severe hemolytic transfusion reactions. *Transfusion.* 2009;49(9):1845–1849.
133. Heal JM, Masel D, Rowe JM, Blumberg N. Circulating immune complexes involving the ABO system after platelet transfusion. *Br J Haematol.* 1993;85(3):566–572.
134. Hendrickson JE. Platelet transfusion refractory patients. In: Shaz BH, ed. *Transfusion Medicine and Hemostasis: Clincial and Laboratory Aspects.* 2nd ed. Amsterdam: Elsevier; 2013.
135. Triulzi DJ, Assmann SF, Strauss RG, et al. The impact of platelet transfusion characteristics on posttransfusion platelet increments and clinical bleeding in patients with hypoproliferative thrombocytopenia. *Blood.* 2012;119(23):5553–5562.
136. Aster RH. Effect of anticoagulant and ABO incompatibility on recovery of transfused human platelets. *Blood.* 1965;26(6):732–743.
137. Duguesnoy RJ, Anderson AJ, Tomasulo PA, Aster RH. ABO compatibility and platelet transfusions of alloimmunized thrombocytopenic patients. *Blood.* 1979;54(3):595–599.
138. Klumpp TR, Herman JH, Innis S, et al. Factors associated with response to platelet transfusion following hematopoietic stem cell transplantation. *Bone Marrow Transplant.* 1996;17(6):1035–1041.
139. Pavenski K, Warkentin TE, Shen H, Liu Y, Heddle NM. Posttransfusion platelet count increments after ABO-compatible versus ABO-incompatible platelet transfusions in noncancer patients: an observational study. *Transfusion.* 2010;50(7):1552–1560.
140. Shehata N, Tinmouth A, Naglie G, Freedman J, Wilson K. ABO-identical versus nonidentical platelet transfusion: a systematic review. *Transfusion.* 2009;49(11):2442–2453.
141. Refaai MA, Carter J, Henrichs KF, et al. Alterations of platelet function and clot formation kinetics after in vitro exposure to anti-A and -B. *Transfusion.* 2013;53(2):382–393.

142. Lee EJ, Schiffer CA. ABO compatibility can influence the results of platelet transfusion. Results of a randomized trial. *Transfusion*. 1989;29(5):384–389.

143. Heal JM, Rowe JM, Blumberg N. ABO and platelet transfusion revisited. *Ann Hematol*. 1993;66(6):309–314.

144. Carr R, Hutton JL, Jenkins JA, Lucas GF, Amphlett NW. Transfusion of ABO-mismatched platelets leads to early platelet refractoriness. *Br J Haematol*. 1990;75(3):408–413.

145. Kiefel V, Konig C, Kroll H, Santoso S. Platelet alloantibodies in transfused patients. *Transfusion*. 2001;41(6):766–770.

146. Stanworth SJ, Navarrete C, Estcourt L, Marsh J. Platelet refractoriness–practical approaches and ongoing dilemmas in patient management. *Br J Haematol*. 2015; 171(3):297–305.

147. Vassallo RR. Recognition and management of antibodies to human platelet antigens in platelet transfusion-refractory patients. *Immunohematology*. 2009;25(3):119–124.

148. Doughty HA, Murphy MF, Metcalfe P, Rohatiner AZ, Lister TA, Waters AH. Relative importance of immune and non-immune causes of platelet refractoriness. *Vox Sang*. 1994;66(3):200–205.

149. Sanz C, Freire C, Alcorta I, Ordinas A, Pereira A. Platelet-specific antibodies in HLA-immunized patients receiving chronic platelet support. *Transfusion*. 2001;41(6): 762–765.

150. Kopko PM, Warner P, Kresie L, Pancoska C. Methods for the selection of platelet products for alloimmune-refractory patients. *Transfusion*. 2015;55(2):235–244.

151. Elhence P, Chaudhary RK, Nityanand S. Cross-match-compatible platelets improve corrected count increments in patients who are refractory to randomly selected platelets. *Blood Transfus*. 2014;12(2):180–186.

152. Fontao-Wendel R, Silva LC, Saviolo CB, Primavera B, Wendel S. Incidence of transfusion-induced platelet-reactive antibodies evaluated by specific assays for the detection of human leucocyte antigen and human platelet antigen antibodies. *Vox Sang*. 2007;93(3):241–249.

153. Lim J, Kim Y, Han K, et al. Flow cytometric monocyte phagocytic assay for predicting platelet transfusion outcome. *Transfusion*. 2002;42(3):309–316.

154. Arthur CM, Patel SR, Sullivan HC, et al. CD8+ T cells mediate antibody-independent platelet clearance in mice. *Blood*. 2016;127(14):1823–1827.

155. Nahirniak S, Slichter SJ, Tanael S, et al. Guidance on platelet transfusion for patients with hypoproliferative thrombocytopenia. *Transfus Med Rev*. 2015;29(1):3–13.

156. Juskewitch JE, Norgan AP, De Goey SR, et al. How do I... manage the platelet transfusion-refractory patient? *Transfusion*. 2017;57(12):2828–2835.

157. Moroff G, Garratty G, Heal JM, et al. Selection of platelets for refractory patients by HLA matching and prospective crossmatching. *Transfusion*. 1992;32(7):633–640.

158. Petz LD, Garratty G, Calhoun L, et al. Selecting donors of platelets for refractory patients on the basis of HLA antibody specificity. *Transfusion*. 2000;40(12):1446–1456.

159. Bolgiano DC, Larson EB, Slichter SJ. A model to determine required pool size for HLA-typed community donor apheresis programs. *Transfusion*. 1989;29(4): 306–310.

160. Vassallo R, F M. Management of the platelet transfusion refractory patient. In: Sweeney JLM, ed. *Platelet Transfusion Therapy*. Bethesda: AABB Press; 2013.

161. Rachel JM, Summers TC, Sinor LT, Plapp FV. Use of a solid phase red blood cell adherence method for pre-transfusion platelet compatibility testing. *Am J Clin Pathol*. 1988;90(1):63–68.

162. Heal JM, Mullin A, Blumberg N. The importance of ABH antigens in platelet crossmatching. *Transfusion*. 1989; 29(6):514–520.

163. Heal JM, Blumberg N, Masel D. An evaluation of crossmatching, HLA, and ABO matching for platelet transfusions to refractory patients. *Blood*. 1987;70(1):23–30.

164. Vassallo RR, Fung M, Rebulla P, et al. Utility of cross-matched platelet transfusions in patients with hypoproliferative thrombocytopenia: a systematic review. *Transfusion*. 2014;54(4):1180–1191.

165. Wiita AP, Nambiar A. Longitudinal management with crossmatch-compatible platelets for refractory patients: alloimmunization, response to transfusion, and clinical outcomes (CME). *Transfusion*. 2012;52(10):2146–2154.

166. Pappalardo PA, Secord AR, Quitevis P, Haimowitz MD, Goldfinger D. Platelet transfusion refractoriness associated with HPA-1a (Pl(A1)) alloantibody without coexistent HLA antibodies successfully treated with antigen-negative platelet transfusions. *Transfusion*. 2001; 41(8):984–987.

167. Dahlke MB, Weiss KL. Platelet transfusion from donors mismatched for crossreactive HLA antigens. *Transfusion*. 1984;24(4):299–302.

168. McVey M, Cserti-Gazdewich CM. Platelet transfusion refractoriness responding preferentially to single donor aphaeresis platelets compatible for both ABO and HLA. *Transfus Med*. 2010;20(5):346–353.

169. Pavenski K, Rebulla P, Duquesnoy R, et al. Efficacy of HLA-matched platelet transfusions for patients with hypoproliferative thrombocytopenia: a systematic review. *Transfusion*. 2013;53(10):2230–2242.

170. Murphy ME. Manging the platelet refractory patient. *ISBT Sci Ser*. 2014;9:234–238.

171. Messerschmidt GL, Makuch R, Appelbaum F, et al. A prospective randomized trial of HLA-matched versus mismatched single-donor platelet transfusions in cancer patients. *Cancer*. 1988;62(4):795–801.

172. Atlas E, Freedman J, Blanchette V, Kazatchkine MD, Semple JW. Downregulation of the anti-HLA alloimmune response by variable region-reactive (anti-idiotypic) antibodies in leukemic patients transfused with platelet concentrates. *Blood*. 1993;81(2): 538–542.

173. Lee EJ, Schiffer CA. Serial measurement of lymphocytotoxic antibody and response to nonmatched platelet transfusions in alloimmunized patients. *Blood*. 1987; 70(6):1727–1729.

174. van de Watering L, Hermans J, Witvliet M, Versteegh M, Brand A. HLA and RBC immunization after filtered and

buffy coat-depleted blood transfusion in cardiac surgery: a randomized controlled trial. *Transfusion*. 2003;43(6): 765−771.

175. van Marwijk Kooy M, van Prooijen HC, Moes M, Bosma-Stants I, Akkerman JW. Use of leukocyte-depleted platelet concentrates for the prevention of refractoriness and primary HLA alloimmunization: a prospective, randomized trial. *Blood*. 1991;77(1):201−205.

176. Fast LD, Dileone G, Li J, Goodrich R. Functional inactivation of white blood cells by Mirasol treatment. *Transfusion*. 2006;46(4):642−648.

177. Jackman RP, Muench MO, Inglis H, et al. Reduced MHC alloimmunization and partial tolerance protection with pathogen reduction of whole blood. *Transfusion*. 2017; 57(2):337−348.

178. Jackman RP, Deng X, Bolgiano D, et al. Low-level HLA antibodies do not predict platelet transfusion failure in TRAP study participants. *Blood*. 2013;121(16): 3261−3266. quiz 3299.

179. Aster RH, Szatkowski N, Liebert M, Duquesnoy RJ. Expression of HLA-B12, HLA-B8, w4, and w5 on platelets. *Transplant Proc*. 1977;9(4):1695−1696.

180. Schiffer CA, O'Connell B, Lee EJ. Platelet transfusion therapy for alloimmunized patients: selective mismatching for HLA B12, an antigen with variable expression on platelets. *Blood*. 1989;74(3):1172−1176.

181. Rioux-Masse B, Cohn C, Lindgren B, Pulkrabek S, McCullough J. Utilization of cross-matched or HLA-matched platelets for patients refractory to platelet transfusion. *Transfusion*. 2014;54(12):3080−3087.

181a. Ishida A, Handa M, Wakui M, Okamoto S, Kamakura M, Ikeda Y. Clinical factors influencing posttransfusion platelet increment in patients undergoing hematopoietic progenitor cell transplantation−a prospective analysis. *Transfusion*. 1998 Sep;38(9):839−847. PubMed PMID: 9738624.

182. Mazzara R, Escolar G, Garrido M, et al. Procoagulant effect of incompatible platelet transfusions in alloimmunized refractory patients. *Vox Sang*. 1996; 71(2):84−89.

183. Lucas G, Culliford S, Green F, et al. Recipient-derived HPA-1a antibodies: a cause of prolonged thrombocytopenia after unrelated donor stem cell transplantation. *Transfusion*. 2010;50(2):334−339.

184. Tiller H, Husebekk A, Ahlen MT, Stuge TB, Skogen B. Current perspectives on fetal and neonatal alloimmune thrombocytopenia - increasing clinical concerns and new treatment opportunities. *Int J Womens Health*. 2017;9:223−234.

185. Tiller H, Killie MK, Skogen B, Oian P, Husebekk A. Neonatal alloimmune thrombocytopenia in Norway: poor detection rate with nonscreening versus a general screening programme. *BJOG*. 2009;116(4):594−598.

186. Davoren A, Curtis BR, Aster RH, McFarland JG. Human platelet antigen-specific alloantibodies implicated in 1162 cases of neonatal alloimmune thrombocytopenia. *Transfusion*. 2004;44(8):1220−1225.

187. Williamson LM, Hackett G, Rennie J, et al. The natural history of fetomaternal alloimmunization to the platelet-specific antigen HPA-1a (PlA1, Zwa) as determined by antenatal screening. *Blood*. 1998;92(7): 2280−2287.

188. Kjeldsen-Kragh J, Killie MK, Tomter G, et al. A screening and intervention program aimed to reduce mortality and serious morbidity associated with severe neonatal alloimmune thrombocytopenia. *Blood*. 2007;110(3):833−839.

189. Kamphuis MM, Paridaans N, Porcelijn L, et al. Screening in pregnancy for fetal or neonatal alloimmune thrombocytopenia: systematic review. *BJOG*. 2010;117(11): 1335−1343.

190. L'Abbe D, Tremblay L, Filion M, et al. Alloimmunization to platelet antigen HPA-1a (PIA1) is strongly associated with both HLA-DRB3*0101 and HLA-DQB1*0201. *Hum Immunol*. 1992;34(2):107−114.

191. Wienzek-Lischka S, Konig IR, Papenkort EM, et al. HLA-DRB3*01:01 is a predictor of immunization against human platelet antigen-1a but not of the severity of fetal and neonatal alloimmune thrombocytopenia. *Transfusion*. 2017;57(3):533−540.

192. Sainio S, Javela K, Tuimala J, Haimila K. Maternal HLA genotyping is not useful for predicting severity of fetal and neonatal alloimmune thrombocytopenia. *Br J Haematol*. 2017;176(1):111−117.

193. Tiller H, Killie MK, Chen P, et al. Toward a prophylaxis against fetal and neonatal alloimmune thrombocytopenia: induction of antibody-mediated immune suppression and prevention of severe clinical complications in a murine model. *Transfusion*. 2012;52(7):1446−1457.

194. Eksteen M, Tiller H, Averina M, et al. Characterization of a human platelet antigen-1a-specific monoclonal antibody derived from a B cell from a woman alloimmunized in pregnancy. *J Immunol*. 2015;194(12):5751−5760.

195. Mueller-Eckhardt C. Post-transfusion purpura. *Br J Haematol*. 1986;64(3):419−424.

196. Williamson LM, Stainsby D, Jones H, et al. The impact of universal leukodepletion of the blood supply on hemovigilance reports of posttransfusion purpura and transfusion-associated graft-versus-host disease. *Transfusion*. 2007;47(8):1455−1467.

197. Shulman NR, Aster RH, Leitner A, Hiller MC. Immunoreactions involving platelets. V. Post-transfusion purpura due to a complement-fixing antibody against a genetically controlled platelet antigen. A proposed mechanism for thrombocytopenia and its relevance in "autoimmunity". *J Clin Investig*. 1961;40(9):1597−1620.

198. Cushing MM. Post-transfusion purpura. In: Shaz BH, ed. *Transfusion Medicine and Hemostasis: Clincial and Laboratory Aspects*. 2nd ed. Amsterdam: Elsevier; 2013.

199. Wernet D, Sessler M, Dette S, Northoff H, Schnaidt M. Post-transfusion purpura following liver transplantation. *Vox Sang*. 2003;85(2):117−118.

200. Shtalrid M, Shvidel L, Vorst E, Weinmann EE, Berrebi A, Sigler E. Post-transfusion purpura: a challenging diagnosis. *Isr Med Assoc J*. 2006;8(10):672−674.

201. Lubenow N, Eichler P, Albrecht D, et al. Very low platelet counts in post-transfusion purpura falsely diagnosed as heparin-induced thrombocytopenia. Report of four cases and review of literature. *Thromb Res.* 2000;100(3): 115−125.

202. National Healthcare Safety Network Biovigilance Component Hemovigilance Module Surveillance Protocol, v2.5. Division of Healthcare Quality Promotion National Center for Emerging and Zoonotic Infectious Diseases Centers for Disease Control and Prevention Atlanta, GA, USA. January 2018

203. Watkins NA, Smethurst PA, Allen D, Smith GA, Ouwehand WH. Platelet alphaIIbbeta3 recombinant autoantibodies from the B-cell repertoire of a post-transfusion purpura patient. *Br J Haematol.* 2002; 116(3):677−685.

204. Woelke C, Eichler P, Washington G, Flesch BK. Post-transfusion purpura in a patient with HPA-1a and GPIa/IIa antibodies. *Transfus Med.* 2006;16(1):69−72.

205. Stricker RB, Lewis BH, Corash L, Shuman MA. Posttransfusion purpura associated with an autoantibody directed against a previously undefined platelet antigen. *Blood.* 1987;69(5):1458−1463.

206. Taaning E, Tonnesen F. Pan-reactive platelet antibodies in post-transfusion purpura. *Vox Sang.* 1999;76(2): 120−123.

207. Minchinton RM, Cunningham I, Cole-Sinclair M, Van der Weyden M, Vaughan S, McGrath KM. Autoreactive platelet antibody in post transfusion purpura. *Aust N Z J Med.* 1990;20(2):111−115.

208. Lucas GF, Pittman SJ, Davies S, Solanki T, Bruggemann K. Post-transfusion purpura (PTP) associated with anti-HPA-1a, anti-HPA-2b and anti-HPA-3a antibodies. *Transfus Med.* 1997;7(4):295−299.

209. Schwartz J, Padmanabhan A, Aqui N, et al. Guidelines on the use of therapeutic apheresis in clinical practice-evidence-based approach from the writing committee of the American society for apheresis: the seventh special issue. *J Clin Apher.* 2016;31(3):149−162.

210. Brecher ME, Moore SB, Letendre L. Posttransfusion purpura: the therapeutic value of PlA1-negative platelets. *Transfusion.* 1990;30(5):433−435.

211. Loren AW, Abrams CS. Efficacy of HPA-1a (PlA1)-negative platelets in a patient with post-transfusion purpura. *Am J Hematol.* 2004;76(3):258−262.

212. Vogelsang G, Kickler TS, Bell WR. Post-transfusion purpura: a report of five patients and a review of the pathogenesis and management. *Am J Hematol.* 1986;21(3): 259−267.

213. Godeau B, Fromont P, Bettaieb A, Beaujean F, Duedari N, Bierling P. Relapse of posttransfusion purpura after transfusion with frozen-thawed red cells. *Transfusion.* 1991; 31(2):189−190.

214. Cobos E, Gandara DR, Geier LJ, Kirmani S. Post-transfusion purpura and isoimmune neonatal thrombocytopenia in the same family. *Am J Hematol.* 1989; 32(3):235−236.

215. Zucker MB, Ley AB, Borrelli J, Mayer K, Firmat J. Thrombocytopenia with a circulating platelet agglutinin, platelet agglutinin, platelet lysin and clot retraction inhibitor. *Blood.* 1959;14(2):148−161.

216. Pavenski K, Webert KE, Goldman M. Consequences of transfusion of platelet antibody: a case report and literature review. *Transfusion.* 2008;48(9):1981−1989.

217. Brunner-Bolliger S, Kiefel V, Horber FF, Nydegger UE, Berchtold P. Antibody studies in a patient with acute thrombocytopenia following infusion of plasma containing anti-PI(A1). *Am J Hematol.* 1997;56(2):119−121.

218. Brouk H, Ouelaa H. Fetal and neonatal alloimmune thrombocytopenia: advances in laboratory diagnosis and management. *Int J Blood Res Disord.* 2015;2.

219. Hod E, Schwartz J. Platelet transfusion refractoriness. *Br J Haematol.* 2008;142(3):348−360.

CHAPTER 9

Alloimmunization in Pregnancy

MICHELLE L. ERICKSON, MD, MBA

INTRODUCTION

Maternal alloimmunization describes the presence of non-AB red blood cell (RBC) antibodies in a pregnant woman. Alloimmunization during pregnancy has important clinical consequences for the fetus and mother, and imparts a high-risk status on the pregnancy. Some alloantibodies, particularly IgG type, can cross the placenta and enter fetal circulation, causing fetal hemolysis, anemia, and hydrops. Prenatal consequences include fetal demise due to cardiovascular collapse, while postnatal events may include severe hemolysis with kernicterus causing neurodevelopmental delay. Early identification of maternal alloimmunization allows monitoring during pregnancy and timely intervention to prevent poor fetal outcomes and long-term disability. Additionally, steps can be taken to ensure the safety of the mother, who is herself at risk due to the potential delay of care associated with alloantibodies.

Maternal alloimmunization is uncommon and highly variable, leading to confusion among general obstetricians and midwives who may not be familiar with the 50 plus non-AB blood groups implicated in hemolytic disease of the fetus and newborn (HDFN).[1] This author has encountered several misconceptions on maternal alloimmunization that, if not corrected, can lead to poor outcomes. Several of these involve underestimation of fetal risk caused by unfamiliarity with non-RhD antibodies. One of the most pervasive myths is that once HDFN has been ruled out, the pregnancy can then be considered low risk. However, the mother with antibodies is herself at risk due to potential complications should she require transfusion. Postpartum hemorrhage is common, occurring in 3% −5% of deliveries and causing 12% of maternal deaths.[2,3] Up to 20% of these cases will occur in women without known risk factors for hemorrhage[4]; however, many alloimmunized mothers already have known risk factors, such as prior abruption, Caesarean section, or fetal hemorrhage. The presence of alloantibodies delays the blood bank work-up and acquisition of appropriate crossmatched compatible blood, disrupting obstetric surgical scheduling and creating a hazard during hemorrhage events. Upon transfusion, patients with antibodies are at risk of acute and delayed hemolytic transfusion reactions. For mothers considering additional childbearing, prevention of further alloimmunization should also be considered in the provision of matched blood (Table 9.1).

EPIDEMIOLOGY

Alloimmunization Rates

Rhesus D blood antigen has long been recognized as the most immunogenic antigen and dismaying cause of HDFN due to maternal alloimmunization. Studies have demonstrated that up to 80% of healthy Rhesus D-negative adults exposed to D^+ blood will become isoimmunized to the antigen[5−8] while 8%−10% will form antibodies to non-D antigens. Miniscule volumes of 0.03−0.5 mL antigen-positive blood exposure

TABLE 9.1
Misconceptions About Maternal Alloimmunization.
Common Misconceptions on Maternal Alloimmunization
First pregnancies are unaffected
Only anti-D is associated with HDFN
Screening is required only for RhD-negative women
Antibodies form after, not during, pregnancy
Antibody screening should be done only at intake
Anti-M is always benign
Once risk for HDFN is ruled out, the pregnancy is low risk
One titer is sufficient for the duration of pregnancy
The risks associated with the presenting pregnancy will be the same for subsequent pregnancies

Immunologic Concepts in Transfusion Medicine. https://doi.org/10.1016/B978-0-323-67509-3.00009-3

suffices to induce antibody formation,[9,10] meaning that even minor fetal maternal hemorrhage or the amount of blood in a shared needle can stimulate maternal isoimmunization.[11] Surprisingly, in a study evaluating the impact of phenotypic matching of blood units, several patients developed antibodies via platelet transfusion only.[12] Although overall rates of maternal alloimmunization are low at about 0.1% for anti-D isoimmunization and 0.3% for other antigens[13] about 20% of these affected women may form two or more antibodies.[14] Although RhD isoimmunization may still be the most frequent cause of HDFN requiring intrauterine transfusion (IUT) at 90%,[15] in some studies, anti-Kell (K) and anti-E have surpassed anti-D as the most frequent antibodies detected.[16]

Most young women of childbearing age presenting with pregnancy are *not* chronically transfused and in fact have no known transfusion exposure. Not surprisingly, research evaluating alloimmunization mitigation and antibody exposure rates has found that the majority, up to 83%, of maternal alloimmunization and HDFN were not attributable to a prior transfusion.[17] It is reasonable and consistent with published literature to conclude that most of these immunization events occurred after exposure to a prior pregnancy. Despite this, transfusion remains one of the most important predictive risk factors for alloimmunization, followed by parity, surgery, and hematologic disease.[18] With the as little as 0.03 mL of RBCs sufficient for isoimmunization, unrecognized early pregnancy loss, intravenous drug abuse, and other minor exposures likely account for the remainder. When surveying published literature and the clinical situation, it is important to account for potential occult RBC exposures in affected patients.[19] Other studies, especially when focusing on non-RhD, non-ABO alloimmunization, have shown that up to 50% of these cases were attributed to transfusion, often to pregnancy-related transfusion.[18]

Unfortunately, the opioid epidemic has exploded over the past 20 years, causing 6 times the fatalities in 2017 as 1999, and accounting for 68% of over 70,200 drug overdose deaths.[20] The rise in the opioid epidemic can be attributed to three waves of narcotic abuse. The first involved prescription opiates with steadily increasing use beginning in 1999. The second was heroin abuse beginning in 2010, and the third is a rise in synthetic opiates beginning in 2013 and continuing today.[21] Heroin alone has caused a 400% increase in rate of death from 2010 until 2017,[22] and is particularly concerning because of the morbidity associated with needle sharing. As well as causing hepatitis and HIV, intravenous drug abuse (IVDA) during pregnancy is associated with poor prenatal care, social and financial disadvantage, incarceration, intrauterine growth restriction, fetal demise, and higher rates of maternal alloimmunization. The combined deterioration of health, behavior, and social stability due to drug abuse makes providing care to this population particularly difficult. One early study by Bowmen et al. identified five cases of IVDA leading to RhD isoimmunization with only one fetus surviving.[23] In the IVDA population, rates of alloimmunization are high at 3.6%, with 1:30 women affected. RhD alloimmunization is common, likely due to a combination of IV blood exposure, unrecognized early pregnancy loss, and noncompliance with routine obstetric care including Rh-D-immune globulin (RhIg) administration.[24]

For those women who are chronically transfused due to hemoglobinopathy or other chronic anemias, screening for blood antibodies is essential and often routine. Known patient groups prone to alloimmunization, such as those with sickle cell anemia or thalassemia, may already be on an extended phenotypic antigen match protocol. These patients are at high risk for alloimmunization. Some patient groups, such as those with AIDS, other immunodeficiency syndromes, and enzymatic deficiencies may be unlikely to form antibodies even after repeated transfusion exposures.

Antigens Implicated in HDFN

Although there are over 330 known blood group antigens with more than 50 antigens documented in the literature as having caused HDFN, Rhesus D is by far the best recognized and most historically relevant. Most antigens implicated in clinically significant alloimmunization are polypeptide antigens. The carbohydrate antigens are usually associated with anti-IgM antibodies as they are T-cell independent.[25] Risk of developing alloimmunization and subsequent HDFN depends partially upon the population in question due to differing rates of antigen frequency and chances of exposure via pregnancy, transfusion, transplant, or IVDA.

ABO

ABO incompatibility is the most commonly occurring HDFN, although usually mild. Antibodies to A and B are predominantly type IgM; however, IgA and IgG class antibodies are also present, especially in type O individuals.[26] In cases of ABO incompatibility, IgG class antibodies are transported via the placenta to the fetal circulation, causing hemolysis of fetal RBCs. In the Caucasian population, 15%–20% of pregnancies are impacted by ABO discrepancy between a type O mother and type A or B fetus. 10% of these develop HDFN, usually affecting the type A infant of a type O mother.[26] Overall, ABO hemolytic disease is seen in 0.3%–0.8% of Caucasian pregnancies but is more severe and more frequent at 3%–5% in Asian or African pregnancies.[27] Blood type prevalence is variable among different ethnic groups. For example, Native American populations have a high frequency of type O blood, ranging from 79% to 100%, while Oceanic populations show <1% type B (and AB). African and Asian populations show the highest rates of type B blood at 25% and 20%, respectively.[28] As populations migrate, the medical facilities in their new homeland must adapt to differing rates of ABO incompatibility.[29] Only about 1.5%–2% of ABO HDFN affected infants have hemolysis severe enough to require neonatal transfusion. There are several theories as to why ABO incompatibility causes typically mild HDFN. Fetal RBCs express antigens A and B poorly, making them less of a target, whereas the endothelial and epithelial lining of the placenta expresses A and B antigens profusely, potentially clearing IgG from circulation and lowering the titer within fetal circulation. Additionally, the subclass of implicated IgG, IgG_2, is less efficiently transported across the placental barrier, again providing some fetal protection. Thus, despite the ubiquitous production of IgG anti-A and B in type O mothers, only rarely is severe HDFN seen in their neonates.[30]

Although ABO incompatibility is responsible for the most common cause of HDFN, it is also responsible for mitigating the rates of alloimmunization to non-AB antigens. The reduced rates of isoimmunization in Rh-negative mothers with ABO incompatibility were noted years ago in 1943 by Levine.[31] More recent studies have demonstrated that the same protective effect of incompatibility extends to non-RhD isoimmunization, with lower rates than expected based on population at risk.[32] This may be due to rapid clearance of the incompatible fetal cells from maternal circulation before an immunogenic response can be launched.

Rhesus D
RhD, an erythroid-specific transmembrane transporter, is the most immunogenic of all the antigens and has been associated with HDFN as first described by Levine and Stetson in 1939. Before initiation of RhIg therapy in the 1960s, incidence of maternal alloimmunization to RhD in Western countries was 14% with associated HDFN affecting 1% of newborns, causing fetal mortality at rates of 1:2200.[33] After initiation of routine blood transfusion matching for ABO and RhD and the standardization of administration of RhIg during pregnancy and at delivery, the rates of RhD alloimmunization

have dropped to below 0.2% in developed countries.[34] In developing countries, rates of anti-RhD alloimmunization remain higher, between 2.9% and 6.5%, likely due to limited access to perinatal care including RhIg.[35,36] Western studies on incidence may not be applicable to developing countries or even to minority populations within developed countries, as antigen prevalence varies between populations. For example, in Indian populations, 93% of the population is D-positive, with 5% of pregnancies at risk; whereas, Asians and Native Americans are 99% RhD-positive and blacks are 92% positive.[37,38]

Expression of the D antigen is variable, with 10–33,000 antigen sites per RBC on common D, up to 200,000 on exalted D phenotypes, and only 100–10,000 on weak D phenotypes.[39] The expression of even a small amount of the complete D protein is protective against alloimmunization. For women of childbearing age, it is essential to differentiate the weak D phenotype from a partial D phenotype. Partial D occurs when a section of the *RHD* gene has undergone gene recombination with the homologous and closely approximated *RHCE* gene, replacing part of the D molecule with CE protein. Partial D patients may test as D^+ with monoclonal anti-D, but are susceptible to alloimmunization against the missing part of the protein. Dozens of variant D types have been described, and molecular phenotyping is available at reference laboratories. Although serologic testing has traditionally been used to differentiate weak D from partial D, with monoclonal antibodies, this methodology may not be reliable. Individuals identified as partial D should be treated as Rh-negative patients and Rh-positive blood donors to prevent inadvertent exposure and alloimmunization. These mothers should receive anti-D-immune globulin, as their fetus may inherit the fragment of D antigen they lack. Individuals identified as weak D should be treated as Rh-positive patients and blood donors, as any amount of D antigen can induce immunization in Rh-negative blood recipients.[40,41] The confirmed weak D mother does not need RhIg administration.

Non-D, Non-ABO Alloimmunization
The rates of alloimmunization to other antigens, although low at 0.15%–1.1%, have become a greater percentage of maternal alloimmunization cases and causes of HDFN. Among alloimmunized women, over 80% of antibodies are non-RhD.[42,43] Rates of isoimmunization are skewed toward those antigens that are most immunogenic, especially the Rhesus and Kel1 blood groups (Table 9.2).

| TABLE 9.2 |
| Immunogenicity. |
| **Immunogenicity** |
| D > K > E, c > e > Jka, Fya, C > S > Jkb, Fyb > s |

Rhesus non-D

Besides D, the other Rhesus antigens, especially c and E, are highly immunogenic. The RHCE gene is homologous with the RHD gene, encoding a similar transmembrane erythroid polypeptide. Four common alleles, *RHCE*01, RHCE*02, RHCE*03 and RHCE*04* encode the proteins we refer to as ce, Ce, cE, and CE, respectively. In alloimmunized women, antibodies to the Rhesus antigens are well represented, with 14%–23% showing anti-E; 5.8%–10% showing anti-c; and 4.7% anti-C.[16,43] As with D, partial phenotypes abound. However, due to the antithetical nature of the gene, finding matched blood for these becomes significantly more difficult. Antibodies to c and E are IgG class antibodies capable of crossing the placenta to cause moderate-to-severe HDFN.[39] Anti C also can be associated with HDFN but is usually mild. The e antigen is high frequency in the population, present on 98% –99%, and therefore cases of anti-e HDFN are extremely rare as well as mild.[39]

Kell

The Kell system is a group of related blood antigens carried on a 93 kD single-pass zinc endopeptidase membranous protein.[44] The protein is not specific to RBCs, but is found on both erythroid and myeloid progenitors as well as on other tissues. Significantly, the antigen was first described in 1946 and was named after Mrs. Kelleher, an anti-K alloimmunized mother whose fetus was affected by HDFN. After RhD, the Kell blood groups are the most immunogenic antigens. Antibodies directed against them have been implicated in autoimmune hemolytic anemia as well as HDFN, with anti-K responsible for about 18%–22% of maternal alloimmunization[43] and affecting 3.2 of 1000 pregnancies.[42] Within the blood group, Kel1 is of the most concern due to its frequency and severity, causing severe HDFN in up to 38% of susceptible pregnancies.[45] About 9% of Caucasians, 2% of blacks, and up to 25% of Arabs are positive for Kel1 while the antithetical antigen, k (Cellano) is almost ubiquitous. Anti-K is known to cause severe fetal anemia, sometimes with prolonged suppression of erythropoiesis.

Duffy

The Duffy blood group consists of polypeptides present on the multipass membrane protein DARC, which is a chemokine receptor as well as the receptor for some *Plasmodium* species.[46] Not surprisingly then, Africans and Arabs have the highest frequency of being Fy(a-b-) as this confers resistance to malaria. The GATA box mutation present in Fy[b]-negative blacks affects Duffy b expression on RBCs only, while other tissues continue to express the antigen. These patients are therefore protected from alloimmunization.[47] Asians have the highest frequencies of Fy(a+b-), while 50% of Caucasians are Fy(a+b+). Duffy antigens are much less immunogenic than the Rhesus and Kell blood groups, with Fy[b] about 20 times less immunogenic than its antithetical antigen Fy[a]. Of alloimmunized women, about 5% have anti-Fy[a] antibodies.[43] When isoimmunization does occur, antibodies of the IgG class are produced. Although Fy[a] is expressed on fetal RBCs, the antigen density is low, increasing to adult levels by about 3 months old. Anti-Fy[a] is associated with mild-to-severe HDFN, while anti-Fy[b] is rarely associated with mild HDFN.[39]

Kidd

The Kidd blood groups are antigens present on a multipass transmembrane urea transporter molecule extant on RBCs and the endothelial cells of the renal vasa recta. The blood group and Jk[a] antigen was named for John Kidd in 1951, a newborn who died of severe HDFN due to anti-Jk[a]. Jk[a] and Jk[b] are antithetical, with four possible phenotypes: Jk(a+b−), Jk(a−b+), Jk(a+b+), and Jk(a−b−). The third antigen in the group, Jk3 is almost ubiquitous, missing only in the rare few (usually Polynesians or Finns) who are Jk null.[48] Any of the Kidd antibodies can be associated with mild HDFN, but Jk[a] shows higher levels of clinical impact contributing 1.5% of alloimmunization.[43] Rare severe cases are reported in the literature.[49–51]

MNS

The MNS blood groups are glycophorin antigens, single-pass carbohydrate-bearing transmembrane glycoproteins. M and N antigens are present in roughly 75% of black and Caucasian populations, little s is present in about 90%, while S is present in 55% of Caucasian and 33% of black populations. Generally, anti-M and anti-N are naturally occurring, and can be found in patients without any possible prior exposure. These antibodies are typically cold reacting IgM class and are not associated with transfusion reactions or with HDFN. However, there are cases of antigen-induced

IgG class anti-M. These IgG class anti-Ms present as warm antibodies, reacting at 37°F and at Coombs instead of immediate spin. Such cases have been described in both the pregnant population and in the veteran population.[14] Similar to other IgG antibodies, the IgG class anti-M antibody does efficiently cross the placenta and has been associated with severe HDFN. Furthermore, because M antigen is expressed on membrane proteins such as glycophorin A of erythroid precursors, anti-M in the IgG form suppresses erythropoiesis. About half of anti-M induced HDFN cases have late onset anemia with delayed recovery.[52] Although these cases are reportedly rare in European and African populations, a recent report by Li et al. notes that in China, anti-M is second only to Rhesus alloimmunization, and is known to cause severe HDFN with hyporegenerative anemia. Titers are reportedly unreliable for predicting severity of disease. Li's review of the literature shows that 88% of anti-M caused HDFN occurred in Asian patients, and documents three case studies in China.[53]

Due to the N-like epitope of glycophorin B, M + N-individuals are very unlikely to become alloimmunized, and thus anti-N is extremely rare. Anti-S, -s, and -U have been reported as causing mild-to-severe HDFN. These all have the potential to be IgG class antibodies, but are less commonly identified. Although anti-S is rare in Caucasians at less than 5% of clinically significant antibody specificities, in the African population it is much more common, comprising 17%–32% of alloimmunization.[54] Some alloimmunization, such as anti-Mur and anti-Mi[a] are particularly prevalent in the Asian population, causing severe HDFN.[53]

Others

Due to the fact that there is a plethora of blood group antigens, with over 50 described as contributing to HDFN, they are not all described here. When faced with an unusual maternal antigen, it is best to consult with transfusion medicine and maternal–fetal medicine specialists to determine the risk for that particular pregnancy rather than assume the antibody is harmless. Rare antibodies with risk of HDFN include anti -U, Mi[a], Mur, Vw, Hut, Hil, and En[a] from the MNS blood group, Hr, Cw, f, G, and Rh32 from the Rhesus blood group, k, Kpa, Kpa, Jsa, and Jsb, from the Kell group, and Di[a], Wr[a], Co[a], PP1P[k], Vel, and Bi from other various blood groups.[16]

There are, however, several clinically insignificant antibodies that may be commonly encountered in pregnant women yet have never been implicated in causing HDFN. Some antigens are not expressed on fetal RBCs, and thus cannot be a target for maternal antibody.

These include Lewis a/b and Chido/Rodgers, which are not intrinsic to the RBC membrane, but are adsorbed onto it, AnWj, and Sd[a]. Other blood groups not associated with HDFN include P1, Cartwright, I, JMH, and Knops.[39]

Multiple Alloimmunization

About 13% of alloimmunized mothers will form multiple antibodies to various RBC groups. Multiple immunization carries increased risk for HDFN, especially when anti-D is compounded with additional antibodies, as it is in 40% of cases.[55] Frequent antibody combinations seen included anti-D plus -C, and anti-D plus -E, about 50% of which showed severe HDFN.[56] Other combinations reported included anti-c plus -E, anti-K plus Fy[a], anti-K plus -E, and anti-E plus Jk[a]. Patients with multiple alloimmunization were shown to have an overall 5.6 times increased odds of HDFN.[56] These patients may be considered "hyperresponders," as described later, and are at elevated risk for multiple alloimmunization. Moreover, 78% of patients with multiple antibodies have formed antibodies to more than one blood group system (Table 9.3).[57]

CLINICAL IMPACT

Fetal Impact: Hemolytic Disease of the Fetus and Newborn

Hemolytic disease of the fetus and newborn occurs as IgG class antibodies are actively transported across the placenta and enter fetal circulation. In the United States, the risk for HDFN is 35/10,000, of which 20% are at risk to be severely affected.[56] Ordinarily, the passive transfer of antibodies is highly protective against disease for the newborn with an immature immune system, but is pathologic in the case of maternal alloimmunization. IgM class antibodies are too large to cross the placenta and thus these are not associated with HDFN. Antibodies directed toward antigens that are present in abundance on the placenta itself may be cleared by the placental barrier, providing fetal protection. For example, anti-P1 is an IgG class antibody, but is removed from circulation by the abundance of placental antigen.

If the fetus carries the antigen to which the mother has alloimmunized, then the IgG antibody binds the fetal RBC marking them for destruction via the endoreticulum in the spleen. Fetal anemia stimulates increased rates of hematopoiesis, but the level of compensation may be insufficient to mitigate anemia. Antibodies directed against antigens present on erythrocyte precursor cells, such as antigens in the Kell and glycoprotein

TABLE 9.3
Common Maternal Antibodies.

Blood Group	Antigen	Antigen Prevalence	Immunogenicity	Class II HLA Restriction	Antibody	Risk for HDFN	Critical Titer	Clinical Course	Notes:	References
ABO	A, B	High, naturally occurring			IgM and IgG	Low		Mild	Rarely severe	26–32
Rhesus	D	85%	Strongest, 80%–90%	DRB1*01, DQB1*02, DRB1*11, DRB1*15	IgG	High	1:16	Severe		33–41;58–62
	C	65%	Strong		IgG	Medium	1:32	Mild—moderate	Rarely severe	16,39,43
	c	80%	Strong		IgG	High	1:32	7%–10% severe	Yes	16,39,43
	E	29%	Strong, 8%–10%	DRB1*09	IgG	Medium	1:32	Mild	2% severe	16,39,43,62
	e	98%	Strong		IgG	Medium	1:32	Mild	Sometimes	16,39,43
	Cw	2%	Strong		IgG	Medium	1:32	Mild	Sometimes	39
Kell	K	9%	Strong, 8%–10%	DRB1*11 and DRB1*13	IgG	High	1:8	26%–38% severe	Yes	42–45;58,60
	k	99%			IgG		1:32		Rarely severe	39
Duffy	Fya	66%	Moderate—weak	DRB1*04, DRB1*15	IgG	Medium	1:32	16% severe	No	58,59
	Fyb	83%	Very weak		IgG	Medium	1:32	Mild	No	39,43,46,47
Kidd	Jka	77%	Strong—moderate	DRB1*01	IgG	Low	1:32	Mild	Rarely severe	39,43,46,47,61
	Jkb	72%	Weak		IgG	Low	1:32	Mild—moderate	Rarely severe	48–51
	Jk3	0.1%					1:16—1:32	Mild—moderate	Rarely severe. Polynesians, Mennnonite	48

System	Antigen	Frequency	Nature	HLA	Ig class	Titer/Incidence	Serologic note	Severity	Comment	References
MNS	M	78%	Naturally occurring		IgM Rare IgG	Low	Unreliable for IgG	Mild	Rare, IgG-related HDFN. DAT negative. Erythroblastosis suppression.	52–54
	N	72%	Naturally occurring		IgM	Low		Mild		39
	S	55%	Weak	DRB1*07	IgM and IgG	Low	1:32	Mild		54,62
	s	99%	Weak		IgG	Low		Mild		39
	U	99%			IgG	Low		Mild-severe		39
Others	I		Cold agglutinin		IgM	None		None		16,39
	P1	79%			IgM	None		None		16,39
	Lub	99%			IgG	Rare		Mild		16,39
	Yt					None		None		16,39
	Lewis		Pregnancy induced		IgM	None		None	No	16,39
Multiple			Strong		IgG	High		Severe	Close clinical monitoring required	55–57

MNS system, may be particularly problematic, as this antibody-mediated destruction both directly and indirectly causes anemia through hemolysis of fetal RBCs and suppression of erythroid precursors.[27]

The development of severe uncompensated fetal anemia leads to rapid vascular flow rates, with cardiomegaly and congestive failure. Fetal hydrops develops, including edematous tissue and skin, hepatosplenomegaly, heart failure, and serous fluid retention (ascites, pleural effusion, pericardial effusion). Hemolysis leads to elevated bilirubin that is cleared from fetal circulation via the placenta, but can be detected in the amniotic fluid. Severe fetal anemia and hydrops can lead to fetal demise with subsequent spontaneous abortion or stillbirth.[63]

For the newborn surviving delivery, the process of hemolysis continues as long as passively transferred maternal antibodies are present in the serum. Neonates remain at risk of demise due to hydrops, anemia, and heart failure.[52] Laboratory blood bank testing often reveals a positive antibody screen, direct Coombs (DAT) testing, and if tested, eluate. As hemolysis continues, the neonate suffers ongoing worsening anemia and hyperbilirubinemia. Due to immaturity of the blood brain barrier in neonates, bilirubin crosses into the brain putting the infant at risk of kernicterus and permanent brain injury or death.[64] Treatment includes phototherapy to allow the skin to process the excess bilirubin that the immature liver cannot, and exchange transfusions to replace the RBCs with antigen-negative donor blood.

Maternal Impact

If fetal risk for HDFN is ruled out due to a low risk antibody or homozygous negative paternal testing, the remaining *maternal* risk cannot be neglected. The presence of even nonspecific antibodies in maternal serum can confound the blood bank testing, delaying care in the case of obstetric surgery or maternal hemorrhage. It is important to classify pregnant mothers with antibodies as high risk in the blood bank, and to anticipate when possible the chance of peripartum hemorrhage. Consideration should be given to routine type and crossmatch upon registration to prevent delay, especially if other known risk factors are present. Mitigation of the chances for transfusion via prenatal anemia screening and iron therapy, expectant management, and a conservative transfusion strategy may reduce transfusions to this patient population.

Transfusion reaction risk

Patients with known antibodies have confirmed prior exposure to blood antigens and have proven themselves

to be responders, if not hyperresponders. Research has shown that rates of alloimmunization may be underestimated due to evanescence.[6] Multiple alloimmunization is seen in over 20% of isoimmunizations, but these cases are also prone to evanescence, and therefore equally likely to evade detection.[14] Alloimmunized mothers are therefore at risk for delayed hemolytic transfusion reactions as well as acute hemolytic transfusion reactions. As studies have shown that 20% of responders form additional antibodies, alloimmunized mothers should be transfused conservatively to prevent exposure to additional antigens.

Risk of delayed care during delivery

Patients with maternal alloimmunization face a higher risk for delay of care should transfusion support be needed during their delivery. With the complications of a high-risk pregnancy and concern for the well-being of the fetus, the difficulties in attaining blood for the mother may be overlooked. However, the presence of antibodies complicates both the antibody screening process and the acquisition of compatible crossmatched units. Should a facility wish to provide additional phenotypic matching, the case becomes even more complex and the preparation lengthier. Depending on the desired antigen combination, some patients are a phenotypic match to less than 5% of the donor population. Different from routine surgical patients, the alloimmunized mother is continuously at risk for additional antibody formation. Therefore a current specimen is required for testing.

Impact on future childbearing

The impact of a high-risk pregnancy is both emotionally and financially taxing to affected families, as additional testing and treatment may be required throughout and after perinatal care and delivery. In considering future childbearing, families should be advised as to the risks associated with the antibody in question and the chances for paternal antigen inheritance by additional offspring. For example, in the case of anti-D HDFN, a previously affected child increases the risk to over 80% that a subsequent antigen-positive sibling will be affected. In these cases, middle cerebral artery peak systolic velocity testing is recommended starting at 18 weeks gestation regardless of titers.[65]

IMMUNOHEMATOLOGY
Factors Increasing Risk of Alloimmunization

Women of childbearing age are not typically a population undergoing routine transfusion. Much of the alloimmunization occurring in this group is pregnancy related, either due to fetal RBC exposure or due to pregnancy-related transfusion.[18] Conditions increasing risks of alloimmunization correspond to increased fetal maternal hemorrhage, including miscarriage and termination of pregnancy, invasive diagnostic procedures, external version, Cesarean section, assisted vaginal delivery, surgical removal of the placenta, and transfusion for peripartum anemia. Patients with known hemoglobinopathies such as sickle cell disease or thalassemia are at well-documented increased risk due to exposure from chronic transfusion, with up to 47% of adult sickle cell patients forming antibodies.[66] Other risk factors include multiple parity, multiple gravidity, IVDA, prior major surgeries, and other blood exposures. Patients with immunosuppression, such as from AIDS, are much less likely to become alloimmunized.[5] The differences between ethnic antigen frequencies, antigen frequencies in the donor population, and individual variance between the mother and father of baby also drive rates of exposure to novel antigens.

Antigen epitopes are not exclusive to the extracellular exposed protein loops on the RBC surface, as would be expected in a solely B-cell-mediated immune reaction. Studies have demonstrated that immunogenic epitopes include intracellular, membrane spanning, and extracellular domains, indicating that these antigens are being processed and displayed by antigen presenting cells before being recognized by T cells. Four particular Rh-D peptides elicited a response in over 50% of immunized volunteers, confirming that certain peptides are stimulatory. Primed T cells remain in the circulation for years.[67] Within the highly polymorphic RH genes, variant alleles are common, especially in the African populations. Between 65% and 90% of sickle cell patients, for example, have been shown to carry at least one variant RH allele.[68,69] Common Rh stimulatory epitopes may be missing or altered, and "partial" expression is seen regularly in the D, C, and e proteins and less often in the c and E proteins as well. The variation among these Rh alloreactive peptides complicates serologic phenotyping and is associated with high rates of alloimmunization even when phenotypic matching is attempted.[70] For some populations, especially of African descent, this poses a particular challenge as both patients and donors may show misleading serologic testing results that do not fully represent their antigen status. These findings further demonstrate the clinical relevance of small stimulatory epitopes in the process of alloimmunization.

However, these known risks are insufficient to explain why some patients exposed to minuscule amounts of foreign antigen launch an aggressive immune reaction, while others do not, even after a large exposure. Furthermore, it is clear that some antigens are more immunogenic than others, for example, as shown in the REDS III study with 75% of the alloimmunized patients having antibodies to the Rh and Kell families.[71] Contrary to other alloimmunized populations, the antibodies implicated in HDFN after maternal alloimmunization to fetal antigens have been documented to be more persistent with lower rates of evanescence. In fact, antibodies causing HDFN remained detectable in the entire population evaluated, whereas the other antibodies induced by fetal antigens were less persistent, and those not directed against antigens present in the child showed even higher rates of evanescence.[72] The tenacity of these antibodies correlated to their titer and specificity. It is well known that some patients are more prone to alloimmunization than others. In fact, transfusion recipients have been categorized as "nonresponders," "responders," and "hyperresponders" based on their proclivity to alloimmunization.[14]

Patients with thalassemia, sickle cell disease, and myelodysplastic syndromes are especially prone to alloimmunization, with incidences up to 37%, 47%, and 58.6%, respectively.[6] Patients with hematologic malignancies show much higher rates of alloimmunization than those with other oncologic disease.[73,74] Hospitalized patients show rates of alloimmunization of 20%–30%.[7,8] The general population is much less susceptible with rates of isoimmunization between 1% and 10%, while young children and infants very rarely show isoimmunization. Up to 22% of alloimmunized patients develop more than one alloantibody, while an additional 12% of them form three or more and may be considered "hyperresponders."[14,75] Inflammation, genetics, and underlying hematologic pathology predispose the formation of alloantibodies. Inflammatory conditions potentiating antibody formation include systemic lupus erythematosus, rheumatoid arthritis, ulcerative colitis, and infection.[71] Literature is now elucidating how HLA class II restriction impacts the presentation of various noncarbohydrate blood antigens to antigen-specific CD4+ T cells.

Both population studies and basic science are shedding light on the mechanisms of immunogenicity of the blood antigens. A growing body of literature is implicating certain class II HLA alleles as potentiating alloimmunization. The HLA-DR molecules differ among their β-chain residues within a binding grove. Pockets within the binding grove impact the presentation of peptides, influencing the recognition and response of T cells.

Several RBC antigens appear to be HLA restricted, for example a study on Caucasians alloimmunized to Fy^a found them to all share the DRB1*04 restriction model, whereas anti-K immunized patients showed a variety of HLA-DRB1* molecules,[58] including DRB1*11 and *13.[60] Additional studies have confirmed Fy^a to be restricted to DRB1*04 and DRB1*15.[59] Kel1 immunization has been associated with a variety of DRB1* alleles, but especially with DRB1*11 and DRB1*13.[60] HLA-DRB1*01 is seen more frequently in Jk^a immunization than in controls.[61] Anti-E is now known to be associated with DRB1*09, while anti-S with DRB1*07.[62]

Additionally, patients immunized to more than one blood antigen have also been shown to have certain HLA restrictions, with about 40% of these "hyper-responders" positive for HLA-DRB1*15[73] in a European population, and over 15% positive in a Brazilian sickle cell patient population.[76] A study of the Czech population revealed that alloimmunization to C and D was associated with HLA-DRB1*15 and DRB1*06; anti-E and -c was associated with the DRB1*13 and DQB1*06 allelic groups, and those immunized against E and C^w showed the DRB1*03 and DQB1*02 alleles.[77] Conversely, studies have also shown some alleles, for example HLA-DQ2, -3, and -5, confer a protective effect against alloimmunization in multiply transfused sickle cell patients. Some combinations, such as HLA-DQ2/6 and HLA-DQ5/5 impart additional resistance.[78]

In addition to the well-described HLA-Class II associations with alloimmunization, other potentiating and protective immune factors are being evaluated. Cytokine gene polymorphisms are now also known to be associated with higher risks for RBC alloimmunization. Specific allelic polymorphisms of both tumor necrosis factor A and interleukin 1B impart statistically significant increased risks for blood group immunization in sickle cell patients.[76] The levels of fucosylation on the IgG antibodies themselves seem to impact HDFN, with less fucosylation driving increased severity for anti-D. For anti-D IgG, low levels of fucosylation increase the affinity to IgG-Fc receptors IIIa and IIIb. Other blood group antibodies, however, have shown mixed findings, with levels of Fc-glycosylation increasing or decreasing levels of hemolysis depending on the specificity of the antibody.[79,80] Clearly, the Fc glycosylation of anti-RBC antibodies impacts their potency and affinity to receptors, but additional research is needed to clarify these models.

The spleen seems to play an essential role in alloimmunization to RBC antigens. Data extracted from the Risk Factors for Alloimmunization to Red Blood Cell Transfusion (R-FACT) study has shown that

splenectomized patients only rarely become alloimmunized.[81,82] Patel et al. showed that, in a murine model, transfused Kel1-positive RBCs are captured within the marginal sinuses of the spleen, localizing with marginal zone B cells. The removal of these B cells eradicates immunization to Kel1 antigen following exposure.[83] Follicular dendritic cells are also known to participate in antigen presentation to follicular B cells; however, removal of CD4 T cells and follicular B cells do not prevent immunization,[83] demonstrating that the marginal zone B cells are playing an essential and possibly independent role.

A set of experimental transgenic mouse models has been developed, expressing model antigens, human RBC antigens, and hybrid mouse–human antigens. Studies using these murine models have shown that transfusion can induce RBC alloimmunization, especially in the presence of inflammation, similar to that seen in humans.[84] Murine models have been used to demonstrate that immune priming to one RBC alloantigen directly enhances a humoral response to disparate RBC antigens. Patel et al. showed that induced inflammation enhances anti-K antibody formation to Kel1-positive transfusion via a $CD4^+$ T-cell-dependent process, while also directly facilitating second anti-Duffy antibodies upon subsequent exposure.[85] Not only is RBC immunization enhanced after initial alloimmunization, but also Verduin et al. have shown that mothers treated for HDFN with intrauterine transfusion have a high risk of forming both additional RBC alloantibodies as well as HLA class 1 antibodies. These hyperresponders had higher titers, formed more antibodies with 76% developing at least 2, and had longer persistence of detectable antibodies than controls.[86]

Murine models are further elucidating the impact of the complement system upon T-cell-mediated alloimmunization, especially for KEL1. $CD4^+$ T-cells are known to play an important role in immunization; however, Mener et al. have now shown that depletion and deletion of these failed to prevent anti-K formation. Surprisingly, complement specifically C3 and the complement receptors 1 and 2 dictate either a $CD4^+$ dependent or an independent antibody formation.[87] The absence of C3 in the C3 knockout mouse model unexpectedly results in enhanced levels of anti-K formation, whereas the Duffy-like antibody response was not affected. C3 showed enhanced deposition on the Kel1-positive RBCs, resulting in removal of the antigen from the RBC surface and depressed antibody formation.[88]

The immune system can be manipulated to mitigate rates of alloimmunization. Within 20 years of discovering anti-RhD alloimmunization, polyclonal RhIg was developed and administered to postpartum RhD-negative women, drastically reducing the rates of immunization and HDFN. The mechanisms for how passive antibody administration reduces immunization remain incompletely understood. Postulated theories include the following: (1) induction of rapid clearance of tagged RBCs, (2) steric hindrance of B cells, causing antigen masking, (3) inhibition of Fyc receptors inhibiting B-cell response, and (4) direct antigen modulation/removal from the RBC surface.[89] The lower risk of alloimmunization in mothers with ABO discrepancy supports the mechanism of rapid RBC removal but studies have shown that each of these mechanisms may play a role, and may be antigen dependent.[88] To date, anti-D immunoglobulin is the only available prophylaxis against alloimmunization.

PREVENTION, MITIGATION, TREATMENT
Screening Protocols
Unfortunately, there is no known method to completely prevent alloimmunization in any population, including pregnant women. Risk reduction, early detection, and HDFN mitigation are the modalities used to reduce morbidity and mortality associated with maternal alloimmunization. Most obstetric practices include blood typing and RBC antibody screening with their prenatal work-up at intake evaluation of pregnant women, as is recommended by the American College of Obstetrics and Gynecology.[90] Studies have shown that due to late alloimmunization, up to 37% of anti-D antibodies and 27% of severe non-D antibodies were missed at first trimester screening but detectable by late second to early third trimester screening.[91] First trimester screening has been shown to be only about 75% sensitive, with excellent outcomes in those cases detected but mixed outcomes in those that are missed.[92,93] Therefore, many protocols recommend screening for all pregnant woman at 28 weeks in addition to intake.[34,94]

Immunoprophylaxis: RhD-Immune Globulin
Use of polyclonal antigen-directed immune globulin postdelivery as a means to reduce the rates of alloimmunization was developed in the 1960s in an effort to mediate the risks of HDFN in Rh-negative women, reducing the incidence of RhD alloimmunization from about 14% to 1%–2%.[95] In the 1970s, an additional antenatal dose was added to the protocol during the late second trimester/early third trimester, bringing rates of alloimmunization down to less than

0.1%,[16,96] and rates of HDFN to less than 0.08%.[97] The administration of RhD-immune globulin as a means of antibody-mediated immune suppression has been highly successful in reducing rates of anti-D immunization from about 14% to less than 0.2% in countries where it is used routinely,[33,34] but has not been expanded to other antibodies implicated in HDFN. There is some evidence that anti-D administration may protect against additional alloimmunization to other blood antigens and groups, as well as to RhD.[32]

To provide adequate protection, a dose of 300 μg RhIg should be administered routinely to all nonsensitized RhD-negative women at 28 weeks gestation (or alternatively smaller doses at 28 and 34 weeks), unless the fetus is confirmed as RhD-negative. An additional administration of 300 μg of RhD immune globulin is recommended within 72 hours of delivery for all nonimmunized RhD-negative mothers of RhD-positive infants. Studies have shown than even the single dose of RhIg given at 28 weeks (in addition to a delivery dose) halves the risk of subsequent sensitization and HDFN.[98] If fetal maternal hemorrhage is greater than 30 mL of fetal whole blood (15 mL of RBCs), additional anti-D Ig should be administered. Moreover, 300 μg RhIg is also recommended in cases of abortion or miscarriage after 12 weeks (a smaller dose of 120 μg can be administered before 12 weeks), ectopic pregnancy, partial molar pregnancy, amniocentesis, chorionic villous sampling, cordocentesis, and placental trauma. In cases of placental trauma, quantitative testing for fetal maternal hemorrhage should be done as additional RhIg is required for fetal maternal hemorrhage over 30 mL whole blood. If RhIg is not administered within the 72 hours, it should be given as soon as possible within 28 days of the exposure.[34]

Paternal Testing
Once maternal alloimmunization has been confirmed and is of a type associated with HDFN, an assessment of fetal risk is initiated, usually starting with paternal testing for the implicated antigen. If paternity is certain, paternal antigens can be serologically or molecularly phenotyped to ascertain the risk of fetal inheritance.[42] Should the father be heterozygous or paternity uncertain, fetal testing by amniocentesis or by cell-free fetal DNA analysis can be initiated to definitively determine fetal antigen status. Fetal DNA is well represented in maternal plasma, at 3.4% of total plasma DNA during the first trimester and increasing to 6.2% by the third trimester of pregnancy.[42] The preferred testing methodology is noninvasive, as chorionic villous sampling and amniocentesis have risks of increasing fetal–maternal

hemorrhage and inducing multiple alloimmunizations, as well as direct fetal risks of amniotic fluid leak and preterm rupture of membranes.[65]

Fetal Monitoring

Once antibodies are detected and identified, if the fetus is at risk for inheriting the offending antigen, antibody titers should be followed over time to detect a rise. Anti-D titers rising above 16 or 32 are generally considered critical. Anti-K titers are critical earlier, with titers of eight raising concern for critical levels. Most clinically significant antigens have critical titers of 32, however, for some, like the IgG class anti-M antibody, titers are reportedly unreliable.[53] In very high-risk cases, especially where there is a history of severe HDFN in a prior pregnancy, titers may also be suspect and clinical suspicion should remain high.

Critical titers should prompt notification of the clinical team so an assessment of fetal anemia and well-being can be initiated. Prior methodology included serial amniocentesis to detect fetal bilirubin levels by spectrophotometry. The value of the ΔOD 450 as compared to that of baseline amniotic fluid was analyzed using Liley's or Freda's graphs. This testing was invasive with inherent risk to both mother and fetus, as amniocentesis carries risks of fetal maternal hemorrhage and multiple maternal alloimmunizations, preterm premature rupture of membranes, and miscarriage. Additionally, the technique may fail to detect fetal anemia mediated through suppression of fetal erythropoiesis, such as is seen with anti-K. Instead, most centers now use middle cerebral artery Doppler assessment to evaluate peak MCA velocity as a measure of fetal anemia, using multiples of the median normalized against gestational velocities in nonaffected pregnancies.[99,100]

Intrauterine Transfusion and Postnatal Treatment

For the fetus with life-threatening anemia and or hydrops, IUT is the preferred treatment but comes with associated risks and side effects. About half of pregnancies affected by severe HDFN due to anti-D will require antenatal intrauterine transfusion whereas the rest may be delivered and treated as a newborn.[47] Regardless, the benefits of the procedure outweigh the morbidity and mortality associated with severe fetal anemia and hydrops. Moreover, 25% of women undergoing IUT develop additional alloimmunization, increasing to 70% after delivery.[101] Fetal transfusion is lifesaving, with survival rates of about 90%,[102] and mitigates neurodevelopmental impairment, including cerebral palsy, developmental delay, and deafness for about

95% of children as shown in the LOTUS study.[63] Early detection, referral, and IUT prevent the onset of fetal hydrops, a strong predictor of morbidity. IUT is usually performed through week 35.[103]

After week 35, the fetus can usually be safely delivered, and treatment of a neonate becomes preferable to the risks associated with IUT. Neonates lose the benefit of placental removal of bilirubin and are therefore monitored for both hyperbilirubinemia and anemia. In mild cases of hemolysis, phototherapy may be sufficient, but others require exchange transfusion with antigen-negative blood. As discussed earlier, some antigens are associated with suppression of fetal erythropoiesis and may present with late and persistent anemia.

Case studies and small series have described attempts at using antenatal intravenous immune globulin (IVIg) for treatment of alloimmunization, to reduce levels of maternal IgG being produced and to delay or prevent the need for IUT. These studies are insufficient to make recommendations, as per the 2013 Cochrane Pregnancy and Childbirth group.[104]

Partial or Extended Phenotypic Matching

Several countries provide limited phenotypic matching to all transfused women of childbearing age, for example, matching for Kell or for K, c, and E as in the Netherlands.[32] In multiply transfused patients, the literature supports programs to reduce antigen exposure, and for sickle cell patients, at least C, E, and K are matched at most major centers. Studies have shown, however, that up to 83% maternal alloimmunization is due to prior exposure via pregnancy.[17] Thus, routine phenotypic matching of maternal antigens is not recommended.[12] However, in defined high-risk situations, there may be benefit to extending matching. Some studies have shown that phenotyping and matching in specific high-risk populations lowers rates of alloimmunization. With evidence that the alloimmunized mother is at least a "responder," mitigation of risk due to transfusion may lower rates of multiple alloimmunization by up to 60%.[105] A Dutch study estimated that matching for C, c, E, K, and Jka would have reduced the alloimmunization rate in their general population by 78%, but notes that their data likely applies only to Caucasian populations.[82] Known "hyperresponders" with multiple alloimmunizations should receive phenotypically matched blood, although this will not prevent immunization to fetal antigens. For other mothers with known immune deficiency disorders who are at a very low risk of alloimmunization, matching makes little sense. Although the cost of universal matching is likely prohibitive and shows limited value,[106] for those mothers with known alloimmunization at high risk for HDFN, phenotypic matching may mitigate the risks of additional exposure. This is consistent with matching protocols for other high-risk populations, such as the chronically transfused.[75] In patients with multiple transfusions, extended matching for C, c, E, e, and K has been shown to reduce the incidence of alloimmunization from 34% to 17.5%.[107] For the sickle cell population, limited matching is predicted to reduce immunization by over 50% and extended matching (although not always possible) by up to 70%.[108] As the cost and complexity of genotyping decreases, it may become more practical to perform molecular phenotypic typing of donors and extended matching for high-risk patient populations (Table 9.4).[109]

Additional and practical reduction in risk comes with management of prenatal anemia, planning for known risk factors for peripartum hemorrhage, and maintaining a conservative transfusion policy. By remedying underlying prenatal anemia and recognizing peripartum hemorrhage risks, transfusions can be minimized. When transfusion is needed, if time allows the "responder" and "hyperresponder" type mother may receive partial or extended phenotypic matching. All mothers should also receive leukoreduced blood.[110]

In conclusion, maternal alloimmunization remains a clinically significant problem for both the mother and fetus, as the pregnancy involved becomes high risk. However, with appropriate RhD-immune prophylaxis, early detection, and fetal monitoring, most cases of HDFN can be adequately treated to prevent morbidity and mortality. As it is clear from population studies and recent immunohematologic studies, some patients will be at particularly high risk for alloimmunization and multiple alloimmunization. Identification of these responders and extra care during pregnancy and transfusions may mitigate their risk.

REFERENCES

1. Hendrickson JE, Delaney M. Hemolytic disease of the fetus and newborn: modern practice and future investigations. *Transfus Med Rev.* 2016;30:159−164.
2. Evensen A, Anderson JM, Fontaine P. Postpartum hemorrhage: prevention and treatment. *Am Fam Physician.* 2017; 95(7):442−449.
3. Knight M, Callaghan WM, Berg C, et al. Trends in postpartum hemorrhage in high resource countries: a review and recommendations from the International Postpartum Hemorrhage Collaborative Group. *BMC Pregnancy Childbirth.* 2009;9:55.
4. Say L, Chou D, Gemmill A, et al. Global causes of maternal death: a WHO systematic analysis. *Lancet Glob Health.* 2014;2(6):e323−e333.
5. Boctor FN, Ali NM, Mohandas K, Uehlinger J. Absence of D- alloimmunization in AIDS patients receiving D-mismatched RBCs. *Transfusion.* 2003;43:173−176.
6. Gehrie EA, Tormey CA. The influence of clinical and biological factors on transfusion-associated non-ABO antigen alloimmunization: responders, hyper-responders, and non-responders. *Transfus Med Hemotherapy.* 2014; 41:420−429.
7. Frohn C, Dumbgen L, Brand JM, Gorg S, Luhm J, Kirchner H. Probability of anti-D development in D- patients receiving D+ RBCs. *Transfusion.* 2003;43:893−898.
8. Yazer MH, Triulzi DJ. Detection of anti-D in D- recipients transfused with D+ red blood cells. *Transfusion.* 2007;47: 2197−2201.
9. Lozano M, Cid J. The clinical implications of platelet transfusions associated with ABO of Rh(D) incompatibility. *Transfus Med Rev.* 2003;17:57−68.
10. Bowman JM. The prevention of RH immunization. *Transfus Med Rev.* 1988;2(3):129−150.
11. Markham KB, Scrape SR, Prasad M, Rossi KQ, O'Shaughnessy RW. Hemolytic disease of the fetus and newborn due to intravenous drug use. *Am J Perinatol Rep.* 2016;6:e129−132.
12. Schonewille H, Honohan A, van der Watering LMG, et al. Incidence of alloantibody formation after ABO-D or extended matched red blood cell transfusions: a randomized trial (MATCH study). *Transfusion.* 2016;56: 311−320.
13. Solheim B. Provision of K- (Kel1-) blood to women not more than 50 years of age. *Transfusion.* 2015;55: 468−469.

TABLE 9.4
Alloimmunization Risk Mitigation Strategies.

Maternal Alloimmunization Mitigation Strategies
Early detection and treatment of anemia
Routine universal prenatal antibody screening, at intake and 28 weeks
Rhogam administration at 28 weeks and delivery
Identification of mothers at high risk for peripartum hemorrhage
Consider limited phenotypic matching for Rh and Kell antigens
Consider extended phenotypic matching for "hyperresponders"
Conservative transfusion strategy
Leukoreduction of RBC units
Communication between blood banks and treating teams.

14. Tormey CA, Stack G. The characterization and classification of concurrent blood group antibodies. *Transfusion.* 2009;49:2709−2718.

15. Van Kemp IL. *Review of the Literature on Red Cell Alloimmunization in Pregnancy.* Dordrecht, Boston: Kluwer Academic Publishers; 2004.

16. Eder AF. Update on HDFN: new information on long-standing controversies. *Immunohematology.* 2006;22(4):188−195.

17. Delaney M, Wikman A, van der Watering L, et al. Blood group antigen matching influence on gestational outcomes (AMIGO) study. *Transfusion.* 2017;57:525−532.

18. Koelewijn JM, Vrijkotte TGM, de Haas M, van der Shoot, Bonsel GJ. Risk factors for the presence of non-rhesus D red blood cell antibodies in pregnancy. *BJOG.* 2009;116:655−664.

19. Brunker PAR. Consider the source: the importance of including all transfused product and exposures in red blood cell alloimmunization research. *Transfusion.* 2016;56:290−293.

20. www.cdc.gov/drugoverdose/epidemic/index.html.

21. Scholl L, Seth P, Kariisa M, Wilson N, Baldwin G. Drug and opioid-involved overdose deaths − United States, 2013−2017. *WR Morb Mortal Wkly Rep.* 2019;67:1419−1427.

22. Hedegaard H, Miniño AM, Warner M. *Drug Overdose Deaths in the United States, 1999−2017.* NCHS Data Brief, no 329. Hyattsville, MD: National Center for Health Statistics; 2018.

23. Bowman J, Harman C, Manning F, Menticoglou S, Pollock J. Intravenous drug abuse causes Rh immunization. *Vox Sang.* 1991;61(2):96−98.

24. Lappen JR, Stark S, Gibson KS, Prasad M, Bailit JL. Intravenous drug use is associated with alloimmunization in pregnancy. *Am J Obstet Gynecol.* 2016;215(3):344.e1−344.e6.

25. Kormoczi GF, Mayr WR. Responder individuality in red blood cell alloimmunization. *Transfus Med Hemotherapy.* 2014;41:446−451.

26. Kattimani VS, Ushakiran CB. Hemolytic disease of the newborn due to ABO incompatibility. *Int J Contemp Pediatrics.* 2018;5(2):605−611.

27. De Haas M, Thurik FF, Koelewijn JM, van der Schoot CE. Haemolytic disease of the fetus and newborn. *Vox Sang.* 2015;109:99−113.

28. Margaglione M, Grandone E. Population genetics of venous thromboembolism. A narrative review. *Thromb Haemostasis.* 2011;105(2):221−231.

29. Basu S, Kuar R, Kuar G. Hemolytic disease of the fetus and newborn: current trends and perspectives. *Asian J Transfus Sci.* 2011;5(1):3−7.

30. Bennardello F, Coluzzi S, Gurciarello G, Todros T, Villa S. Recommendations for the prevention and treatment of hemolytic disease of the foetus and newborn. *Blood Transfus.* 2015;13:109−134.

31. Levine P. Serological factors as possible causes in spontaneous abortions. *J Hered.* 1943;34:71−80.

32. Zwiers C, Koelewijn JM, Vermij L, et al. ABO incompatibility and RhIG immunoprophylaxis protect against non-D alloimmunization by pregnancy. *Transfusion.* 2018;58:1611−1617.

33. Moise KJ. Management of rhesus alloimmunization in pregnancy. *Obstet Gynecol.* 2002;100:600−611.

34. Fung FK, Eason E, Crane J, et al. Prevention of Rh alloimmunization. *J Obstet Gynaecol Can.* 2003;25:765−773.

35. Karim F, Moiz B, Kamran N. Risk of maternal alloimmunization in Southern Pakistan − a study in a cohort of 1000 pregnant women. *Transfus Apher Sci.* 2015;52:99−102.

36. Altuntas N, Yenicesu I, Himmetoglu O, et al. The risk assessment study for hemolytic disease of the fetus and newborn in a university hospital in Turkey. *Transfus Apher Sci.* 2013;48(3):377−380.

37. Agarwal K, Rana A, Ravi AK. Treatment and prevention of Rh isoimmunization. *J Fetal Med.* 2014;1:81−88.

38. Dean L. *Blood Groups and Red Cell Antigens.* Bethesda (MD): National Center for Biotechnology Information (US); 2005 (Chapter 7), The Rh blood group. Available from: https://www.ncbi.nlm.nih.gov/books/NBK2269/.

39. Reid ME, Lomas-Francis C, Olsson ML. *The Blood Group Antigen Facts Book.* 3rd ed. Amsterdam, Netherlands: Elsevier Academic Press; 2012.

40. Wagner T, Kormoczi GF, Buchta C, et al. Anti-D immunization by DEL red blood cells. *Transfusion.* 2005;45:520−526.

41. Kormoczi GF, Gassner C, Shao CP, Uchikawa M, Legler TJ. A comprehensive analysis of DEL types: partial DEL individuals are prone to anti-D alloimmunization. *Transfusion.* 2005;45:1561−1567.

42. Ven der Schoot CE, Tax GH, Rijnders RJ, de Haas M, Christiaens GC. Prenatal typing of Rh and Kell blood groups antigens: the edge of a watershed. *Transfus Med Rev.* 2003;17:31−44.

43. Geifman-Holtzman O, Wojtowycz M, Kosmas E, Artal R. Female alloimmunization with antibodies known to cause hemolytic disease. *Obstet Gyncol.* 1997;89:272−275.

44. Lee S, Wu X, Reid M, Zelinski T, Redman C, et al. Molecular basis for the Kel1 (K1) phenotype. *Blood.* 1995;85:912−916.

45. Moise KJ. Red blood cell alloimmunization in pregnancy. *Semin Hematol.* 2005;42:169−178.

46. Pogo AO, Chaudhuri A. The Duffy protein: a malarial and chemokine receptor. *Semin Hematol.* 2000;37:122−129.

47. Tournamille C, Colin Y, Cartron JP, Le Van Kim. C, et al. Disruption of a GATA motif in the Duffy gene promoter abolishes erythroid gene expression in Duffy-negative individuals. *Nat Genet.* 1995;10:224−228.

48. Lawicki S, Coberly EA, Lee LA, Johnson M, Eichbaum Q. Jk3 alloantibodies during pregnancy-blood bank management and hemolytic disease of the fetus and newborn risk. *Transfusion.* 2018;58:1157−1162.

49. Lawicki S, Covin RB, Powers AA. The Kidd (JK) blood group system. *Transfus Med Rev.* 2017;31(3):165−172.

50. Baek EJ, Park SC, Kwon YH, Kim CR. Hemolytic disease of newborn due to anti-Jka and the duration of antibody persistence, 2013 *J Pediatr Child Health*. 2013;49: e101–102.

51. Mittal K, Sood T, Bansal N, Bedi RK, Kaur P, Kaur G. Clinical significance of rare maternal anti-Jka antibody. *Indian J Hematol Blood Transfus*. 2016;32(4):497–499.

52. Yasuda H, Ohto H, Nollet KE, et al. Hemolytic disease of the fetus and newborn with late-onset anemia due to anti-M: a case report and review of Japanese literature. *Transfus Med Rev*. 2014;28:1–6.

53. Li S, Mo C, Huang L, et al. Hemolytic disease of the fetus and newborn due to alloanti-M: three Chinese case reports and a review of the literature. *Transfusion*. 2019; 59:385–395.

54. Natukunda B, Mugyenyi G, Brand A, et al. Maternal red blood cell alloimmunization in south western Uganda. *Transfus Med*. 2011;21:262–266.

55. Spong CY, Porter AE, Queenan JT. Management of isoimmunization in the presence of multiple maternal antibodies. *Am J Obstet Gynecol*. 2001;185(2):481–484.

56. Markham KB, Rossi KQ, Nagaraja HNN, O'Shaughnessy RW. Hemolytic disease of the fetus and newborn due to multiple maternal antibodies. *Am J Obstet Gynecol*. 2015;213, 68.e1-5.

57. Schonewille H, Brand A. Does an alloimmune respond to strong immunogenic red blood cell antigens enhance a response to weaker antigens? *Transfusion*. 2008;48: 958–963.

58. Noizat-Pirenne F, Tournamille C, Bierlinng P, et al. Relative immunogenicity of Fya and K antigens in a Caucasian population, based on HLA class II restriction analysis. *Transfusion*. 2006;46:1328–1333.

59. Picard C, Frassati C, Basire A, et al. Positive association of DRB1*04 and DRB1*15 alleles with Fya immunization in a Southern European population. *Transfusion*. 2009; 49:2412–2417.

60. Chiaronni J, Dettori I, Ferrera V, et al. HLA-DRB1 polymorphism is associated with Kell immunization. *Br J Haematol*. 2005;132:374–378.

61. Reviron D, Dettori I, Ferrera V, et al. HLA-DRB1 alleles and Jka immunization. *Transfusion*. 2005;45:956–959.

62. Schonewille H, Doxiadis IIN, Levering WHBM, Roelen DL, Claas FHJ, Brand A. HLA-DRB1 associations in individuals with single and multiple clinically relevant red blood cell antibodies. *Transfusion*. 2014;54: 1971–1980.

63. Lindenburg IT, Smits-Wintjens VE, van Klink JM, et al. Long-term neurodevelopmental outcome after intrauterine transfusion for hemolytic disease of the fetus/newborn: the LOTUS study. *Am J Obstet Gynecol*. 2012; 206:141.e1–141.e8.

64. Dean L. *Blood Groups and Red Cell Antigens*. Bethesda (MD): National Center for Biotechnology Information (US); 2005 (Chapter 4), Hemolytic disease of the newborn. Available from: https://www.ncbi.nlm.nih.gov/books/NBK2269/.

65. Cacciatore A, Rapiti S, Carrara S, et al. Obstetric management in Rh alloimminized pregnancy. *J Prenatal Med.* 2009;3(2):25–27.

66. Aygun A, Padmanabhan S, Paley C, Chandrasekaran V. Clinical significance of RBC alloantibodies and autoantibodies in sickle cell patients who received transfusions. *Transfusion*. 2002;42:37–43.

67. Stott LM, Barker RN, Urbaniak SJ. Identification of alloreactive T-cell epitopes on the Rhesus D protein. *Blood*. 2000;96:4011–4019.

68. Sippert E, Fujita CR, Machado D, et al. Variant RH alleles and Rh immunization in patients with sickle cell disease. *Blood Transfus*. 2015;13:72–77.

69. Chou ST, Jackson T, Vege S, Smith-Whitely K, Friedman DF, Westhoff CM. High prevalence of red blood cell alloimmunization in sickle cell disease despite transfusion from RH matched minority donors. *Blood*. 2013;122(6):1062–1071.

70. Chou ST, Flanagan JM, Vege S, et al. Whole-exome sequencing for RH genotyping and alloimmunization risk in children with sickle cell anemia. *Blood Advances*. 2017;1(18):1414–1422.

71. Karafin MS, Westlake M, Hauser RG, et al. Risk factors for red blood cell alloimmunization in the recipient epidemiology and donor evaluation study (REDS-III) database. *Br J Haematol*. 2018;181:672–681.

72. Verduin EP, Brannd A, van der Watering LMG, et al. Factors associated with persistence of red blood cell antibodies in women after pregnancies complicated by fetal alloimmune hemolytic disease treated with intrauterine transfusions. *Br J Haematol*. 2014;168: 443–451.

73. Gonzalez-Porras JR, Graciani IF, Perez-Simon JA, et al. Prospective evaluation of a transfusion policy of D+ red blood cells into D- patients. *Transfusion*. 2008;48: 1318–1324.

74. Evans D, Zwaginga JJ, Tijmensen J, et al. Treatments for hematologic malignancies in contrast to those for solid cancers are associated with reduced red cell alloimmunizationn. *Haematologica*. 2017;102(1):52–59.

75. Schonewille H, van de Watering LM, Brand A. Additional red blood cell alloantibodies after blood transfusions in a nonhematologic alloimmunized patient cohort: is it time to take precautionary measures? *Transfusion*. 2006;46: 630–635.

76. Sippert EA, Visentainer JEL, Alves HV, et al. Red blood cell alloimmunization in patients with sickle cell disease: correlation with HLA and cytokine gene polymorphisms. *Transfusion*. 2017;57:379–389.

77. Maluskova A, Mrazek F, Pauloskova P, Koristka M, Jindra P, Cermakova Z. Association of HLA-DRB1 and HLA-DQB1 with red-blood cell alloimmunization in the Czech population. *Vox Sang*. 2017;112:156–162.

78. Tatari-Calderone Z, Gordish-Dressman H, Fasano R, et al. Protective effect of HLA-DQB1 alleles against alloimmunization in patients with sickle cell disease. *Hum Immunol*. 2016;77(1):35–40.

79. Kapur R, Della Valle L, Sonneveld M, et al. Low anti RhD IgG-fc-fucosylation in pregnancy: a new variable predicting severity in haemolytic disease of the fetus and newborn. *Br J Haematol.* 2014;166:936−945.

80. Sonneveld ME, Koelewijn J, de Haas M, et al. Antigen specificity determines anti-red blood cell IgG-fc alloantibody glycosylation and thereby severity of haemolytic disease of the fetus and newborn. *Br J Haematol.* 2017; 176:651−660.

81. Evers D, Van Der Bom JG, Tijmensen J, et al. Absence of the spleen and the occurrence of primary red cell alloimmunization in humans. *Haematologica.* 2007;102:289−292.

82. Evers D, Middleburg RA, de Haas M, et al. Red blood cell alloimmunization in relation to antigens' exposure and their immunogenicity; a cohort study. *Lancet Haematol.* 2016;3(6):284−292.

83. Patel SR, Gibb DR, Girard-Pierce K, et al. Marginal zone B cells induce alloantibody formation following RBC transfusion. *Front Immunol.* 2018;9(2516):1−15.

84. Stowell SR, Girard-Pierce KR, Smith NH, et al. Transfusion of murine red blood cells expressing the human KEL glycoprotein induces clinically significant alloantibodies. *Transfusion.* 2014;54:179−189.

85. Patel SR, Bennett A, Girard-Pierce K, et al. Recipient priming to one RBC alloantigen directly enhances subsequent alloimmunization in mice. *Blood Advances.* 2018;2(2): 105−115.

86. Verduin EP, Schonewille H, Brand A, et al. High anti-HLA response in women exposed to intrauterine transfusions for severe alloimmune hemolytic disease is associated with mother-child HLA triplet mismatches, high anti-D titer, and new red blood cell antibody formation. *Transfusion.* 2013;53:939−947.

87. Mener A, Patel SR, Arthur CM, et al. Complement serves as a switch between CD4+ T-cell independent and dependent RBC antibody responses. *JCI Insight.* 2018; 3(22):e121631.

88. Mener A, Arthur CM, Patel SR, Liu J, Hendrickson JE, Stowell SR. Complement component 3 negatively regulates antibody response by modulation of red blood cell antigen. *Front Immunol.* 2018;9(676):1−18.

89. Maier CL, Mener A, Patel SR, et al. Antibody-mediated immune suppression by antigen modulation is antigen specific. *Blood Advances.* 2018;2(21):2986−3000.

90. ACOG Practice bulletin No. 192 Management of alloimmunization during pregnancy. *Obstet Gynecol.* 2018; 131(3):e82−90.

91. Dajak S, Stefanovic V, Capkun V. Severe hemolytic disease of the fetus and newborn caused by red cell antibodies not detected at the first trimester screening. *Transfusion.* 2011;51:1380−1388.

92. Koelewijn JM, Vrijkotte TGM, van der Schoot CE, Bonsel GJ, de Haas M. Effect of screening for red cell antibodies, other than anti-D to detect hemolytic disease of the fetus and newborn: a population study in the Netherlands. *Transfusion.* 2008;48:941−952.

93. Slootweg YM, Koelewijn JM, van Kemp IL, van der Bom JG, Oepkes D, de Haas M. Third trimester screening for alloimmunization in Rhc-negative pregnant women: evaluation of the Dutch national screening programme. *Br J Obstet Gynecol.* 2016;123:955−963.

94. White J, Qureshi H, Massey E, et al. British Committee for Standards in Hematology. Guideline for blood grouping and red cell antibody testing in pregnancy. *Transfus Med.* 2016;26(4):246−263.

95. Crowther C, Middleton P. Anti-D administration after childbirth for preventing Rhesus alloimmunization. *Cochrane Database Syst Rev.* 2000;(2).

96. Bowman JM, Chown B, Lewis M, Pollock JM. Rh isoimmunization during pregnancy: antenatal prophylaxis. *Can Med Assoc J.* 1978;118:623−627.

97. Geaghan SM. Diagnostic laboratory technologies for the fetus and neonate with isoimmunization. *Semin Perinatol.* 2011;35:148−154.

98. Koelewijn JK, de Haas M, Vrijkotte TGM, Bonsel GJ, van der Shoot CE. One single dose of 200 μg of antenatal RhIg halves the risk of anti-D immunization and hemolytic disease of the fetus and newborn in the next pregnancy. *Transfusion.* 2008;48:1720−1729.

99. Moise KJ. The usefulness of middle cerebral artery Doppler assessment I the treatment of the fetus at risk for anemia. *Am J Obstet Gynecol.* 2008;198: 161.e1−161.e4.

100. Bullock R, Martin WL, Coomarasamy A, et al. Prediction of fetal anemia in pregnancies with red cell alloimmunization: comparison of middle cerebral artery peak systolic velocity and amniotic fluid OD450. *Ultrasound Obstet Gynecol.* 2005;25(4):331−334.

101. Vietor HE, Kanhai HH, Brand A. Induction of additional red cell antibodies after intrauterine transfusions. *Transfusion.* 1994;34:970−974.

102. Van Kamp IL, Klumper FJ, Oepkes D, et al. Complications of intrauterine intravascular transfusion for fetal anemia due to maternal red-cell alloimmunization. *Am J Obstet Gynecol.* 2005;192:171−177.

103. Webb J, Delaney M. Red blood cell alloimmunization in the pregnant patient. *Transfus Med Rev.* 2018;32: 213−219.

104. Wong KS, Connan K, Rowlands S, Kornman LH, Savoia HF. Antenatal immunoglobulin for fetal red blood cell alloimmunization. *Cochrane Database Syst Rev.* 2013;5. Art.No.CD008267.

105. Schonewille H, Prinsen-Zander KJ, Reijnnart M, et al. Extended matched intrauterine transfusions reduce maternal Duffy, Kidd and S antibody formation. *Transfusion.* 2015;55:2912−2919.

106. O'Brien KL, Kim YA, Haspel RL, Uhl L. Provision of Kel1-negative blood to obstetric patients: a 3-year single

institution retrospective review. *Transfusion*. 2015;55:
599—604.

107. Makarovska-Bojadzieva T, Velkova E, Blagoevska M. The
impact of extended typing on red blood cell alloimmunization in transfused patients. *Basic Science*. 2017;5(2):
107—111.

108. Castro O, Sandler SG, Houston-Yu P, Rana S. Predicting
the effect of transfusion only phenotype-matched RBCs
to patients with sickle cell disease: theoretical and practical implications. *Transfusion*. 2002;42:684—690.

109. Flegel WA, Gottschall JL, Denomme GA. Implementing
mass-scale red cell genotyping at a blood center. *Transfusion*. 2015;55(11):2610—2615.

110. Hendrickson JE, Tormey CA, Shaz BH. Red blood cell
alloimmunization mitigation strategies. *Transfus Med
Rev*. 2014;28:137—144.

CHAPTER 10

Immune-Mediated Cytopenia in the Pediatric Setting

HOLLIE M. REEVES, DO

FETAL AND NEONATAL ALLOIMMUNE THROMBOCYTOPENIA

Fetal and neonatal alloimmune thrombocytopenia (FNAIT) occurs when there is an incompatibility or mismatch between mother and fetus for (most commonly) a human platelet antigen (HPA) and the mother produces immunoglobulin G (IgG) antibodies that cross the placenta and lead to fetal and/or neonatal platelet clearance and thrombocytopenia.[1] FNAIT occurs in approximately 1 in 1000 live births.[2] It is a common cause of severe thrombocytopenia (platelet count less than 25×10^9/L) and complications such as intracranial hemorrhage (ICH) in fetuses and term neonates.[3–5] The first cases of FNAIT were described in the 1950s and 1960s[6,7] and since then much progress has been made in the identification and characterization of the various HPA implicated.[2] Additionally, testing for platelet antibodies and antigens has improved as well as new developments in prenatal interventions.[2]

Pathogenesis

As mentioned earlier, pregnancies in which there is an incompatibility between the mother and the fetus for HPA are at risk for developing FNAIT. This occurs when the fetus inherits an HPA antigen(s) from the father that the mother's platelets lack. As antigen-positive platelets enter the maternal circulation, this may result in maternal alloimmunization. This alloimmunization leads to IgG alloantibody production against the fetal platelets. These antibodies can cross the placenta making their way into the fetal circulation where they bind to fetal platelets. The antigen-coated platelets then get removed by the reticuloendothelial system. See Fig. 10.1. This resulting thrombocytopenia can then lead to clinical sequelae, with ICH in severe cases. In addition to advances in the diagnosis, testing, and prenatal management of FNAIT, recent research has led to progress in four key areas thought to contribute to its pathogenesis.[2]

These important contributors to the pathogenesis of FNAIT include the following:[2]
- HPA incompatibility between the fetus and mother
- Maternal exposure to incompatible fetal HPA
- Maternal alloimmunization—mother produces IgG antibodies against foreign antigen
- Maternal–fetal antibody transfer—maternal IgG antibodies cross the placenta and enter the fetal circulation resulting in clearance of fetal (and neonatal) platelets

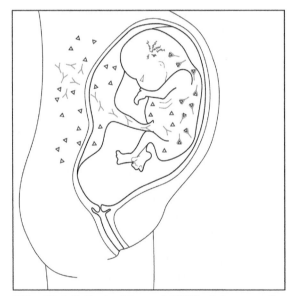

FIG. 10.1 Pathophysiology of FNAIT. Antigen-negative mother is exposed to antigen-positive fetal platelets (Δ). The mother becomes alloimmunized, developing IgG antibodies (ʎ) that cross the placenta sensitizing the fetal platelets. This leads to accelerated destruction of fetal (and neonatal) platelets resulting in thrombocytopenia and in some cases intracranial hemorrhage (ICH).

Immunologic Concepts in Transfusion Medicine. https://doi.org/10.1016/B978-0-323-67509-3.00010-X

HPA incompatibility between the fetus and mother

To date, 35 HPAs located on platelet glycoproteins (GP) and GP complexes have been described (http://www.ebi.ac.uk/ipd/hpa/table1.html last accessed 03/01/2019). These GPs coat the platelet membrane surface and are important for carrying out the platelet's biological functions, such as fibrinogen and von Willebrand factor binding sites. Single nucleotide polymorphisms (SNPs) in the genes that encode these platelet GPs lead to amino acid changes that can alter the GP structure, creating the HPA epitopes.[2] When an individual lacking an HPA antigen is homozygous for the opposite HPA, they can become alloimmunized when exposed to that missing antigen. The most commonly cited example of this is an individual who is HPA-1b/b (and therefore lacks HPA-1a) producing anti-HPA-1a antibodies.

Antibodies to platelet antigen HPA-1a (also known as Pl^{A1}) are the most commonly implicated antibodies in FNAIT in the Caucasian population, accounting for approximately 80%−85% of cases in this population.[2,8] Approximately 2%−2.5% of the Caucasian population lack the HPA-1a antigen putting them at risk for alloimmunization.[9] Furthermore, there is a well-documented association with HLA-DRB3*0101, with over 90% of HPA-1a antibodies made by women who express this allele.[10−12] Much of our understanding of the pathogenesis of FNAIT comes from studies of HPA-1a.

HPA-1a and the anti-HPA-1a immune response

The HPA-1a antigen is located on platelet membrane GPIIIa (the β3 integrin subunit of the αIIb/β3 platelet fibrinogen receptor).[13] A leucine to proline SNP at amino acid 33 (Leu33Pro) encoded by a T196C DNA base substitution in *ITGB3* defines the HPA-1 system [HPA-1a/b (Leu33/Pro33)].[14,15] Amino acid 33 is located within a disulfide-bond rich, knot-like structure known as the plexin−semaphorin−integrin (PSI) domain.[13] The PSI domain lies between the hybrid and integrin epidermal growth factor 1 (EGF, I-EGF1) domains of the GPIIIa.[13,16]

Early studies looking at the structure of the HPA-1a epitope on the β3 integrin showed that the Leu33Pro polymorphism is necessary for expression but is not sufficient by itself and that the anti-HPA-1a humoral response is heterogeneous and complex.[17−20] Using site-directed mutagenesis, Valentin et al. disrupted the disulfide bond linking the PSI domain to the EGF1 domain of GPIIIa and found that nearly one third of anti-HPA-1a antibodies lost some or all reactivity with the mutant protein. Based on these findings, the authors proposed that HPA-1a antibodies can be classified as type I or type II based upon their dependence on noncontiguous linear sequences present in the PSI and EGF1 domains.[18] Supporting this work, Stafford and coworkers found that in approximately 20% of FNAIT samples, anti-HPA-1a antibodies reacted with recombinant fragments of GPIIIa only when the fragment contained both the PSI and EGF1 domains (type II antibodies); however, type I antibodies are present in most FNAIT cases.[21] A correlation between antibody category and clinical severity of FNAIT could not be established.[21]

The β3-chain forms heterodimers either with αIIb or with αv on the surface of platelets, and these heterodimers function as fibrinogen or vitronectin receptors, respectively.[22,23] To what degree the αIIb and αv subunits contribute to the HPA-1a epitopes is unknown. It has been demonstrated that among anti-HPA-1a antibodies, some bind discretely to the β3-chain and others recognize compound epitopes formed by αIIb and β3.[17−19,24]

Different from αIIbβ3, αvβ3 is expressed on cells other than platelets, including endothelial cells[25] with documentation that HPA-1a is constitutively expressed on endothelial αvβ3.[26,27] Previous studies have implicated a role for β3 in angiogenesis, however, what that exact role is remains undetermined.[28−33] Whether or not anti-HPA-1a antibodies affect vascular integrity, possibly contributing to the pathogenesis of FNAIT, particularly ICH, is controversial.[34,35] Using both active and passive murine models of FNAIT, Yougbare and colleagues showed that ICH only occurred in anti-β3-mediated (target includes HPA-1a antigen), but not anti-GPIbα-mediated FNAIT despite similar thrombocytopenia in both groups. These results suggest that impaired angiogenesis and not thrombocytopenia is the key cause of ICH in FNAIT.[36] In this same study, the authors also looked at the ability of maternal intravenous immunoglobulin (IVIG) administration to stop impairment of vascular development in the brain and retina of anti-β3-mediated FNAIT mice pups. Similarly, they found that IVIG treatment decreased endothelial cell apoptosis and restored vascular development when compared to controls, suggesting a second mechanism of IVIG in FNAIT treatment besides improving thrombocytopenia.[36]

In human studies, Santoso and colleagues published their findings on whether a specific anti-HPA-1a antibody subtype exists in FNAIT cases with ICH, versus those without ICH. In this study, the authors investigated antibodies from mothers with ICH-positive and

ICH-negative FNAIT to identify any serological or functional differences between the two groups.[23] Using an antigen capture assay, stronger binding of antibodies from ICH-positive mothers to endothelial cell-derived $\alpha v\beta 3$ was observed. Further experiments using absorption techniques identified anti-HPA-1a antibodies of anti-$\alpha v\beta 3$ specificity in the ICH-positive, but not the ICH-negative group.[23] With identification of this new anti-HPA-1a antibody subtype, it is proposed that three different anti-HPA-1a subtypes may exist, see Table 10.1.

Identification of the maternal anti-HPA-1a antibody subtype(s) may determine whether ICH occurs providing diagnostic predictive potential, allowing for risk stratification and prophylactic treatment.[23]

Recent structural studies of the $\beta 3$ integrin suggest that anti-HPA-1a antibodies may also have a conformation-dependent feature.[15] Zhou and colleagues observed that there were local conformational changes at the PSI and EGF1 domains upon $\beta 3$ extension that may be responsible for the differences in anti-HPA-1a binding.[15] The authors proposed that these findings provide a structure-based interpretation for why some but not all anti-HPA-1a antibodies have been found to block the function of $\alpha IIb\beta 3$ and/or $\alpha v\beta 3$ integrins as previously described.[23,37]

Zhi et al. used transgenic mice expressing murine GPIIIa (muGPIIIa) isoforms that contained select humanized residues within the PSI and EGF1 domains to study binding of monoclonal and polyclonal HPA-1a-specific antibodies.[13] Their results revealed additional unsuspected complexity in the specificities of antibody subpopulations found in polyclonal maternal anti-HPA-1a alloantisera.[13] The authors suggest that high-resolution mapping of the polyclonal immune response to HPA-1a and analysis of the antibody subpopulations may provide a predictive diagnostic benefit.[13] Thus far, preliminary studies indicate that type I and type II antibodies have unique effects on the ability of platelets to interact with their ligand with additional studies planned in this area.[13,15]

TABLE 10.1
Proposed HPA-1a Antibody Subtypes.[23]

Antibody	Specificity
Anti-$\alpha IIb\beta 3$	Platelets only
Anti-$\beta 3$	Platelets and endothelial cells
Anti-$\alpha v\beta 3$	Endothelial cells (predominantly)

Other HPA and non-HPA incompatibilities implicated in FNAIT

In Caucasian patients, greater than 95% of FNAIT cases confirmed by serology are caused by maternal alloimmunization against antigens belonging to five HPA systems: HPA-1, HPA-2, HPA-3, HPA-5, and HPA-15.[9] See Fig. 10.2. Each of these antigen systems consists of two alleles that are relatively common in most populations. Alloantibodies to HPA-5b are implicated in approximately 10%–15% of FNAIT cases[38,39] followed by anti-HPA-1b in approximately 6%.[39] Multiple anti-HPA-specific alloantibodies detected in maternal sera occurs in approximately 3% of FNAIT cases.[39]

In FNAIT cases where antibodies to the common HPA antigen systems listed earlier are not detected, less common HPA antigens have been identified and reported. Interestingly though, Ghevaert et al. reported that after studying 1054 FNAIT referral cases, minor alleles of HPA-4 and -6bw to -17bw are exceedingly rare in the Caucasian population and did not explain the large number of FNAIT cases that test negative for the common HPA antibodies.[40] More recent reports, however, have identified additional low frequency platelet-specific antigens responsible for cases of FNAIT, some severe,[41−48] see Fig. 10.2. Of these rare HPA alloantigens, HPA-9b (Maxa) that is located near the HPA-3 antigen site on GPIIb appears to be the most immunogenic.[9,49]

Due to the rarity of the HPA-1b/1b type in non-Caucasians, antibodies to HPA-1a are a rare cause of FNAIT. In Asian populations, HPA-4 antibodies are more likely the cause.[50,51] HPA-6b and HPA-21b are also significantly more common in Asian versus Caucasian populations.[43,52]

Glycoprotein IV

Isoantibodies to glycoprotein IV (CD36) causing FNAIT have been described in African and Asian populations[53−55] as approximately 5% of persons with these ancestral backgrounds are CD36 deficient and upon exposure through transfusion or pregnancy can become alloimmunized.[9] Glycoprotein IV is a member of the class B scavenger receptor family of proteins and is expressed not only on platelets, but also on red cells, endothelial cells, and other tissues.[9] Two types of human CD36 deficiency have been described: Type I in which persons lack the protein on platelets, monocytes, and other tissues and are homozygous or compound heterozygous for mutant CD36 genes and Type II (more common) where only platelets are CD36 deficient and usually only one mutant CD36 gene is identified.[53] The clinical presentation in these patients with

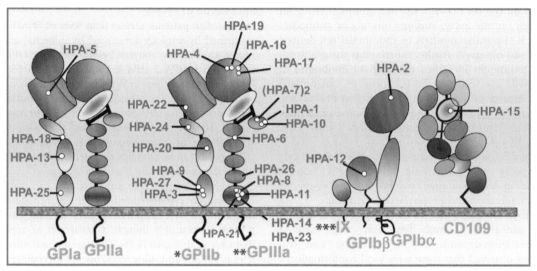

FIG. 10.2 Human platelet antigens (HPA) on platelet surface glycoproteins (GP) and GP complexes responsible for cases of fetal and neonatal alloimmune thrombocytopenia (FNAIT); common HPAs are highlighted. In addition to those HPA pictured, recently discovered platelet antigens implicated in FNAIT cases include *HPA-28bw[48] and Lap(a)[45] on GPIIb, **HPA-29bw[44] and Dom(b)[47] on GPIIIa, and ***Cab4b[46] on GPIX. (Modified from Peterson JA, McFarland JG, Curtis BR, Aster RH. Neonatal alloimmune thrombocytopenia: pathogenesis, diagnosis and management. *Br J Haematol* 2013;161(1):3−14. Peterson JA, Pechauer SM, Gitter ML, et al. New platelet glycoprotein polymorphisms causing maternal immunization and neonatal alloimmune thrombocytopenia. *Transfusion* 2012;52(5):1117−1124. with permission.)

anti-CD36 antibodies is similar to those with HPA-mediated disease and can include severe thrombocytopenia.[53]

Human leukocyte antigens

In addition to HPAs, human platelets express class I human leukocyte antigens (HLAs) and account for most HLA antigens present in circulating blood.[56] Estimates vary depending on parity and detection methods, but anti-class I HLA antibodies are found in as many as 30%−60% of all pregnant women.[57] Maternal anti-HLA class I antibodies have been found in cases of FNAIT in which no anti-HPA antibodies are found.[58−63] A recent retrospective study by Dahl and colleagues found that in suspected FNAIT cases where no platelet specific antibodies were found, maternal sera possessed anti-HLA class I antibodies that were specific toward fetal/paternal HLA antigens and their reactivity was significantly higher compared to controls.[57] Their results did not link immunization to a particular antigen but interestingly, they did observe that in pregnancies where HLA-B*27 was the most probable cause of maternal immunization, platelet count nadirs in the neonates were significantly lower when compared to the

rest of the case group.[57] This study highlights the importance of additional investigation into the role of anti-HLA class I antibodies and neonatal thrombocytopenia.

ABO antigens

Platelets normally express low levels of A and B antigens on their surface. Very rarely, cases of FNAIT not explained by HPA incompatibility may be due to ABO incompatibility between the fetus/neonate and the mother.[64]

Maternal exposure to incompatible fetal HPA

Much of what is known regarding fetal−maternal blood exchange comes from the literature on hemolytic disease of the fetus and newborn (HDFN) studying maternal red blood cell alloimmunization during pregnancy. The risk of fetal−maternal hemorrhage is greatest at time of delivery when it is likely that a small amount of fetal blood (0.5−1 mL) enters the maternal circulation, even in uncomplicated deliveries.[65] However, if a normal platelet count is assumed at 15 weeks gestation, experts postulate that there would be too few platelets, even for the highly immunogenic HPA-1a (which is expressed on platelets as early as 18 weeks gestation[66]) to immunize the mother.[2] FNAIT due to anti-HPA-1a, different from HDFN, occurs more frequently in first pregnancies indicating that previous maternal exposure to fetal platelets has occurred through blood transfusion, prior failed or undetected pregnancies, or fetal platelets during the current pregnancy.[2] Under normal circumstances, fetal and maternal blood do not mix except at the time of delivery. However, if there is a loss in trophoblast membrane integrity, which could occur from trauma, obstetrical interventions, infections, or other placental abnormalities, fetal blood cells including platelets could pass through and enter the maternal circulation.[67] In the absence of such interventions or trauma that may allow for exposure to fetal platelets, the fetal trophoblast itself has been proposed as an alternative explanation for the source of maternal alloimmunization to HPA-1a.

Fetal trophoblast cells express the β3 integrin (GPIIIa) as part of the αvβ3 complex.[68] Kumpel et al. demonstrated binding of GPIIIa monoclonal antibody (mAb) to the microvilli on the apical surface of syncytiotrophoblast cells in first trimester and term placentas. These cells are bathed by maternal blood and shed senescent parts into the maternal circulation during pregnancy.[68] The authors concluded that this trophoblast-derived fetal HPA-1a-positive GPIIIa could be the source of maternal alloimmunization, particularly in the first pregnancy.[68] As further support of this, in 2015, a mAb specific for HPA-1a named 26.4 was developed from the sera of a woman sensitized during pregnancy. This mAb bound to platelets and to purified integrins αIIbβ3 from platelets and αvβ3 from trophoblasts.[69] This model however does not explain maternal alloimmunization to HPA not expressed on the β3 integrin and additional research is therefore needed.

Until recently, placental pathology in FNAIT has not been well studied. An early report did find chronic villitis in untreated cases of FNAIT (no maternal receipt of IVIG) compared to those cases in which antenatal IVIG was administered.[70] In these untreated cases, it was also found that intrauterine growth restriction and fetal demise occurred as frequently as ICH.[70] Since then, two separate groups have reported on the likelihood that maternal alloimmunization to HPA-1a can affect normal placental development and contributes to placental dysfunction and miscarriages in FNAIT, possibly via activation of uterine natural killer (NK) cells.[71,72] To date, this has not been confirmed in human studies and remains an area in need of more research.

Maternal alloimmunization

Why do only some HPA-1a-negative mothers who are exposed to incompatible HPA become alloimmunized? In Caucasian populations, the HPA-1b/1b phenotype frequency is 2%, meaning that approximately 1 in 50 women could be susceptible to HPA-1a alloimmunization during pregnancy.[2] However, as mentioned earlier, the frequency of FNAIT is less, approximately 1 in every 1000 live births. It has been well documented that the anti-HPA-1a immune response is strongly associated with the human MHC class II allele, HLA-DRB3*0101.[10-12,73,74] In a large, prospective study of greater than 100,000 pregnant women of which 2% were HPA-1a-negative, approximately 10% of those had anti-HPA-1a detected.[12] Among those sensitized women who also underwent typing for the presence of HLA DRB3*0101, greater than 90% were positive.[12]

The B-cell response in FNAIT has been extensively studied. Realizing a high degree of HLA restriction, however, has led others to look at the contribution of T cells to the immune response in FNAIT. There is documented preference for binding of β3 peptides with HPA-1a (Leu33) in the peptide binding groove of DRB3*0101 over peptides with HPA-1b (Pro33) and presentation to antigen-presenting cells.[75,76] The Leu33 polymorphism serves as an anchor residue for stable binding of the HPA-1a peptide to the HLA-DRB3*0101 molecule[77] allowing for indirect HPA-1a-specific T-cell recognition.[78] Additionally, HPA-1a-specific DRB3*0101-restricted CD4 T cells have been isolated from alloimmunized women who have had FNAIT affected pregnancies[78-80] supporting that HPA-1a antigen presentation and the subsequent immune response is optimum when in the context of class II that is DRB3*0101.[2]

Bacterial and viral infections have been causally linked with the pathogenesis of immune-mediated thrombocytopenia (ITP). Could this be similar in FNAIT? In 2013, Li et al. examined the role of infection on the maternal immune response to incompatible platelets using a mouse model of fetal and neonatal isoimmune thrombocytopenia (FNIT). In this model, β3[−/−] and GP1bα[−/−] mice were injected with lipopolysaccharides or polyinosinic:polycytidylic acid (Poly I:C) to mimic bacterial and viral infections, respectively, following wild-type mouse platelet transfusion.[81] These mice produced significantly higher levels of β3 and GP1bα antibodies compared to controls.[81] Interestingly, they also found a higher rate of miscarriage in these female mice.[81]

Traditional serologic diagnosis of FNAIT is based on the detection of anti-HPA-1a antibodies using monoclonal antibody-based antigen-capture assays (MAIPA assay).[82] There are cases of FNAIT in HPA-1b/1b mothers, however, in which no anti-HPA-1a was detected using this method.[83] Studies utilizing alternative techniques such as a highly sensitive surface plasmon resonance (SPR) assay[82,84] or modified antigen capture enzyme-linked immunosorbent assays (ELISA)[85] found previously undetected low-avidity anti-HPA-1a antibodies in maternal sera in 9%–50% of FNAIT cases. The ability of these low-avidity anti-HPA-1a antibodies to cause platelet destruction in vivo has been studied in murine models. Bakchoul et al. demonstrated that low-avidity anti-HPA-1a does induce specific clearance of HPA-1a-positive platelets; however, this occurs at a slower rate than the platelet clearance produced by high-avidity (traditionally detected) anti-HPA-1a.[84] Similarly, Peterson and colleagues, using a nonobese diabetic/severe combined immunodeficiency mouse model, confirmed that low-avidity HPA-1a antibodies can cause FNAIT but the presence of such does not predict that an infant will be clinically affected.[85]

Maternal–fetal antibody transfer

Maternal immunoglobulins (mostly IgG_1 and IgG_3) are transported across the placenta to the fetal circulation via the MHC class I-related neonatal Fc receptor (FcRn).[80] The FcRn are expressed on placental syncytiotrophoblasts that are in contact with maternal blood and contain endosomes that internalize maternal IgG. The maternal IgG is transferred to the fetal circulation through a pH-dependent process of transcytosis.[2] To examine the role of FcRn in the pathogenesis and treatment of isoimmune thrombocytopenia in murine models, Chen et al. used combined β3/FcRn-deficient mice (FNIT model) to demonstrate that FcRn is critical for the induction of FNIT.[86] They also found that anti-FcRn antibody and IVIG prevented FNIT suggesting that therapies targeting FcRn in human FNAIT may have potential.[86]

The thrombocytopenia in FNAIT occurs when maternal anti-platelet IgG alloantibodies cross the placenta and bind to IgG-Fc receptors (FcγR) on phagocytes in the fetal spleen and liver.[87] The strength of the interaction between IgG and FcγR depends on several factors:[87]

- IgG subclass formed during the immune response
- IgG relative affinity to FcγRs
- Expression levels of FcγR allotypes
- FcγR copy number variation

- Cytokines influencing the expression of FcγR
- IgG-Fc glycosylation pattern

Using mass spectrometry to investigate the IgG-Fc glycosylation profiles of total and HPA-1a-specific IgG1 antibodies from the sera of 48 women with anti-HPA-1a and fetuses affected by FNAIT, Kapur and colleagues found markedly decreased levels of core fucosylation of anti-HPA-1a-specific IgG1 compared to total serum IgG1.[87] Additionally, antibodies with low amounts of fucose had higher binding affinity for receptors and enhanced neutrophil phagocytosis of platelets.[2,87] This group also concluded that lower anti-HPA-1a Fc core fucose levels correlate with decreased neonatal platelet counts and increased severity in their FNAIT cohort.[87] Sonneveld and colleagues reported similar findings, demonstrating a significant correlation between anti-HPA-1a antibodies with decreased fucosylation combined with antibody level and bleeding severity.[88] Whether these parameters can be used in screening for severe cases of FNAIT remains to be determined.

Diagnosis

In the newborn period, FNAIT is typically suspected when the neonate presents with petechiae or bleeding in the setting of thrombocytopenia, most with platelet counts below 50×10^9/L.[80] Maternal platelet counts are generally in the normal range separating this diagnosis from ITP. After ruling out other causes of thrombocytopenia, such as sepsis, the diagnosis of FNAIT is supported by the accurate detection of maternal antibodies to fetal/neonatal platelet antigen(s) that the mother lacks. Currently, the gold standard for the detection of platelet-specific antibodies is the MAIPA assay.[89] See Fig. 10.3. Although MAIPA is a sensitive and specific capture immunoassay,[90,91] it is time consuming and complicated requiring highly skilled technicians to perform and a panel of phenotyped platelets.[92] Quantification of anti-HPA-1a antibodies can be performed using a modified MAIPA assay.[93] Over the last 10–15 years, other technologies have been developed to detect platelet-specific antibodies including modified antigen-capture ELISA, Luminex bead assays, flow cytometry, and as an alternative to using platelet panels, techniques employing captured platelet antigens or cells transfected with cDNA encoding specific HPA.[92,94] These non-MAIPA methods, however, have limited sensitivity or lack the ability to confirm antibody identification.[95–98] As mentioned earlier, SPR technology can be used to identify low-avidity anti-HPA-1a antibodies.[82]

Molecular testing, including genotyping patients, their parents, or both can be useful in supporting the

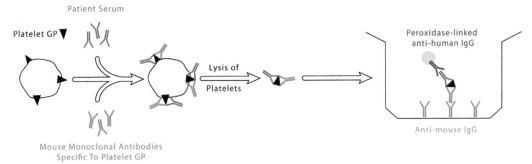

FIG. 10.3 Monoclonal antibody immobilization of platelet antigens (MAIPA) assay. (Modified from Brouk H, Ouelaa H. Fetal and neonatal alloimmune thrombocytopenia: advances in laboratory diagnosis and management. *Int J Blood Res Disorders* 2015;2.)

diagnosis of FNAIT. In cases of a previously affected fetus or neonate, it is common practice in the United States to genotype the father for HPA-1a status. If the father is HPA-1ab heterozygous then the risk of the fetus being HPA-1ab is 50% and fetal HPA-1a typing is performed on a sample obtained via amniocentesis.[99] This invasive procedure is not without risk, including fetal loss, bleeding, and potential increase in the maternal antibody response.[99]

Assays for noninvasive prenatal testing to detect fetal HPA-1a DNA in maternal plasma have been developed but are not routine practice in most countries.[100–102] Recently, Ferro and colleagues reported development of a noninvasive test using high resolution melting (HRM) polymerase chain reaction (PCR) to determine the maternal HPA-1a type and using DNA isolated from that same maternal plasma sample for fetal HPA-1a typing using coamplification at lower denaturation temperature HRM PCR.[103] This method still requires validation in larger clinical trials.[99]

Management and Progress Toward Prophylaxis
Prenatal management
Currently, no defined biomarker(s) or parameters can predict the risk of bleeding complications in FNAIT.[104] Therefore, previous pregnancy affected by severe FNAIT, with or without bleeding complications, is the most reliable parameter used to determine the risk of severe FNAIT in subsequent pregnancies, and serves as the basis for antenatal management.[80] Some centers monitor the maternal HPA-1a antibody levels and recommend delivery if the antibody level is ≥3 IU/mL[80]; however, reliable cut-off values to guide individual management have not been widely accepted.[105] In a recent review including three prospective studies and 10 retrospective studies, the authors concluded that HPA-1a antibody

level has the potential to predict the severity of FNAIT but due to the low positive predictive values is less suited for the final diagnosis or for guiding antenatal treatment.[106] Other promising markers or mechanisms include the fucosylation patterns of the anti-HPA-1a antibodies[87,88] and/or the subtype of HPA-1a antibody,[23] as described in detail earlier in the chapter.

A recent systematic review suggests that first-line antenatal management in FNAIT is weekly maternal IVIG administration, with or without the addition of corticosteroids.[107] With the assumption that FNAIT severity increases in subsequent pregnancies, the aim of antenatal IVIG therapy to increase neonatal platelet count or avoidance of ICH in the current pregnancy compared to the previous.[80] This assumption has recently been challenged with Tiller and colleagues reporting higher neonatal platelet counts in subsequent pregnancies without the use of antenatal treatment.[108] Other studies have suggested that IVIG may not work only by increasing the platelet count but may offer a protective benefit of lowering the risk of ICH recurrence, possibly by restoring angiogenesis in the fetal brain.[36,109]

Serial fetal blood sampling and intrauterine platelet transfusion have largely been abandoned due to the risk associated with this invasive procedure and the overall effectiveness of maternal IVIG administration.[107,110] The mode and timing of delivery is not currently standardized and may depend on the clinical scenario, for example, if the previous pregnancy was affected by ICH, or may vary by country.[80] In the event of a planned delivery, either by caesarean section or by vaginal, early communication with the blood bank/transfusion service is essential (Table 10.2).

Postnatal management
Management of a newborn affected by FNAIT will depend on the clinical condition and the severity of

TABLE 10.2
Overview of Recommendations for Antenatal Management of Pregnancies Complicated by FNAIT[105,107].

CURRENT PREGNANCY COMPLICATED BY FNAIT, I.E., FETUS WITH ICH

1. Weekly maternal IVIG administration ± corticosteroids
2. Fetal brain imaging with MRI and multidisciplinary meeting
3. Intrauterine platelet transfusion
4. Early delivery at 34 weeks by cesarean section

PREVENTATIVE IN A MOTHER WITH A PRIOR PREGNANCY AFFECTED BY FNAIT

Standard Risk (No ICH in Sibling)	High Risk (Sibling with ICH)
1. Weekly maternal IVIG administration, starting around 24 weeks ± corticosteroids	1. Weekly maternal IVIG administration, starting earlier than in standard risk cases (12–16 weeks) and At a higher dose ± corticosteroids
2. Ultrasound monitoring of fetal brain every 2–4 weeks	2. Ultrasound monitoring of fetal brain every 2–4 weeks
3. Planned delivery at 37 weeks	3. Planned delivery at 36 weeks

the thrombocytopenia.[111] Platelet transfusion is the first choice of treatment and can be used prophylactically[112] based on platelet count or therapeutically in a bleeding neonate.[105] The most appropriate threshold for prophylactic platelet transfusion has not been established. In most centers, the threshold for stable non-bleeding neonates is between $20 \times 10^9/L$ and $30 \times 10^9/L$.[105] Additional risk factors such as a sibling previously affected by ICH, a planned invasive procedure or operation, recovery from a large hemorrhage, gestational age <32 weeks, low birth weight, or a clinically unstable neonate may indicate the need for a higher threshold of $50 \times 10^9/L$.[105] In a bleeding infant, $50-100 \times 10^9/L$ may be necessary.[113]

Antigen-negative platelets are preferred for transfusion; however, this is usually only possible in a case of FNAIT diagnosed antenatally or in a subsequent pregnancy, if the alloantibody specificity is known and there is enough time to order the appropriate

platelets. Otherwise, washed maternal platelets or random platelets should be transfused. Arranging the transfusion of washed and irradiated maternal platelets can be logistically challenging and time consuming. Therefore, when matched donor platelets or washed maternal platelets are not available, studies support the use of random donor platelets. Kiefel et al. showed that multiple random donor platelet transfusions result in increased platelet counts in most cases of FNAIT and is an acceptable strategy.[113] Neonatal treatment with IVIG can be used to supplement platelet transfusion and is generally given for 1–3 days depending on response of platelet count to transfusion.[114–116]

Prophylaxis

To date, national screening programs for FNAIT have not been implemented in any country, although this has been advocated for by many groups and national health authorities.[110,117,118] One reason for this is the lack of an effective prophylactic treatment.

Animal studies have helped set the stage for human studies in FNAIT prophylaxis. Two groups developed antibodies (B2G1Δnab[119] and NGM-SZ21[120]) that effectively blocked HPA-1a-positive platelet clearance using two separate mouse models. In both studies, it was found that these HPA-1a blocking antibodies could displace polyclonal anti-HPA-1a attached to platelet β3,[119,120] providing a potential therapy in those severely affected FNAIT cases to reverse thrombocytopenia.[2] In 2012, Tiller and colleagues found that they could induce antibody-mediated immune suppression (AMIS), the name given to the inhibitory effect of passive anti-D IgG administration in HDFN prophylaxis, in an FNIT mouse model.[2,121] Prophylactic administration of human anti-HPA-1a or mouse mAb SZ21 significantly reduced the β3 antibody response in $\beta3^{-/-}$ female mice that were transfused with human HPA-1a-positive platelets and showed improved pregnancy outcomes.[121]

Using the human recombinant high-affinity HPA-1a antibody (B2G1Δnab) developed in earlier murine studies, Ghevaert et al. demonstrated that injection of this antibody protected platelets from destruction by anti-HPA-1a in the circulation of HPA-1ab human volunteers[122] and Eksteen and colleagues recently developed a monoclonal antibody specific for HPA-1a derived from an immortalized B cell from an alloimmunized woman who had an infant affected by FNAIT.[69] Such monoclonal antibodies may serve as a future source of human passive immunoprophylaxis to prevent development of FNAIT, and/or for therapeutic treatment of pregnant women who have already formed anti-HPA-1a to minimize fetal thrombocytopenia. An upcoming trial of passive polyclonal immune prophylaxis in pregnant women at-risk of FNAIT (HPA-1a-negative, HLA DRB3*01:01 positive) is planned in Europe (http://www.profnait.eu).

NEONATAL ALLOIMMUNE NEUTROPENIA

Neonatal alloimmune neutropenia (NAIN) is similar to FNAIT, except that it results from a fetal—maternal incompatibility to human neutrophil antigens (HNA) rather than HPAs. The incidence of NAIN is reported to be less than 1 in 1000 live births, and similar to FNAIT, NAIN may occur in the first pregnancy.[123] Typically, affected neonates present with absolute neutrophil counts (ANCs) of less than 500 per μL.[124] Skin infections and omphalitis are the most commonly seen infections, with severe infections such as meningitis or pneumonia being rare.[124,125] Interestingly, neutropenia in the fetus does not appear to cause deleterious effects, likely due to the protection provided by the amniotic sac.[126] The neutropenia usually resolves within 3—28 weeks, and antibiotics along with recombinant human granulocyte-colony-stimulating factor can be used as treatment for affected infants.[123]

Pathogenesis

NAIN occurs when a mother becomes immunized to a paternally inherited antigen present on the infant's neutrophils that she lacks. This immunization leads to the formation of IgG antibodies that cross the placenta and react with the newborn's neutrophils.[127] These antibody-coated neutrophils are then removed by the spleen, liver, and lungs resulting in neutropenia.[128] Reported cases of NAIN include alloantibodies to the antigens HNA-1a, HNA-1b, HNA-1c, HNA-1d, HNA-2, HNA-3a, HNA-4a, HNA-4b, HNA-5a, and most recently HNA-3b.[123] Isoantibodies to FcγRIIIb have also been reported to cause NAIN in mothers that are FcγRIII null.[1]

Human neutrophil antigens are a group of glycoproteins located on the surface of neutrophil granulocytes and are clinically relevant in allo- and autoimmunity.[129,130] The antigen nomenclature is based on the serologically defined epitope(s) on the glycoproteins and each antigen system is coded by a number, for example HNA-1.[129] All HNAs are expressed on neutrophils; however, some may also be expressed on other tissues, including HNA-3 that is also expressed on lymphocytes, platelets, and various tissues.[129] There are five HNA antigen systems (see Table 10.3).

Interestingly, neutrophil-specific antibodies are present in approximately 20% of pregnant and postpartum

TABLE 10.3
Human Neutrophil Antigen Systems and Associated Glycoproteins.[129]

Antigen System	Glycoprotein
HNA-1	FcγRIIIb, CD16
HNA-2	CD177
HNA-3	CTL2
HNA-4	CD11b
HNA-5	CD11a

CTL2, choline transporter-like protein 2.

women but less than 2% of newborns are affected by NAIN.[1] Reasons for this low detection rate may include the following: (1) many cases of NAIN do not show any symptoms; (2) other possible causes of neutropenia may make NAIN harder to detect; and (3) clinicians may be unaware of the need for a serological investigation or deem it unnecessary.[131]

Glycoproteins carrying HNAs are not expressed in placental tissue, yet as many as 40% of NAIN cases are diagnosed in first pregnancies.[132] Neutrophil-specific antibodies have been detected in females that have no alloexposure by pregnancy or transfusion and in males with no exposure to transfusion and experts postulate that these likely represent autoantibodies or naturally occurring antibodies, likely triggered by pathogens.[131]

DIAGNOSIS

Neonatal neutropenia is defined as an ANC of $<1.0 \times 10^9/L$ and severe neutropenia as an ANC of $<0.5 \times 10^9/L$[131]; however, neutrophil counts can vary depending on ethnicity and gestational age, with neutropenia more common in premature infants.[128] In a newborn with isolated neutropenia and a high level of clinical suspicion, the diagnosis of NAIN is made by demonstrating antineutrophil antibodies in both the infant and the mother. Genotyping of both parents for HNA helps to confirm the diagnosis.[127] Over the last 2 decades, the molecular basis of the five HNA antigen systems has been rigorously studied. This has enabled the development of reliable in-house and commercial assays for genotyping and antibody detection to aid in the confirmation of clinically suspected cases of NAIN; however, this is still very much limited to a few research laboratories.[130] The current recommended method for HNA antibody screening is the combination of the granulocyte aggregation test and the granulocyte immunofluorescence test.[133,134] This method uses a panel of freshly isolated and typed granulocytes but is time consuming and technically challenging.[133] The addition of flow cytometry-based methods such as the Flow-WIFT (flow cytometric white blood cell immunofluorescence test) may aid in increasing the sensitivity of screening for these antibodies.[133] Monoclonal antibody-specific immobilization of granulocyte antigens (MAIGA) is a glycoprotein-specific assay that can be used to confirm the antibody specificities responsible for the panel reactivity in the screening tests.[133] MAIGA does have limitations; antibodies to the HNA-3 system cannot be detected because no monoclonal antibodies are available against the CTL2 glycoprotein.[123]

MANAGEMENT

Due to the passive nature of these antibodies, the neutropenia usually resolves during the first 6 weeks of life but can last as long as 6 months.[128] The management of NAIN is lacking large observational studies or randomized clinical trials and mainly focuses on antibiotic therapy.[128] Some report the use of IVIG or recombinant human granulocyte-colony-stimulating factor to elevate the neutrophil levels[124]; however, this is often not necessary due to the transient nature of the neutropenia.[128]

SUMMARY

Alloimmune-mediated cytopenias in the fetal and neonatal period are rare but can be life threatening. Many advances in the mechanism underlying FNAIT, especially those cases caused by alloantibodies to HPA-1a, have been made. Despite these advances, however, additional research is needed. Future research directions include study on the relationship between maternal anti-platelet antibodies and miscarriage, further evaluating the role of anti-HPA-1a antibody subtypes, particularly related to angiogenesis and ICH, the ability to use antibody-mediated immune suppression as prophylaxis similar to the HDFN model, and the potential therapeutic role of anti-FcRn antibodies.

IVIG is a mainstay of antenatal management in pregnancies affected by FNAIT or in those mothers with a history of a previously affected pregnancy/child but identifying pregnancies at risk without a prior history of FNAIT remains a challenge. To date, no national screening programs exist. Platelet transfusion is used in neonates with thrombocytopenia and/or bleeding, although thresholds may vary. Antigen-negative platelets are preferred; however, unmatched platelets do offer hemostatic benefit and should be given if antigen-negative platelets are not available. In any

case of platelet transfusion, early communication with the transfusion service is key.

NAIN is a rare entity that may be under recognized; however, the molecular basis of the HNA system is being rigorously studied and diagnostic methods continue to improve. Fortunately, most cases of neutropenia are self-limited and no additional treatment or transfusion support is necessary.

REFERENCES

1. Lewin S, Bussel JB. Review of fetal and neonatal immune cytopenias. *Clin Adv Hematol Oncol.* 2015;13(1):35–43.
2. Curtis BR. Recent progress in understanding the pathogenesis of fetal and neonatal alloimmune thrombocytopenia. *Br J Haematol.* 2015;171(5):671–682.
3. Dreyfus M, Kaplan C, Verdy E, Schlegel N, Durand-Zaleski I, Tchernia G. Frequency of immune thrombocytopenia in newborns: a prospective study. Immune Thrombocytopenia Working Group. *Blood.* 1997; 89(12):4402–4406.
4. Berkowitz RL, Bussel JB, McFarland JG. Alloimmune thrombocytopenia: state of the art 2006. *Am J Obstet Gynecol.* 2006;195(4):907–913.
5. Gunnink SF, Vlug R, Fijnvandraat K, van der Bom JG, Stanworth SJ, Lopriore E. Neonatal thrombocytopenia: etiology, management and outcome. *Expert Rev Hematol.* 2014;7(3):387–395.
6. Harrington WJ, Sprague CC, Minnich V, Moore CV, Aulvin RC, Dubach R. Immunologic mechanisms in idiopathic and neonatal thrombocytopenic purpura. *Ann Intern Med.* 1953;38(3):433–469.
7. Shulman NR, Aster RH, Pearson HA, Hiller MC. Immunoreactions involving platelet. VI. Reactions of maternal isoantibodies responsible for neonatal purpura. Differentiation of a second platelet antigen system. *J Clin Investig.* 1962;41:1059–1069.
8. Strong NK, Eddleman KA. Diagnosis and management of neonatal alloimmune thrombocytopenia in pregnancy. *Clin Lab Med.* 2013;33(2):311–325.
9. Peterson JA, McFarland JG, Curtis BR, Aster RH. Neonatal alloimmune thrombocytopenia: pathogenesis, diagnosis and management. *Br J Haematol.* 2013;161(1):3–14.
10. L'Abbe D, Tremblay L, Filion M, et al. Alloimmunization to platelet antigen HPA-1a (PIA1) is strongly associated with both HLA-DRB3*0101 and HLA-DQB1*0201. *Hum Immunol.* 1992;34(2):107–114.
11. Williamson LM, Hackett G, Rennie J, et al. The natural history of fetomaternal alloimmunization to the platelet-specific antigen HPA-1a (PlA1, Zwa) as determined by antenatal screening. *Blood.* 1998;92(7): 2280–2287.
12. Kjeldsen-Kragh J, Killie MK, Tomter G, et al. A screening and intervention program aimed to reduce mortality and serious morbidity associated with severe neonatal alloimmune thrombocytopenia. *Blood.* 2007;110(3): 833–839.

13. Zhi H, Ahlen MT, Thinn AMM, et al. High-resolution mapping of the polyclonal immune response to the human platelet alloantigen HPA-1a (Pl(A1)). *Blood Adv.* 2018;2(21):3001–3011.

14. Newman PJ, Derbes RS, Aster RH. The human platelet alloantigens, PlA1 and PlA2, are associated with a leucine33/proline33 amino acid polymorphism in membrane glycoprotein IIIa, and are distinguishable by DNA typing. *J Clin Investig.* 1989;83(5):1778–1781.

15. Zhou D, Thinn AMM, Zhao Y, Wang Z, Zhu J. Structure of an extended beta 3 integrin. *Blood.* 2018;132(9):962–972.

16. Xiao T, Takagi J, Coller BS, Wang JH, Springer TA. Structural basis for allostery in integrins and binding to fibrinogen-mimetic therapeutics. *Nature.* 2004; 432(7013):59–67.

17. Honda S, Honda Y, Bauer B, Ruan C, Kunicki TJ. The impact of three-dimensional structure on the expression of PlA alloantigens on human integrin beta 3. *Blood.* 1995;86(1):234–242.

18. Valentin N, Visentin GP, Newman PJ. Involvement of the cysteine-rich domain of glycoprotein IIIa in the expression of the human platelet alloantigen, PlA1: evidence for heterogeneity in the humoral response. *Blood.* 1995;85(11):3028–3033.

19. Liu LX, Nardi MA, Casella JF, Karpatkin S. Inhibition of binding of anti-PLA1 antibodies to platelets with monoclonal antibody LK-4. Evidence for multiple PLA1 receptor sites on platelet GPIIIa. *Blood.* 1996;88(9): 3601–3607.

20. Barron-Casella EA, Nebbia G, Rogers OC, King KE, Kickler TS, Casella JF. Construction of a human platelet alloantigen-1a epitope(s) within murine glycoprotein IIIa: identification of residues critical to the conformation of the antibody binding site(s). *Blood.* 1999;93(9): 2959–2967.

21. Stafford P, Ghevaert C, Campbell K, et al. Immunologic and structural analysis of eight novel domain-deletion beta3 integrin peptides designed for detection of HPA-1 antibodies. *J Thromb Haemost.* 2008;6(2):366–375.

22. Bennett JS, Berger BW, Billings PC. The structure and function of platelet integrins. *J Thromb Haemost.* 2009; 7(Suppl 1):200–205.

23. Santoso S, Wihadmadyatami H, Bakchoul T, et al. Antiendothelial alpha v beta 3 antibodies are a major cause of intracranial bleeding in fetal/neonatal alloimmune thrombocytopenia. *Arterioscler Thromb Vasc Biol.* 2016;36(8):1517–1524.

24. Allen DL, Abrahamsson S, Murphy MF, Roberts DJ. Human platelet antigen 1a epitopes are dependent on the cation-regulated conformation of integrin alpha(IIb)beta(3) (GPIIb/IIIa). *J Immunol Methods.* 2012;375(1–2):166–175.

25. Cheresh DA, Smith JW, Cooper HM, Quaranta V. A novel vitronectin receptor integrin (alpha v beta x) is responsible for distinct adhesive properties of carcinoma cells. *Cell.* 1989;57(1):59–69.

26. Leeksma OC, Giltay JC, Zandbergen-Spaargaren J, Modderman PW, van Mourik JA, von dem Borne AE. The platelet alloantigen Zwa or PlA1 is expressed by cultured endothelial cells. *Br J Haematol.* 1987;66(3): 369–373.

27. Giltay JC, Leeksma OC, von dem Borne AE, van Mourik JA. Alloantigenic composition of the endothelial vitronectin receptor. *Blood.* 1988;72(1):230–233.

28. Brooks PC, Clark RA, Cheresh DA. Requirement of vascular integrin alpha v beta 3 for angiogenesis. *Science.* 1994;264(5158):569–571.

29. Brooks PC, Montgomery AM, Rosenfeld M, et al. Integrin alpha v beta 3 antagonists promote tumor regression by inducing apoptosis of angiogenic blood vessels. *Cell.* 1994;79(7):1157–1164.

30. Di Q, Cheng Z, Kim W, et al. Impaired cross-activation of beta3 integrin and VEGFR-2 on endothelial progenitor cells with aging decreases angiogenesis in response to hypoxia. *Int J Cardiol.* 2013;168(3):2167–2176.

31. Stupack DG, Cheresh DA. Integrins and angiogenesis. *Curr Top Dev Biol.* 2004;64:207–238.

32. Hynes RO. A reevaluation of integrins as regulators of angiogenesis. *Nat Med.* 2002;8(9):918–921.

33. Robinson SD, Reynolds LE, Kostourou V, et al. Alpha v beta3 integrin limits the contribution of neuropilin-1 to vascular endothelial growth factor-induced angiogenesis. *J Biol Chem.* 2009;284(49):33966–33981.

34. van Gils JM, Stutterheim J, van Duijn TJ, et al. HPA-1a alloantibodies reduce endothelial cell spreading and monolayer integrity. *Mol Immunol.* 2009;46(3):406–415.

35. Radder CM, Beekhuizen H, Kanhai HH, Brand A. Effect of maternal anti-HPA-1a antibodies and polyclonal IVIG on the activation status of vascular endothelial cells. *Clin Exp Immunol.* 2004;137(1):216–222.

36. Yougbare I, Lang S, Yang H, et al. Maternal anti-platelet beta3 integrins impair angiogenesis and cause intracranial hemorrhage. *J Clin Investig.* 2015;125(4): 1545–1556.

37. Kroll H, Penke G, Santoso S. Functional heterogeneity of alloantibodies against the human platelet antigen (HPA)-1a. *Thromb Haemostasis.* 2005;94(6):1224–1229.

38. Kaplan C, Morel-Kopp MC, Kroll H, et al. HPA-5b (Br(a)) neonatal alloimmune thrombocytopenia: clinical and immunological analysis of 39 cases. *Br J Haematol.* 1991;78(3):425–429.

39. Davoren A, Curtis BR, Aster RH, McFarland JG. Human platelet antigen-specific alloantibodies implicated in 1162 cases of neonatal alloimmune thrombocytopenia. *Transfusion.* 2004;44(8):1220–1225.

40. Ghevaert C, Rankin A, Huiskes E, et al. Alloantibodies against low-frequency human platelet antigens do not account for a significant proportion of cases of fetomaternal alloimmune thrombocytopenia: evidence from 1054 cases. *Transfusion.* 2009;49(10):2084–2089.

41. Peterson JA, Gitter ML, Kanack A, et al. New low-frequency platelet glycoprotein polymorphisms associated with neonatal alloimmune thrombocytopenia. *Transfusion.* 2010;50(2):324–333.

42. Peterson JA, Pechauer SM, Gitter ML, et al. New platelet glycoprotein polymorphisms causing maternal

immunization and neonatal alloimmune thrombocytopenia. *Transfusion.* 2012;52(5):1117–1124.

43. Peterson JA, Pechauer SM, Gitter ML, Szabo A, Curtis BR, Aster RH. The human platelet antigen-21bw is relatively common among Asians and is a potential trigger for neonatal alloimmune thrombocytopenia. *Transfusion.* 2012;52(4):915–916.

44. Sullivan MJ, Peterson J, McFarland JG, Bougie D, Aster RH, Curtis BR. A new low-frequency alloantigen (Kha(b)) located on platelet glycoprotein IIIa as a cause of maternal sensitization leading to neonatal alloimmune thrombocytopenia. *Transfusion.* 2015;55(6 Pt 2):1584–1585.

45. Wihadmadyatami H, Heidinger K, Roder L, et al. Alloantibody against new platelet alloantigen (Lap(a)) on glycoprotein IIb is responsible for a case of fetal and neonatal alloimmune thrombocytopenia. *Transfusion.* 2015;55(12):2920–2929.

46. Jallu V, Beranger T, Bianchi F, et al. Cab4b, the first human platelet antigen carried by glycoprotein IX discovered in a context of severe neonatal thrombocytopenia. *J Thromb Haemost.* 2017;15(8):1646–1654.

47. Sullivan MJ, Kuhlmann R, Peterson JA, Curtis BR. Severe neonatal alloimmune thrombocytopenia caused by maternal sensitization against a new low-frequency alloantigen (Dom(b)) located on platelet glycoprotein IIIa. *Transfusion.* 2017;57(7):1847–1848.

48. Poles A, Wozniak MJ, Walser P, et al. A V740L mutation in glycoprotein IIb defines a novel epitope (War) associated with fetomaternal alloimmune thrombocytopenia. *Transfusion.* 2013;53(9):1965–1973.

49. Peterson JA, Balthazor SM, Curtis BR, McFarland JG, Aster RH. Maternal alloimmunization against the rare platelet-specific antigen HPA-9b (Max a) is an important cause of neonatal alloimmune thrombocytopenia. *Transfusion.* 2005;45(9):1487–1495.

50. Ohto H, Miura S, Ariga H, et al. The natural history of maternal immunization against foetal platelet alloantigens. *Transfus Med.* 2004;14(6):399–408.

51. Curtis BR, McFarland JG. Detection and identification of platelet antibodies and antigens in the clinical laboratory. *Immunohematology.* 2009;25(3):125–135.

52. Tanaka S, Taniue A, Nagao N, et al. Genotype frequencies of the human platelet antigen, Ca/Tu, in Japanese, determined by a PCR-RFLP method. *Vox Sang.* 1996;70(1):40–44.

53. Curtis BR, Ali S, Glazier AM, Ebert DD, Aitman TJ, Aster RH. Isoimmunization against CD36 (glycoprotein IV): description of four cases of neonatal isoimmune thrombocytopenia and brief review of the literature. *Transfusion.* 2002;42(9):1173–1179.

54. Kankirawatana S, Kupatawintu P, Juji T, et al. Neonatal alloimmune thrombocytopenia due to anti-Nak(a). *Transfusion.* 2001;41(3):375–377.

55. Lin M, Xu X, Lee HL, Liang DC, Santoso S. Fetal/neonatal alloimmune thrombocytopenia due to anti-CD36

antibodies: antibody evaluations by CD36-transfected cell lines. *Transfusion.* 2018;58(1):189–195.

56. Pereira J, Cretney C, Aster RH. Variation of class I HLA antigen expression among platelet density cohorts: a possible index of platelet age? *Blood.* 1988;71(2):516–519.

57. Dahl J, Refsum E, Ahlen MT, et al. Unraveling the role of maternal anti-HLA class I antibodies in fetal and neonatal thrombocytopenia-Antibody specificity analysis using epitope data. *J Reprod Immunol.* 2017;122:1–9.

58. Saito S, Ota M, Komatsu Y, et al. Serologic analysis of three cases of neonatal alloimmune thrombocytopenia associated with HLA antibodies. *Transfusion.* 2003;43(7):908–917.

59. Moncharmont P, Dubois V, Obegi C, et al. HLA antibodies and neonatal alloimmune thrombocytopenia. *Acta Haematol.* 2004;111(4):215–220.

60. Thude H, Schorner U, Helfricht C, Loth M, Maak B, Barz D. Neonatal alloimmune thrombocytopenia caused by human leucocyte antigen-B27 antibody. *Transfus Med.* 2006;16(2):143–149.

61. Gramatges MM, Fani P, Nadeau K, Pereira S, Jeng MR. Neonatal alloimmune thrombocytopenia and neutropenia associated with maternal human leukocyte antigen antibodies. *Pediatr Blood Canc.* 2009;53(1):97–99.

62. Starcevic M, Tomicic M, Malenica M, Zah-Matakovic V. Neonatal alloimmune thrombocytopenia caused by anti-HLA-A24 alloantibodies. *Acta Paediatr.* 2010;99(4):630–632.

63. Meler E, Porta R, Canals C, Serra B, Lozano M. Fatal alloimmune thrombocytopenia due to anti-HLA alloimmunization in a twin pregnancy: a very infrequent complication of assisted reproduction. *Transfus Apher Sci.* 2017;56(2):165–167.

64. Curtis BR, Fick A, Lochowicz AJ, et al. Neonatal alloimmune thrombocytopenia associated with maternal-fetal incompatibility for blood group B. *Transfusion.* 2008;48(2):358–364.

65. Solomonia N, Playforth K, Reynolds EW. Fetal-maternal hemorrhage: a case and literature review. *AJP Rep.* 2012;2(1):7–14.

66. Gruel Y, Boizard B, Daffos F, Forestier F, Caen J, Wautier JL. Determination of platelet antigens and glycoproteins in the human fetus. *Blood.* 1986;68(2):488–492.

67. Dawe GS, Tan XW, Xiao ZC. Cell migration from baby to mother. *Cell Adhes Migrat.* 2007;1(1):19–27.

68. Kumpel BM, Sibley K, Jackson DJ, White G, Soothill PW. Ultrastructural localization of glycoprotein IIIa (GPIIIa, beta 3 integrin) on placental syncytiotrophoblast microvilli: implications for platelet alloimmunization during pregnancy. *Transfusion.* 2008;48(10):2077–2086.

69. Eksteen M, Tiller H, Averina M, et al. Characterization of a human platelet antigen-1a-specific monoclonal antibody derived from a B cell from a woman alloimmunized in pregnancy. *J Immunol.* 2015;194(12):5751–5760.

70. Althaus J, Weir EG, Askin F, Kickler TS, Blakemore K. Chronic villitis in untreated neonatal alloimmune

thrombocytopenia: an etiology for severe early intrauterine growth restriction and the effect of intravenous immunoglobulin therapy. *Am J Obstet Gynecol.* 2005; 193(3 Pt 2):1100−1104.

71. Eksteen M, Heide G, Tiller H, et al. Anti-human platelet antigen (HPA)-1a antibodies may affect trophoblast functions crucial for placental development: a laboratory study using an in vitro model. *Reprod Biol Endocrinol.* 2017;15(1):28.

72. Yougbare I, Tai WS, Zdravic D, et al. Activated NK cells cause placental dysfunction and miscarriages in fetal alloimmune thrombocytopenia. *Nat Commun.* 2017; 8(1):224.

73. Mueller-Eckhardt C, Mueller-Eckhardt G, Willen-Ohff H, et al. Immunogenicity of and immune response to the human platelet antigen Zwa is strongly associated with HLA-B8 and DR3. *Tissue Antigens.* 1985;26(1):71−76.

74. Valentin N, Vergracht A, Bignon JD, et al. HLA-DRw52a is involved in alloimmunization against PL-A1 antigen. *Hum Immunol.* 1990;27(2):73−79.

75. Maslanka K, Yassai M, Gorski J. Molecular identification of T cells that respond in a primary bulk culture to a peptide derived from a platelet glycoprotein implicated in neonatal alloimmune thrombocytopenia. *J Clin Investig.* 1996;98(8):1802−1808.

76. Anani Sarab G, Moss M, Barker RN, Urbaniak SJ. Naturally processed peptides spanning the HPA-1a polymorphism are efficiently generated and displayed from platelet glycoprotein by HLA-DRB3*0101-positive antigen-presenting cells. *Blood.* 2009;114(9): 1954−1957.

77. Wu S, Maslanka K, Gorski J. An integrin polymorphism that defines reactivity with alloantibodies generates an anchor for MHC class II peptide binding: a model for unidirectional alloimmune responses. *J Immunol.* 1997; 158(7):3221−3226.

78. Ahlen MT, Husebekk A, Killie IL, Skogen B, Stuge TB. T cell responses to human platelet antigen-1a involve a unique form of indirect allorecognition. *JCI Insight.* 2016;1(14):e86558.

79. Rayment R, Kooij TW, Zhang W, et al. Evidence for the specificity for platelet HPA-1a alloepitope and the presenting HLA-DR52a of diverse antigen-specific helper T cell clones from alloimmunized mothers. *J Immunol.* 2009;183(1):677−686.

80. Tiller H, Husebekk A, Ahlen MT, Stuge TB, Skogen B. Current perspectives on fetal and neonatal alloimmune thrombocytopenia − increasing clinical concerns and new treatment opportunities. *Int J Womens Health.* 2017;9:223−234.

81. Li C, Chen P, Vadasz B, et al. Co-stimulation with LPS or Poly I:C markedly enhances the anti-platelet immune response and severity of fetal and neonatal alloimmune thrombocytopenia. *Thromb Haemostasis.* 2013;110(6): 1250−1258.

82. Socher I, Andrei-Selmer C, Bein G, Kroll H, Santoso S. Low-avidity HPA-1a alloantibodies in severe neonatal alloimmune thrombocytopenia are detectable with surface plasmon resonance technology. *Transfusion.* 2009;49(5):943−952.

83. Bussel JB, Zacharoulis S, Kramer K, McFarland JG, Pauliny J, Kaplan C. Clinical and diagnostic comparison of neonatal alloimmune thrombocytopenia to nonimmune cases of thrombocytopenia. *Pediatr Blood Canc.* 2005;45(2):176−183.

84. Bakchoul T, Kubiak S, Krautwurst A, et al. Low-avidity anti-HPA-1a alloantibodies are capable of antigen-positive platelet destruction in the NOD/SCID mouse model of alloimmune thrombocytopenia. *Transfusion.* 2011;51(11):2455−2461.

85. Peterson JA, Kanack A, Nayak D, et al. Prevalence and clinical significance of low-avidity HPA-1a antibodies in women exposed to HPA-1a during pregnancy. *Transfusion.* 2013;53(6):1309−1318.

86. Chen P, Li C, Lang S, et al. Animal model of fetal and neonatal immune thrombocytopenia: role of neonatal Fc receptor in the pathogenesis and therapy. *Blood.* 2010;116(18):3660−3668.

87. Kapur R, Kustiawan I, Vestrheim A, et al. A prominent lack of IgG1-Fc fucosylation of platelet alloantibodies in pregnancy. *Blood.* 2014;123(4):471−480.

88. Sonneveld ME, Natunen S, Sainio S, et al. Glycosylation pattern of anti-platelet IgG is stable during pregnancy and predicts clinical outcome in alloimmune thrombocytopenia. *Br J Haematol.* 2016;174(2): 310−320.

89. Kiefel V, Santoso S, Weisheit M, Mueller-Eckhardt C. Monoclonal antibody−specific immobilization of platelet antigens (MAIPA): a new tool for the identification of platelet-reactive antibodies. *Blood.* 1987;70(6): 1722−1726.

90. Metcalfe P, Allen D, Chapman J, Ouwehand WH. Interlaboratory variation in the detection of clinically significant alloantibodies against human platelet alloantigens. *Br J Haematol.* 1997;97(1):204−207.

91. Metcalfe P, Allen D, Kekomaki R, Kaplan C, de Haas M, Ouwehand WH. An International Reference Reagent (minimum sensitivity) for the detection of anti-human platelet antigen 1a. *Vox Sang.* 2009;96(2):146−152.

92. Bonstein L, Haddad N. Taking a wider view on fetal/neonatal alloimmune thrombocytopenia. *Thromb Res.* 2017;151(Suppl 1):S100−S102.

93. Bertrand G, Jallu V, Gouet M, et al. Quantification of human platelet antigen-1a antibodies with the monoclonal antibody immobilization of platelet antigens procedure. *Transfusion.* 2005;45(8):1319−1323.

94. Hayashi T, Hirayama F. Advances in alloimmune thrombocytopenia: perspectives on current concepts of human platelet antigens, antibody detection strategies, and genotyping. *Blood Transfus.* 2015;13(3):380−390.

95. Nguyen XD, Goebel M, Schober M, Kluter H, Panzer S. The detection of platelet antibodies by simultaneous analysis of specific platelet antibodies and the monoclonal antibody-specific immobilization of platelet antigens: an interlaboratory comparison. *Transfusion.* 2010; 50(7):1429−1434.

96. Rockenbauer L, Eichelberger B, Panzer S. Comparison of the bead-based simultaneous analysis of specific platelet antibodies assay (SASPA) and Pak Lx Luminex technology with the monoclonal antibody immobilization of platelet antigens assay (MAIPA) to detect platelet alloantibodies. *Clin Chem Lab Med.* 2015;53(11):1779–1783.

97. Mortberg A, Meinke S, Berg P, et al. Sensitive detection of platelet-specific antibodies with a modified MAIPA using biotinylated antibodies and streptavidin-coated beads. *J Immunol Methods.* 2016;434:9–15.

98. Cooper N, Bein G, Heidinger K, Santoso S, Sachs UJ. A bead-based assay in the work-up of suspected platelet alloimmunization. *Transfusion.* 2016;56(1):115–118.

99. Kjeldsen-Kragh J. New elegant methods for maternal and fetal HPA-1a typing. *Transfusion.* 2018;58(10):2253–2254.

100. Le Toriellec E, Chenet C, Kaplan C. Safe fetal platelet genotyping: new developments. *Transfusion.* 2013;53(8):1755–1762.

101. van der Schoot CE, Thurik FF, Veldhuisen B, de Haas M. Noninvasive prenatal blood group and HPA-1a genotyping: the current European experience. *Transfusion.* 2013;53(11 Suppl 2):2834–2836.

102. Wienzek-Lischka S, Krautwurst A, Frohner V, et al. Noninvasive fetal genotyping of human platelet antigen-1a using targeted massively parallel sequencing. *Transfusion.* 2015;55(6 Pt 2):1538–1544.

103. Ferro M, Macher HC, Fornes G, et al. Noninvasive prenatal diagnosis by cell-free DNA screening for fetomaternal HPA-1a platelet incompatibility. *Transfusion.* 2018;58(10):2272–2279.

104. Lakkaraja M, Berkowitz RL, Vinograd CA, et al. Omission of fetal sampling in treatment of subsequent pregnancies in fetal-neonatal alloimmune thrombocytopenia. *Am J Obstet Gynecol.* 2016;215(4):471. e471-479.

105. Winkelhorst D, Oepkes D, Lopriore E. Fetal and neonatal alloimmune thrombocytopenia: evidence based antenatal and postnatal management strategies. *Expert Rev Hematol.* 2017;10(8):729–737.

106. Kjaer M, Bertrand G, Bakchoul T, et al. Maternal HPA-1a antibody level and its role in predicting the severity of Fetal/Neonatal Alloimmune Thrombocytopenia: a systematic review. *Vox Sang.* 2019;114(1):79–94.

107. Winkelhorst D, Murphy MF, Greinacher A, et al. Antenatal management in fetal and neonatal alloimmune thrombocytopenia: a systematic review. *Blood.* 2017;129(11):1538–1547.

108. Tiller H, Husebekk A, Skogen B, Kjeldsen-Kragh J, Kjaer M. True risk of fetal/neonatal alloimmune thrombocytopenia in subsequent pregnancies: a prospective observational follow-up study. *BJOG.* 2016;123(5):738–744.

109. Ni H, Chen P, Spring CM, et al. A novel murine model of fetal and neonatal alloimmune thrombocytopenia: response to intravenous IgG therapy. *Blood.* 2006;107(7):2976–2983.

110. Kamphuis MM, Paridaans N, Porcelijn L, et al. Screening in pregnancy for fetal or neonatal alloimmune thrombocytopenia: systematic review. *BJOG.* 2010;117(11):1335–1343.

111. Bertrand G, Kaplan C. How do we treat fetal and neonatal alloimmune thrombocytopenia? *Transfusion.* 2014;54(7):1698–1703.

112. Stanworth SJ, Clarke P, Watts T, et al. Prospective, observational study of outcomes in neonates with severe thrombocytopenia. *Pediatrics.* 2009;124(5):e826–834.

113. Kiefel V, Bassler D, Kroll H, et al. Antigen-positive platelet transfusion in neonatal alloimmune thrombocytopenia (NAIT). *Blood.* 2006;107(9):3761–3763.

114. Bussel J. Diagnosis and management of the fetus and neonate with alloimmune thrombocytopenia. *J Thromb Haemost.* 2009;7(Suppl 1):253–257.

115. Kanhai HH, Porcelijn L, Engelfriet CP, et al. Management of alloimmune thrombocytopenia. *Vox Sang.* 2007;93(4):370–385.

116. te Pas AB, Lopriore E, van den Akker ES, et al. Postnatal management of fetal and neonatal alloimmune thrombocytopenia: the role of matched platelet transfusion and IVIG. *Eur J Pediatr.* 2007;166(10):1057–1063.

117. Madsen C, Prahm KP, Nilsson C, Pedersen LH, Dziegiel MH, Hedegaard M. [Establishing a screening programme in Denmark for foetal and neonatal alloimmune thrombocytopenia]. *Ugeskr Laeger.* 2018;180(17).

118. Skogen B, Killie MK, Kjeldsen-Kragh J, et al. Reconsidering fetal and neonatal alloimmune thrombocytopenia with a focus on screening and prevention. *Expert Rev Hematol.* 2010;3(5):559–566.

119. Ghevaert C, Wilcox DA, Fang J, et al. Developing recombinant HPA-1a-specific antibodies with abrogated Fcgamma receptor binding for the treatment of fetomaternal alloimmune thrombocytopenia. *J Clin Investig.* 2008;118(8):2929–2938.

120. Bakchoul T, Boylan B, Sachs UJ, et al. Blockade of maternal anti-HPA-1a-mediated platelet clearance by an HPA-1a epitope-specific F(ab') in an in vivo mouse model of alloimmune thrombocytopenia. *Transfusion.* 2009;49(2):265–270.

121. Tiller H, Killie MK, Chen P, et al. Toward a prophylaxis against fetal and neonatal alloimmune thrombocytopenia: induction of antibody-mediated immune suppression and prevention of severe clinical complications in a murine model. *Transfusion.* 2012;52(7):1446–1457.

122. Ghevaert C, Herbert N, Hawkins L, et al. Recombinant HPA-1a antibody therapy for treatment of fetomaternal alloimmune thrombocytopenia: proof of principle in human volunteers. *Blood.* 2013;122(3):313–320.

123. Lopes LB, Abbas SA, Moritz E, et al. Antibodies to human neutrophil antigen HNA-3b implicated in cases of neonatal alloimmune neutropenia. *Transfusion.* 2018;58(5):1264–1270.

124. Curtis BR, Reno C, Aster RH. Neonatal alloimmune neutropenia attributed to maternal immunoglobulin G antibodies against the neutrophil alloantigen HNA-1c (SH): a report of five cases. *Transfusion.* 2005;45(8):1308–1313.

125. Bux J, Jung KD, Kauth T, Mueller-Eckhardt C. Serological and clinical aspects of granulocyte antibodies leading to alloimmune neonatal neutropenia. *Transfus Med.* 1992; 2(2):143−149.
126. Reil A, Sachs UJ, Siahanidou T, Flesch BK, Bux J. HNA-1d: a new human neutrophil antigen located on Fcgamma receptor IIIb associated with neonatal immune neutropenia. *Transfusion.* 2013;53(10):2145−2151.
127. Agueda S, Rocha G, Ferreira F, Vitor B, Lima M, Guimaraes H. Neonatal alloimmune neutropenia: still a diagnostic and therapeutical challenge. *J Pediatr Hematol Oncol.* 2012;34(7):497−499.
128. Dale DC. How I manage children with neutropenia. *Br J Haematol.* 2017;178(3):351−363.
129. Flesch BK, Curtis BR, de Haas M, Lucas G, Sachs UJ. Update on the nomenclature of human neutrophil antigens and alleles. *Transfusion.* 2016;56(6):1477−1479.
130. Flesch BK, Reil A. Molecular genetics of the human neutrophil antigens. *Transfus Med Hemotherapy.* 2018; 45(5):300−309.

131. van den Tooren-de Groot R, Ottink M, Huiskes E, et al. Management and outcome of 35 cases with foetal/ neonatal alloimmune neutropenia. *Acta Paediatr.* 2014; 103(11):e467−474.
132. Lalezari P, Radel E. Neutrophil-specific antigens: immunology and clinical significance. *Semin Hematol.* 1974; 11(3):281−290.
133. Heinzl MW, Schonbacher M, Dauber EM, Panzer S, Mayr WR, Kormoczi GF. Detection of granulocyte-reactive antibodies: a comparison of different methods. *Vox Sang.* 2015;108(3):287−293.
134. Immunobiology IWPoG, Bierling P, Bux J, et al. Recommendations of the ISBT Working Party on Granulocyte Immunobiology for leucocyte antibody screening in the investigation and prevention of antibody-mediated transfusion-related acute lung injury. *Vox Sang.* 2009; 96(3):266−269.
135. Brouk H, Ouelaa H. Fetal and neonatal alloimmune thrombocytopenia: advances in laboratory diagnosis and management. *Int J Blood Res Disorders.* 2015;2.

CHAPTER 11

Alloimmunization in Chronically Transfused Patients and Those With Malignancies

SALLY A. CAMPBELL–LEE, MD

ALLOIMMUNIZATION IN CHRONICALLY TRANSFUSED PATIENTS

Hemoglobinopathies

Thalassemia

The thalassemias are a group of disorders caused by inherited mutations in the genes for the globin chains of hemoglobin, leading to reduced or absent synthesis of normal hemoglobin. Mutations of the γ-, ε-, or ζ-globin genes are considered lethal, and therefore not observed in clinical medicine. Those surviving to birth are persons with mutations of the α- or β-globin genes. Thalassemia has been seen in every geographic region, with 1.5% of the world population as carriers, but is most common among those with Mediterranean, Asian, or African ancestry or any region where malaria is endemic, similar to sickle cell disease (SCD).[1] There is a broad spectrum of clinical presentation and severity, and thus diagnosis requires thorough evaluation of red blood cell (RBC) indices, hemoglobin profile, and DNA analysis. Severe forms of the α-thalassemia syndromes may include transfusion as part of their treatment.[2] Transfusion also plays a major role in the treatment of β-thalassemia, with the exception of thalassemia minor (also referred to as thalassemia trait), where transfusions are generally not required. Until 2012, β-thalassemias were classified as thalassemia major or thalassemia intermedia; these entities are now referred to as either non–transfusion-dependent thalassemia (NTDT, which includes what was previously called thalassemia intermedia) or transfusion-dependent thalassemia (TDT, most often referring to thalassemia major) based upon the role of transfusion which ranges from occasional and intermittent (NTDT) to lifelong chronic therapy (TDT).[3]

Chronic transfusion.

Patients with Hb Barts, who have deletions of all four α-globin genes, require transfusion beginning in utero to prevent fetal hydrops, and continuing after birth. TDT patients who have β-thalassemia usually present between 6 months and 2 years of age, once hemoglobin F production ceases. Their presentation can be marked by severe anemia (Hb < 7 g/dL), pallor, jaundice, and growth failure. Without transfusion their condition will progress to skeletal deformities, and ineffective erythropoiesis resulting in abdominal enlargement due to hepatomegaly and splenomegaly.[3] Thus, since recognition of its ability to reduce these complications, chronic simple transfusion has been a major part of therapy for these patients.[4] The goal of chronic transfusion in this setting is to allow normal growth and development while preventing complications related to ineffective erythropoiesis. Patients are often begun on chronic transfusion if the hemoglobin is at or less than 7 g/dL, with a goal to maintain the hemoglobin at 9–10 g/dL. This requires monthly transfusion in children, and usually must be done more frequently in adults, generally every 3 weeks.[5] For adult patients, chronic transfusion is also used to prevent or manage the development of pulmonary hypertension, thromboses, and extramedullary hematopoietic pseudotumors in patients at high risk. The major complication for all TDT patients is the development of iron overload, which can result in damage and failure of the heart, liver, and endocrine glands. Patients require strict monitoring and management with iron chelation therapy.[6] Iron overload develops due to the continued deposition of iron from transfusions. Chronic exposure to RBC components also increases the risk of alloimmunization to foreign blood group antigens.

Immunologic Concepts in Transfusion Medicine. https://doi.org/10.1016/B978-0-323-67509-3.00011-1

The likelihood of RBC alloimmunization is determined by multiple factors, both recipient and component related. The largest RBC alloimmunized patient cohort studied in the United States was evaluated as part of the Recipient Epidemiology and Donor Evaluation Study (REDS-III). This study included over 319,000 alloimmunized recipients and demonstrated that older age, female sex, and Rh(D) negative status were associated with increased risk of being a responder to RBC alloantigens.[7] In addition, antigenic differences between the recipient and donor and recipient immune status are also known to impact immune response to allogeneic RBC antigens.

In one of the first detailed studies of RBC alloimmunization in multiply transfused thalassemia patients, Economidou and colleagues studied pretransfusion specimens from 147 Greek patients with TDT aged 3–24 years. The patients had received red cell transfusions over a period ranging from 2 to 18 years. 6.1% (9 out of 147) had detectable red cell alloantibodies: three anti-K1, four anti-Rh, and two with anti-I specific cold agglutinin. The patients who formed anti-Rh antibodies were all RhD negative; four made anti-RhD while two of these patients also made anti-C and one other also made both anti-C and anti-E. The authors determined the rate of alloimmunization which was surprisingly low, even in patients receiving over 200 transfusions. They concluded that the heavy load of transfusions at a young age led to immune tolerance.[8] Although not specifically studied in TDT patients, there does appear to be evidence that chronic transfusions started at a younger age in other hemoglobinopathy patients (SCD) result in reduced susceptibility to alloimmunization, and have been associated with recipients with certain immunogenetic profiles.[9] However, in the Economidou et al. study, the similarity between the recipient and donor RBC antigen profiles likely is the main reason for the low prevalence of alloimmunization. Another cohort of TDT patients receiving transfusion from donors with similar RBC phenotypes, this time from Oman, was retrospectively reviewed. The study included 268 patients seen over 25 years. The alloimmunization prevalence here was 9.3%, with anti-E and anti-K1 antibodies most common (48%).[10] This group was older (age range 2–43 years) than the Economidou study group but had a mean age at the start of transfusion of 10 months. Another interesting finding in the Oman cohort is that prior to 1991, Oman imported its blood supply mainly from the United States. Subanalysis of patients who were transfused between 1985 and 1990 showed a higher prevalence of alloimmunization. Alloantibody prevalence was 20% for patients born before 1985, 44% for those born between 1985 and 1990, 24% for patients born between 1991 and 1996, and 12% for patients born between 1997 and 2015.

In Thailand, thalassemia constitutes a large public health problem, with a disease prevalence of 1%.[11] RBC alloimmunization among TDT patients at Srinagarind Hospital in northeast Thailand was evaluated by Romphruk and colleagues.[12] 16.9% of 383 transfused patients had alloantibodies identified, higher than some other centers with similar RBC phenotypes in donors and recipients. The mean age of recipients was 10 years with a range of 1–45 years. Ninety-nine percent were RhD positive. Anti-E, anti-c, and anti-Mia were the most common alloantibodies. Thedsawad et al. studied alloimmunization among 59 TDT patients at their center in Bangkok.[13] This cohort had a mean age of 32 years (range 17–64 years), with a mean age at first transfusion of 7 years. The prevalence of alloimmunization was 33.9%. The most common antibodies seen in this group were anti-E, anti-Mia, anti-Dia, and anti-c.

Chronically transfused thalassemia patients receiving blood from donors of different ethnicities with disparate RBC phenotypes tend to have much higher rates of alloimmunization. Worldwide, thalassemia is most common among those of Asian descent, and in Western countries such as the United States, many TDT patients are of Asian ancestry. Singer et al. demonstrated that in a largely Asian (75%) population of 64 transfused thalassemia patients at their center in Northern California, 22% had become alloimmunized. Thirty patients had β-thalassemia major, 24 patients had E-β-thalassemia, and 10 had hemoglobin H constant spring. The age range of this group (2–39 years, mean age 15 years) was somewhat older than the Economidou study. Of note, the greatest antigen disparity between the recipients and donors was found for K1, c, S, and Fy^b antigens, which represented 38% of alloantibodies found in recipients.[14] The Thalassemia Western Consortium comprises 11 referral centers providing care for thalassemia patients in the Western United States. Lal et al. have documented their transfusion practice, which includes over 700 patients.[2] Approximately 35% of this group was transfusion dependent. Of the 314 intermittently or chronically transfused patients, 17% of patients had alloantibodies; when clinically insignificant antibodies were removed, 12% of patients had antibodies to clinically significant blood group antigens. The most common antibody specificities were anti-K1, anti-E, and anti-c.

Splenectomy and alloimmunization.

Splenomegaly is seen in thalassemia as a result of ineffective erythropoiesis and extramedullary hematopoiesis. In addition to worsening of anemia, thrombocytopenia and neutropenia can develop. Splenomegaly usually decreases with regular transfusions but can persist in spite of appropriate transfusion therapy. When transfusion requirements increase due to splenomegaly, surgical splenectomy is often considered. The transfusion requirements of 11 patients studied at least 6 months before and after splenectomy decreased 24%–74% when compared to weight-based transfusion volumes prior to splenectomy ($P < .001$).[15]

Because the spleen puts transfused RBCs directly in contact with cells which can present antigen to the immune system, its presence has been postulated to have an impact on RBC alloimmunization. In a murine model of RBC alloimmunization, it was noted that simulation of an inflammatory environment with polyinosinic:polycytidylic acid (poly I:C) increased alloimmunization. When inflammation was not present, transfused RBCs were consumed by macrophages with trace consumption by dendritic cells. With induction of inflammation, there was a significant increase in consumption by dendritic cells as well as proliferation of $CD4^+$ T cells specific for the RBC antigen. Enhancement of RBC alloimmunization with inflammation was removed by splenectomy.[16] As part of a multicenter study in the Netherlands evaluating risk factors for RBC alloimmunization, 505 alloimmunized cases and 1010 nonalloimmunized controls were included. Twenty patients were identified who had received splenectomy, mainly due to trauma or complicated abdominal surgery. RBC transfusions subsequent to splenectomy were estimated to have a 20-fold lower risk of alloimmunization (RR 0.05, 95% CI 0.01–0.55). There were no patients with hemoglobinopathies included in the study.[17] 20 patients in the series of TDT studied by Thedsawad et al. had their spleen removed and did not have increased frequency of RBC alloimmunization, but did have an increased frequency of nonspecific IgG bound to their RBCs.[13] Al-Riyami and colleagues also did not find an increase in alloimmunization among splenectomized TDT patients.[10] However, these data are in contrast to the majority of retrospective studies in thalassemia, which show an association of increased prevalence of RBC alloimmunization in splenectomized thalassemia patients. Hussein et al. evaluated 272 patients in Egypt with TDT.[18] The overall alloimmunization incidence was 22.8%. Splenectomized patients had a higher rate of alloimmunization at 32% versus 16% of patients

who did not undergo splenectomy ($P = .003$). A study of 697 patients by the Thalassemia Clinical Research Network Investigators found that 49% of patients had been splenectomized. These patients were more likely to have alloantibodies (OR 2.528, $P < .0001$); 21% of patients who had no spleen were alloimmunized compared to only 7.7% of patients who still had spleens. Splenectomy preceded alloimmunization in most cases.[19] Additional studies have demonstrated an association between splenectomy and increased prevalence of alloimmunization[11,12,14]; but it should be cautioned that patients requiring splenectomy often have higher RBC exposure, and the timing of when alloimmunization occurs, pre- or postsplenectomy, should be considered among other factors.

Transfusion protocols in thalassemia.

Prophylactic antigen matching is used to either reduce the risk of initial alloimmunization or prevent additional alloimmunization in chronically transfused patients with hemoglobinopathies since the principal risk is discrepancy in RBC phenotype between donor and recipient. In this strategy, RBCs for transfusions are matched for recipient RBC antigens beyond ABO and RhD, usually for C/c/E/e antigens of Rh blood group and the K1 of the Kell blood group since these are the most common alloantibodies in most series. Additional antigens are occasionally matched, which is referred to as extended matching. Belsito et al. performed a prospective study of extended prophylactic antigen matching in patients with β-thalassemia in Italy.[20] The alloimmunization rate while receiving extended prophylactic antigen matching was compared to the rate while matching for Rh and Kell antigens. Donors were typed using serologic and molecular methods. Eighteen nonalloimmunized patients were included in the study and were monitored for 2 years (receiving Rh and Kell matched the first year, and extended matched the second year), with a similar number of units transfused both years. No new alloantibodies were detected during receipt of either antigen matching protocol. Patients transfused in Romphruk et al.'s study in Thailand received Rh C/c/E/e and Mi^a-matched RBC; of note only 3.5% of patients receiving antigen-matched RBCs became alloimmunized.[12] However, anti-E and anti-Mi^a were identified in these patients, but these antibodies are often found in never transfused or pregnant donors in their population. Outside of these potential naturally occurring antibodies no other antibodies were identified in the prophylactic antigen-matched group during the 10-year observation period. In the survey of transfusion practices performed by Lal et al.[2] at 11 thalassemia centers in the United States, all centers provided prophylactic Rh and Kell-matched RBCs, with one center providing Duffy matching in addition, and one center providing extended antigen matching (addition of Duffy, Kid, S/s antigens). Patients with alloantibodies received extended antigen matching.

In an attempt to provide guidance for transfusion protocols for patients with hemoglobinopathies, an international consensus panel performed a systematic review and developed recommendations.[21] The panel recommended use of Rh C/c/E/e and Kell-matched RBCs for thalassemia patients to reduce the risk of alloimmunization, transfusion of RBC negative for antigens to which a patient had become alloimmunized, and use of extended antigen matching for patients who have one or more alloantibodies. All recommendations were felt by the panel to be based upon low-quality evidence according to GRADE criteria. Thus, additional well-designed studies are needed in this area (Table 11.1).

Sickle cell disease

SCD is not just one disease but a collection of disorders caused by inheritance of abnormal β-globin alleles with the sickle mutation. The mutation is a substitution of a single amino acid, valine for glutamine, which results in sickle hemoglobin (HbS) instead of normal hemoglobin A (HbA). SCD is most common in those with ancestry from geographic regions where malaria is endemic. Due to codominant expression, a number of compound heterozygous conditions, such as hemoglobin SC (HbSC), or HbS with β-thalassemia (HbSβ⁰-thalassemia or HbSβ⁺-thalassemia) are seen. Homozygous expression of HbS occurs due to inheritance of one HbS gene from each parent and results in sickle cell anemia (HbSS), which is the most common form of the disease. Therefore, there is a wide spectrum of clinical disease characteristics. In addition, the carrier state, sickle trait (HbAS), is seen in approximately 8% of African Americans but is not associated with actual disease.[22] Nearly 100,000 Americans have SCD, but this is dwarfed by a birthrate of babies with SCD of 120,000 annually in Africa.[23] When sickle hemoglobin is present, the hemoglobin polymerizes and transforms RBC from easily malleable concave discs to rigid, sickle shapes. This leads to vaso-occlusion, but there are many other cellular factors such as an enhanced inflammatory state, abnormal endothelial interactions, and other features which lead to vaso-occlusive crises, infections, and renal, cardiopulmonary and vascular complications.

The goals of RBC transfusion in SCD are to treat anemia and to reduce the proportion of HbS to levels that decrease the risk of complications. Usually this equates to a posttransfusion hematocrit of 30% or a HbS fraction of 30% or lower. There are indications for transfusion which are both acute and chronic. Acute indications include treatment of acute chest syndrome

TABLE 11.1
Prevalence of Red Blood Cell Alloimmunization in Transfusion-Dependent Thalassemia.

	Alloantibody Prevalence (%)	Common Alloantibodies	Prophylactic Antigen Matching (Y/N)	Percent Splenectomized
Economidou et al.[8]	4.8	D, K1	N	30
Al-Riyami et al.[10]	9.3	E, K1	Y (Rh, K1)	19
Romphruk et al.[12]	19.3	E, Mi[a], c	Y (Rh, Mi[a])	34.5
Thedsawad et al.[13]	33.9	E, Mi[a], Di[a], c	N	33.9
Singer et al.[14]	22	K, E, c	Y*	36
Thompson et al.[19]	16.5	E, C, K1	Y** (5 out of 28 sites—Rh, K1)	21
Lal et al.[2]	16.9	C, E, K1	Y	Not stated
Belsito et al.[20]	0	None	Y (Rh, K1 then extended)	Not stated

or acute stroke. Patients may be placed on a chronic transfusion regimen for prevention of first or recurrent stroke or for reduction of the risk of recurrent acute chest syndrome. Allogeneic RBC can be provided either by simple transfusion, where 1–2 units are infused, or by exchange transfusion, which often requires 5–10 units of RBC. Exchange transfusion can be performed as a manual exchange (more commonly used in small children) or as an automated exchange, which is more typical for older children and adults. RBC transfusion is an important part of therapy for SCD[24]; however, the risks of transfusion-related complications such as iron overload, hemolytic reactions, and RBC alloimmunization must be acknowledged.

Alloimmunization prevalence.

RBC alloimmunization has been known to be a significant problem in the transfusion management of patients with SCD for some time. Vichinsky et al. chronicled the development of alloimmunization among patients seen at Children's Hospital Oakland between 1978 and 1985.[25] Thirty percent of 107 patients who had been transfused had developed alloantibodies. Of 42 children (mean age 10 years, range 1–17 years), 24% had produced antibodies. Among the 65 adults (mean age 24 years, range 18–41 years), 34% had alloantibodies. Both children and adults with antibodies had received a greater number of transfusions than nonalloimmunized patients. Of note, 66% of the antibodies detected were against C, E, and K1 antigens. This study also evaluated the difference in antigen expression between donors and recipients. The most significant differences in antigen expression were for C, E, K1, Fy^a, Fy^b, S, and Jk^b. The authors noted that alloimmunization resulted in delayed availability of blood components for transfusion and delayed hemolytic transfusion reactions. In the same year that Vichinsky's group published the above description, the Cooperative Study of Sickle Cell Disease (CSSCD) published the findings of their evaluation of alloimmunization in SCD patients.[26] In this large study, which included 1814 transfused SCD patients, a somewhat lower overall rate of alloimmunization, 18.6%, was found. Parallel to Vichinsky et al., the CSSCD study found that patients who were alloimmunized had received more transfusions than those patients who were not alloimmunized. In fact, the amount transfused was felt to the primary determinant for alloimmunization. Additionally, there was a slightly lower rate among children less than 10 years, which was even less than expected for the amount transfused. Women were more frequently alloimmunized than men; however, this

was also possibly due to pregnancy. Antibodies to C, E, K1, and Lewis were most common in this series. Nonpersistent antibodies were defined as those that were not detectable on two occasions at a time more than 1 year after the initial detection. Approximately 40% of anti-C, anti-S, and anti-Jkb were nonpersistent. Twenty-six percent of anti-D, 32% of anti-E, and 30% of anti-K1 were also nonpersistent.

Differences in red cell antigen expression between donor and recipient and volume of transfusions appear to be among the most influential indicators of whether or not a patient with SCD will become alloimmunized. Jamaican patients with SCD who were transfused at the University Hospital of the West Indies in Kingston were compared to patients treated at the Manchester Royal Infirmary in the United Kingdom.[27] Only 2.6% of transfused Jamaican patients had clinically significant antibodies, the lowest reported rate in the literature for patients with SCD, as compared to 76% of patients treated in Manchester. The Jamaican cohort received significantly fewer transfusions (median 2 units, range 1–22) than patients in Manchester (median 14 units, range 4–24). Eighty percent of donors in the National Blood Service for Jamaica matched the commonest RBC phenotype for Jamaican SCD patients, while the majority of blood donors in the United Kingdom had some phenotypic discrepancy with recipients (66% of donors were Fy^a positive with most exhibiting the R^{1}r Rh haplotype). In Nigeria, which has the highest prevalence of SCD in the world, two studies of transfused SCD patients are of note here. Ugwu et al.[28] found an alloimmunization prevalence of 9.3% of 86 transfused patients. The majority of antibodies were anti-E (37.5%), anti-C (25%), anti-D (12.5%), and anti-e (also 12.5%). Notably in this study, there was no relationship between alloimmunization and the number of transfusions received. Kangiwa and colleagues[29] found an overall alloimmunization frequency of 18.7% among recently transfused SCD patients, with 86% of antibodies against Rh and Kell antigens. However overall, the alloimmunization prevalence was 5%. Similarly in Uganda, at the Mulago National Referral Hospital in Kampala, 6.1% of 428 transfused patients with SCD had alloantibodies, predominately against Rh and the S antigen.[30] Thus, as in thalassemia patients, patients with SCD receiving RBCs from ethnically similar donors have a lower prevalence of RBC alloimmunization (Table 11.2).

Chronic RBC transfusion has been used for many years in the treatment of SCD,[31] but its use became more widespread once the results of a randomized trial (referred to as the Stroke Prevention Trial in Sickle Cell

TABLE 11.2
Prevalence of Red Blood Cell Alloimmunization in Sickle Cell Disease.

Study	Alloantibody Prevalence (%)	Common Antibodies	Prophylactic Antigen Matching (Y/N)
Vichinsky et al. 1990[25]	30	C, E, K1, Jk[b]	N
Rosse et al.[26]	18.6	C, E, K1	N
Kangiwa et al.[29]	18.7	c E, e	N
Olujohungbe et al.[27]	2.6 (Jamaicans)	E, Le[a]	N
	76 (UK)	C, E, K1	N
Campbell-Lee et al.[39]	37.5	C, E, K1	N
	26.2	C, E, K1	Y (extended for alloimmunized)
LaSalle-Williams et al.[38]	7	Le[a], Kp[a], M, D	Y (Rh, K1, Jk, Fy[a])
O'Suoji et al.[40]	14	C, E, Jk	Y (C, E, K1)
Tahhan et al.[34]	34.8	C, E, K1	N
	0	None	Y (C, E, K1, S, Fy[a], Fy[b])

Anemia or STOP study) of chronic transfusion for prevention of a first stroke in children with abnormal transcranial dopplers was published.[32] One hundred and thirty children with a mean age of 8 years were included in the study. Sixty-three were randomized to receive RBC transfusions every 3 to 4 weeks; the comparison arm of 67 received standard therapy. There were 10 strokes in the standard therapy group compared to one in the transfusion group ($P < .001$), and the study was terminated early. The authors understood that RBC alloimmunization would be a potentially limiting factor in utilization of this therapy. Consequently, prophylactic phenotype-matching protocols have been utilized in many centers as a means of preventing alloimmunization in patients with SCD receiving chronic transfusion.

Prophylactic phenotype matching.

The most common alloantibodies formed by chronically transfused patients with SCD are to the C and E antigens of the Rh blood group, and the K1 antigen of the Kell blood group. The majority of patients with SCD are of African descent. Rh D positive people of African descent most frequently have an Rh phenotype of R^0r, where cDe is one haplotype and ce the other. Thus, when exposed to the common Rh phenotypes of Caucasian donors, who more commonly express the C and E antigens, anti-C and anti-E can result.[33] As a preventative strategy, some centers caring for patients with SCD began providing C, E, and K1 negative RBCs

to prevent alloimmunization. Other centers began providing more extensively matched RBCs.

Tahhan et al.[34] provided RBCs matched for C, E, K1, S, Fy[a], and Fy[b] antigens to patients with SCD on chronic transfusion programs between 1980 and 1993. Eighty-six patients who received antigen-matched RBCs were included in the study. Forty patients only received antigen-matched RBCs, while 46 had received a mixture of both antigen-matched and non-antigen-matched. None of the 40 patients receiving only antigen-matched RBCs developed clinically significant alloantibodies, while 34% of patients who had received non-antigen-matched RBCs became alloimmunized. In contrast, the children transfused in the STOP study received RBC matched for only C, E, and K1 antigens. Five of the sixty-three (8%) transfused patients developed new clinically significant antibodies (two were sensitized to E, two to K1, and one produced antibodies against Fy[a], Le[a], Le[b], and S), with the anti-E immunization due to non-compliance with the study design early on in the protocol.[35,36] In addition to the breakthrough demonstration of chronic transfusions preventing strokes in at-risk children with SCD, the STOP study was a multicenter study which showed that prophylactic antigen matching could be implemented on a wide scale. Prophylactic antigen matching for C, E, and K1 antigens for transfusions in SCD became a recommended strategy for prevention of alloimmunization as its effectiveness was demonstrated in several other studies.[21,36,37]

Later publications evaluated long-term utilization of extended matching protocols. LaSalle-Williams and colleagues studied 99 SCD patients who were transfused only with ABO-compatible RBC matched for Rh C, D, and E; K1, Jk[a], and Jk[b]; and Fy[a] antigens between 1993 and 2006. Only seven (7%) patients developed alloantibodies, each patient becoming sensitized to one blood group antigen. One patient made anti-Le[a], one made anti-Kp[a], and two persons made anti-M. Three patients produced anti-D; each was later identified as having an Rh variant D antigen. This is in contrast to a period when only ABO-/D-matched RBCs were transfused to SCD patients at the same center; 34% of patients were alloimmunized during this period.[38] Campbell-Lee and collaborators evaluated 476 patients with SCD for prevalence of RBC alloimmunization occurring over two contiguous 5-year periods.[39] In the first time period, only ABO-/D-matched RBCs were transfused, resulting in a 38% prevalence of alloantibodies. In the second time period, RBCs matched for Rh, Kell, S, Duffy, and Kidd antigens were provided only for patients who had made antibodies after their initial ABO-/D-matched transfusions. This lowered the prevalence of alloantibodies to 26%, but there was no significant difference between the two time periods after adjusting for number of units transfused, percentage of leukoreduced units, gender, and age. Thus, actual prophylactic antigen matching, provided prior to the development of any alloantibodies, is currently the best strategy for limiting sensitization in SCD patients.

Recipient Risk Factors
Rh variants

Even with the expansion of the use of prophylactic antigen matching in SCD, alloimmunization still occurs. In many instances a patient on chronic transfusion receiving antigen-matched RBCs at one institution may be emergently admitted to a second hospital and may not receive the same level of antigen matching, or even any antigen matching beyond ABO/D at all. That patient may present back to their home institution with a new alloantibody. O'Suoji et al. identified that over half of the patients at their institution who became alloimmunized despite their provision of C, E, and K1 negative RBCs had been transfused at another hospital.[40] They also found five patients who had produced antibodies against Rh antigens to which the patient typed serologically positive. Genotyping revealed these patients to have variant Rh antigens, including two previously unidentified Rh(e) variants.

Further examination of this specific aspect of alloimmunization by Chou et al. yielded surprising results.[41] The effects of matching for C, E, and K1 in 182 patients with SCD were studied. Fifty-eight percent of chronically transfused patients had become alloimmunized, as had 15% of the occasionally transfused. In addition, 45% of chronically transfused patients and 12% of episodically transfused had produced alloantibodies against Rh antigens. An astonishingly high 91 out of 146 Rh antibodies were unexplained: 56 of the antibodies were in recipients who were phenotypically positive by serologic methods, and 35 of the antibodies were in those who were serologically antigen negative and had received only correspondingly antigen negative transfusions. Eighty-seven percent of those examined in the study had RH variants identified by high-resolution genotyping. Over one-half of both RHD and RHCE alleles were variants. 30%, 40%, and 36% of patients had altered D, c, or e antigens, respectively. Of the 117 RhD positive patients, 17% who had only a variant RHD, 26% with heterozygosity for conventional and variant RHD, and 23% with conventional RHD only, had produced anti-D.

Obtaining Rh and K1-matched RBCs for transfusion recipients with SCD is recommended, but not always easy due to low number of donors of African ancestry; the reasons for low participation in blood donation are multifactorial but include a distrust of medical institutions.[42] There have been successful programs aimed at recruiting African American blood donors in support of chronic transfusion programs for patients with SCD.[43] However, with alloimmunization still occurring due to high expression of RH variants among both recipients and donors of African ancestry, consideration has been given to matching RBC antigens not just for serologic phenotype but genotype. The practicality and outcomes of molecular matching have been examined by Castilho and Dinardo.[44] At their blood center in Brazil, molecular matching of transfusions for patients with SCD was performed at three levels: RH and K matching (level 1); extended matching (RH, KEL, FY, JK, MNS, DI) (level 2); and extended matching including RHD and RHCE variant alleles (level 3). Recipients of level 1 matching had an alloimmunization prevalence of 5% −10%; less than 1% of those with level 2 of matching became sensitized. Both level 1 and level 2 matching recipients also had improved posttransfusion RBC survival. The authors state that level 3−matched transfusions have been difficult to procure due to limited numbers of RH genotyped donors. An alternative approach may be to use next-generation sequencing to identify important RH variants in both donors and recipients,[45] but the feasibility of this approach remains to be seen.

Patient age

Patients with SCD begin chronic transfusion programs at relatively young ages. This is due to the proficiency of RBC transfusions at preventing first and subsequent strokes. However, exposure to allogeneic antigens at younger ages has been thought to result in lower immune response. In both the early studies of Vichinsky et al.[25] and Rosse et al.[26] of transfused SCD patients, there was lower prevalence of alloimmunization in younger patients. Twenty-four percent of patients with a mean age of 10 years were alloimmunized in the Vichinsky study; in the Rosse study, there was a slightly lower rate of antibody formation among those less than 10 years old and the rate was lower than expected for the amount transfused. Campbell-Lee et al.[39] showed that when comparing patients aged less than 16 years to those older, there was a greater likelihood of a lower prevalence of alloimmunization in the younger age group, even after regression analysis adjusting for whether or not any prophylactic antigen matching was used, sex, transfusion amount, percentage of leukoreduced RBCs or presence or absence of acute febrile illness [OR 0.44 (CI 0.25−0.78), $P = .005$].

Tatari-Calderone et al.[9] studied the incidence of RBC alloimmunization in SCD patients related to a polymorphism in rs660 C/T in the nearby Ro52 gene, suggesting that the rs660 polymorphism is a marker of efficiency of immune competence development to RBC antigens in SCD patients. Fifty percent of T/T homozygous and 42.9% of C/T heterozygous patients had RBC alloantibodies. Increased expression of Ro52 was associated with the T/T genotype. A relationship of the polymorphism to age at first transfusion and RBC alloimmunization was noted as 75% of C/T heterozygous, and only 30.8% of T/T homozygous patients who developed antibodies were first transfused before the age of 5 years; this combined with an inverse correlation between time of exposure to antigen or number of transfusions received were felt by the authors to indicate the development of immune competence to RBC transfusions.

Inflammation

SCD is a chronic hemolytic anemia, but inflammation is also an important part of the pathophysiology of SCD. Cell-free heme and ischemia-reperfusion injury result in the generation of reactive oxygen species and neutrophil extracellular traps, along with release of tissue- or cell-derived DAMPs and multiple other agents. This inflammatory environment promotes adhesion of neutrophils, platelets, and endothelial cells, contributing to vas-occlusion.[46] Concern has been raised that this inflammatory environment also contributes to an SCD patient's predisposition to alloimmunization. In a murine model of RBC alloimmunization using a hen-egg-lysozyme antigen, immune responsiveness to transfusion was relatively weak until recipients were also infused with polycytidylic acid, which enhanced the alloantibody response.[47] A retrospective study of alloimmunized SCD patients evaluated the clinical state at the time of transfusions resulting in alloimmunization.[48] Patients who received transfusions during clinical events such as acute febrile illness, splenic sequestration, or vaso-occlusive crisis, but in particular during acute chest syndrome had significantly increased odds of becoming alloimmunized versus being transfused for acute stroke or aplastic crisis. However, Campbell-Lee et al.[39] did not replicate this finding; in their study, alloimmunized patients were no more likely to have been transfused during vaso-occlusive crisis, acute chest syndrome, or other clinical scenarios when compared to nonalloimmunized patients.

Genetic influences

Although the primary drivers for alloimmunization are the differences in donor-recipient RBC antigen expression and overall number of transfusions, it has long been postulated that there are SCD patients with a genetic predisposition to RBC alloimmunization. Information on how to predict which patients are immune responders as opposed to nonresponders has been sought with an eye toward being used to determine which patents should receive more extensively antigen-matched or even molecularly antigen-matched RBCs.

The antigen presentation process involves T regulatory cell activity, cytokine production, and human leukocyte antigens (HLAs). Several studies have found gene polymorphisms associated with alloimmunization related to this process. When examining HLAs in transfused patients, 67% of antibody responders were shown in one early study to express HLA-B35 versus only 25% of nonresponders.[49] More recently, evaluation of cytokine gene polymorphisms and HLA Class I genotyping was performed in a cohort of Brazilian patients with SCD. TNF-α, IL-1β, and HLA-DRB1 gene polymorphisms were found to be represented significantly more in alloimmunized patients.[50] A lower percentage of CD4+ T cells in nonalloimmunized than alloimmunized SCD patients, along with spontaneous expression of IL-10 by $CD4^+$ T cells and low Tbet expression among alloimmunized patients were identified by Vingert et al.[51] The cytotoxic T-lymphocyte-associated antigen-4 (CTLA-4) is a costimulatory molecule expressed on T regulatory cells. As a receptor for B7-1 and B7-2 of antigen presenting cells, it downgrades activated CD4 T cells. SCD patients heterozygous for the −318T allele of the CTLA-4 gene had an increased risk of alloimmunization.[52] A protective effect of HLA DQ2, DQ3, and DQ5 alleles against alloimmunization in SCD patients was found by Tatari-Calderone and colleagues.[53]

Polymorphisms in genes controlling other aspects of the immune response have also been identified. Fc γ receptors are found on immune effector cells such as macrophages and monocytes, and bind to the Fc portion of IgG. SCD patients with a polymorphism in the FCGR2C.nc-ORF were identified as having over a threefold lower risk for RBC alloimmunization compared to patients without this mutation. The association was strongest for exposure to antigens other than Rh or K1.[54] A genome-wide association study of African American adult SCD chronically transfused patients found a single nucleotide polymorphism on chromosome 5 surpassing genome-wide significance (rs75853687, Pmeta = 6.6×10^{-9}) for alloimmunized patients and was included in high-responders with three or more RBC alloantibodies.[55] The locus is rare outside of populations of African descent and includes genes involved in immune regulation.

Together, the results of the above studies demonstrate that in all likelihood there are multiple genes which both enhance and reduce the risk of RBC alloimmunization in SCD. The ability to predict who will become an immune responder will most probably be dependent upon development of genetic panels taking multiple most significant loci into account; obviously many further studies are due in this regard.

Component Factors

SCD patients requiring transfusion can receive simple transfusion of one to two units. Alternatively, automated RBC exchange has become increasingly used due to the procedure's ability to slow and even sometimes somewhat reverse iron overload which is exceptionally problematic for chronically transfused SCD patients receiving simple transfusion. A concern with automated RBC exchange is that multiple units of RBCs are required for each procedure, increasing exposure to allogeneic RBC antigens. The expectation has been that there would be higher rates of alloimmunization among patients receiving chronic RBC exchange.

This was reported by Rosse et al.,[26] although more recent studies directly examining chronic RBC exchange as a risk for alloimmunization have found the opposite. Wahl et al. retrospectively compared 45 pediatric SCD patients, 22 of whom received chronic RBC exchange and 23 received chronic simple transfusions between 1994 and 2010.[56] The chronic exchange patients received a mean of 338 RBC units per patient, versus 152 units per patient in the simple transfusion group (P = .001). The alloimmunization rate was 0.013 antibodies per 100 units in chronic exchange group; the simple transfusion group was alloimmunized at a significantly higher rate at 0.143 antibodies per 100 units (P = .03). In a study of adult SCD patients comparing alloimmunization between chronic exchange and chronic simple transfusion patients, even though the chronic exchange patients received 10-fold more RBC per patient, their rate of alloimmunization was significantly lower.[57] In both studies, RBCs matched for recipient C, E, and K1 antigens were used. Potential mechanisms for this difference include removal of inflammatory cytokines by automated exchange, or the overwhelming of the recipient immune system by large amounts of allogenic RBCs.

During storage of RBCs, changes in the RBC membrane occur and lead to the release of microparticles; there is also increased plasma nontransferrin bound iron, increased intracellular heme, and a variety of other changes collectively referred to as the RBC storage lesion. Transfusion of 14-day stored RBCs in mice led to a 10- to 100-fold increase over fresh RBCs in the alloimmunization response.[58] In a retrospective study of 166 SCD patients followed for 7 years, 19 (11%) developed new alloantibodies. Alloimmunization was strongly associated with older age of implicated RBC units. Seven-day-old units had a hazard ratio of 3.5 (95% CI 1.71−7.11), while 35-day-old RBCs had a hazard ratio of 9.8 (95% CI 2.66−35.97) (P = .002). All units transfused had been matched for C, E, and K1 antigens.[59]

Murine models of transfusion have also demonstrated that leukoreduction of RBC components decreases the propensity for development of alloimmunization.[60] This has been more difficult to demonstrate in transfused SCD patients as most hospital systems with comprehensive sickle cell centers now provide universally leukoreduced cellular components. Campbell-Lee et al.[39] did demonstrate a correlation between receipt of a lower percentage of leukoreduced RBCs and increased prevalence of alloimmunization (P = .0004), when comparing transfusions provided during one time period when leukoreduced RBCs were not required for patients with a diagnosis of

SCD, versus institution of a transfusion protocol requiring leukoreduction. The authors recommended provision of HbS negative; leukoreduced; C-, E-, and K1-matched RBCs for patients with SCD requiring transfusion.

ALLOIMMUNIZATION IN PATIENTS WITH MALIGNANCIES

Myelodysplastic Syndrome

Myelodysplastic syndrome (MDS) is a clonal disorder of hematopoietic stem cells which causes peripheral cytopenias and has the potential to transform into marrow failure and acute leukemia. Anemia is a prominent feature in this disorder, which is one of the most common hematologic malignances in people above 70 years.[61] Eighty to ninety percent of patients require RBC transfusions and a large proportion, as high as 45%, become transfusion dependent. Because these patients have a need for chronic RBC transfusion they are at increased risk of RBC alloimmunization.

The proliferation of lymphoid stem cells can lead to B cell dysfunction, and an increase in immunologic abnormalities including alloantibody and autoantibody production. Stiegler et al.[62] hypothesized that this may be the reason for the increased frequency of alloimmunization in MDS. Their retrospective study compared the incidence of RBC alloimmunization in transfused MDS patients to those with other hematologic disorders and patients with end-stage renal disease. Although there was a higher incidence in MDS patients (21%) compared to all other hematologic diseases included in the study (11%), there was no statistically significant difference between the two groups. However, there was a significant difference between alloimmunization incidence in MDS and end-stage renal disease patients, of whom only 3% were alloimmunized. Of note, antibodies were detected after transfusion at a median of 5 months in MDS, versus 2–3 years in the other hematologic diseases, and after 1 year in end-stage renal disease. It was postulated that the reason for the increased alloimmunization incidence in both MDS and hematologic diseases was the increased immune responsiveness, while chronic uremia tends toward decreased immune response. Kim et al.[63] compared RBC alloimmunization incidence in transfused Korean MDS and liver cirrhosis patients, since cirrhosis patients also routinely require RBC transfusions. Of 115 MDS patients, in contrast to other studies, only 4.3% became alloimmunized, versus 7% of liver cirrhosis patients who were deemed to have a cumulatively higher risk than MDS patients in this

study. Sanz and colleagues[64] studied 272 MDS and chronic myelomonocytic leukemia (CMML) patients over a 20-year period. Eleven percent had refractory anemia, 42% were categorized as refractory cytopenia with multilinear dysplasia, 26% were refractory anemia with excess blasts, and 18% of the patients had been diagnosed with CMML. Fifteen percent had made RBC alloantibodies, most commonly against Kell and Rh E. The factor which most predisposed patients to alloantibody formation was the number of RBC units transfused. In the most comprehensive study to date, Singhal et al.[61] reviewed the incidence of alloimmunization among 817 MDS patients from the South Australian MDS Registry, who had been diagnosed between 1990 and 2015. Ninety-eight patients (12%) had made RBC alloantibodies posttransfusion. Although the most important predictor of alloimmunization was the number of RBC units transfused, with alloimmunized patients receiving significantly more units (4.1 vs. 2.8 units per month, $P < .001$), 73% made antibodies after less than 20 RBC units. Antibodies to Rh and Kell antigens were most frequent. Attesting to the potentially devastating consequences of RBC alloimmunization, the authors described one patient, a 51-year-old man, who developed alloantibodies and proceeded to suffer a life-threatening delayed hemolytic transfusion reaction, cardiac arrest, multiorgan failure, and a prolonged intensive care unit stay. Lastly, of note, the study evaluated patients by treatment category. Patients who received disease modifying therapy (which could include azacitidine, lenalidomide, intensive chemotherapy, and/or allogeneic hematopoietic stem cell transplant) had a lower incidence of alloimmunization which was also unrelated to the amount transfused. This lower rate due to immunosuppressive effects of therapy was also believed to be a factor in the alloimmunization rate in MDS patients seen in Kim et al.'s study.[63] Nonetheless, it may be prudent to consider prophylactic antigen matching for Rh and Kell antigens for MDS patients about to start a chronic transfusion regimen.

Leukemia and Lymphoma

In patients with hematologic malignancies, the primary concern with posttransfusion alloimmunization has been with the development of HLA alloantibodies. This is due to the increased incidence of platelet refractoriness in HLA-alloimmunized platelet transfusion recipients, which places them at increased risk for adverse events including hemorrhage. Nineteen to forty-five percent of patients receiving non-leukoreduced platelets develop HLA alloantibodies. Leukoreduction of platelet components reduces this to 7%–18%.[65] Concerns with RBC alloimmunization were related to contaminating RBCs in platelet components, which is higher in whole blood derived or random donor platelets compared to apheresis or single donor platelets. Since only 15% of most populations are negative for the Rh D antigen, these patients often must receive platelet components from Rh D positive donors. Previous studies have shown an anti-D alloimmunization rate in this setting ranging from 0% to 19%. Cid et al.[66] found that of 22 Rh D negative patients with hematologic malignancies, after receiving pooled platelets from Rh D positive donors who were prepared by the buffy coat method with a mean RBC contamination of 4 mL, none produced anti-D after an 8-week median follow-up period. The majority of patients in this study had acute leukemia or non-Hodgkin's lymphoma and were receiving immunosuppressive therapy.

The incidence of RBC alloimmunization in patients with hematologic malignancies after receiving RBC transfusion is a concern not just for its impact on the ability to supply compatible RBCs for transfusion, but because of the potential for impact on outcomes with hematopoietic stem cell transplant. The rate of alloimmunization may be impacted by the patient's primary disease. Blumberg et al.[67] retrospectively evaluated 703 patients receiving chronic transfusions. Of the 99 patients with lymphocytic leukemia, who received an average of 13 transfusions per patient, none developed alloantibodies. Sixteen percent of the 123 patients with myelogenous leukemia became alloimmunized after an average of 23 transfusions, and 29% of 52 patients with hemoglobinopathies became alloimmunized after 40 transfusions. Patients with myelogenous leukemia receiving immunosuppressive chemotherapy, often cited as a reason for low rates of alloimmunization in such patients, did not have a reduced rate of alloimmunization in this study. In the study performed by Abou-Elella and colleagues,[68] 193 patients receiving bone marrow transplant were evaluated for RBC alloantibodies. This cohort included 57 patients with leukemia, 54 patients with lymphoma, as well as 68 with breast cancer. The rate of alloimmunization was low at 2%. Of the four alloimmunized patients, one patient with MDS made two alloantibodies, one patient with leukemia, and two patients with breast cancer each made one antibody. The RBC alloimmunization rate was 0.1% per unit. This was in contrast to a much higher HLA alloimmunization rate of 5%–10%.

The potential correlation between concurrent immunosuppressive therapy and the risk of RBC alloimmunization was examined in a study from Austria. Leisch and colleagues[69] retrospectively assessed 184 patients with myeloid neoplasms treated with azacitidine. RBC transfusions were prospectively matched for Rh D, C, and E antigens and Kell. There was a direct correlation between increased amount of RBC transfusion and alloimmunization. Eleven percent of patients developed alloantibodies, with 55% from patients with MDS and 45% of those with acute myelogenous leukemia. There was no significant difference in incidence of alloimmunization between those receiving immunomodulatory therapy (including lenalidomide, thalidomide, or cyclosporine) versus immunosuppressive therapy (cytotoxic chemotherapy, hydroxyurea, or Ara C).

Solid Tumors

The focus of most studies evaluating transfusion in the treatment of patients with solid tumors has been on perioperative transfusion and the risks of recurrence or metastases. Perioperative transfusion has been associated with decreased overall and/or recurrence-free survival rates in colorectal cancer,[70] head and neck squamous cell carcinoma,[71] non-small cell lung cancer,[72] and prostate cancer[73]; while in other studies the results have shown no impact on survival.[74] The mechanistic pathway by which transfusion impacts survival in this setting has not been established; however, transfusion-related immunomodulation has been speculated to be the cause. The immunosuppressive effects of transfusion are likely mediated by many components of blood components, thus making examination of their impact on patient outcomes complex. Donor white blood cells elaborate soluble FAS-L, TGF-β, and HLA molecules. RBCs release cell-free heme, iron, and ubiquitin during degradation. All of these factors can have direct effects on recipient immune cells, leading to increased production of anti-inflammatory cytokines, decreased production of cytokines from monocytes and macrophages, and decreased neutrophil and NK cell activity.[75]

There are few studies evaluating the incidence of RBC alloimmunization in patients with solid tumors following transfusion. In one case-control study,[76] disease severity and inflammatory background, represented by measures of performance status, metastasis and BMI, and C-reactive protein, respectively, in alloimmunized oncology patients were compared with a nonalloimmunized control group. Twenty-two alloimmunized patients were compared with 44 control patients. The alloimmunized patients had made anti-E and anti-K1 most commonly, with 36% making multiple antibodies. Alloimmunized patients received a mean of four transfusions per patient which was not different from the control group. There were no significant differences between any of the disease severity or inflammatory indicators in either group in this small study. The risk of alloimmunization in hematologic malignancies and nonhematologic malignances was compared by Evers et al. in 505 alloimmunized cases and 1010 controls.[77] Nonhematologic malignancies included 295 patients with colorectal (71 patients), lung (41), prostate (21), and breast (21) tumors. Hematologic malignancies were seen in 270 patients, and included acute myeloid leukemia (76 patients), MDS (63), and lymphomas (40). Patients with acute myeloid or lymphoid leukemia and mature B or T cell lymphomas had a significantly reduced risk of alloimmunization compared to patients with nonhematologic malignancies. This was likely due to the type of treatment, since patients receiving chemotherapy, chemotherapy with immunotherapy, or stem cell transplant similarly had a significantly reduced risk compared to patients receiving no chemotherapy.

SUMMARY

RBC transfusion is a key component of therapy for patients with hemoglobinopathies and malignancies. Many of these patients require chronic transfusion, which exposes them to large numbers of allogeneic RBCs, often over the course of many years. When alloimmunization to non-ABO blood group antigens occurs, this can limit availability of this therapy to the patient. The primary risk factor for alloimmunization is the volume of exposure to allogeneic RBCs. However, the presence of other factors such as ancestry-related discrepancies in blood group antigen expression between patients and donors, as well as recently described genetic factors affecting immune response in some patient groups can provide added risk for alloimmunization. These appear to be of greatest impact in patients with SCD. Patients with some hematologic malignancies and solid tumors appear to have a much lower risk of alloimmunization due in part to immunosuppressant chemotherapeutic agents used in their treatment. Due to the complex nature of the interaction between blood component contents and recipient clinical condition, treatment, and potential genetic risk factors for alloimmunization, further studies are necessary to better define these influences.

REFERENCES

1. Galanello R, Origa R. Beta-thalassemia. *Orphanet J Rare Dis*. 2010;5:11. https://doi.org/10.1186/1750-1172-5-11.
2. Lal A, Wong TE, Andrews J, et al. Transfusion practices and complications in thalassemia. *Transfusion*. 2018;58: 2826−2835.
3. Viprakasit V, Ekwattanakit S. Clinical classification, screening and diagnosis for Thalassemia. *Hematol Oncol Clin N Am*. 2018;32:193−211.
4. Wolman IJ. Transfusion therapy in Cooley's anemia: growth and health as related to long-range hemoglobin levels. A progress report. *Annals of the NY Acad of Sciences*. 1964;119(2):736−747.
5. Cazzola M. A moderate transfusion regimen may reduce iron loading in beta thalassemia major without producing excessive expansion of erythropoiesis. *Transfusion*. 1997; 37:135−140.
6. Taher AT, Capellini MD. How I manage medical complications of B-thalassemia in adults. *Blood*. 2018;132(17): 1781−1791.
7. Karafin MS, Westlake M, Hauser RG, et al. Risk factors for red blood cell alloimmunization in the Recipient Epidemiology and Donor Evaluation Study (REDS-III) database. *Br J Haematol*. 2018;181:672−681.
8. Economidou J, Constantoulakis M, Augoustaki O, Adinolfu M. Frequency of Antibodies to various antigenic determinants in polytransfused patients with homozygous thalassaemia in Greece. *Vox Sang*. 1971;20:252−258.
9. Tatari-Calderone Z, Minniti C, Kratovil T, et al. rs660 polymorphism in Ro52(SSA1;TRIM 21) is a marker for age-dependent tolerance induction and efficiency of alloimmunization in sickle cell disease. *Mol Immunol*. 2009;47:64−70.
10. Al-Riyami AZ, Al-Muqbali A, Al-Sudiri S, et al. Risks of red blood cell alloimmunization in transfusion dependent B-thalassemia in Oman: a 25 year experience of a university tertiary care reference center and a literature review. *Transfusion*. 2018;58:871−878.
11. Chaibunruang A, Sornkayasit K, Chewasateanchai M, et al. Prevalence of thalassemia among newborns: a Re-visited after 20 Years of a prevention and control program in northeast Thailand. *Mediterr J Hematol Infect Dis*. 2018;10(1): e2018054. https://doi.org/10.4084/MJHID.2018.054. eCollection 2018.
12. Romphruk AV, Simtong P, Butryojantho C, et al. The prevalence, alloimmunization risk factors, antigenic exposure, and evaluation of antigen-matched red blood cells for thalassemia transfusions: a 10-year experience at a tertiary care hospital. *Transfusion*. 2018. https://doi.org/10.1111/trf.15002.
13. Thedsawad A, Taka O, Wanachiwanawin W. Prevalence and clinical significances of red cell alloimmunization and red cell bound immunoglobulin G in polytransfused patients with thalassemias. *Hematology*. 2019;24(1): 208−214.
14. Singer ST, Wu V, Mignacca R, et al. Alloimmunization and erythrocyte autoimmunization in transfusion-dependent

thalassemia patients of predominantly Asian descent. *Blood.* 2000;96:3369–3373.

15. Cohen A, Markenson AL, Schwartz E. Transfusion requirements and splenectomy in thalassemia Major. *J Pediatr.* 1980;97(1):100–102.

16. Hendrickson JE, Chadwick TE, Roback JD, et al. Inflammation enhances consumption and presentation of transfused RBC antigens by dendritic cells. *Blood.* 2007;110:2736–2743.

17. Evers D, van der Bom JG, Tijmensen J, et al. Absence of the spleen and the occurrence of primary red cell alloimmunization in humans. *Haematologica.* 2017;102:e292.

18. Hussein E, et al. Predictors of red cell alloimmunization in multitransfused Egyptian patients with B-thalassemia. *Arch Pathol Lab Med.* 2014;138:684–688.

19. Thompson AA, et al. Red cell alloimmunization in a diverse population of transfused patietns with thalassaemia. *BJH.* 2011;153:121–128.

20. Belsito A, et al. Clinical outcome of transfusions with extended red blood cel matching in B thalassemia patients: a single-center experience. *Transfus Apher Sci.* 2018. https://doi.org/10.1016/j.transci.2018.11.006.

21. Compernolle V, Chou ST, Tanael S, et al. Red blood cell specifications for patients with hemoglobinopathies: a systematic review and guideline. *Transfusion.* June 2018;58(6):1555–1566.

22. Ware RE, de Montalembert M, et al. Sickle cell disease. *Lancet.* 2017;390:311–323.

23. US Centers for Disease Control and Prevention. Sickle Cell Disease: Data and Statistics.http://www.cdc.gov/ncbddd/sicklecell/data.html. Accessed 1/14/19.

24. Yawn BP, Buchanan GR, Afenyi-Annan AN, et al. Management of sickle cell disease summary of the 2014 evidence based report by expert panel members. *J Am Med Assoc.* 2014;312:1033–1048.

25. Vichinsky EP, Earles A, Johnson RA, et al. Alloimmunization in sickle cell anemia and transfusion of racially unmatched blood. *NEJM.* 1990;322:1617–1621.

26. Rosse WF, Gallagher D, Kinney TR, et al. Transfusion and alloimmunization in sickle cell disease. *Blood.* 1990;76(7):1431–1437.

27. Olujohungbe A, Hambleton I, Stephens L, et al. Red cell antibodies in patients with homozygous sickle cell disease: a comparison of patients in Jamaica and the United Kingdom. *Br J Haematol.* 2001;113:661–665.

28. Ugwu NI, Awodu OA, Bazuaye GN, Okoye AE. Red cell alloimmunization in multi transfused patients with sickle cell anemia in Benin city, Nigeria. *Niger J Clin Pract.* 2015;18(4):522–526.

29. Kangiwa U, Ibegbulam O, Ocheni S, et al. Pattern and Prevalence of Alloimmunization in Multiply Transfused Patients with Sickle Cell Disease in Nigeria.

30. Natukunda B, Schonewille H, Ndugwa C, Brand A. Red blood cell alloimmunization in sickle cell disease patients in Uganda. *Transfusion.* 2010;50:20–25.

31. Piomelli S. Chronic transfusions in patients with sickle cell disease. Indications and problems. *Am J Pediatr Hematol Oncol.* 1985;7(1):51–55. Spring.

32. Adams RJ, McKie VC, Hsu L, et al. Prevention of a first stroke by transfusions in children with sickle cell anemia and abnormal results on transcranial Doppler ultrasonography. *NEJM.* 1998;339:5–11.

33. AABB Technical Manual.

34. Tahhan HR, Holbrook CT, Braddy LR, et al. Antigen-matched donor blood in the transfusion management of patients with sickle cell disease. *Transfusion.* 1994;34:562–569.

35. Vichinsky EP, Luban NLC, Wright E, et al. Prospective RBC phenotype matching in a stroke prevention trial in sickle cell anemia: a multicenter trial. *Transfusion.* 2001;41:1086–1092.

36. Sakhalkar VS, Roberts K, Hawthorne LM, et al. Allosensitization in patients receiving multiple blood transfusions. *Ann N Y Acad Sci.* 2005;1054:495–499.

37. Aygun B, Padmanabhan S, Paley C, Chandrasekaran V. Clinical significance of RBC alloantibodies and autoantibodies in sickle cell patients who received transfusions. *Transfusion.* 2002;42:37–43.

38. LaSalle-Williams M, Nuss R, Le T, et al. Extended RBC antigen matching for transfusions in SCD: a review of a 14 year experience in a single center. *Transfusion.* 2011;51:1732–1739.

39. Campbell-Lee SA, Gvozdjan K, Choi KM, et al. RBC alloimmunization in SCD: assessment of transfusion protocols during two time periods. *Transfusion.* 2018;58:1588–1596.

40. O'Suoji C, Liem RI, Mack K, et al. Alloimmunization in sickle cell anemia in the era of extended RBC typing. *Pediatr Blood Canc.* 2013;60:1487–1491.

41. Chou ST, Jackson T, Vege S, et al. High prevalence of RBC alloimmunization in SCD despite transfusion from Rh-matched minority donors. *Blood.* 2013;122(6):1062–1071.

42. Boulware LE, Ratner LE, Ness PM, et al. The contribution of sociodemographic, medical, and attitudinal factors to blood donation among the general public. *Transfusion.* 2002;42(6):669–678.

43. Price CL, Boyd JH, Watkins AR, et al. Mailing of a sickle cell disease educational packet increases blood donors within an African American community. *Transfusion.* 2006;46(8):1388–1393.

44. Castilho L, Dinardo CL. Optimized antigen-matched in sickle cell disease patients: chances and challenges in molecular times - the Brazilian way. *Transfus Med Hemotherapy.* 2018;45(4):258–262.

45. Chou ST, Flanagan JM, Vege S, et al. Whole-exome sequencing for RH genotyping and alloimmunization risk in children with sickle cell anemia. *Blood Advances.* 2017;1(18):1414–1422.

46. Sundd P, Gladwin MT, Novelli EM. Pathophysiology of sickle cell disease. *Annu Rev Pathol.* 2018. https://doi.org/10.1146/annurev-pathmechdis-012418-012838.

47. Hendrickson JE, Desmarets M, Deshpande SS, et al. Recipient inflammation affects the frequency and magnitude of immunization to transfused red blood cells. *Transfusion.* 2006;46(9):1526–1536.

48. Fasano RM, Booth GS, Miles M, et al. Red blood cell alloimmunization is influenced by recipient inflammatory state at time of transfusion in patients with sickle cell disease. *Br J Haematol*. 2015;168:291–300.

49. Alarif L, Castro O, Ofosu M, et al. HLA-B35 is associated with red cell alloimmunization in sickle cell disease. *Clin Immunol Immunopathol*. 1986;38:178–183.

50. Sippert EA, Visentainer JEL, Alves HV, et al. Red blood cell alloimmunization in patients with sickle cell disease: correlation with HLA and cytokine gene polymorphisms. *Transfusion*. 2017;57:379–389.

51. Vingert B, Tamagne M, Habibi A, et al. Phenotypic differences of CD4(+) T cells in response to red blood cell immunization in transfused sickle cell disease patients. *Eur J Immunol*. 2015;45:1868–1879.

52. Oliveira VB Dezan MR, Gomes FCA, et al. -318C/T polymorphism of the CTLA-4 gene is an independent risk factor for RBC alloimmunization among sickle cell disease patients. *Int J Immunogenet*. 2017;44:219–224.

53. Tatari-Calderone Z, Gordish-Dressman H, Fasano R, et al. Protective effect of HLA-DQB1 alleles against alloimmunization in patients with sickle cell disease. *Hum Immunol*. 2016;77:35–40.

54. Meinderts SM, sins JWR, Fijnvandraat K, et al. Nonclassical FCGR2C haplotype is associated with protection from red blood cell alloimmunization in sickle cell disease. *Blood*. 2017. https://doi.org/10.1182/blood-2017-05-784876.

55. Williams LM, Qi Z, Batai K, et al. A locus on chromosome 5 shows African ancestry–limited association with alloimmunization in sickle cell disease. *Blood Adv*. 2018. https://doi.org/10.1182/bloodadvances.2018020594.

56. Wahl SK, Garcia A, Hagar W, et al. Lower alloimmunization rates in pediatric sickle cell patients on chronic erythrocytapheresis compared to chronic simple transfusions. *Transfusion*. 2012;52:2671–2676.

57. Michot JM, Driss F, Guitton C, et al. Immunohematologic tolerance of chronic transfusion exchanges with erythrocytapheresis in sickle cell disease. *Transfusion*. 2015;55: 357–363.

58. Hendrickson JE, Hod EA, Spitalnik SL, et al. Immunohematology: storage of murine red blood cells enhances alloantibody responses to an erythroid-specific model antigen. *Transfusion*. 2010;50:642–648.

59. Desai PC, Deal AM, Pfaff ER, et al. Alloimmunization is associated with older age of transfused red blood cells in sickle cell disease. *Am J Hematol*. 2015;90(8):691–695.

60. Ryder AB, Zimring JC, Hendrickson JE. Factors influencing RBC alloimmunization: lessons learned from murine models. *Transfus Med Hemotherapy*. 2014;41:406–419.

61. Singhal D, Kutyna MM, Chhetri R, et al. Red cell alloimmunization is associated with development of autoantibodies and increased red cell transfusion requirements in myelodysplastic syndrome. *Haematologica*. 2017;102(12): 2021–2029.

62. Stiegler G, Sperr W, Lorber C, et al. Red cell antibodies in frequently transfused patients with myelodysplastic syndrome. *Ann Hematol*. 2001;80:330–333.

63. Kim HY, Cho EJ, Chun S, et al. Red blood cell alloimmunization in Korean patients with myelodysplastic syndrome and liver cirrhosis. *Ann Lab Med*. 2019;39: 218–222.

64. Sanz C, Nomdedeu M, Belkaid M, et al. Red blood cell alloimmunization in transfused patients with myelodysplastic syndrome or chronic myelomonocytic leukemia. *Transfusion*. 2013;53:710–715.

65. Stanworth SJ, Navarrete C, Estcourt L, Marsh J. Platelet refractoriness-practical approaches and ongoing dilemmas in patients management. *Br J Haematol*. 2015;171: 297–305.

66. Cid J, Ortin X, Elies E, et al. Absence of anti-D alloimmunization in hematologic patients after D-incompatible platelet transfusions. *Transfusion*. 2002;42:173–176.

67. Blumberg N, Peck K, Ross K, Avila E. Immune response to chronic red blood cell transfusion. *Vox Sang*. 1983;44: 212–217.

68. Abou-Elella AA, Camarillo TA, Allenn MB, et al. Low incidence of red cell and HLA antibody formation by bone marrow transplant patients. *Transfusion*. 1995;35:931–935.

69. Leisch M, Weiss L, Lindlbauer N, et al. Red blood cell alloimmunization in 184 patients with myeloid neoplasms treated with azacitidine-a retrospective single center experience. *Leuk Res*. 2017;59:12–19.

70. Pang QY, An R, Liu HL. Perioperative transfusion and the prognosis of colorectal cancer surgery: a systematic review and meta-analysis. *World J Surg Oncol*. 2019;17(1):7. https://doi.org/10.1186/s12957-018-1551-y.

71. Baumeister P, Canis M, Reiter M. Preoperative anemia and perioperative blood transfusion in head and neck squamous cell carcinoma. *PLoS One*. 2018;13(10):e0205712. https://doi.org/10.1371/journal.pone.0205712.

72. Cata JP, Gutierrez C, Mehran RJ, et al. Preoperative anemia, blood transfusion, and neutrophil-to-lymphocyte ratio in patients with stage i non-small cell lung cancer. *Cancer Cell Microenviron*. 2016;3(1):e1116.

73. Kim JK, Kim HS, Park J, et al. Perioperative blood transfusion as a significant predictor of biochemical recurrence and survival after radical prostatectomy in patients with prostate cancer. *PLoS One*. 2016;11(5):e0154918. https://doi.org/10.1371/journal.pone.0154918. eCollection 2016.

74. Abt NB, Puram SV, Sinha S, et al. Transfusion in head and neck cancer patients undergoing pedicled flap reconstruction. *The Laryngoscope*. 2018;128(12): E409–E415. https://doi.org/10.1002/lary.27393.

75. Remy KE, Hall MW, Cholette J, et al. Mechanisms of red blood cell transfusion-related immunomodulation. *Transfusion*. 2018;58(3):804–815.

76. Dinardo CL, Ito GM, Sampaio LR, Junior AM. Study of possible clinical and laboratory predictors of alloimmunization against red blood cell antigens in cancer patients. *Rev Bras Hematol Hemoter*. 2013;35(6):414–416.

77. Evers D, Zwaginga JJ, Tijmensen J, et al. Treatments for hematologic malignancies in contrast to those for solid cancers are associated with reduced red cell alloimmunization. *Haematologica*. 2017;102(1):52–59.

CHAPTER 12

Graft-Versus-Host Disease and Transfusion-Associated Graft-Versus-Host Disease

ALEX B. RYDER, MD, PHD • YAN ZHENG, MD, PHD

INTRODUCTION

In order to maintain safe and effective transfusion practices, it is imperative to identify risks associated with transfusion and employ strategies to minimize these risks. Many transfusion-related complications are due to recipient immune responses to transfused blood components. However, this chapter focuses on a well-recognized clinical complication in which donor immune cells mediate a profound response against recipient tissues. Transfusion-associated graft-versus-host disease (TA-GVHD) is a severe immune-mediated complication associated with the transfusion of cellular blood components to susceptible immunocompetent and immunocompromised recipients. Because of the high mortality associated with TA-GVHD, blood banks and transfusion services devote considerable efforts to prevent its occurrence, which fortunately is quite rare.

The history of the recognition of clinical symptoms that likely represent manifestations of TA-GVHD is both extensive and interesting.[1,2] The first reports of classical clinical presentations consistent with TA-GVHD in transfused immunocompromised infants and fetuses were published during the 1960s.[3,4] An even earlier description of "postoperative erythroderma" associated with high mortality in transfused immunocompetent Japanese surgical patients was published in 1955.[5] Many experts believe this to be the earliest published report of TA-GVHD.

This chapter describes the immune pathophysiology of TA-GVHD; provides clinically relevant information, including recognized donor-/component- and recipient-related risk factors associated with the development of TA-GVHD; and explores both long-standing and emerging interventions that reduce the risk of TA-GVHD from transfused cellular blood components. Some clinical and mechanistic similarities

exist between TA-GVHD and GVHD that are associated with allogeneic bone marrow and stem cell transplantations, as well as between TA-GVHD and passenger lymphocyte syndrome (PLS) that are associated with solid organ transplants. Therefore, this chapter also compares classical GVHD and PLS with TA-GVHD to provide an overview of the spectrum of immune-mediated complications of engrafted donor lymphocytes associated with transfusion and transplantation.

PATHOPHYSIOLOGY OF TA-GVHD

The development of TA-GVHD is primarily dependent on the inability of transfusion recipients to eliminate transfused donor T lymphocytes. Although the inability to eliminate donor T lymphocytes alone is not sufficient for TA-GVHD to develop, it does underscore that TA-GVHD can occur in both immunocompromised patients with diminished cellular immunity against donor T lymphocytes and in immunocompetent patients unable to recognize transfused lymphocytes as "nonself" (Fig. 12.1).

Classically, three conditions are required for the development of TA-GVHD: (1) transfusion of viable donor T lymphocytes, (2) activation of donor lymphocytes by the recognition of recipient cell surface antigens as nonself, and (3) recipient inability to effectively eliminate donor T lymphocytes, allowing for their proliferation, engraftment, and subsequent attack.[6] If these three conditions are sufficiently met, it is possible for donor lymphocytes to engraft in the transfusion recipient, attack recipient tissues based on recognition of nonself cell surface antigens, namely human leukocyte antigen (HLA), and eventually eliminate recipient bone marrow components. Generally, the result of this sequence is death due to either bone marrow aplasia or its

Immunologic Concepts in Transfusion Medicine. https://doi.org/10.1016/B978-0-323-67509-3.00012-3

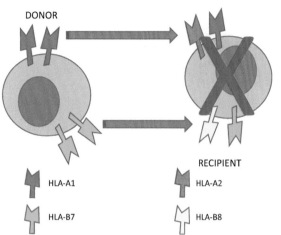

FIG. 12.1 TA-GVHD as a consequence of immune tolerance. In this case, the donor is homozygous for an HLA haplotype that is shared with the recipient. The recipient is heterozygous for the HLA haplotype: one recipient HLA-A/HLA-B haplotype is shared with the donor, and the other recipient haplotype is unique. Due to the unique recipient HLA haplotype, donor lymphocytes recognize recipient cells as "nonself," leading to donor lymphocyte activation, proliferation, and attack on host tissues. Conversely, recipient immune cells recognize donor lymphocytes as "self" due to the shared haplotype and do not mediate a response to eliminate these donor cells. *TA-GVHD*, Transfusion-associated graft-versus-host disease; *HLA*, Human leukocyte antigen.

associated complications (e.g., overwhelming infections). Attack on recipient bone marrow distinguishes TA-GVHD as a much more severe and feared complication than GVHD. Because donor hematopoietic stem cells in GVHD have ideally reconstituted functional marrow elements, they attack only recipient nonmarrow tissues. Conversely, in TA-GVHD, the recipient marrow is as susceptible to destruction as are other tissue types, without the possibility of reconstitution by donor hematopoietic stem cells.

Although it is mechanistically simple to understand that transfusion recipients with severely compromised cellular immunity may be at risk for development of TA-GVHD because of their inability to "counterattack" donor T lymphocytes, it is also possible for immunocompetent transfusion recipients to develop TA-GVHD when recipient immune cells recognize donor HLA antigens as "self" (Fig. 12.1). This immune tolerance may occur when a transfusion donor possesses a homozygous compliment of HLA antigens (i.e., both haplotypes homozygous for each allele) and the recipient expresses each of the donor HLA antigens, as well

as additional antigens (i.e., haplotypes heterozygous for *HLA* alleles) (Fig. 12.1). In this context, donor lymphocytes are recognized as self by recipient immune cells because each HLA antigen expressed on the donor lymphocytes is also expressed by the recipient. Conversely, the donor lymphocytes see recipient tissues as nonself due to their expression of additional HLA antigens. This immune tolerance can result in the activation of donor T lymphocytes to mediate an immune attack on recipient tissues, including hematopoietic tissues. Although this is a rare occurrence in populations with marked HLA diversity, it can be a considerable risk in populations lacking such diversity. In Japan, for example, the risk for such a complication is higher because of decreased HLA diversity among the population. Due to early recognition of TA-GVHD as a devastating complication of transfusion, Japan has historically practiced irradiation of blood components in many clinical scenarios and began a practice of universal irradiation of transfused cellular blood components in 2000 to mitigate this risk.[7]

The degree and extent of HLA antigen matching between transfusion donors and immunocompetent recipients necessary for the development of TA-GVHD is not well established. Although some cases have occurred in the context of full matches among HLA-A and HLA-B, and occasionally HLA-DR, this is not consistent.[8] A recent analysis of published cases of TA-GVHD revealed that they are more frequent when donor HLA-I and HLA-II antigens are not recognized as nonself by the recipient but that cases also occur when nonself donor HLA antigens are present.[9] The picture is even more complex when considering that the incidence of TA-GVHD is considerably lower than the calculated frequency of transfusion events in which the donor is homozygous for one recipient HLA antigen haplotype (theoretically, a potential situation of tolerance).[10] Therefore, other mechanisms not yet fully understood must contribute to TA-GVHD susceptibility.

TA-GVHD is thought to depend on the contributions of both CD4+ and CD8+ donor T lymphocytes.[2] Initially, donor CD4+ T lymphocytes become activated upon recognition of foreign recipient tissues expressing nonself HLA molecules. These activated CD4+ T lymphocytes, in turn, release inflammatory cytokines that promote, among other cell types, cytotoxic CD8+ T lymphocytes to mediate substantial tissue destruction, including against recipient hematopoietic cells, which express histocompatibility antigens.[8,11] An interesting characteristic of TA-GVHD is that HIV/AIDS is generally not considered to be a risk factor for its development, despite severely compromised cellular immunity in this population. Donor leukocytes do not appear to proliferate or persist long term in patients with HIV/AIDS, perhaps due to viral infection of donor $CD4^+$ T lymphocytes, mitigating their ability to promote a robust attack.[12]

The dose of viable transfused T lymphocytes required to produce TA-GVHD is difficult to determine, with reports ranging from as low as 10^4/kg to as high as 10^7/kg.[8] The dose of T lymphocytes required to induce TA-GVHD varies depending on many factors and is therefore challenging to establish definitively.

CLINICAL CHARACTERISTICS OF TA-GVHD

TA-GVHD is characterized by the development of symptoms, such as fever, rash, diarrhea, nausea, vomiting, and hepatitis, which are similar to those of GVHD. Distinguishing TA-GVHD from GVHD is the frequent development of pancytopenia due to the mechanism of TA-GVHD attack, although this complication occurred in only 65% of recently reviewed cases.[9] The time from transfusion to symptom onset is generally within 2−30 days after transfusion, and symptoms are generally followed by a characteristically high mortality rate due to targeting of transfusion recipient bone marrow.

Although diagnosis of TA-GVHD is largely based on its clinical presentation, establishing a definitive diagnosis depends on the identification of cell populations that can be linked to a transfusion donor. This may be established through cytogenetic analysis or by molecular studies, such as restriction fragment length polymorphisms and short tandem repeats.[1,13] However, more sensitive molecular techniques that are currently available may play a role in diagnosing TA-GVHD in the future.

Because of the patient populations most prone to experiencing TA-GVHD, it is possible that this complication may go underrecognized and underreported in formal monitors of hemovigilance. Severely immunocompromised transfusion recipients experience overwhelming infections much more frequently than TA-GVHD; therefore, identifying such cases may be a challenge. Given the increase in irradiation of cellular blood components for susceptible transfusion recipients, however, it is unlikely that this number is large. Additionally, because the symptoms of TA-GVHD are similar to those of GVHD, and GVHD occurs more frequently, it is possible that TA-GVHD is not considered during diagnosis. Finally, TA-GVHD may go undiagnosed in immunocompetent patients because of its rarity and relatively rapid course, and is instead confounded with other more common causes of its characteristic symptoms.

A number of conditions of immunocompromise are associated with an increased risk of developing TA-GVHD. As previously mentioned, HIV/AIDS is not among these conditions, perhaps due to virus-donor T lymphocyte interaction. Table 12.1 depicts the recipient- and product-related factors associated with TA-GVHD risk. The conditions generally considered high risk for TA-GVHD development include congenital cellular immunodeficiencies, such as DiGeorge syndrome, stem cell/bone marrow transplant recipients, fetuses requiring intrauterine transfusions, premature low birth weight neonates, patients with acute leukemia, and patients with Hodgkin lymphoma. Relatively immunocompromised patients, including those receiving high-dose purine analogues (e.g., antithymocyte globulin) or alemtuzumab (anti-CD52) therapy, term neonates, and patients with chronic leukemia or lymphoma may also be at risk. Solid organ transplant recipients are generally believed to be at lower risk, but many centers consider them a susceptible patient population as well.

In patient populations that are not generally considered immunocompromised, many additional risk factors have been identified. These include patients undergoing cardiac surgery[14]; transfusion of directed blood donations, particularly from relatives[15]; and the transfusion of fresh blood components.[16] Interestingly, transfusion of red blood cells (RBCs) and whole blood units stored >14 days are not linked to cases of TA-GVHD, whereas fresh units transfused shortly after collection are significantly more likely to be implicated.[9] Older units are proposed to be less likely to cause TA-GVHD because of decreasing T lymphocyte functional and proliferative ability over the duration of storage.[17] The implications for this finding on prophylaxis are not yet clear.

Although TA-GVHD may develop after the transfusion of any nonirradiated cellular blood component (e.g., RBCs, whole blood, platelets, granulocytes, and liquid never-frozen plasma), it is most commonly linked to RBCs (38%), whole blood (26%), and platelets (6%).[9] Risk for developing TA-GVHD is not associated with transfusion of previously frozen RBCs, plasma, or cryoprecipitate because the freezing process destroys donor lymphocytes.[18]

In contrast to GVHD, for which various treatments have proven modestly successful, no well-established treatments are available for TA-GVHD, and consequently, mortality is high. Reports of some patients who do survive despite TA-GVHD are known, but no unifying treatment was described in these instances.[19,20]

TABLE 12.1
Risk Factors for Development of Transfusion-Associated Graft-Versus-Host Disease.

RECIPIENT FACTORS

Immunocompromised

    Cellular immunodeficiencies (DiGeorge, SCID)

    Stem cell/bone marrow transplant recipients

    Acute leukemia

    Aplastic anemia

    Intrauterine transfusions

    Premature, low birth weight neonate

    Term neonate

    Hodgkin lymphoma

    Chronic leukemia

    Solid organ transplant

    Solid tumor

    Non-Hodgkin lymphoma

    Purine analogues

    ATG therapy

    Alemtuzumab (anti-CD52) therapy

Immunocompetent

    Cardiac surgery

    Trauma/Massive transfusion

    Low HLA diversity populations

COMPONENT FACTORS

Freshness

Cellularity: RBCs, whole blood, platelets, liquid plasma, granulocytes

Directed donations, particularly relatives

HLA, Human leukocyte antigen; *RBCs*, Red blood cells.

PREVENTION OF TA-GVHD

Because no effective treatments for TA-GVHD are available, efforts are focused on the prevention of TA-GVHD. It is well accepted that the number of donor functional T lymphocytes in blood components is associated with the development of TA-GVHD; therefore, approaches that reduce the number of donor lymphocytes or inhibit the function of donor lymphocytes have been explored.

Up to 1 to 2×10^9 white blood cells (WBCs) are present in blood components,[2] and leukoreduction filters typically remove 99.9% of the WBCs. Per AABB standards, the WBC number in a blood component unit should be less than 5×10^6/unit in 95% of the units tested.[21] However, cases of TA-GVHD occur despite leukoreduction.[9] It appears that leukoreduction reduces but does not prevent the development of TA-GVHD. With the development of new filtration technologies, the current generation of leukoreduction filters can remove 99.99% (4 $\log_{10}$ reduction) of WBCs; however, it is unknown if this is sufficient to eliminate TA-GVHD.[22]

The current practice for the prevention of TA-GVHD is to irradiate blood components with γ-rays or X-rays. The AABB standard recommends a minimal 2500 cGy to the central portion of the unit and a minimal of 1500 cGy to any point of the unit.[21] Ionizing irradiation can induce various types of DNA damage, including cross-linking and single-strand and double-strand breaks, of which double-strand breaks are the most deleterious types of lesions and can be unrepairable.[23] Cells that accumulate unrepairable DNA damage cease to proliferate and undergo apoptosis. The minimal γ-irradiation dose for blood components was established by Pelszynski et al. by using an in vitro mixed lymphocyte culture (MLC) with limiting dilution analysis (LDA).[24] MLC or mixed lymphocyte reaction is used to test the allogeneic reactivity of T lymphocytes. T lymphocytes from one individual (responder cells) are mixed with lymphocytes from a second individual (stimulator cells). The stimulator cells are usually treated such that they are nonreactive to the responder cells. Because 1%−10% T lymphocytes from an individual can recognize nonself major histocompatibility complex (MHC) molecules, this exposure leads to substantial proliferation and cytokine production of the responder cells. Proliferation of the responder cells can be quantified by microscopic examination of cell cluster formation and incorporation of [^{3}H] thymidine or 5-bromo-2′-deoxyuridine upon DNA replication. MLC is sensitive for detecting the presence of the responder cells in a population of mixed cells but is limited in determining the absolute number/concentration of the responder cells, particularly if the frequency is low. The absolute number/concentration of the responder cells in a specimen can be determined by LDA. Specifically, the responder cells are subjected to a series of dilutions, and the diluted responder cells are added to the stimulator cells with a number of replicate cultures prepared at each dilution. The cultures are then assessed as responding or nonresponding. Mathematical analysis of the percentage of nonresponding cultures at each dilution allows the estimation of the responder cell number/concentration in the original cell population.

Initially, MLC was used to determine the appropriate dose of irradiation for TA-GVHD prevention. On the basis of data derived from MLCs, many blood banks irradiated blood components with 1500 to 2000 cGy. However, TA-GVHD remained problematic, as isolated cases of TA-GVHD continued to occur.[25–27] To investigate the effect of higher than 2000 cGy irradiation in suppressing T lymphocyte function, Pelszynski et al. used LDA.[24] Furthermore, to maximize the allogenic response, the authors activated the responder cells with a mixture of stimulator cells from multiple individuals, followed by extended expansion in the presence of excess cytokines. Specifically, mononuclear cells were isolated from irradiated RBC units, quantified, and subjected to serial dilution. The diluted cells were seeded and activated by a pool of buffy coats (stimulator cells) from 11 different individuals, followed by expansion in the presence of supplemented T lymphocyte growth factors and cytokines for 28 days. T lymphocyte growth was then evaluated by microscopic identification of T lymphocyte cluster formation. By using the numbers of cells seeded per well and the fractions of wells without growth, they calculated the number and concentration of T lymphocytes in the original samples. This modified LDA permits identification of 1 T lymphocyte in 10^6 cells and thereby can detect a >5 $\log_{10}$ reduction of functional T lymphocytes. With this approach, they showed that a >5 $\log_{10}$ reduction of functional T lymphocytes can be achieved by 2500 cGy, and a >4 $\log_{10}$ of functional T lymphocyte reduction can be achieved by 1500 cGy. Because of the findings, 2500 to 3000 cGy is now the standard dose used to inactivate T lymphocytes in blood components. However, irradiation of blood components introduces numerous challenges, including the high cost of purchasing and maintaining irradiation instruments, high security requirement for the irradiation sources, delays in transfusion of blood due to irradiation, and irradiation-associated RBC membrane damage.[28] Therefore, alternative approaches for TA-GVHD prevention are the focus of current research studies.

Concerns for transfusion-transmitted disease, despite infectious disease screening of blood donors, led to the development of pathogen reduction processes.[29] These pathogen reduction processes block replication of contaminating microbes in blood components by modifying their DNA and RNA.[30] By the same mechanisms, pathogen reduction also inhibits T lymphocyte proliferation, reducing the risk of TA-GVHD. Two pathogen reduction processes have been extensively studied in the context of TA-GVHD,

amotosalen plus ultraviolet A (UVA) light (i.e., the INTERCEPT blood system marketed by the Cerus Corporation), and riboflavin plus UV light (i.e., the Mirasol pathogen reduction technology system marketed by Terumo BCT, Inc.).

The INTERCEPT system uses a combination of the photochemical amotosalen and UVA light. Amotosalen, a synthetic form of psoralen, intercalates initially between strands of DNA or RNA.[31] Upon exposure to UVA light, amotosalen is activated, binds covalently to pyrimidine bases, and then forms cross-links between the two nucleic acid strands. The cross-links prevent replication of the nucleic acids, rendering the cell inactive. The efficacy of amotosalen for inactivating T lymphocytes in platelet concentrates has been evaluated in vitro. Grass et al. demonstrated with the modified LDA that treatment with 150 µM of amotosalen and 3 J/cm² UVA light (the recommended dosage by INTERCEPT) results in a >5 $\log_{10}$ reduction of functional T lymphocytes. Various cytokines are produced by residual leukocytes, including T lymphocytes, during platelet storage such as IL-1β, IL-6, TNF-α, IL-8, and others. Amotosalen treatment completely inhibits IL-8 production during the 5-day platelet storage period. DNA isolated from the amotosalen-treated leukocytes had an average of 12 ± 3 amotosalen-DNA adducts per 1000 bp, which resulted in failed PCR amplification of even small genomic DNA sequences of 242–439 bp. In comparison, irradiation with 2500 cGy minimally affects IL-8 production and induces one DNA break per 37,000 bp, which does not interfere with amplification of small DNA sequences.

Amotosalen treatment was also examined in a parent into F1 murine GVHD model. In this well-characterized murine GVHD model, the parental mice, strain A, are homologous at the *H2* locus (i.e., the mouse *MHC* locus), and the offspring mice B6AF1 (C57BL/6 × A) are heterozygous at the *H2* locus with one haplotype shared with the parental mice. When parental splenocytes are infused into the offspring mice, the offspring/recipient T lymphocytes recognize the parent/donor cells as "self" and fail to react; whereas, the parent/donor T lymphocytes recognize the offspring/recipient cells as "nonself" and become activated, causing a phenotype similar to the clinical findings of TA-GVHD.[32] However, transfusion of parental splenocytes treated with 150 µM of amotosalen and 2.1 J/cm² UVA did not result in detectable signs of GVHD in the offspring/recipient mice. The INTERCEPT pathogen reduction system for platelets was approved in Europe in 2002 and in the United States in 2014. Postmarketing hemovigilance programs have been implemented to monitor adverse events associated with INTERCEPT-treated platelets, including rare adverse events such as TA-GVHD. In an observational study, Knutson et al. reported that from 2003 to 2010, 4067 patients received 19,175 INTERCEPT-treated platelet transfusions, and no cases of TA-GVHD were reported.[33] Therefore, amotosalen treatment can potentially replace irradiation for the prevention of TA-GVHD.

The Mirasol is an alternative pathogen reduction method and uses riboflavin and UV light. Riboflavin interacts with and induces oxidative damages to nucleotides, resulting in strand breaks and fragmentation.[31] Riboflavin treatment is known to inactivate T lymphocytes in platelets.[34,35] Furthermore, riboflavin treatment has been shown to be effective for inhibiting T lymphocytes in whole blood as well.[36]

The treatment of whole blood and RBCs by pathogen reduction processes is nevertheless challenging. Hemoglobin in RBCs absorbs UV light; therefore, the energy dose of UV light must be normalized according to the number of RBCs in the units. In addition, UV light doses must be balanced between the efficacy of pathogen reduction and the quality of the blood components.[37,38] Riboflavin treatment of whole blood has been assessed in vitro and in vivo. Fast et al. treated whole blood with riboflavin (35 mL of riboflavin mixed with 470 mL of whole blood) and 80 J UV light/mL RBCs and found that peripheral blood mononuclear cells (PBMCs) isolated from riboflavin-treated whole blood failed to proliferate in response to various stimuli (e.g., T lymphocyte mitogen phytohemagglutinin, anti-CD3 and anti-CD28, and allogeneic stimulator cells in MLCs).[36] They further showed by the modified LDA that riboflavin treatment results in a 4.7 $\log_{10}$ reduction of functional T lymphocytes. The authors next tested the riboflavin-treated PBMCs in an in vivo xenogeneic GVHD mouse model. In this model, human PBMCs are injected intravenously into severely immunodeficient NOD-SCID IL2γ^{null} (NSG) mice. NSG mice lack mature T lymphocytes, B lymphocytes, and natural killer cells and are deficient in multiple cytokine signaling pathways.[39] The profound immunodeficiency of these mice permits engraftment of human hematopoietic stem cells, which in turn recognize murine MHC molecules as foreign/xenoantigens and mediate attack of murine tissues. The affected mice develop signs of GVHD including weight loss and a hunched appearance with ruffled fur. By using this model, Fast et al. showed that PBMCs isolated from riboflavin-treated whole blood do not cause GVHD in NSG recipient mice.[36] The Mirasol system was approved for platelets in Europe in 2009 and for whole blood recently.

Hemovigilance data on more than 190,000 transfusions in multiple European centers from 2010 to 2015 showed low adverse reaction rates, with no cases of TA-GVHD identified.[40] Therefore, riboflavin treatment may represent a second alternative method for TA-GVHD prevention, in addition to amotosalen.

COMPARISON OF TA-GVHD TO GVHD AND PASSENGER LYMPHOCYTE SYNDROME

GVHD develops in the context of engrafted allogeneic bone marrow constituents that mediate an immune attack on host tissues, predominantly the liver, skin, and gastrointestinal tract. TA-GVHD is more devastating because of the additional destruction of host bone marrow by engrafted transfused donor lymphocytes. The high mortality associated with TA-GVHD is generally related to bone marrow aplasia and its associated complications that result from this destructive process. GVHD is a relatively common complication of allogeneic bone marrow and stem cell transplant and is recognized to have a spectrum of severity, with multiple treatment options of varying efficacy. Conversely, TA-GVHD is more rare than GVHD but has a mortality rate approaching 90% due to a lack of recognized treatment options.

PLS is an immune-mediated disorder resulting from the persistence of RBC antigen-specific B lymphocytes contained within a transplanted solid organ, particularly the liver or other lymphoid-rich organs.[41] Rather than causing a direct attack on recipient tissues, however, PLS is an antibody-mediated complication in which donor B lymphocytes expressing antibodies directed against recipient RBC antigens cause considerable and prolonged hemolytic anemia. Although most frequently directed against ABO antigens, other RBC antibodies implicated in PLS have been reported.[41] The outcome of PLS is variable, with some patients experiencing only mild, transient anemia, and others requiring long-duration transfusion support and sometimes therapeutic plasma exchange.

NEW DEVELOPMENTS IN TA-GVHD

Recent studies have explored whether TA-GVHD is always a fatal complication of transfusion or if its symptoms fall along a spectrum of severity and what factors may contribute to a milder course of disease. TA-GVHD is historically associated with mortality rates of approximately 90%, but recent evidence indicates that mortality may be decreasing in recent years.[8,9] This may be attributed, in part, to improved and more widespread use of leukoreduction,[8,42] although this is certainly not a substitute for methods, such as irradiation, that inactivate donor lymphocytes. It is hypothesized that a number of factors, including incomplete inactivation by irradiation and partial donor-recipient HLA mismatches, may contribute to a milder course of disease.[8]

In some transfusion cases, particularly those associated with trauma, low-level proliferation and persistent engraftment of a small population of donor lymphocytes occurs, which is a phenomenon known as transfusion-associated microchimerism.[43,44] Understanding mechanisms of transfusion-associated microchimerism may provide useful information regarding the spectrum of transfusion-related donor lymphocyte engraftment and pathogenesis.

Additionally, there has been a shift in the immune status of patients with recently identified cases of TA-GVHD, with approximately half of newly identified cases occurring in patients without classical risk factors for TA-GVHD.[9] It is possible that this is due to more widespread practices of irradiation of transfusion components for patients with immunologic risk factors. These recent observations are areas that warrant further investigation.

CONCLUSION

TA-GVHD represents a serious immune-mediated complication of transfusion because of the high mortality associated with documented cases. Although other related lymphocyte-mediated complications of stem cell/bone marrow and solid organ transplants are important considerations, TA-GVHD is distinguished by its lack of effective treatment and considerably higher mortality. New interest in determining previously unrecognized mechanisms by which TA-GVHD develops, identifying the patient populations at highest risk, and developing new methods for mitigating this risk are promising ongoing areas of investigation.

REFERENCES

1. Schroeder ML. Transfusion-associated graft-versus-host disease. *Br J Haematol.* 2002;117(2):275–287.
2. Bahar B, Tormey CA. Prevention of transfusion-associated graft-versus-host disease with blood product irradiation: the past, present, and future. *Arch Pathol Lab Med.* 2018;142(5):662–667.
3. Naiman JL, et al. Possible graft-versus-host reaction after intrauterine transfusion for Rh erythroblastosis fetalis. *N Engl J Med.* 1969;281(13):697–701.
4. Hathaway WE, et al. Aplastic anemia, histiocytosis and erythrodermia in immunologically deficient children.

5. Shimoda T. On postoperative erythroderma. (Japanese). *Geka.* 1955;17:487–492.
6. Billingham RE. The biology of graft-versus-host reactions. *Harvey Lect.* 1966;62:21–78.
7. Uchida S, et al. Analysis of 66 patients definitive with transfusion-associated graft-versus-host disease and the effect of universal irradiation of blood. *Transfus Med.* 2013;23(6):416–422.
8. Kleinman S, Stassinopoulos A. Transfusion-associated graft-versus-host disease reexamined: potential for improved prevention using a universally applied intervention. *Transfusion.* 2018;58(11):2545–2563.
9. Kopolovic I, et al. A systematic review of transfusion-associated graft-versus-host disease. *Blood.* 2015;126(3):406–414.
10. Wagner FF, Flegel WA. Transfusion-associated graft-versus-host disease: risk due to homozygous HLA haplotypes. *Transfusion.* 1995;35(4):284–291.
11. Bahar B, et al. The perils of storing thawed cryoprecipitate in the refrigerator. *Transfusion.* 2017;57(12):2826–2827.
12. Kruskall MS, et al. Survival of transfused donor white blood cells in HIV-infected recipients. *Blood.* 2001;98(2):272–279.
13. Sage D, et al. Diagnosis of transfusion-associated graft-vs.-host disease: the importance of short tandem repeat analysis. *Transfus Med.* 2005;15(6):481–485.
14. Juji T, et al. Post-transfusion graft-versus-host disease in immunocompetent patients after cardiac surgery in Japan. *N Engl J Med.* 1989;321(1):56.
15. Ohto H, et al. Risk of transfusion-associated graft-versus-host disease as a result of directed donations from relatives. *Transfusion.* 1992;32(7):691–693.
16. Ohto H, Anderson KC. Survey of transfusion-associated graft-versus-host disease in immunocompetent recipients. *Transfus Med Rev.* 1996;10(1):31–43.
17. Chang H, et al. Irreversible loss of donor blood leucocyte activation may explain a paucity of transfusion-associated graft-versus-host disease from stored blood. *Br J Haematol.* 2000;111(1):146–156.
18. Treleaven J, et al. Guidelines on the use of irradiated blood components prepared by the British Committee for Standards in Haematology blood transfusion task force. *Br J Haematol.* 2011;152(1):35–51.
19. Murakami T, et al. OKT3 therapy for transfusion-associated graft-versus-host disease in a neonate. *Acta Paediatr Jpn.* 1997;39(4):462–465.
20. Hutchinson K, et al. Early diagnosis and successful treatment of a patient with transfusion-associated GVHD with autologous peripheral blood progenitor cell transplantation. *Transfusion.* 2002;42(12):1567–1572.
21. AABB. *Standards for Blood Banks and Transfusion Services.* 31st. AABB; 2016.
22. Sharma RR, Marwaha N. Leukoreduced blood components: advantages and strategies for its implementation in developing countries. *Asian J Transfus Sci.* 2010;4(1):3–8.

Probable human runt disease. *N Engl J Med.* 1965;273(18):953–958.

23. Jackson SP, Bartek J. The DNA-damage response in human biology and disease. *Nature.* 2009;461:1071.

24. Pelszynski MM, et al. Effect of gamma irradiation of red blood cell units on T-cell inactivation as assessed by limiting dilution analysis: implications for preventing transfusion-associated graft-versus-host disease. *Blood.* 1994;83(6):1683–1689.

25. Drobyski W, et al. Third-party-mediated graft rejection and graft-versus-host disease after T-cell-depleted bone marrow transplantation, as demonstrated by hypervariable DNA probes and HLA-DR polymorphism. *Blood.* 1989;74(6): 2285–2294.

26. Lowenthal RM, et al. Transfusion-associated graft-versus-host disease: report of an occurrence following the administration of irradiated blood. *Transfusion.* 1993;33(6):524–529.

27. Sproul AM, et al. Third party mediated graft rejection despite irradiation of blood products. *Br J Haematol.* 1992;80(2):251–252.

28. Mintz PD, Wehrli G. Irradiation eradication and pathogen reduction. Ceasing cesium irradiation of blood products. *Bone Marrow Transplant.* 2009;44(4):205–211.

29. Fast LD. Developments in the prevention of transfusion-associated graft-versus-host disease. *Br J Haematol.* 2012; 158(5):563–568.

30. Salunkhe V, et al. Development of blood transfusion product pathogen reduction treatments: a review of methods, current applications and demands. *Transfus Apher Sci.* 2015;52(1):19–34.

31. Pelletier JP, Transue S, Snyder EL. Pathogen inactivation techniques. *Best Pract Res Clin Haematol.* 2006;19(1): 205–242.

32. Hakim F, et al. Animal models of acute and chronic graft-versus-host disease. *Curr Protoc Im.* 1998;27(1): 4.3.1–4.3.21.

33. Knutson F, et al. A prospective, active haemovigilance study with combined cohort analysis of 19,175 transfusions of platelet components prepared with amotosalen-UVA photochemical treatment. *Vox Sang.* 2015;109(4): 343–352.

34. Fast LD, et al. Mirasol PRT treatment of donor white blood cells prevents the development of xenogeneic graft-versus-host disease in Rag2-/-gamma c-/- double knockout mice. *Transfusion.* 2006;46(9):1553–1560.

35. Fast LD, et al. Functional inactivation of white blood cells by Mirasol treatment. *Transfusion.* 2006;46(4):642–648.

36. Fast LD, et al. Treatment of whole blood with riboflavin plus ultraviolet light, an alternative to gamma irradiation in the prevention of transfusion-associated graft-versus-host disease? *Transfusion.* 2013;53(2):373–381.

37. Cancelas JA, et al. Red blood cells derived from whole blood treated with riboflavin and ultraviolet light maintain adequate survival in vivo after 21 days of storage. *Transfusion.* 2017;57(5):1218–1225.

38. Cancelas JA, et al. In vivo viability of stored red blood cells derived from riboflavin plus ultraviolet light-treated whole blood. *Transfusion.* 2011;51(7):1460–1468.

39. Shultz LD, et al. Human lymphoid and myeloid cell development in NOD/LtSz-scid IL2R gamma null mice engrafted with mobilized human hemopoietic stem cells. *J Immunol.* 2005;174(10):6477–6489.

40. Piotrowski D, et al. Passive haemovigilance of blood components treated with a riboflavin-based pathogen reduction technology. *Blood Transfus.* 2018;16(4):348–351.

41. Cserti-Gazdewich CM, et al. Passenger lymphocyte syndrome with or without immune hemolytic anemia in all Rh-positive recipients of lungs from rhesus alloimmunized donors: three new cases and a review of the literature. *Transfus Med Rev.* 2009;23(2):134–145.

42. Williamson LM, et al. The impact of universal leukodepletion of the blood supply on hemovigilance reports of posttransfusion purpura and transfusion-associated graft-versus-host disease. *Transfusion.* 2007;47(8): 1455–1467.

43. Reed W, et al. Transfusion-associated microchimerism: a new complication of blood transfusions in severely injured patients. *Semin Hematol.* 2007;44(1):24–31.

44. Utter GH, et al. Transfusion-associated microchimerism. *Vox Sang.* 2007;93(3):188–195.

CHAPTER 13

Complications of ABO- and Non-ABO-incompatible Stem Cell Transplantations

SABRINA EWA RACINE-BRZOSTEK, MD, PHD • RUCHIKA GOEL, MD, MPH • LJILJANA V. VASOVIC, MD

BLOOD GROUP INCOMPATIBILITY IN HEMATOPOIETIC PROGENITOR CELL TRANSPLANTATION

Hematopoietic progenitor cell transplantation (HPCT) is a potentially curative treatment for a variety of malignant and nonmalignant hematological and congenital diseases, including acute myeloid leukemia, lymphoid leukemias, multiple myeloma, and sickle cell disease (SCD).[1-3] Human leukocyte antigen (HLA) matching is critical and plays a dominant role in allogeneic HPCT donor selection.[4,5] In contrast to solid organ transplantation, crossing the donor-recipient ABO incompatibility barrier has been feasible in HPCT, effectively expanding the donor pool multifold.[6,7]

Despite the general consensus that ABO incompatibility is not a prohibitive barrier and has a lesser effect on overall HPCT outcomes,[8,9] immune and hematological complications frequently do arise. Appropriate therapeutic and supportive management of ABO, as well as non-ABO, blood group—incompatible HPCT recipients can become critical and challenging during the posttransplantation time period.[10] Understanding the immunologic basis of the blood group antigen (Ag) and the characteristic primary antibody (Ab) responses might allow for a better appreciation of the underlying mechanism, of the hemolytic complications, delayed engraftment, and its impact on graft-versus-host disease (GVHD) and transplant-related mortality (TRM). It may also aid in the early detection of hemolysis and proper therapeutic management during the transplantation process. As such, this chapter discusses the immune concepts related to blood group Ag and Ab, and the laboratory testing for the early diagnosis and decision-making process while managing HPCT recipients.

Blood group Ag, both ABO and certain non-ABO, are expressed not only on hematopoietic cells but may display a tissue-wide distribution. In fact, the Ag that make up the ABO(H) Ag grouping are also termed histo-blood group Ag due to their body-wide distribution on a variety of human tissues and expression on epithelial and endothelial cells.[11] As such, the ABO group is of fundamental significance in not only determining compatibility for transfusion but also solid organ transplantation. ABO incompatibility can lead to risk of massive hemolysis with potential for fatal consequences or significant morbidity including acute renal failure, disseminated intravascular coagulation, or thrombosis. These dramatic responses to blood group incompatibility can be successfully overcome in ABO- and non-ABO-incompatible HPCT due to the recognition of unique immunological circumstances of an HPCT and with proper management.

As HLA matching is a crucial clinical prerequisite for a successful HPCT, it is estimated that 20% −50% of HLA-matched HPCT are ABO incompatible.[12] The geographically variable incidence of ABO Ag further highlights the difficulty that may occur if both HLA and ABO matching were equally imperative. Although there are numerous reports on ABO incompatibility in HPCT, the exact incidence of non-ABO red blood cell (RBC) Ag disparities within the transplant population remains unreported in any large investigation. As such, the standard doctrine of matching in HPCT is to minimize, as much as possible, the effect of the mismatch based on the following: ABO, then Rh, then other human erythrocyte Ag (HEA), particularly in pretransplant immunized recipients.

Immunologic Concepts in Transfusion Medicine. https://doi.org/10.1016/B978-0-323-67509-3.00013-5

Due to the separate chromosomal locations, HLA is inherited independently of the ABO blood group systems. The HLA system is found on chromosome 6p21, and the donor-recipient matching in this system is crucial for engraftment and clinical outcomes, while ABO system rendering carbohydrate glycosyltransferases are located on chromosome 9q34. Furthermore, ABO-incompatible HPCT are feasible due to the lack of ABO Ag expression on hematopoietic stem cells (HPCs), early pluripotent stem cells, and early committed HPC.[13] Also, the relatively low expression of RBC Ags on platelets (ABO antigens are generally absorbed from the plasma onto the platelet surface), and the mature cells of the myeloid and lymphoid lineages, allows for a permissive environment for successful posttransplant engraftment. In addition to the natural characteristics of the RBC Ag, posttransplant tolerance induction and therapeutic interventions like transfusion support, cellular therapy product (CTP) modification, and supportive immunomodulatory therapy aid in enabling RBC Ag–incompatible transplantation.

Blood Group Incompatibility Definitions

In broad terms, donor compatibility is traditionally defined, per Landsteiner law, by an absence of Ag when the recipient has preexisting Ab or has a potential to produce corresponding Ab. This definition is consistently applied to the ABO system due to the invariable presence of naturally occurring Ab. This compatibility definition has been adequately used for providing RBC transfusions and matching solid organ transplants. However, when discussing HPCT, the concept of "compatibility" is too narrow due to significant donor antirecipient reactivity as a form of GVH blood Ag.[14] Donor preformed Ab either anti-ABO isohemagglutinins (IH) or Ab from prior HEA immunization may be directly infused, produced upon stimulation of passenger lymphocytes, or by de-novo immunized stem cell–derived naïve lymphocytes, due to an impaired tolerance mechanism.[15] Those donor-derived Ab can target residual host RBC or constitutively expressed host Ag on endothelial and epithelial cells, or soluble proteins, resulting in a variety of clinical complications. As such, it is more fitting to describe HPCT in terms of matched or identical HPCT and mismatched HPCT being further recognized as major and minor incompatible transplants.

Based on the ABO matching between the donor and recipient, allogeneic HPCT can be categorized into four groups:
(1) ABO identical
(2) Major ABO incompatible: group A, B, or AB donors to group O recipients, and group AB donors to

group A or B recipients (A→O, B→O, AB→O, AB→A, AB→B)
(3) Minor ABO incompatible: group O donors to group A or B or AB recipients and group A or B donors to group AB recipients (O→A, O→B, O→AB, A→AB, B→AB)
(4) Bidirectional ABO mismatch is both major and minor incompatible: group A donors to group B recipients or group B donors to group A recipients (A→B, B→A)

Based on the Rh(D) matching between the donor and recipient, allogeneic HPCT can be categorized as:
(1) Rh(D) identical
(2) Major Rh(D) incompatibility: Rh(D) positive donors to Rh(D) negative recipients
(3) Minor Rh(D) incompatibility: Rh(D) negative donors to Rh(D) positive recipients

The same paradigm may be applied to other non-ABO blood groups; however, routine qualification and matching is not standard of care.

The major ABO incompatible group accounts for 20%–25% of transplants of HPCT[16] and is characterized by the recipient's preformed IH or residual lymphocytes producing anti-A and/or anti-B Ab directed against the donor's infused and/or newly engrafted RBCs. Similarly, 20%–25% of transplants of HPCT are of the minor ABO incompatible group. These HPCT transplants are characterized by the presence of anti-A and/or anti-B against the recipient's RBCs and ABO Ag expressed throughout the body. Bidirectional ABO incompatibility is the rarest of the HPCT ABO-incompatible group, accounting for <5% of all HPCT.[16]

An immunized recipient to non-ABO blood requires additional level of consideration and if possible search for HEA phenotypically matched donors. A successful HPCT can be achieved by mitigating transplant-related complications, immunosuppression, anticipatory adverse reaction management, and ultimately achieving chimerism and long-term tolerance. Furthermore, there are additional ABO and HEA mismatch considerations that are unique to allogeneic HPCT that must be taken into account. For example, the temporal relationship between the CTP infusion and postinfusion test result interpretation that can dictate the short-term and long-term management strategies.

IMMUNE RESPONSE TO RED BLOOD CELL AG

The cardinal role of the immune system is to protect against infectious agents, and its primary mechanism of operation is to distinguish self from nonself.[17]

Self-Ag recognized during early development is subject to tolerance. Nonself Ag recognition leads to activation of the immune cells, including effector and regulatory cell subsets.[18] The immune mechanisms underlying RBC alloimmunization are poorly understood. The primary characterization of immune response is focused on the humoral immune response and supporting helper T cell responses that drive Ab production.[19,20] The immunogenicity of a blood group antigen is an important factor determined by nature of the antigen Ags carbohydrate or protein, Ag density on RBC surface, presence of T helper epitopes, among other factors.[21,22] The Ag immunogenicity predicts if a person exposed to RBCs expressing that antigen during adult life will develop the corresponding allo-Ab.[23,24] Generally, the expression of blood group Ag during early fetal and neonatal life causes tolerance of self-reactive lymphocytes to these Ag, shaping the immune repertoire. Blood group Ags constitute interactive members of the human and primate mucosal innate immune system.[25,26] Surface glycoproteins are principal receptors used by pathogens to invade target cells. The blood group glycoproteins can serve as a pathogen decoy.[27] Those Ags are also expressed by numerous microorganisms. Consequently, absence of anti-ABO and anti-non-ABO Ab in the immune repertoire limits adaptive immunity toward pathogens bearing cognate blood group Ag or biosimilar cross-reactive Ag.[28] The innate immune response incorporates defense lectins, which can provide immunity against pathogens that express blood group-like Ag on their surfaces. Defense lectins, such as galectin-4 and galectin-8, are expressed in the intestinal tract, and recognize and kill independent of complement *Escherichia coli* expressing human blood group Ag–B.[28] Similarly, blood group antigens play a role in pathogen cell entry like MNS glycophorins.[29] Duffy (Fya/Fyb), a receptor for malaria, is an evolutionary driver of Ag expression and geographic distribution of HEA.[30,31] Also, RBCs exert modulatory activity on innate and adaptive immune cells.[32–35]

Humoral Immune Response to RBC Ag
Naturally occurring Ab
Two distinct subsets of B lymphocytes, the B1 subset (CD51) and the B2 subset (CD52), produce a "naturally occurring" Ab response "without prior stimulation" in a T cell–independent manner. This type of response is termed the innate immune system and includes the ABO IH and other Ab produced against carbohydrate Ag as part of the innate immune system.[36] Some investigators believe that ABO IH are initially produced "spontaneously" from a fixed set of ancestral germline genes found in B1 B lymphocytes.[37,38] Newborns have mostly B1 B lymphocytes and produce only IgM Ab, including ABO IH, early in life.[39]

The B2 or conventional B lymphocyte subset function within the humoral response of the adaptive immune system and are dependent on T cells for their activation. It is known that IgG IH, like anti-A, anti-B, can be further stimulated, in response to bacterial and/or food Ag and may be boosted during pregnancy, transfusion, or transplant.[40] Capacity to provide help during response to T cell–dependent ABO system antigens is restricted to individuals of blood group O.[41]

Unexpected or irregular Ab
The terms unexpected or irregular Ab traditionally refer to Ab stimulated by pregnancy, transfusion, or transplant to non-ABO Ags. In general, those are protein Ags that require presence of alloreactive T cell epitopes.[42,22] Upon exposure to another person's RBC, through either transfusion or pregnancy, the primary immune response can be initiated, culminating in the formation of new Ab.[23] This may take up to several months, and the Ab may remain detectable, or may disappear over time without further stimulation. If reexposed to the Ag, the secondary anamnestic immune response can begin, with rapid development of an IgG Ab. This may be 3–14 days post reexposure. This scenario is relevant to post HPCT developed hemolysis as well.

Tolerance to RBC Ag
Exposure to antigens early in life may lead to tolerance rather than immunogenicity. However tolerance to incompatible A and B blood group antigens does not occur following placement of ABO-incompatible homografts in late childhood and adult life.[43] The mechanisms responsible for immune tolerance induction via mixed chimerism after hematopoietic stem cell transplantation (HSCT) are not well established. ABO(H) histo-blood group antigens, expressed on recipient endothelial cells did not demonstrate evidence of chimerism after ABO-incompatible HSCT, contributing to tolerance.[44] ABO blood group Ags are covalently attached to plasma von Willebrand factor (vWF). vWF is synthesized exclusively by endothelial cells and megakaryocytes, and is constitutively secreted into plasma. In ABO-mismatched HSCT, the ABO(H) blood group Ags on the vWF are consistent with the recipient's blood group. Furthermore, independent of the donor-derived erythrocytes, it is possible that persistence of the recipient's blood group Ag on plasma glycoproteins, such as vWF, may influence the immunological system

in the production of anti-blood group Ab, resulting in the establishment of immunological tolerance in the recipient plasma.[45]

BLOOD GROUP AG AND CORRESPONDING AB CHARACTERISTICS

At present, 36 blood group systems representing over 350 Ags are listed by International Standard for Blood and Transplant (ISBT),[46] the scientific society that defines and classifies the RBC Ag. HEAs are characterized utilizing both serologic and molecular evidence. Important and clinically significant Ags are discussed here as they relate to complications of non-ABO-incompatible stem cell transplantations. However, a review of all 36 blood groups is beyond the scope of this chapter. A summary of some of the clinically significant Ag and their biochemical composition are found in Table 13.1. For a more detailed description of RBC Ag and the Ab characteristics,[47] the ISBT and the *Blood Group Antigen FactsBook* are excellent resources.[48]

ABO Blood Group System

Blood group A, group B, and group AB were originally discovered by Dr. Karl Landsteiner in the early 1900s.[49] The function of the ABO blood group Ag are not definitively known and those lacking the A and B Ag, namely blood type O, are considered otherwise healthy genetic variants. This blood group system consists of the four distinct antigens A, A1, B, and A,B Ag

that vary in expression on the RBC surface, other cells and structures. They are complex carbohydrate structures synthetized in a stepwise addition of common sugars. The carbohydrate backbone on which A and B are synthesized is the H Ag (Fig. 13.1). Blood type O individuals have only H Ag and, therefore, the ABO(H) terminology also has been used in the literature. While the antigenic activity is determined by the sugars residing on the carbohydrate structures, the genes that determine an individual's ABO blood group Ag, in fact, codes for the sugar-transferring glycosyltransferases.

The gene encoding the glycosyltransferase enabling the attachment of the L-fucose to the polypeptide backbone is found on chromosome 19. If no A or B functional gene is present, this backbone is the basis for the O blood group. The genes encoding the ABO carbohydrate glycosyltransferases are located on chromosome 9q34. The ABO locus has three main allelic forms: A, B, and O. The A allele encodes a glycosyltransferase (ABO, α-1-3-N-acetylgalactosaminyltransferase)[50] that produces the A Ag (N-acetylgalactosamine as the immunodominant sugar). Similarly, the B allele encodes a glycosyltransferase (α-1-3-galactosyltransferase) that creates the B Ag (D-galactose as the immunodominant sugar). The O allele is similar to the A but has a one base deletion, forming a frame shift with a premature transcriptional stop. This results in the lack of a functional glycosyltransferase and the generation of the O blood type null phenotype.[51]

TABLE 13.1
Summary of Selected Clinically Significant RBC Antigens In Transplant.

Blood Group System	Gene Function	Antigen Physical and Chemical Nature	Number of Antigens	Major Antigens
ABO	Glycosyltransferases	Carbohydrate	4	A, B, A'B, A1
H	Fucosyltransferases	Carbohydrate	1	H
Lewis (Le)	Fucosyltransferases	Carbohydrate	6	Lea, Leb
MNS	Negative charge on sialic acid	Carbohydrate	46	M, N, S, s, U
P1PK	Galactosyltransferase	Glucoside	3	P1, pk, NOR
Rh (004)	Structural link	Protein	52	D, C, E, c, e,
RHAG (030)	Ammonia transport	Protein		
Kell (K)	Enzyme, role in vasoconstrictor	Protein	34	K, K, Kpa, Kpb, Jsa, Jsb
Duffy (Fy)	Chemokine receptor	Protein	5	Fya, Fyb, Fy3, Fy6
Kidd (Jk)	Urea transport	Protein	3	Jka, Jkb, Jk3

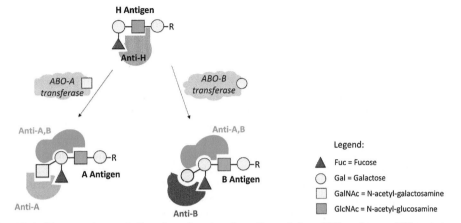

FIG. 13.1 Diagram demonstrating the stepwise formation of the ABO antigens. Different terminal immunodominant sugars are attached by the various types of glycosyltransferases and specifically recognized by antibodies. The addition of L-fucose by its fucosyl-transfurase generates O red cell antigen and the precursor backbone for the A, and B antigens. The ABO-A, alpha 1-3-N-acetylgalactosaminyltransferase produces the A antigen with the N-acetylgalactosamine is its immunodominant sugar. Similarly, ABO-B, alpha 1-3-galactosyltransferase creates the B antigen, with D-galactose is its immunodominant sugar. There is no functional glycosyltransferase that is encoded by the O allele. Therefore the O blood group antigen is simply the precursor backbone that was generated by the fucosyl-transfurase.

Fucosylated glycans, including H-Ag, may play critical roles in hematopoietic progenitor cell homing, adhesion, growth, and differentiation. H-active Ag, which are strongly expressed on CD34$^+$ progenitor cells and committed megakaryocytic progenitors, may mediate adhesion to marrow stromal fibroblasts.[52] The ABO blood group also may influence the composition of human intestinal microbiota.[53,54]

The A and B alleles of the ABO system are codominant, whereas the null O alleles are recessive.[51] The ABO blood group is the first molecular polymorphism to be characterized in humans. The ABO gene was cloned in 1990 following purification of A transferase; since then, over 300 different alleles have been described. Two amino acids at positions 266 and 268 in exon 7 are responsible for the A and B enzymatic specificity in humans. ABO Ags circulate in body fluids and are attached to lipids at the surface of various gastrointestinal tract epithelial cells and endothelial cells; however, they are present in RBCs only in hominids.[55,56] The phylogenetic origin of hominids—Old and New World monkey—have diverged many times in the millions of years under a model of convergent evolution. These data suggest that A is the ancestral allele and a major turnover with a neutral substitution occurred on the branch leading to Old World monkey.[57] This finding also argues that the benefit of IH in antimicrobial immunity was influenced by

geographical location. The frequency of the ABO Ag and its worldwide distribution pattern follows a complex evolutionary history.[58] In general, group O blood type is the most common around the world in humans, with about 65% of the world's population phenotypically typing as group O. This is particularly true for the indigenous populations in South America, where it approaches 100%. The lowest frequency of O is found in Asian countries, where group A or B blood types are more common. The group A blood type is more common worldwide than group B, with about 20% of the world's population typing as group A. Finally, the group B blood type is the rarest worldwide, with only 15% of the world's population typing as B. This diversity in ABO group distribution can influence the frequency of ABO mismatch.[59]

Anti-ABO Antibodies

Ab to the ABO Ag, anti-A, anti-A1, anti-B, and anti-A,B are clinically significant as they are naturally occurring, universally found, and strongly reactive with a strong propensity for causing acute hemolysis through complement activation. These Ab consist of immunoglobulin (IgM, IgG, and IgA classes). Anti-H (IgM) is seen in a null phenotype Bombay Oh (Fig. 13.1, Table 13.2).

ABH Ags are developed in utero early in fetal life and establish tolerance toward the expressed Ag. The early production of "noncorresponding" anti-ABO Ab is stimulated when the immune system encounters the "nonself" ABO blood group Ag. ABH-like Ags are ubiquitously found in the environment, present in food and microbiota. The very early exposure to the ABH Ag results in the development of Ab early in neonatal life, with ABO Ab formation within the first 3 months of age and peaking at 10 years.[60] Therefore, anti-A and anti-B of IgM class are found in the plasma of individuals lacking the corresponding A and B Ag: namely group A have anti-B, group B have anti-A, while group AB have neither Ab. Group O have anti-A, anti-B, and in addition a high affinity IgG anti-A,B that can be especially significant in developing a high titer in HPCT. Glycoprotein blood Ag akin to protein epitopes might have a high immunogenicity, and they may elicit anti-A,B IgG in a T helper cell–dependent fashion.[41] (Table 13.2).

The combination of the high level of ABO Ag expression on RBC and the potent high affinity Ab present in circulation leads to the destruction of transfused incompatible RBC. This manifests as acute intravascular hemolysis or delayed hemolysis, due to the destruction of the erythroid membrane adjacent to the Ab-Ag complex, or by frank hemophagocytosis.[61,62]

Non-ABO RBC Ag and Ab Considerations

As discussed throughout this chapter, despite their relative immunosuppressed state, HPCT patients are at risk for alloimmunization.[63–65] Outside of the ABO blood

group system, the non-ABO Ag generally may not be taken in consideration when selecting an allogeneic donor, unless there is a preexisting recipient and/or donor immunization. Mismatching of the non-ABO systems has different implications compared to the ABO Ag system and has differing clinical significance in HPCT matching. This rationale primarily stems from the fact that non-ABO system allo-Abs are relatively rare in comparison to the ABO system, and incompatibility (major or minor) is taken into consideration only if the recipient or donor have had previous exposure to the Ag, such as in pregnancy or prior transfusion (Table 13.1). It has been estimated that between 1% and 8% of HPCT patients develop non-ABO red cell allo-Ab in the post HPCT period.[66,67] Furthermore, the literature has described relatively few non-ABO Ag clinically significant Abs that have led to acute major and minor hemolysis, delayed RBC engraftment, pure red cell aplasia (PRCA), or passenger lymphocyte syndrome (PLS). These cases included mismatches in the Rh, Kell, Kidd, Lewis, MNS, Diego, and other RBC Ag systems.[66,68] Therefore, when unexpected allo-Ab are developed, extended phenotypically matched RBCs that are compatible with both recipient and donor can then be provided.

One of the most commonly encountered non-ABO Ag involved with hemolysis in HPCT is the Rh system, particularly Rh-D incompatibility.[69,70] If either recipient or donor is Rh negative, a common approach to

TABLE 13.2
Basic ABO Blood Group System Summarizing The Genetic Basis of The ABO Groups, Their Antigens and Resulting Naturally Occurring Antibodies.

Genes	ABO Group	Antigens	Phenotypes/Subgroups	Allo Antibodies
A transferase FUT1	A	H, A, A1, A'B H, A, A'B	A1 A2	Anti-B (IgM)
B transferase FUT1	B	H, B A'B	B	Anti-A (IgM) Anti-A1(IgM)
A transferase B transferase FUT1	AB	H, A, A1, B, A'B H, A, B, A'B	A1B A2B	None
None* FUT1	O	H		Anti-A (IgM) Anti-A1 (IgM) Anti-B (IgM) Anti-A'B (IgG)
None* or A transferase and/or B transferase	Bombay Oh	None		Anti-H (IgM) Anti-A (IgM) Anti-A1 (IgM) Anti-B (IgM) Anti-A'B (IgG)

transfusion practice would dictate Rh negative RBCs be provided until which point the blood type has converted to that of the donor. This practice aims in preventing the generation of de novo anti-D; however, there are little to no reports of severe clinical consequences with this Ab.[71] Furthermore, the literature has suggested that due to the immunocompromised state of HPCT recipients, there is an incidence of only 5% of anti-D alloimmunization in Rh D−mismatched HPCT.[71] Therefore, weighing the individual institutions' blood component resources against the clinical importance of these Abs (as with those patients of childbearing age), the decision may be made to not provide Rh D negative RBCs during the engraftment period. Regardless, as Rh D alloimmunization can result in hemolysis, HPCT patients with a preexisting Ab against Rh D should be transfused with Rh D negative RBC until the Ab is no longer detected on screening and on crossmatch.

The Kidd (Jk^a/Jk^b) system has also been implicated in causing hemolysis in HPCT recipients. These reports often fault the severe intravascular hemolysis to a passenger lymphocyte mechanism, which is discussed in more detail below.[72] Lastly, the Lewis Ag system is a curious system implicated in HPCT hemolysis, in that the Ag is not part of the red cell membrane, but a soluble Ag found in body fluids and the phenotype is acquired by Lewis substance absorption from the plasma. As such, the recipient continues to express the Ag even after engraftment of a Lewis-mismatched HPCT, and reports have attributed hemolysis to anti-Lewis Ab of donor origin.[73]

CLINICAL COMPLICATIONS OF BLOOD AG−MISMATCHED TRANSPLANT

The unique immunological circumstances that arise when crossing the ABO blood group barrier in ABO-incompatible HPCT can lead to a variety of immunohematological complications. These include hemolytic anemia (HA), delayed erythroid engraftment, GVHD, transplant-associated thrombotic microangiopathy (TAM), among others.

Although the underlying disease, conditioning and immunosuppressant agents, infection, and GVHD are major cause of transplant-related morbidity, blood group−mismatched transplant might contribute to unfavorable transplant-related outcomes, including TRM, and overall survival.

Immune-Mediated Hemolysis

Hemolysis is a cardinal symptom of blood group incompatibility and is predominantly complement mediated or RBCs are lyzed by antibody-dependent cell-mediated cytotoxicity.[74,75] Hemolysis can present during or immediately postinfusion of CTPs or as a delayed hemolysis. Immediate hemolysis is especially a concern in major ABO-incompatible HPCT due to presence of incompatible RBC in the infused product. However, immediate hemolysis may also be encountered in minor ABO-incompatible HPCT with high IH titers.

Delayed hemolysis in major incompatible transplant presents as a delayed erythroid engraftment/PRCA. Delayed hemolysis in minor incompatible transplant usually presents as a transient HA due to an expansion of passenger lymphocytes.

Acute hemolytic reaction due to major ABO incompatibility

Acute hemolytic reactions may occur due to a major ABO incompatibility as the CTP may contain significant amounts of donor RBCs. For the most part, the source of the CTP, or HPC, determines the volume of contaminating RBC in the stem cell product. For example, HPCs derived from bone marrow (HPC-M) generally produce a large, 1−1.5 L product. It is not uncommon for these products to contain donor-derived Ab and a hematocrit of 20%−30%. These collections significantly increase the risk of immediate immune-mediated hemolysis and, despite RBC and plasma volume reduction during HPC processing, the HPC-M products continue to possess an inherent risk of hemolysis. In recent decades, HPCT have been increasingly collected from peripheral blood by apheresis (HPC-A), after the mobilization of hematopoietic progenitor cells by agents such as granulocyte colony stimulating factor (G-CSF) or plerixafor, a small molecule that selectively inhibits the chemokine receptor CXCR4. Compared to HPC-M, HPC-A products contain smaller RBC and plasma volumes, 20−40 mL and 150−300 mL, respectively. This alone can minimize the risk of immediate immune-mediated hemolysis. Similarly, after standard RBC and plasma reduction, cord blood product total volume is about 20 mL, resulting in minimal to no risk of acute hemolysis during infusion. Of note, older processing technique of "RBC replete" cord blood can produce acute hemolysis even in ABO-matched units due to a cryopreservation injury of RBC. Current standard practice for a major ABO incompatibility dictates 0.4 mL RBC/kg of the adult recipient's weight, or approximately 20−40 mL, as a tolerable limit of donor RBC contamination. RBC depletion may also be done on an ABO-identical or autologous bone marrow product to alleviate a nonimmune hemolysis due to damage of erythrocytes during cryopreservation and thawing. Treatment for postinfusion hemolysis includes hydration, acidification, and symptomatic support. When multiple CTPs are to be infused, postponing the remainder of the HPCT infusion may also be a management option.

Delayed engraftment/pure red cell aplasia due to major ABO incompatibility

High-recipient Ab titers in major ABO-incompatible HPCT can cause chronic hemolysis of donor RBCs, leading to delayed engraftment and, in severe cases, development of PRCA. PRCA is characterized by the by a failure of erythropoiesis but with preservation of the myeloid and megakaryocytic cell lineages (Fig 13.2). HA seen in major incompatible HPCT can persist for months, or even years posttransplant.

It is most frequently observed in Group O recipients receiving group A HPCT and is the result of residual recipient B lymphocytes/plasma cells producing Ab directed against the donor RBC. Red cell lineage engraftment is defined as the number of days required for a reticulocyte count $\geq 25 \times 10^9$/L. It may take up to 3—4 months before recipient's Ab titer declines sufficiently, allowing the engraftment of newly emerging donor reticulocytes to occur. During this time period, the patient is often transfusion dependent, and laboratory testing may reveal direct antiglobulin test (DAT) positivity, with anti-A or anti-B Ab in the eluate. A persistence of a high titer IgG anti-A,B Ab detected plays a significant role in duration of hemolysis. As the RBC engraftment proceeds, DAT may become negative and transfusion dependence decreases due to the sustained RBC production by the new graft. Time to red cell engraftment may be further prolonged if nonmyeloablative regimens or reduced intensity conditioning are used.

Delayed engraftment with remaining reticulocytes <1% for more than 28 days after transplantation, and relative absence or erythroid precursors in bone marrow (Fig. 13.2),[76] is defined as PRCA. Various therapeutic modalities may be used as treatment, including high-dose corticosteroids and rituximab.[77,78] Efficacy of therapeutic plasma exchange (TPE) for PRCA treatment has been established, but it is currently reserved only for severe cases. However, these therapies may not be any more successful than sustained transfusions for the patient. In fact, severe pancytopenia associated with PRCA may require a second HPCT. Although not currently approved for use in the United States, an additional option in refractory cases is the use of Ig-Therasorb immunoadsorption for

the removal of residual persistent IH Ab.[77,79,80] Factors that complicate the diagnosis of PRCA are the determination of stem cell dose appropriateness, extent of disease, and the chemotherapy conditioning regimen effect on the bone marrow niche. Concurrent iron deficiency and presence of microangiopathic hemolytic anemia (MAHA) processes also need to be considered during PRCA diagnosis and are discussed below.

Acute hemolytic reaction due to minor ABO incompatibility

Acute hemolytic reactions may also occur due to minor ABO incompatibility. If Ab titers in an HPC collection product exceed 1:256, acute infusion-related hemolysis attributable to ABO incompatibility may be seen.[81] HPC products from donors with known high-plasma Ab titers may be plasma reduced so that the risk of minor incompatibility may be minimized. In fact, this type of HPC plasma reduction is performed routinely as part of standard cryopreservation protocols. This is analogous to RBC depletion in major incompatible HPCT described previously.

Passenger lymphocyte syndrome

During a minor ABO-incompatible HPCT, mature memory lymphocytes in the CTP may recognize recipient RBC, producing significant IH titers or Ab titers against non-ABO RBC Ag. This phenomenon is termed PLS and is seen most often in HPCT involving a group O donor receiving a group A CTP due to the presence of Anti-A,B IgG. HA of PLS manifests itself typically 7—15 days post HPCT, with the recipient experiencing potentially life-threatening acute hemolysis. Laboratory testing will indicate signs of intravascular hemolysis, such as elevated levels of lactate dehydrogenase (LDH), hemoglobinuria, and hemoglobinemia, as well as a positive DAT. Most cases eventually subside upon the clearance of recipient RBC and as the HPCT progresses to engraftment. Ab developed during PLS frequently does not persist and present only as an ABO discrepancy during HPCT engraftment phase.[82] If the hemolysis is especially severe, automated RBC exchange may aid in the removal of the recipient RBC. Of note, CD34 selected products devoid of immune lymphocytes do not pose a risk for PLS development.

Blood Group Incompatibility as an Adverse Risk Factor for Transplant Outcome
Graft rejection

Allogeneic HSC graft rejection can manifest as the lack of initial engraftment, primary graft failure, or as a

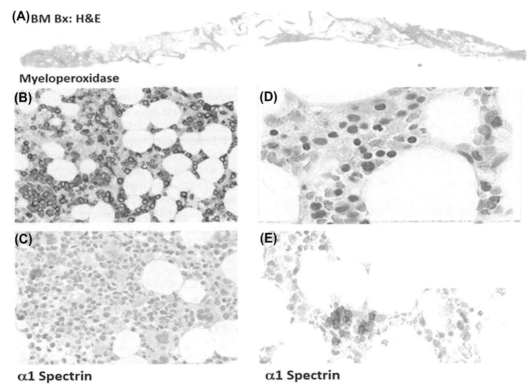

FIG. 13.2 Bone marrow biopsy demonstrating Pure Red Cell Aplasia (PRCA) secondary to HSCT selected erythroid engraftment failure. This bone marrow biopsy was taken from an adult patient after receiving a HSCT due to diffuse lard B cell lymphoma. **(A)** Hematoxylin and eosin stain, 2x. and **(B)** 100x demonstrating a paucity of erythroid precurors. Note in **(D** and **E)** only 1 area of an erythroid precursor cluster was identified within the entire biopsy. **(B)** 40x; myeloperoxidase staining demonstrates the myeloid lineage within the bone marrow, which stains abundantly. Immunohistochemical staining for alpha-1 Spectrin in **(C)** 40x and **(E)** 100x, highlights the lack of erythroid precursors within this marrow, with only one cluster identified in **(E)**, which correlates with the image in **(B)**.

secondary graft loss after initial engraftment. The immunologic mechanism against the donor HPCT is believed to be due to a cellular rather than a humoral mediated response. The response may be mounted by recipient T lymphocytes, but other mechanisms have been proposed, such as a natural killer cell–mediated rejection or Ab-mediated rejection.[83] The major risk factor for graft failure is an HLA mismatch, while blood group incompatibility can be a modulating factor.

The role of major ABO mismatch in graft failure remains controversial,[84] and there has been literature suggesting that the use of ABO major incompatible graft increases the risk of graft failure after unrelated donor HPCT.[85,59] One study had observed a graft failure of 7.5% in major ABO-incompatible HPCT compared to the 0.6% in minor ABO-incompatible HPCT.[86] Blood group O individuals are known to have larger amounts

of immune anti-A,B IgG Ab that can contribute to overall graft failure.[87] Some individuals have higher levels of ABO Ag expression on platelets that can contribute to delayed platelet engraftment.[88,59] It is believed that additional factors beyond the ABO incompatibility may have influenced the graft failure observed in these studies as further studies have not found such high incidence of graft failure.[16,83,89]

Graft-versus-host disease
GVHD is a common complication of allogeneic CTPs containing mature memory lymphocytes against minor histocompatibility Ag.[90] Interestingly, there is a higher risk of GVHD associated with minor ABO incompatibility. One explanation is the association of Ab reacting to the ABO Ag on the recipient endothelium, leading to intravascular cell damage and upregulation of HLA,

culminating in cytokines potentiation and immune cell activation. Another possible explanation describes the formation of immune complexes between the Ab and soluble ABO Ag, which contributes to the amplification of a bystander effect. An interesting observation in major ABO incompatibility is the expression or passive adsorption of ABO on donor lymphocytes, possibly allowing the removal of GVHD reactive lymphocytes from circulation. The rate of disappearance of recipients IH was positively correlated with the rate of acute GVHD.[91] This is consistent with the observation that IgG-producing cells of host origin persisted only in patients without clinical evidence of GVHD.[92]

Transplant-related mortality
ABO incompatibility can play a role in graft rejection and overall survival.[93,94] Both ABO minor and major incompatibilities in HPCT are risk factors for worse transplantation outcomes.[95] However, the associated hazards may not be uniform across different transplantation populations.[96,45,97] Likewise, challenge in providing adequately matched transfusion components might be another confounding factor.[98,99]

Relapse
As proposed in some studies, risk of relapse may be associated with ABO group mismatch due to graft versus tumor effect.[100–102] However, larger studies failed to confirm these findings.[8,59,88,103]

Transplant-associated thrombotic microangiopathy
TAM is characterized by MAHA, thrombocytopenia, and microvascular thrombosis. This entity is rarely seen in HPCT; however, it must be considered in the differential diagnosis of a posttransplant HA.[104] TAM usually has poor prognosis and is refractory to standard treatments such as TPE. Unlike thrombotic thrombocytopenic purpura (TTP), wherein there is an inborn or acquired deficiency of ADAMTS13, the exact pathophysiology of TAM remains unclear. Veno-occlusive disease (VOD), with or without multiorgan dysfunction, after HPCT can be influenced by platelet transfusion containing ABO-incompatible plasma and is a major limiting factor of high-dose chemotherapy in children. TAM and VOD should be always considered in the differential diagnosis of anemia and thrombocytopenia in the posttransplant period. The typical intravascular hemolysis laboratory values, such as elevated LDH, bilirubin, serum creatinine, and decreased haptoglobin, will be observed. Although rarely performed, diagnosis may be confirmed by renal biopsy.

Reduced intensity conditioning
Use of RIC regimen pretransplant is associated with an increased incidence, up to 30%, of severe delayed immune hemolysis in minor ABO-mismatched HSCT.[81] Nonmyeloablative regimens for allo-HPCT are increasingly used as graft-versus-leukemia and/or tumor effects can be achieved with minimal additional toxicities and lower risk of TRM than with standard myeloablative transplants. Following RIC regimens, mixed chimerism of both hematopoietic myeloid and lymphoid subsets are observed. The immune response observed are both of host and donor in origin for variable periods after transplant, with a delayed disappearance of host allo-Ab-producing plasma cells. Thus, the risks of hemolytic reactions, delayed RBC engraftment, and PRCA may be higher in cases of donor-recipient ABO incompatibility when RIC regimens are used.[88,105]

LABORATORY TESTING
Outside of the clinical setting of HPCT, a patient's anemia typically is uncovered through history and physical, followed by laboratory testing in order to rule out hemolysis. By comparison, hemolysis often does occur during and after ABO-incompatible HPCT, and a high index of suspicion is required during the engraftment process. As discussed above, a variety of immune-hematological complications may arise during HPCT; however, other nonimmune causes of hemolysis should also be considered. Laboratory testing is mentioned while discussing complications of blood Ag–mismatched HPCT. The following will briefly summarize relevant laboratory testing used while monitoring the engraftment process in HPCT.

In general, the standard laboratory testing is performed in patients undergoing HPCT as would be with any patient with a suspicion of HA. Assessment of hemoglobin, a complete blood count, blood smears and blood chemistries of bilirubin, LDH, and creatinine are standard and essential. Monitoring for the decrease of haptoglobin and hemoglobinuria can be of use as well. If there is a suspicion of TAM, ADAMTS13 measurement may also be performed. One of the most useful standard tests in evaluating immune-mediated hemolysis are ABO forward and reverse typing for evaluation of blood group conversion,[106] the DAT, the elution testing, and Ab titrations. Other common blood back techniques like serologic phenotyping or autologous adsorption are not appropriate due to different levels of chimerism posttransplant. Differential allogeneic adsorption is frequently utilized. Tests unique to the HPCT patient population include genomic DNA analysis of both recipient and donor. DNA extracted from circulating (nucleated) white blood cells is used for HEA and HPA genotyping, to aid transfusion strategy.

Direct Antiglobulin Test

DAT testing, also known as the direct Coombs test, detects in vivo coating of RBC by Ab or complement, and evaluates for the resulting agglutination. It is one of the most useful tests in distinguishing immune from nonimmune causes of hemolysis, although its interpretation must always be made within proper clinical context. IgM or IgG Ab against RBC Ag may bind RBC, causing agglutination, although IgG Ab usually do not produce direct agglutination. In order to detect IgG Ab on RBCs via agglutination, the DAT requires the addition of a secondary Ab that can bind human globulin (the anti-human globulin, or AHG). AHG reagents may be specific against the IgG Ab or the complement Ab, such as C3b/d.

Once it is determined that an Ab is bound to the RBC (i.e., a positive DAT), an eluate may be performed. As the name suggests, the bound Abs are eluted from the sensitized RBCs using a variety of techniques, such as acid washes or heat. Once the Abs are removed, they may be identified by standard practices, and the results may be utilized in determining appropriate transfusion strategy.

Isohemagglutinin Titer Testing

Once the presence of an Ab is detected and it is identified, the Ab titer can measure the relative amount of the Ab within the patient's (or donor's) plasma. In general, the titer can correlate to the strength of the Ab response. The Ab titer is useful throughout the HPCT process. For example, it may be used prior to transplantation for Ab level assessment in either the donor or recipient in an ABO or non-ABO-incompatible HPCT. Additionally, prior to transplant, some institutions may attempt to prevent complications of major ABO-incompatible HPCT and reduce the Ab titers of the recipient via TPE. However, there is no consensus within the literature on this strategy. Ab titers may be followed during the engraftment period, allowing the monitoring of the recipient's Ab titer as they decline, an indication of the engraftment of newly emerging donor reticulocytes.

Pretransplant Genotyping

The molecular basis of the RBC Ag, or the HEA, has been established, and molecular gene polymorphisms responsible for >300 blood-groups Ag have been identified.[51] When serological RBC phenotyping cannot be performed, the phenotype can be reliably predicted from genotype results.[107] Interestingly, genotyping can be more challenging for the ABO and Rh systems due to the ABO system consisting of genes encoding ABO transferases and the Rh system's association with a large number of insertions, deletions, and hybrid gene formation.

Post-HPCT patient phenotype prediction based on genotype is complicated by a mixed chimerism that can present as an indeterminate result. Of note, leukocytes from transfused units do not interfere with this determination. However, if there is a discrepant engraftment of myeloid and erythroid lineage especially when evaluating blood group–mismatched transplant, it might be challenging to delineate predicted HEA from recipient and donor.[108] Pretransplant samples from both recipient and donor or a buccal swab of recipient could aid in the result resolution.[109]

Methodologies for genotyping, such as multiplex systems, have been optimized for the simultaneous detection of multiple HLA, HEA, and human platelets Ag (HPA). This type of testing has become invaluable in coordinating transplant and transfusion management. In this regard, it can be foreseen that RBC genotyping may be implemented for routine pre-transplant testing of transplant recipients and donors. Furthermore, multiplex genotyping systems that simultaneously detect of RBC, HPA, and molecular HLA can potentially allow the screening of individuals and large populations of donors. This practice shows promise for improving the efficiency, reliability, and extent of RBC matching in transplant-recipient population, especially if it could be coimplemented with informatics systems, allowing matching of transplant patients' Ag profiles with available Ag-negative and/or rare blood-typed donors.

THERAPEUTICS SUPPORT

As alloimmunization may lead to hemolysis and other severe clinical consequences during HPCT, mitigation strategies limiting the development of alloimmunization can be undertaken.[110] Additionally, steps may be taken to limit the damage that can occur as ABO and non-ABO Ab develop in the HSC recipient.

Transfusion Support of Transplant Patients

The transfusion requirements before, during, and after an HPCT can be significant and can affect transplant-related morbidity and long-term survival outcomes.[111] Transfusion strategies in ABO-incompatible HPCT can become complicated, as there is need to focus on the compatibility of both the recipient and the donor, while at the same time avoiding transfusion of Ab directed against residual recipient's RBC.[112] Furthermore, decisions as to when to change the donor blood type may vary from institution to institution.

Providing transfusion support during HPCT takes into account both the aforementioned major and minor ABO incompatibilities and the phase of HPCT. Transfusion during HPCT can be separated into three phases: phase I occurring during the preparative regimen, phase II during engraftment, and phase III as postengraftment.

During phase I of HPCT, transfusion support and indications are similar to those of other hematologic malignancies, namely focusing on irradiation and leukoreduction of blood components. The blood components received by the patient can be of the recipient type. Additionally, there may be avoidance of donations from family members to prevent alloimmunization against minor histocompatibility and low-incidence Ag, which may increase the risk of graft rejection.

Transfusion during phase II of the HPCT requires careful attention to the ABO compatibility of both the recipient and donor, as the composition of cells may be arising from the patient's original bone marrow while transitioning to that of the donor. Also, the recipient's anti-A or anti-B may persist within the recipient's circulation. As discussed in the laboratory testing above, there also may be ABO discrepancies in pretransfusion testing during this phase. During this phase, the type of ABO incompatibility must be taken into consideration when selecting blood components.

As mentioned previously, a major ABO incompatibility is present if the recipient possesses or has the potential to possess preformed Ab directed against the donor graft. This occurs in all group O recipients who receive non–group O HPCT. It may also occur in group A or group B recipients who receiving a group AB HPCT. The most significant complications that can occur in this type of incompatibility are hemolysis, delayed RBC engraftment, or PRCA. Therefore, the major focus of transfusion support in major ABO-incompatible HPCT is the compatibility of the RBC transfused and the avoidance of Ab directed against the newly engrafting RBCs. This is accomplished by transfusing RBC of the recipient type and, in order to prevent delayed engraftment of donor cells, plasma components of the donor type. Other considerations include RBC depletion of plasma components during processing; however, products collected by apheresis usually have less than 30 mL of RBC and rarely are cause for severe

hemolysis. Also, TPE can be considered prior to HPC product infusion if the recipient has very high anti-A or anti-B titers.

Conversely, a minor ABO incompatibility is present if the donor's plasma contains Ab directed against the recipients RBC. This occurs, for example, when recipient is group A, B, or AB and donor is type O. A similar scenario occurs when the recipient is group AB and receives an HPCT from a group A or B donor. The most significant complications that can occur in this type of incompatibility are hemolysis of the recipient's RBC at the time of the infusion, followed by delayed hemolysis of the recipient's RBC secondary to the stimulation of the donor B lymphocytes. As such, the transfusion strategy during phase II in minor ABO-incompatible HPCT should focus on RBC compatibility with both the donor and recipient, in addition to the avoidance of Ab directed against the residual RBC of recipient origin. Therefore, the RBC transfused should be that of the donor's type and platelets and/or plasma must be of the recipient. Other considerations include the plasma depletion of HPC products during processing in order to avoid hemolysis of incompatible circulating recipient RBC.

Finally, bidirectional ABO incompatibility, or the presence of both major and minor ABO incompatibilities in the same HPCT, occurs when a group A recipient receives a group B HPCT (or vice versa). The complications mentioned in the major and minor incompatibilities apply to bidirectional ABO incompatibility. When devising a transfusion strategy in phase II of a bidirectional ABO-incompatible HPCT, only group O RBC can be transfused as all other types of RBC would be incompatible. Similarly, AB plasma components would be first choice, as all other types would contain Ab incompatible with the RBC. Another strategy to consider includes the RBC and plasma depletion of the HPC-M products to minimize hemolysis.

Once the donor RBC have engrafted in phase III of the HPCT, the patient may receive transfusion of all components of the donor type. However, some institutions prefer to also consider the fact that there is expression of ABO Ag of the recipient type on cells other than RBC, for instance, the endothelial lining. Therefore, transfusion of plasma components compatible with both the donor and recipient in phase II may also be considered. Namely, in major ABO incompatibility, platelets and plasma can be of donor type while in minor ABO-incompatible/bidirectional incompatible HPCT, platelets and plasma can be of the recipient type.

Iron overload, a complication arising from frequent transfusions before and during engraftment, may lead to hemosiderosis-related adverse effects. As such, transfusions should be minimized and iron chelation should be provided to prevent such complications. Of note, thalassemia major, myelodysplastic syndrome, or SCD patients, having received multiple lifetime RBC transfusions and showing evidence of hepatic iron overload, often have poor HPCT outcomes.

Therapeutic Apheresis

The use of TPE has been discussed throughout this chapter in terms of overall management and support of HPCT patients. The success of TPE requires that the source or substance to be removed from the plasma be removed efficiently enough to allow resolution. Therefore, TPE has been utilized only in very specific situations during the course of an HPCT. Hemolysis in major ABO-incompatible HPCT has been minimized by limiting the RBC within the CTP, either via the RBC reduction of HPC-M products or the use of HPC-A. If an RBC-reduced HPC product cannot be used, TPE may be utilized before HPCT in order to reduce recipient anti-A and/or anti-B titers. In these situations, the intravascular IgM will be more effectively removed than the IgG Ab, as IgG is found in both the intravascular and extravascular compartments. TPE also has become an established treatment for severe PRCA cases.[113,114]

Whereas TPE can dramatically improve the prognosis in TTP, it has limited to no clinical effectiveness for TAM. This is despite the similar clinical picture of the two entities—namely MAHA, thrombocytopenia, and microvascular thrombosis—and primarily stems from their pathophysiology. TPE allows the efficient removal of large vWF multimers and the anti-ADAMTS13 Ab while restoring ADAMTS13 with plasma replacement. On the other hand, the exact pathophysiology of TAM remains unclear, and the utility of TPE remains uncertain.

Plasma Adsorption

The removal of anti-RBC Ab directed against the donor graft in the recipient may be achieved by nonselectively removing plasma via large volume TPE prior or after transplantation. Another strategy involves the selective removal of anti-A and anti-B Ab via in vivo immunoadsorption on immobilized blood group Ag. Although an older technique, studies in the 1970 and 1980s began to reexamine the procedure as a means to prevent hemolysis in ABO-incompatible allogeneic HPCT.[110,115,116] Recently, Ig-Therasorb, an immunoadsorption method originally designed for the elimination of acquired

Factor VIII Ab, has been utilized in Europe for the removal of anti-donor RBC Ab in the post-HPCT setting, especially in refractory cases that may lead to PRCA. This novel immunoadsorption technique passes recipient plasma through columns filled with sepharose-coupled polyclonal sheep Ab raised against human immunoglobulins, thus removing the anti-donor RBC Ab before returning the plasma to the HPCT recipient. The authors claim that this selective process was able to remove the Ab effectively and restore erythropoiesis without the use of replacement fluids such as albumin or fresh frozen plasma.[117-119]

Immunosuppressive Therapy, Steroids, Rituximab, Bortezomib

Successful allogeneic HPCT has major challenges in trying to balance and overcome the immunological systems of both the recipient and the donor. During allogeneic HPCT, the use of systemic immunosuppression is used to impair the recipient's immune competence but at the same time prevent GVHD. Many immunosuppressive regimens include systemic glucocorticosteroids, such as methylprednisolone and prednisone, may act as a means to suppress the immune pathways broadly. Other agents, such as cyclosporine and tacrolimus, calcineurin inhibitors, may affect T-cell proliferation. A drawback to long-term immunosuppression is its associated toxicities and long-term side effects such as the risk of infection and severe osteoporosis. However, attempts to taper off the immunosuppression can increase the risk of GVHD recurrence.

As discussed previously, PRCA is attributed to the presence of recipient Ab-producing plasma cells that had survived the conditioning regimen, causing inhibition of the donor graft. Recently, there has been success in the use of new drug therapies that help mediate the residual host Ab-producing cells. Two such therapies are rituximab and bortezomib. Rituximab, an anti-CD20 monoclonal Ab approved for use in the treatment of B-cell lymphomas, has been utilized in PRCA for its potential to mediate the Ab-dependent, cell-mediated cytotoxicity by its targeting and removal of CD20-positive B lymphocytes.

Bortezomib, a proteasome inhibitor approved for the treatment of multiple myeloma and mantle cell lymphoma, has been documented in the literature for its effectiveness in treating PRCA. Its exact mechanism of action is yet to be fully elucidated, but it is believed it could trigger programmed cell death in the differentiated plasma cells responsible for the persistent production of the anti-donor Ab in ABO-incompatible HPCT.[120,114]

SUMMARY

During HPCT, crossing of the ABO and non-ABO blood group immunological barriers is nonprohibitive toward overall favorable HSCT outcome. Estimates show that 20%–50% of HLA-matched HPCT are ABO incompatible. However, blood group, primarily ABO-incompatible HSCT often do result in distinctive immunohematological complications, such as HA, TAM, PLS, PRCA, and GVHD. The understanding of the immunologic basis of the blood group Ag and the immune responses during HPCT help explain the underlying mechanisms of these complications. With this understanding, the often challenging and complicated therapeutic and supportive management of blood group–incompatible HPCT recipients can be better appreciated during the posttransplantation period. Basic immunehistological testings, such as ABO typing, with Ab titrations, DAT, the elution testing can aid in monitoring the progression of engraftment and the effectiveness of the therapies being provided. Appropriate therapeutic support including blood transfusion during and after an HPCT can tremendously affect transplant-related morbidity and long-term survival outcomes. Interventions such as TPE, in vivo plasma absorption, and immunosuppressive therapies can mitigate the recipient's immune response, providing a more permissive environment for successful posttransplant engraftment.

REFERENCES

1. Kasakura S. Great contributions of E. Donnall Thomas to the development of clinical applications of bone marrow transplantation, leading to the 1990 Nobel Prize in Medicine/Physiology. *Int J Hematol*. 2005; 81(2):87–88.
2. Bortin MM, et al. 25th anniversary of the first successful allogeneic bone marrow transplants. *Bone Marrow Transplant*. 1994;14(2):211–212.
3. Baron F, Storb R, Little MT. Hematopoietic cell transplantation: five decades of progress. *Arch Med Res*. 2003; 34(6):528–544.
4. Molne J, et al. Blood group ABO antigen expression in human embryonic stem cells and in differentiated hepatocyte- and cardiomyocyte-like cells. *Transplantation*. 2008;86(10):1407–1413.
5. Szczepiorkowski ZM, Dumont LJ. Hematopoietic stem cell transplantation: is ABO "a match made in heaven"? *Transfusion*. 2009;49(4):612–614.
6. Rowley SD, Liang PS, Ulz L. Transplantation of ABO-incompatible bone marrow and peripheral blood stem cell components. *Bone Marrow Transplant*. 2000;26(7): 749–757.
7. Sykes M, Spitzer TR. Non-myeloblative induction of mixed hematopoietic chimerism: application to transplantation tolerance and hematologic malignancies in experimental and clinical studies. *Cancer Treat Res*. 2002;110:79–99.
8. Seebach JD, et al. ABO blood group barrier in allogeneic bone marrow transplantation revisited. *Biol Blood Marrow Transplant*. 2005;11(12):1006–1013.
9. Gale RP, et al. ABO blood group system and bone marrow transplantation. *Blood*. 1977;50(2):185–194.
10. Gajewski JL, et al. A review of transfusion practice before, during, and after hematopoietic progenitor cell transplantation. *Blood*. 2008;112(8):3036–3047.
11. de Mattos LC. Structural diversity and biological importance of ABO, H, Lewis and secretor histo-blood group carbohydrates. *Rev Bras Hematol Hemoter*. 2016;38(4): 331–340.
12. Worel N, et al. Transfusion policy in ABO-incompatible allogeneic stem cell transplantation. *Vox Sang*. 2010; 98(3 Pt 2):455–467.
13. Bradley JA, Bolton EM, Pedersen RA. Stem cell medicine encounters the immune system. *Nat Rev Immunol*. 2002; 2(11):859–871.
14. Bray RA, et al. National marrow donor program HLA matching guidelines for unrelated adult donor hematopoietic cell transplants. *Biol Blood Marrow Transplant*. 2008;14(9 Suppl):45–53.
15. Williams KM, Gress RE. Immune reconstitution and implications for immunotherapy following haematopoietic stem cell transplantation. *Best Pract Res Clin Haematol*. 2008;21(3):579–596.
16. Worel N. ABO-mismatched allogeneic hematopoietic stem cell transplantation. *Transfus Med Hemotherapy*. 2016;43(1):3–12.
17. Abbas AK, Lichtman AHH, Pillai S. *Cellular and Molecular Immunology E-Book*. Elsevier Health Sciences; 2014.
18. Noizat-Pirenne F, et al. Relative immunogenicity of Fya and K antigens in a Caucasian population, based on HLA class II restriction analysis. *Transfusion*. 2006; 46(8):1328–1333.
19. Zimring JC, Hudson KE. Cellular immune responses in red blood cell alloimmunization. *Hematology Am Soc Hematol Educ Program*. 2016;2016(1):452–456.
20. Hall AM, et al. Interleukin-10–mediated regulatory T-cell responses to epitopes on a human red blood cell autoantigen. *Blood*. 2002;100(13):4529–4536.
21. Yazdanbakhsh K, Ware RE, Noizat-Pirenne F. Red blood cell alloimmunization in sickle cell disease: pathophysiology, risk factors, and transfusion management. *Blood*. 2012;120(3):528–537.
22. Ansart-Pirenne H, et al. Identification of immunodominant alloreactive T-cell epitopes on the Jka red blood cell protein inducing either Th1 or Th2 cytokine expression. *Blood*. 2004;104(10):3409–3410.
23. Urbaniak SJ. Alloimmunity to human red blood cell antigens. *Vox Sang*. 2002;83(Suppl 1):293–297.
24. Tormey CA, Stack G. Immunogenicity of blood group antigens: a mathematical model corrected for antibody evanescence with exclusion of naturally occurring and pregnancy-related antibodies. *Blood*. 2009;114(19): 4279–4282.

25. Nelson Jr RA. The immune-adherence phenomenon; an immunologically specific reaction between microorganisms and erythrocytes leading to enhanced phagocytosis. *Science*. 1953;118(3077):733−737.

26. Linden S, et al. Role of ABO secretor status in mucosal innate immunity and *H. pylori* infection. *PLoS Pathog*. 2008;4(1):e2.

27. Baum J, Ward RH, Conway DJ. Natural selection on the erythrocyte surface. *Mol Biol Evol*. 2002;19(3):223−229.

28. Stowell SR, et al. Innate immune lectins kill bacteria expressing blood group antigen. *Nat Med*. 2010;16(3): 295−301.

29. Ko WY, et al. Effects of natural selection and gene conversion on the evolution of human glycophorins coding for MNS blood polymorphisms in malaria-endemic African populations. *Am J Hum Genet*. 2011;88(6): 741−754.

30. Ntumngia FB, et al. The role of the human Duffy antigen receptor for chemokines in malaria susceptibility: current opinions and future treatment prospects. *J Recept Ligand Channel Res*. 2016;9:1−11.

31. de Carvalho GB, de Carvalho GB. Duffy Blood Group System and the malaria adaptation process in humans. *Rev Bras Hematol Hemoter*. 2011;33(1):55−64.

32. Gershon H. The anti-inflammatory role of the erythrocyte: impairment in the elderly. *Arch Gerontol Geriatr*. 1997;24(2):157−165.

33. Dzik S, et al. Current research on the immunomodulatory effect of allogeneic blood transfusion. *Vox Sang*. 1996;70(4):187−194.

34. Fonseca AM, et al. Red blood cells inhibit activation-induced cell death and oxidative stress in human peripheral blood T lymphocytes. *Blood*. 2001;97(10): 3152−3160.

35. Arosa FA, Pereira CF, Fonseca AM. Red blood cells as modulators of T cell growth and survival. *Curr Pharmaceut Des*. 2004;10(2):191−201.

36. Montecino-Rodriguez E, Leathers H, Dorshkind K. Identification of a B-1 B cell-specified progenitor. *Nat Immunol*. 2006;7(3):293−301.

37. Panda S, Ding JL. Natural antibodies bridge innate and adaptive immunity. *J Immunol*. 2015;194(1):13−20.

38. Arend P. Ancestral gene and "complementary" antibody dominate early ontogeny. *Immunobiology*. 2013;218(5): 755−761.

39. Merbl Y, et al. Newborn humans manifest autoantibodies to defined self molecules detected by antigen microarray informatics. *J Clin Investig*. 2007;117(3):712−718.

40. Springer GF, Williamson P, Brandes WC. Blood group Activity of gram-negative bacteria. *J Exp Med*. 1961;113(6): 1077−1093.

41. Kay LA. Cellular basis of immune response to antigens of ABO blood-group system. Capacity to provide help during response to T-cell-dependent ABO-system antigens is restricted to individuals of blood group O. *Lancet*. 1984; 2(8416):1369−1371.

42. Stott L-M, Barker RN, Urbaniak SJ. Identification of alloreactive T-cell epitopes on the Rhesus D protein. *Blood*. 2000;96(13):4011−4019.

43. Feingold B, et al. Tolerance to incompatible ABO blood group antigens is not observed following homograft implantation. *Hum Immunol*. 2011;72(10):835−840.

44. Mueller RJ, et al. Major ABO-incompatible hematopoietic stem cell transplantation: study of post-transplant pure red cell aplasia and endothelial cell chimerism. *Xenotransplantation*. 2006;13(2):126−132.

45. Grube M, et al. ABO blood group antigen mismatch has an impact on outcome after allogeneic peripheral blood stem cell transplantation. *Clin Transplant*. 2016;30(11): 1457−1465.

46. Storry JR, et al. International society of blood transfusion working party on red cell immunogenetics and blood group terminology: report of the Dubai, Copenhagen and Toronto meetings. *Vox Sang*. 2019;114(1): 95−102.

47. Denomme GA. The structure and function of the molecules that carry human red blood cell and platelet antigens. *Transfus Med Rev*. 2004;18(3):203−231.

48. Reid ME, Lomas-Francis C, Olsson ML. *The Blood Group Antigen Factsbook*. 3rd ed. Amsterdam: Elsevier/AP; 2012:745.

49. Schwarz HP, Dorner F. Karl landsteiner and his major contributions to haematology. *Br J Haematol*. 2003; 121(4):556−565.

50. Ferguson-Smith MA, et al. Localisation of the human ABO: Np-1: AK-1 linkage group by regional assignment of AK-1 to 9q34. *Hum Genet*. 1976;34(1):35−43.

51. Yamamoto F-i, et al. Molecular genetic basis of the histoblood group ABO system. *Nature*. 1990;345(6272): 229−233.

52. Hoffmann S, et al. Delayed platelet engraftment in group O patients after autologous progenitor cell transplantation. *Transfusion*. 2005;45(6):885−895.

53. Makivuokko H, et al. Association between the ABO blood group and the human intestinal microbiota composition. *BMC Microbiol*. 2012;12:94.

54. Davenport ER, et al. ABO antigen and secretor statuses are not associated with gut microbiota composition in 1,500 twins. *BMC Genomics*. 2016;17(1):941.

55. Szulman AE. The histological distribution of blood group substances A and B in man. *J Exp Med*. 1960;111:785−800.

56. Oriol R, Le Pendu J, Mollicone R. Genetics of ABO, H, Lewis, X and related antigens. *Vox Sang*. 1986;51(3): 161−171.

57. Segurel L, et al. The ABO blood group is a trans-species polymorphism in primates. *Proc Natl Acad Sci U S A*. 2012;109(45):18493−18498.

58. Saitou N, Yamamoto F. Evolution of primate ABO blood group genes and their homologous genes. *Mol Biol Evol*. 1997;14(4):399−411.

59. Kimura F, et al. Impact of ABO-blood group incompatibility on the outcome of recipients of bone marrow transplants from unrelated donors in the Japan Marrow

Donor Program. *Haematologica*. 2008;93(11): 1686–1693.

60. Rieben R, et al. Antibodies to histo-blood group substances A and B: agglutination titers, Ig class, and IgG subclasses in healthy persons of different age categories. *Transfusion*. 1991;31(7):607–615.

61. Iwanaga S, et al. Passenger lymphocyte syndrome with hemophagocytic syndrome after peripheral blood stem-cell transplantation from an HLA-matched full biological sibling: case report. *Transfus Apher Sci*. 2012;47(3): 355–358.

62. Vatsayan A, et al. Post-hematopoietic stem cell transplant hemophagocytic lymphohistiocytosis or an impostor: case report and review of literature. *Pediatr Transplant*. 2018;22(4):e13174.

63. Young PP, et al. Immune hemolysis involving non-ABO/RhD alloantibodies following hematopoietic stem cell transplantation. *Bone Marrow Transplant*. 2001;27:1305.

64. Booth GS, Gehrie EA, Savani BN. Minor RBC Ab and allo-SCT. *Bone Marrow Transplant*. 2014;49(3):456–457.

65. Ting A, et al. Red cell alloantibodies produced after bone marrow transplantation. *Transfusion*. 1987;27(2): 145–147.

66. Franchini M, Gandini G, Aprili G. Non-ABO red blood cell alloantibodies following allogeneic hematopoietic stem cell transplantation. *Bone Marrow Transplant*. 2004; 33(12):1169–1172.

67. Abou-Elella AA, et al. Low incidence of red cell and HLA antibody formation by bone marrow transplant patients. *Transfusion*. 1995;35(11):931–935.

68. Żupańska B, et al. Multiple red cell alloantibodies, including anti-Dib, after allogeneic ABO-matched peripheral blood progenitor cell transplantation. *Transfusion*. 2005;45(1):16–20.

69. Sokol RJ, et al. Cold haemagglutinin disease: clinical significance of serum haemolysins. *Clin Lab Haematol*. 2000; 22(6):337–344.

70. Mijovic A. Alloimmunization to RhD antigen in RhD-incompatible haemopoietic cell transplants with non-myeloablative conditioning. *Vox Sang*. 2002;83(4): 358–362.

71. Cid J, et al. Matching for the D antigen in haematopoietic progenitor cell transplantation: definition and clinical outcomes. *Blood Transfus*. 2014;12(3):301–306.

72. Vucelic D, Savic N, Djordjevic R. Delayed hemolytic transfusion reaction due to anti-Jk(a). *Acta Chir Iugosl*. 2005;52(3):111–115.

73. Myser T, et al. A bone marrow transplant with an acquired anti-Le(a): a case study. *Hum Immunol*. 1986; 17(2):102–106.

74. Garratty G. The James Blundell Award Lecture 2007: do we really understand immune red cell destruction? *Transfus Med*. 2008;18(6):321–334.

75. Flegel WA. Pathogenesis and mechanisms of antibody-mediated hemolysis. *Transfusion*. 2015;55(Suppl 2): S47–S58, 0.

76. Wolgast LR, et al. Spectrin isoforms: differential expression in normal hematopoiesis and alterations in neoplastic bone marrow disorders. *Am J Clin Pathol*. 2011;136(2):300–308.

77. Sharma SK, et al. Oral high dose dexamethasone for pure red cell aplasia following ABO-mismatched allogeneic peripheral blood stem cell transplantation: a case report. *Indian J Hematol Blood Transfus*. 2015;31(2):317–318.

78. Kopinska A, et al. Rituximab is highly effective for pure red cell aplasia and post-transplant lymphoproliferative disorder after unrelated hematopoietic stem cell transplantation. *Contemp Oncol*. 2012;16(3):215–217.

79. Schwartz D, Gotzinger P. Immune-haemolytic anaemia (IHA) after solid organ transplantation due to rhesus antibodies of donor origin: report of 5 cases. *Beitr Infusionsther*. 1992;30:367–369.

80. Park SH, et al. The outcomes of hypertransfusion in major ABO incompatible allogeneic stem sell transplantation. *J Korean Med Sci*. 2004;19(1):79–82.

81. Rowley SD, Donato ML, Bhattacharyya P. Red blood cell-incompatible allogeneic hematopoietic progenitor cell transplantation. *Bone Marrow Transplant*. 2011;46(9): 1167–1185.

82. Raimondi R, et al. ABO-incompatible bone marrow transplantation: a GITMO survey of current practice in Italy and comparison with the literature. *Bone Marrow Transplant*. 2004;34(4):321–329.

83. Mattsson J, Ringden O, Storb R. Graft failure after allogeneic hematopoietic cell transplantation. *Biol Blood Marrow Transplant*. 2008;14(1 Suppl 1):165–170.

84. Aung FM, et al. Incidence and natural history of pure red cell aplasia in major ABO-mismatched haematopoietic cell transplantation. *Br J Haematol*. 2013;160(6): 798–805.

85. Stussi G, et al. Consequences of ABO incompatibility in allogeneic hematopoietic stem cell transplantation. *Bone Marrow Transplant*. 2002;30(2):87–93.

86. Remberger M, et al. Major ABO blood group mismatch increases the risk for graft failure after unrelated donor hematopoietic stem cell transplantation. *Biol Blood Marrow Transplant*. 2007;13(6):675–682.

87. De Santis GC, et al. Higher Anti-A/B isoagglutinin titers of IgG class, but not of IgM, are associated with increased red blood cell transfusion requirements in bone marrow transplantation with major ABO-mismatch. *Clin Transplant*. 2017;31(4).

88. Canals C, et al. Impact of ABO incompatibility on allogeneic peripheral blood progenitor cell transplantation after reduced intensity conditioning. *Transfusion*. 2004; 44(11):1603–1611.

89. Stussi G, et al. Graft-versus-host disease and survival after ABO-incompatible allogeneic bone marrow transplantation: a single-centre experience. *Br J Haematol*. 2001; 113(1):251–253.

90. Mielcarek M, et al. Graft-versus-host disease and donor-directed hemagglutinin titers after ABO-mismatched

related and unrelated marrow allografts: evidence for a graft-versus-plasma cell effect. *Blood.* 2000;96(3):1150–1156.

91. van Tol MJ, et al. The origin of IgG production and homogeneous IgG components after allogeneic bone marrow transplantation. *Blood.* 1996;87(2):818–826.

92. Benjamin RJ, et al. ABO incompatibility as an adverse risk factor for survival after allogeneic bone marrow transplantation. *Transfusion.* 1999;39(2):179–187.

93. Kanda J, et al. Impact of ABO mismatching on the outcomes of allogeneic related and unrelated blood and marrow stem cell transplantations for hematologic malignancies: IPD-based meta-analysis of cohort studies. *Transfusion.* 2009;49(4):624–635.

94. Hefazi M, et al. ABO blood group incompatibility as an adverse risk factor for outcomes in patients with myelodysplastic syndromes and acute myeloid leukemia undergoing HLA-matched peripheral blood hematopoietic cell transplantation after reduced-intensity conditioning. *Transfusion.* 2016;56(2):518–527.

95. Logan AC, et al. ABO mismatch is associated with increased nonrelapse mortality after allogeneic hematopoietic cell transplantation. *Biol Blood Marrow Transplant.* 2015;21(4):746–754.

96. Ozkurt ZN, et al. Impact of ABO-incompatible donor on early and late outcome of hematopoietic stem cell transplantation. *Transplant Proc.* 2009;41(9):3851–3858.

97. Heal JM, et al. What would Karl Landsteiner do? The ABO blood group and stem cell transplantation. *Bone Marrow Transplant.* 2005;36(9):747–755.

98. McRae HL, et al. The effect of ABO immune complexes on endothelial cell integrity as measured by electric cell-substrate impedance sensing (ECIS) and confocal microscopy. *Blood.* 2017;130(suppl 1). pp. 2306–2306.

99. Erker CG, et al. The influence of blood group differences in allogeneic hematopoietic peripheral blood progenitor cell transplantation. *Transfusion.* 2005;45(8):1382–1390.

100. Mehta J, et al. Does donor-recipient ABO incompatibility protect against relapse after allogeneic bone marrow transplantation in first remission acute myeloid leukemia? *Bone Marrow Transplant.* 2002;29(10):853–859.

101. Worel N, et al. ABO mismatch increases transplant-related morbidity and mortality in patients given nonmyeloablative allogeneic HPC transplantation. *Transfusion.* 2003;43(8):1153–1161.

102. Damodar S, et al. Donor-to-Recipient ABO mismatch does not impact outcomes of allogeneic hematopoietic cell transplantation regardless of graft source. *Biol Blood Marrow Transplant.* 2017;23(5):795–804.

103. Worel N, et al. ABO incompatible allogeneic stem-cell transplantation following reduced-intensity conditioning: close association with thrombotic microangiopathy. *Blood.* 2004;104(11). pp. 5042–5042.

104. Liu H, et al. Reduced-intensity conditioning with combined haploidentical and cord blood transplantation results in rapid engraftment, low GVHD, and durable remissions. *Blood.* 2011;118(24):6438–6445.

105. Chan EH, et al. Evaluation of blood group conversion following ABO-incompatible hematopoietic stem cell transplantation (HCT). *Blood.* 2014;124(21). pp. 1557–1557.

106. Daniels G, Reid ME. Blood groups: the past 50 years. *Transfusion.* 2010;50(2):281–289.

107. E Reid M, Lomas-Francis C. *Blood Groups Transf Sci.* 2016:1–10.

108. Rennert H, et al. Avoiding pitfalls in bone marrow engraftment analysis: a case study highlighting the weakness of using buccal cells for determining a patient's constitutional genotype after hematopoietic stem cell transplantation. *Cytotherapy.* 2013;15(3):391–395.

109. Fasano RM, et al. Genotyping applications for transplantation and transfusion management: the emory experience. *Arch Pathol Lab Med.* 2017;141(3):329–340.

110. Cohn CS. Transfusion support issues in hematopoietic stem cell transplantation. *Cancer Control.* 2015;22(1):52–59.

111. O'Donghaile D, et al. Recommendations for transfusion in ABO-incompatible hematopoietic stem cell transplantation. *Transfusion.* 2012;52(2):456–458.

112. Stussi G, et al. Prevention of pure red cell aplasia after major or bidirectional ABO blood group incompatible hematopoietic stem cell transplantation by pretransplant reduction of host anti-donor isoagglutinins. *Haematologica.* 2009;94(2):239–248.

113. Sackett K, et al. Successful treatment of pure red cell aplasia because of ABO major mismatched stem cell transplant. *J Clin Apher.* 2018;33(1):108–112.

114. Tichelli A, et al. ABO-incompatible bone marrow transplantation: in vivo adsorption, an old forgotten method. *Transplant Proc.* 1987;19(6):4632–4637.

115. Bensinger WI, et al. Comparison of techniques for dealing with major ABO-incompatible marrow transplants. *Transplant Proc.* 1987;19(6):4605–4608.

116. Rabitsch W, et al. Prolonged red cell aplasia after major ABO-incompatible allogeneic hematopoietic stem cell transplantation: removal of persisting isohemagglutinins with Ig-Therasorb immunoadsorption. *Bone Marrow Transplant.* 2003;32(10):1015–1019.

117. Knobl P, et al. Elimination of acquired factor VIII antibodies by extracorporal antibody-based immunoadsorption (Ig-Therasorb). *Thromb Haemostasis.* 1995;74(4):1035–1038.

118. Daniele N, et al. The processing of stem cell concentrates from the bone marrow in ABO-incompatible transplants: how and when. *Blood Transfus.* 2014;12(2):150–158.

119. Poon LM, Koh LP. Successful treatment of isohemagglutinin-mediated pure red cell aplasia after ABO-mismatched allogeneic hematopoietic cell transplant using bortezomib. *Bone Marrow Transplant.* 2012;47(6):870–871.

120. Khan F, et al. Subcutaneous bortezomib is highly effective for pure red cell aplasia after ABO-incompatible haematopoietic stem cell transplantation. *Transfus Med.* 2014;24(3):187–188.

CHAPTER 14

Complications of Haploidentical and Mismatched HSC Transplantation

JINGMEI HSU, MD, PHD • ROBERT A. DESIMONE, MD • LJILJANA V. VASOVIC, MD

INTRODUCTION

Allogeneic hematopoietic stem cell transplant (HSCT) provides curative potential for patients with hematologic and nonhematologic diseases. For HSCT to be successful, donor grafts must cross immunologic barriers presented by histocompatibility antigen genetic variabilities. Less than 30% of patients have a human leukocyte antigen (HLA)-identical sibling as a donor. Thus, alternative donors become a major source of allogeneic stem cell transplants. Matched-unrelated, mismatched-unrelated, cord blood units, and more recently haploidentical donors have been explored.

This chapter primarily focuses on complications related to haploidentical stem cell transplants (haplo-SCTs). Additionally, complications of mismatched stem cell transplants will be discussed. As the haploidentical transplantation field evolved, the clinical complications have evolved as well. Herein, we discuss some of the most common problems that arise and their corresponding solutions.

Haplo-SCT requires a donor match at HLA-A, HLA-B, and HLA-DR genotypically and phenotypically. In the majority of the cases, patients have related haploidentical family members that can serve as a donor. Unrelated haploidentical donors are also an option. The feasibility of haplo-SCT was first demonstrated in patients with severe combined immunodeficiency where marrow stem cells were T cell–depleted (TCD) using soybean lectin and erythrocyte (E)-resetting.[1,2] Subsequently, it was adapted to treat patients with acute leukemia.[3] Despite initial successes, graft failure and delayed engraftment and increased high-grade acute graft-versus-host disease (aGVHD) hampered its widespread adoption.[4] To overcome these challenges, the use of TCD "megadose" CD34[+] marrow stem cells resulted in improved engraftment and reduced GVHD.[5,6] However, T cell depletion hampered posttransplant immune reconstitution and caused an increase in posttransplant infections. Several groups developed strategies to selectively remove T cell subsets by targeting T cell receptors (TcRs) such as $\alpha\beta^+$ T cells, as well as CD19[+] B cells from donor grafts, resulting in a lower incidence of GVHD and a more rapid immune reconstitution.[7,8] Adoptive transfer of conventional T cells (Tcon) and regulatory T cells (Treg) without posttransplant immune suppression also yielded lower rates of GVHD with adequate immune reconstitution.[9] A separate approach using a combination of granulocyte-colony stimulating factor (G-CSF) and anti-thymocyte globulin (ATG)-based regimen without T cell depletion was explored in China.[10,11] This approach was thought to lead to induction of immune tolerance through polarization of Th1 and Th2 populations via a complex interplay between Treg, TH17, regulatory B cells, and myeloid-derived suppressors.[12] Development of posttransplant cyclophosphamide (PTCy) without T cell depletion is the latest advancement in the field of haplo-SCT.[13–15] Enhancement of this approach results in excellent immune reconstitution and low infectious complications with clinical outcomes similar to matched-related and matched-unrelated stem cell transplants.[16–20]

ENGRAFTMENT FAILURE

Primary engraftment failure is variably defined as lack of donor hematopoietic recovery with resulting pancytopenia, specifically neutropenia (absolute neutrophil $< 0.5 \times 10^9$/L), post–stem cell transplantation. Secondary engraftment failure is defined as loss of donor cells after initial donor engraftment. We focus on primary engraftment failure here. Risk factors associated with primary graft failure in HLA-matched related/unrelated and umbilical cord donor transplant settings

Immunologic Concepts in Transfusion Medicine. https://doi.org/10.1016/B978-0-323-67509-3.00014-7

include degree of donor graft and recipient HLA compatibility, blood group ABO-mismatch, intensity of conditioning regimen, and stem cell and T cell dose in the donor graft.[21–26] Haploidentical, mismatched donor, or umbilical cord stem cell transplants tend to show an increased engraftment failure, which can be up to 20% in the case of haplo-SCT.[27–29] Several biological mechanisms have been proposed to contribute to primary graft failure. Immunological mechanisms are thought to be one of the main contributing factors.[30]

Cell-Mediated Graft Rejection

Residual host lymphocytes, primarily T and natural killer (NK) cells, are important factors mediating donor graft rejection.[31–33] Early murine stem cell transplant models showed that host T and NK cells mediate acute donor marrow graft rejection through recognition of incompatible MHC determinants.[31,34,35] Using unrelated dog leukocyte antigen and a nonidentical dog transplant model, Raff et al. systematically examined the residual host cells and found lymphocytes and cells with NK activity suppressed donor marrow graft hematopoietic activities.[32] Further studies in murine models showed that both CD4+ and CD8+ subsets of T cells[36–39] and the residual CD8+αβ and γδ TCR+ cells activated by donor antigens play a critical role in graft rejection.[40] Host cytotoxic T cell–mediated rejection involves the perforin and Fas ligand (FasL) pathways.[41] Host CD8 memory T cells can mediate graft rejection without the perforin pathway. In addition to FasL-mediated cytotoxicity, the TNF family ligands TRAIL, TWEAK, and TL1A can also mediate graft rejection in recipients sensitized against donor minor antigens.[42]

Patients who received donor cells with an HLA class I mismatch are predisposed to develop host anti-donor T cell cytotoxicity leading to graft rejection.[43] Both host CD8+ and CD4+ T cells are capable of mediating graft rejection.[44] Interestingly, TCD donor stem cell transplants reduce the incidence of GVHD, but are associated with increased graft failure. Thus, both host and donor T cells play an important role in engraftment. Early recovery of host CD8+ T cells and increased IL-2 producing T helper cells correlated with higher incidence of graft rejection in a nonmyeloablative matched related donor (MRD) transplant followed by donor lymphocyte infusion (DLI).[45] In another HLA-identical stem cell transplant, graft rejection was through cytotoxic T cells against minor HLA antigens.[46] H-Y and DFFRY epitopes on male target cells are identified during graft failure after a sex-mismatched transplant.[47]

An increased degree of HLA disparity is associated with an increase in graft rejection.[4,26,48] With respect to single-allele mismatches, mismatch of HLA-C has the most adverse impact on engraftment.[49] Increased risk of graft failure was associated with mismatching for two or more class I, but not class II HLA-DRB1 or DQB1 alleles.[50] Patients receiving unmodified marrow from a mismatched donor had increased graft failure in 12.3% compared with 2% from a fully HLA-matched related donor.[48] Residual host lymphocytes were detected in 11 of 14 patients with graft failure. A positive crossmatch for anti-donor lymphocytotoxic antibodies was found among 30% of alloimmunized patients and was associated strongly with graft failure.[48]

Host NK cells also cause graft rejection when donor HLA class I-expressing cells fail to inhibit their activation. NK cells are part of the innate immunity, and their reactivity arises from a combination of both inhibitory and activating signals. Host licensed NK cells expressing Killer cell immunoglobulin-like receptors (KIRs) can kill donor graft cells lacking one or more inhibitory KIR ligands or self-MHC class I molecules.[51,52] Unlicensed NK cells that do not express self-MHC class I receptors are also functionally competent in tumor and viral control.[53] Murine experiments depleted different NK cell subsets prior to allogeneic HCT showed that host licensed NK cells were mainly responsible for graft rejection, whereas host unlicensed NK cell subsets had little or no role.[54] The increased risk of engraftment failure is due to an enhanced susceptibility of the graft to conditioning regimen-resistant host NK cell–mediated rejection against mismatched donor cells.[55] De Santis et al. analyzed 104 patients who underwent mismatched-unrelated marrow donor transplant. They found NK cell's HLA-C epitope (C1 and C2) mismatching in the donor direction was associated with an increased graft rejection.[56] Similarly, Beelen et al. also found KIR ligand-incompatible patients had increased graft rejection in unmanipulated myeloablative stem cell transplants[57] but also reduced relapse.

Antibody-Mediated Graft Rejection

Prior alloimmunization is a significant risk factor for graft failure.[48,58] Multiple blood transfusions and pregnancy are known common risk factors for anti-HLA antibody formation.[59–61] Preformed antibodies against donor HLA antigens (DSAs) present at the time of graft infusion have been shown to be a major factor in graft rejection.[62] Antibody-mediated rejection may occur through antibody-dependent cell-mediated cytotoxicity or complement-mediated cytotoxicity.[62,63] Although a small study, DSAs were detected in 21% of 24 patients and accounted for 75% of engraftment failure in patients who underwent T cell−depleted haplo-SCTs.[59] Ciurea et al. examined 122 patients who underwent haplo-SCT with T cell depletion. High anti-HLA antibody titers were detected in 32% of the 22 patients rejecting grafts. DSAs included anti-HLA-A, anti-HLA-B, anti-HLA-DRB1, anti-HLA-DPB1, and anti-HLA-DQB1 antibodies. Patients who had graft rejection also had detectable complement binding antibodies C1q at the time of the transplant.[63] Yoshihara et al. reported detection of DSAs in 11 of 79 patients undergoing unmanipulated haplo-SCT; three of the five patients with high DSA levels had graft failure.[64] Similarly, Chang et al. also reported that the presence of DSAs with mean fluorescence intensity $\geq 10,000$ was associated with engraftment failure.[65] In a cord blood transplant study, 63% of the 294 patients had HLA mismatch and less than 5% patients had DSAs. DSAs were associated with graft failure and poor clinical outcomes.[66]

Antibodies to donor CD34$^+$VEGFR2$^+$ endothelial progenitor stem cell populations[67] and major ABO blood groups[68] have also been reported as causes for graft rejection. Preformed anti-MHC antibodies mediate graft rejection, and neutralizing these antibodies enhanced engraftment.[69]

New Approach to Overcome Immunologic Incompatibility

To ameliorate graft failure and delayed engraftment associated with haplo-SCT, "megadose" CD34$^+$ hematopoietic progenitor cells were introduced to overcome major genetic barriers and enable rapid and durable engraftment through induction of immune tolerance in the host.[70] Aversa et al. successfully performed T cell−depleted haplo-SCTs by infusing G-CSF mobilized peripheral blood progenitor cells.[5] Infusion of CD4$^+$CD25$^+$Foxp3$^+$ Treg induces immune tolerance[71] and effectively promotes donor cell engraftment.[72,73] Steiner et al. showed recently that ex vivo expansion of the naive third-party "off-the shelf" CD4$^+$CD25$^+$ Treg cells can effectively enhance engraftment of T cell−depleted marrow grafts.[74]

Ruggeri et al. initially reported the role of NK cells in facilitating donor stem cell engraftment and NK-alloreactive donor cells, thus enhancing graft-versus-leukemia (GVL) effect with improved survival advantage for patients undergoing haplo-SCT.[75,76] Selective infusion of alloreactive donor NK cells following allogeneic HCT allow for enhanced donor HSC engraftment.[77,78]

DSA levels are not affected by conditioning regimens or immunosuppressive treatments administered in the peritransplant period. Approaches to reduce prestem cell infusion DSAs include therapeutic plasma exchange, intravenous immunoglobulin, rituximab, cyclophosphamide, and proteasome inhibitor Velcade, with combination therapies more effective than monotherapies.[79,80]

GRAFT-VERSUS-HOST DISEASE

The other side of immune incompatibility conflict is GVHD. The main effector cells in GVHD are T lymphocytes.[37,81] The risk of developing acute GVHD has been clearly shown to be associated with the dose of alloreactive T lymphocytes. In unrelated donor transplants, mismatches at HLA-A, HLA-B, HLA-C, and HLA-DR were found to have significant association with grade III−IV acute GVHD and increased mortality, with HLA-A mismatches having the largest impact.[49] Early clinical trials with unmanipulated T cell haplo-SCT had severe GVHD, reaching up to 50%.[4,82] Various methods have been developed to modify T cell−mediated alloreactivity.[83,84]

T Cell Depletion

Bidirectional T cell alloreactivity resulted in severe GVHD and graft failure in early studies of haplo-SCTs. The initial approach to reduce GVHD was to deplete T cells. T cell removal in AML patients undergoing haploidentical HSC was initially achieved using soybean agglutinin binding and sheep E-rosette formation resulting in infused CD34$^+$ selected grafts containing mean T cells $<1 \times 10^4$/kg $(0-4.6)$.[85] None of the evaluable patients developed acute or chronic (c)GVHD. One patient received additional donor T cells 3 months post transplant but did develop and die from acute GVHD.[85] Using CliniMACS for an enhanced positive CD34$^+$ cell selection,[86] 8 of the 100 evaluable patients developed acute GVHD (six grade II and two grade III−IV) and 3 patients developed cGVHD. Even though the incidence of GVHD was reduced, T cell depletion in the CD34$^+$ selected graft resulted in a higher risk of graft rejection or delayed engraftment, increased infection, and higher relapse rate. T cell depletion with megadose CD34$^+$ cells and selective lymphocyte subset depletion was also developed.[83] Aversa et al. were able to curb engraftment failure in the absence of GVHD.[5] However, immune reconstitution lingered and contributed to a high infectious risk. Megadose CD34$^+$ graft cells using G-CSF-mobilized peripheral blood stem cells (PBSCs) had a cumulative incidence of aGVHD (grade II−IV) and cGVHD below 10% in high-risk acute leukemia patients receiving haplo-SCT.[86]

Several studies have shown that depletion of $CD3^+$/$CD19^+$ cells from haplo-SCT grafts can reduce GvHD incidence. The majority of T cells express αβ TCRs, and both CD4 and CD8 αβ T cells are the major mediators of GVHD.[87] Thus, selective depletion of αβ T cells was thought to be able to reduce the incidence of GVHD. With selective αβ T cell depletion, γδ T cells, NK, and Treg cells are still present in the donor grafts, and these cells may contribute to GVL effect without causing GVHD.[83] However, most of the selective αβ TCR/CD19 depletion studies were performed in pediatric patients.[84] In adults, Berthge et al.[88] reported 15 of 28 patients with hematologic malignancies developed acute GVHD (13 grade II and 2 grade III) and 5 patients developed cGVHD (2 limited, 3 extensive). The incidence of grade II–IV aGvHD and cGvHD was 46% and 18%, respectively. This method resulted in a moderate overall increase in GVHD. In another study where only αβ T cells were depleted,[89] 11 (32%) patients developed acute GVHD (9 grade I–II, 2 grade III–IV). Only two patients developed cGVHD (one limited, one extensive). Thus, this study showed a lower incidence of grade II-IV acute GVHD after haplo-SCT with αβ T cell–depleted grafts compared to the reported 46% in patients receiving haplo-SCT with both αβ TCR/CD19-depleted grafts.

Although various graft manipulation strategies have been investigated to deplete T cells or T and B cell subsets from the graft with the goal to selectively eliminate the cells responsible for GVHD and to preserve GVL effects, a higher success rate was seen in pediatric patients with adequate thymic function when compared to adult patients. New approaches using G-CSF-treated grafts and posttransplant cyclophosphamide have developed to reduce GVHD.

Unmanipulated T Cells
G-CSF-primed
In China, combining G-CSF-treated bone marrow with post transplant immune suppression resulted in a high rate of engraftment with tolerable GVHD rates. Huang et al.[10,11] first reported using a combination of G-CSF-primed bone marrow and PBSCs with inclusion of ATG in haploidentical HCTs. With 171 patients treated, 51 (29.8%) patients had grade I and II acute GVHD and 9 and 13 patients had grade III and grade IV aGVHD, respectively. At day 100, 67 of the 150 surviving patients developed cGVHD with 32 patients having limited and 35 having extensive GVHD. When the study was updated in 2013,[90] a total of 756 patients were treated with 752 patients sustaining full donor chimerism, with a median neutrophil engraftment by day 13 posttransplant. The incidence of grade II–IV aGVHD was 43% and 2-year cumulative incidence of chronic GVHD was 53%.

Posttransplant cyclophosphamide-based
Cyclophosphamide selectively kills proliferating lymphocytes and proliferating cancer cells that express low levels of aldehyde dehydrogenase (ALDH1) while $CD34^+$ stem cells and resting lymphocytes express high levels of ALDH1, and thus are spared by cyclophosphamide.[91] Fuches group from Johns Hopkins first applied this approach in haploidentical HCT using unmanipulated T cell grafts with posttransplant cyclophosphamide (PTCy). When Luznik et al.[15] treated 68 patients with hematologic malignancies using nonmyeloablative conditioning and PTCy, the cumulative incidence of aGVHD for grade II–IV was 34% and grade III–IV was 6%. Extensive cGVHD incidence at 1 year was 5% for patients receiving two doses of PTCy and 25% for those who only received one dose. GVHD accounted for 3% of deaths. Using myeloablative conditioning and PTCy haplo-SCT, with 48 evaluable patients for acute GVHD, Raiola et al. reported that 10 patients (21%) developed grade I aGVHD, 3 developed grade II (6%), and 3 developed grade III (6%).[92] The cumulative incidence of grade II–III aGVHD was 12%. For 37 patients evaluable for cGVHD, 6 (16%) had minimal and 4 (10%) had moderate cGVHD. In a multicenter trial, Raj et al. studied peripheral stem cell donor source from related haploidentical donors with nonmyeloablative conditioning and PTCy.[93] Twenty-nine of the 55 patients developed grade II acute GVHD. The cumulative incidence of grades II and grade III aGVHD at 1 year were 53% and 8%, respectively. Nine patients had cGVHD with two severe cases. The cumulative incidence of cGHVD was 16% at 1 year and 18% at 2 years.

In vivo T cell depletion
Rizzieri et al. introduced alemtuzumab for in vivo T cell depletion of both host and donor cells to decrease GVHD in patients with hematologic malignances receiving haplo-SCT.[94] Engraftment was successful in 46 of 49 (94%) patients. Mild skin GVHD was common with a total of 16% patients experiencing grade II–IV GVHD. Severe grade III–IV aGVHD was 8%. Seven patients (14%) experienced cGVHD or failure to thrive, five with limited disease, and two with extensive disease. Encouraging evidence of quantitative lymphocyte recovery through expansion of transplanted T cells was noted by 3–6 months.

Haploidentical hematopoietic stem cell transplantation has made tremendous progress with a decrease in transplant-related mortality and GVHD. Future challenges remain in finding the best approach to reduce the incidence and severity of GVHD while preserving GVL effect to enhance clinical outcomes.

Immune Reconstitution

Immune reconstitution consists of the recovery of different immune cell subsets during engraftment and postengraftment phases. Innate immunity recovery including neutrophil engraftment for peripheral blood, bone marrow, and cord blood stem cells has been reported to occur around 14, 21, and 30 days after stem cell transplantation, respectively.[95,96] Immune reconstitution from donor, recipient or a peaceful coexistence of a chimeric immune repertoire has also been observed.[97–99] For T cell–depleted haplo-SCT, neutrophil engraftment occurred at approximately 11 days. For haplo-SCT that used T cell–repleted marrow, G-CSF-primed bone marrow, and G-CSF-stimulated blood and marrow grafts, neutrophils engrafted at ~15, ~21, and ~13 days, respectively.[100] The recovery of the T cell compartment depends on expansion of the memory T cells and thymic production of naïve T cells.[101] Naïve T cells arise from the thymus and are $CD4^+CD45RA^+$. Elderly patients have thymic atrophy, and thus lack naïve T cells and TCR repertoire diversity.[102] $CD8^+$ T cells recover faster than $CD4^+$ T cells, resulting in an inverted CD4/CD8 ratio. Treg cells are primarily a subset of $CD4^+$ T cells that are either derived from thymus (nTreg)[103] or from secondary lymphoid organs (iTreg).[104] $CD8^+$ Treg cells have been described as well.[105,106] The majority of cytotoxic NK cells are $CD56^{dim}/CD16^+$ and a smaller percentage of NK cells are $CD56^{bright}/CD16^{dim-neg}$.[107] NK cells are the first immune cells to recover posttransplant, and the first detected $CD56^{dim}/CD16^+$ are renamed as unconventional NK cells. In absence of GVHD, NK cells exert strong anti-tumor effects. Recovery of B cells includes recovery of the naïve and memory B cells and can take up to 2 years.[108,109] During the first few months posttransplant, there are very few circulating B cells. The first B cells to recover are $CD19^+CD21^{low}CD38^{high}$ transitional B cells from bone marrow.[110] These cells then give rise to the $CD19^+CD21^{high}CD27^-$ naïve cells with normal B cell number by 6 months.[111] With environmental and vaccine antigen exposure, some of the B cells mature into memory cells. By 3–6 months, the repertoire diversity of naïve B cells, not memory B cells, becomes comparable to normal subjects.[112] Normal levels of serum IgM can be achieved between 3 and 6 months, subsequently IgG and IgA levels will normalize approximately 1 year posttransplant.[113] Factors influencing B cell recovery include delayed T cell recovery,[114] use of ATG,[115] nonmyeloablative conditioning,[116] and development of GVHD.[117]

Immune reconstitution after haplo-SCT differs from HLA-matched related, unrelated, or cord blood HCT in that $CD4^+$ and $CD4^+$ naïve T and dendritic cell (DC) subsets recovery, and anti-CMV immunity are less robust in haplo-SCT.[118] Current technology allows quantitative monitoring of T cell repertoires posttransplant which can provide insight into TCR diversity and T cell immune reconstitution.[102,119] Below, immune reconstitution from distinct haploidentical HCT approaches is discussed.[96,100,120–122]

T Cell–Depleted Grafts
CD34+ selection
Early haplo-SCT experienced a high rate of graft failure and GVHD due to HLA genetic disparities mediated by cytotoxic T cells. Several studies showed that a subpopulation of cells in G-CSF-mobilized peripheral blood or bone marrow grafts can induce immune tolerance and facilitate engraftment.[123] Good engraftment was achieved, but immune reconstitution was delayed with use of "megadose" $CD34^+$ cells using G-CSF-mobilized PBSC.[5] With development of a less toxic myeloablative conditioning regimen, the Aversa group transplanted AML patients with reduced T cells by positively selecting $CD34^+$ cells without posttransplant immunosuppression.[85] The median $CD34^+$ cell dose was 10×10^6/kg, and median T cell dose was 2×10^4/kg. Neutrophil engraftment occurred around day 11 with only 2 of 43 patients experiencing engraftment failure. Natural killer cells normalized by 4 weeks posttransplant. However, there was a delay in CD4 immune reconstitution with $CD4^+$ cell counts still below 200/L at 16 months posttransplant. With simplification of CD34 positive selection using CliniMACS, Aversa led a similar study in 104 patients with AML and ALL.[86] In this study, 91% of patients had neutrophil engraftment by day +11. NK cells normalized by day +30 post transplant and $CD8^+$ cells reached 200/mm^2 by day +60 with a steady rise afterward. However, $CD4^+$ T cell engraftment remained delayed with counts rising above 100–200/mm^3 only after 10 months post transplant.

Selective CD3/CD19 depletion
Positive $CD34^+$ selection leads to delayed immune reconstitution due to depletion of T cells, B cells, non-$CD34^+$ myeloid cells, NK cells, and antigen-presenting cells. Thus, negative selection to specifically deplete

CD3[+] and CD19[+] cells from G-CSF-mobilized PBSCs was developed.[124] Using a reduced intensity conditioning regimen that excludes TBI and ATG, Chen et al. showed rapid recovery of CD3[+] T cells postinfusion of CD3-depleted haploidentical CD34[+] stem cells.[125] This was characterized by a diverse TCRβ repertoire with NK and B cell numbers reaching normal within 1 and 3 months posttransplant, respectively. Bethge et al.[126] from the same German group depleted CD3/CD19 using the same approach without posttransplant immunosuppression.[88,127] Neutrophil engraftment with full donor chimerism was achieved by day +15, and NK cells reached normal levels by day +20. However, T cell reconstitutions remain delayed with median CD4[+] and CD8[+] counts of 70/µL (12−301) and 66/µL (8−170)/mm^3 by day +100, respectively. Both memory and naïve T cells recovery were delayed. Both TCR αβ[+] and γδ T cells were delayed, with most patients demonstrating a restricted TCR repertoire at the end of the study. B cell reconstitution was also delayed, but NK cell reconstitution was early and fast. The shift from positive to negative selection of PBSC also increased GVHD.[88]

Selective TCR αβ +/- CD19 depletion

The majority of T cells express αβ TCRs. The selective depletion of the αβ T cell from the infused CD34[+] donor graft would preserve γδ T and NK cells, and is thought to favor homeostatic immune reconstitution. The γδ TCR expressing T cells belong to the innate immune system and can directly trigger immediate cytotoxic effects without the need for MHC-restricted antigen presentation.[128] Donor γδ T cells were also thought to facilitate engraftment.[129] Most of the studies using selective αβ T/CD19 depletion were in pediatric patients and were initially developed by Locatelli et al.[7] This approach was later adapted in adults. Kaynar et al.[89] reported 34 adult acute leukemia patients who underwent αβ TCD myeloablative haplo-SCT using CliniMACS and anti-TCR αβ antibodies. These patients received a median 12.7×10^6 CD34[+] cells/kg. Median neutrophil engraftment was at day +12. NK cells reached normal range by day +30. By day 30, the median γδ T cells number was 130/uL. The median absolute T cells number was 262/uL by day +90 with median CD4 and CD8 cells at 82/uL and 121/uL, respectively. Median B cell counts reached 162/uL by day +90. Using αβ T cell−depleted grafts, T cell reconstitution appeared to be faster than that with CD3[+]-/CD19[+]-depleted grafts. Likewise, there were also earlier B and CD8[+] reconstitution with improved counts.

Unmanipulated T Cell Grafts
G-CSF/ATG-based

G-CSF is thought to mediate immune tolerance by several mechanisms. G-CSF-mobilized donor CD34[+] stem cells contain myeloid-derived suppressor cells and regulatory B cells that can suppress alloreactive T cell responses.[123] Furthermore, G-CSF can polarize CD4[+] T cells toward the Th2 type and modulate monocytes and DCs. Finally, G-CSF can induce anergy in naïve T cells and stimulate Treg functions.[130] Huang et al.[10,11] first reported using a combination of G-CSF primed bone marrow and PBSCs with inclusion of ATG in haploidentical HCT without depletion of T cell populations. Compared to HLA-matched sibling transplants,[118] total CD4[+], naïve CD45RA[+], and memory CD45RO[+] cells were significantly lower in haplo-SCT patients at day +90 posttransplant. The median number of CD4[+] T cells was <200 cells/µL during the first 3 months in haploidentical recipients and gradually increased to 200 cells/µL by 6 months. On the other hand, CD8[+] T cells, including CD8[+] memory T cells, were significantly higher in haplo-SCT patients at day +90. By 1 year, there were no longer differences between the two groups. Subsets of DC, including myeloid C1, C2, and plasmacytoid DC were lower on days +15 and +30 in haploidentical recipients, but no significant difference in B cell counts at any time point after transplantation in haploidentical and HLA-matched recipients was observed. Thus, this approach resulted in a delayed CD4[+] T cell reconstitution.[118]

Posttransplant cyclophosphamide based

O'Donnell et al.[131] reported an initial experience of PTCy for 10 of 13 patients who received nonmyeloablative conditioning haplo-SCT. The median time to neutrophil engraftment was day +15. NK and CD4[+] T cell recovery was rapid, but B cell reconstitution was delayed. In this setting, the cumulative incidence of graft failure and delayed severe GVHD at 6 months was high.[131] Subsequently, Luznik et al.[15] treated 68 patients with modified PTCy at 50 mg/kg IV on day 3 or days 3 and 4, and increased the frequency of mycophenolate mofetil dosing. Engraftment failure was reduced and occurred in 9 (13%) of the 66 evaluable patients. Median time to neutrophil engraftment was 15 days. CD3[+] T cells and CD33[+] granulocytes showed >95% sustained engraftment by 2 months after transplantation. Thus, achievement of full donor chimerism was rapid. The low observed death rate from opportunistic infections is indicative of effective clinical immune reconstitution after transplantation.

Recently, Retiere et al. compared PTCy in haplo-SCT and ATG usage in matched SCT as GVHD prophylaxis in a reduced conditioning regimen; neutrophil recovery was similar between both groups.[132] Before day +30, αβ T cells, Treg, and CD4[+] T cells were significantly higher in the PTCy group. Conversely, B, NK cells, γδ T cells, and monocytes were higher in the ATG group. Higher median counts of αβ and γδ T cells, CD4[+] and CD8[+] T cells, and NK cells persisted on day +60 in the ATG group. However, profound B cell lymphopenia was observed in both groups. NK cells recovery was rapid and similar for both groups reaching normal counts by day +30. Thus, there were significant immune reconstitution differences between the two approaches. Numerous studies have now shown similar or even better clinical outcomes with PTCy haplo-SCT.[133]

Infectious Complications

Although many different haplo-SCT approaches have allowed us to overcome HLA disparities, delayed immune reconstitution from either T cell depletion or extensive immunosuppression has resulted in various infectious complications.[134–136]

Bacterial infections, most commonly Gram-negative bacteria, occur during the pre- and early engraftment phase after haplo-SCT.[135] They can also occur in patients receiving prolonged immunosuppression and in those experiencing GVHD during postengraftment period. Neutrophil recovery is the most important factor determining the risk of bacterial infection. Bloodstream infection with *Pseudomonas* spp., pulmonary, and gastrointestinal infections (including *Clostridium difficile*) are the most frequent bacterial infections after haplo-SCT.[137] With shorter times to neutrophil engraftment, the rates of bacterial infection have decreased and are comparable to stem cell transplant using matched donors.[135] High CD3[+]CD8[+] T cell count at day +90 correlates with a lower incidence of bacterial infection.[138] Chronic GVHD and associated systemic steroid use also increases the risk of late bacterial infection. Therefore, antibiotic prophylaxis has been used to prevent severe bacterial infections during the preengraftment period.

Infections from various viruses and fungi remain the most commonly reported in a setting of haplo-SCT. In TCD haplo-SCT, the T cell repertoire is very narrow and patients are susceptible to opportunistic infections for several months after transplant. The most common fungal infections are *Aspergillus* and *Candida* spp. The most frequently observed viral pathogens are cytomegalovirus (CMV), herpes simplex virus (HSV), varicella zoster (VZV), herpes human 6, and Epstein-Barr virus (EBV). Both donor and recipient seropositivities for CMV before transplant are a major risk factor for CMV reactivation and CMV disease during the posttransplant period between 4 and 12 months. Late CMV viremia and disease can occur in patients with GVHD requiring steroids and/or with poor or delayed recovery of CMV-specific T cells.[136]

Initial studies in T cell–depleted haplo-SCT using CD34[+] allografts have shown that although NK cells reach normal within 2–4 weeks after transplantation, CD4[+] T cell counts were below 200/mm[3] for as long as 16 months.[85] This led to a high rate of treatment-related mortality largely due to infections. With T cell depletion using e-rossetting, five patients died from systemic bacterial infection (three *Pseudomonas*, two *Staphylococcus*), five from fungal infections (three *Aspergillus*, two *Candida*), and one from CMV-associated pneumonia.[85] Using CliniMACS for enhanced positive CD34 selection,[86] 27 of 104 patients died from infection, 17 patients had viral infections with 14 dying from CMV, 1 adenovirus, 1 HHV6, and 1 EBV-associated posttransplant lymphoproliferative disease (PTLD). Five patients had fungal infections (four *Aspergillus*, one *Candida*) and five bacterial (two *Pseudomonas*, two *Streptococcus viridans*, and one *Escherichia coli*). With selective CD3[+]/19[+] depletion, 10 of the 29 patients died of infection with 1 idiopathic pneumonia syndrome, 2 bacterial pneumonia, 3 viral pneumonia, 1 aspergillosis, 2 toxoplasmosis, 2 meningitis with unknown microorganisms, and 1 patient with EBV-associated PTLD.[126] Eight patients also had CMV and six had HHV6 reactivation. With selective T cell depletion, TCRαβ-depleted haplo-SCT,[89] three patients died from bacterial infection and 2 from fungal infection (1 Blastoschizomyces, one mucormycosis). The cumulative incidence of CMV viremia was 74%, but none had CMV disease. BK uremia was 25% and was treated with cidofovir. None of the patients had EBV viremia or associated PTLD.

Huang et al.[10,11] treated 171 patients with hematological malignancies using a combination of G-CSF-primed bone marrow and PBSC with inclusion of ATG in haplo-SCT. Addition of ATG resulted in *in vivo* T cell depletion. Up to 40% (68/171) of patients had infectious complications. Fourteen patients had VZV and four had HSV skin infections. Fungal infection was significant with seven cases of *Aspergillus*, two of *Candida* and two *of Pneumocystis carinii*. CMV accounted for 3 of the 29 cases of pneumonia. In their updated study with 756 patients treated,[90] the cumulative incidence of CMV viremia at day 100 was 65%. Luznik et al.[15]

treated 68 patients with modified posttransplant cyclophosphamide haplo-SCT and CMV reactivation occurred in 17 patients. *Aspergillus* infection remained significant (n = 5). In unmanipulated haplo-SCT, peripheral T cell expansion is antagonized by the immune suppressive therapy for GVHD prophylaxis. There was a better memory and naïve T cell reconstitution in patients receiving unmanipulated haplo-SCT with PTCy as compared with TCD approaches.[135] A significantly lower incidence of herpesvirus infection and viral infection–related mortality were observed and attributed to a faster T cell recovery and better preserved anti-viral immunities. Trisher et al. compared virus infection in T cell replete haplo-SCT using PTCy and T cell deplete approach using ATG.[139] They found both herpesvirus and CMV reactivation were lower in haplo-SCT with PTCy. Lymphocytes >300/μL, CD3$^+$ T cells >200/μL, and CD4$^+$ T cells >150/μL on day +100 predicted a better overall survival.

Use of fluconazole as primary fungal infection prophylaxis has reduced the risks of invasive fungal infections and systemic candidiasis.[140] Primary prophylaxis using acyclovir against HSV infection is now standard of care,[141] but primary prophylaxis for CMV has not been standardized with valganciclovir[142] and letermovir[143] as effective choices. Adoptive T cell therapies now play an important role in successful treatment of various posttransplant virus infections including EBV, CMV, and adenovirus, and boosting anti-viral immunity without significant risk of GVHD.[144–148]

RELAPSE—MECHANISMS

Genetic disparity in haplo-SCTs should trigger potent graft-versus-tumor effect due to both major and minor histocompatibility antigen differences. Solh et al.[149] recently compared the survival outcomes for 237 patients relapsing after haplo-SCT using PTCy with those relapsing after matched-related donor transplantation or matched-unrelated donor transplantation. The median time to relapse was similar, but 1-year relapse free survival was worse after haplo-SCT. Relapse remains the most common cause of treatment failure for patients with hematologic malignancies after haplo-SCT.[150] T cell–depleted haplo-SCT in its early development had a high relapse rate attributed to significantly diminished alloreactive T cells.[151] Relapse remains high using unmanipulated donor T cells.[150] Several tumor immune escape mechanisms have been described in the transplant settings including decreased expression in MHC I and II molecules, selection of clones resistant to donor T and NK cells, and increased expression of inhibitory cytokines INFγ.[152]

NK cells are the main determinant of the GVL effect after haplo-SCT with T cell depletion. Alloreactive NK cells express KIRs and NKG2A receptors and exert cytotoxic function if engaged HLA class I molecules do not inhibit its function when mismatched. Activation of NK cells is regulated by multiple inhibiting and activating receptors. Donor alloreactive NK cells that eliminate leukemia relapse were first reported by Ruggeri.[75] His group subsequently studied 112 high-risk AML patients who had TCD haplo-SCT. They identified 51 donor/recipient pairs that were alloreactive in the donor-versus-recipient direction. For patients both in complete remission and with active disease prior to transplant, they had a lower relapse rate or better event-free survival if they had NK-alloreactive donors.[76] It needs to be mentioned that both inhibitory and activating NK receptors have specificities. Alloreactive donor NK cells expressing activating KIRs, in particular KIR2DS1, recognize C2 group HLA-Cw antigens and greatly contribute to NK alloreactivity.[153] Thus in choosing donors, provided that a patient's cells express C2 alleles, expression of KIR2DS1 should be a priority. More recently, Symons et al.[154] reported outcomes of 86 patients following nonmyeloablative haplo-SCT with PTCy; patients receiving inhibitory KIR gene-mismatched bone marrow graft had a lower relapse rate and better overall survival. Patients with only one activating KIR encoded by homozygous KIR AA haplotype and received at least one KIR Bx haplotype also had a lower relapse rate and better overall survival.

Minor histocompatibility antigens were initially studied in HLA-identical HCT setting and cytotoxic T cells during GVHD.[155] Subsequently, several minor antigens with their corresponding HLA restrictions and peptides have been identified. Human mHAgs are immunogenic peptides derived from intercellular proteins that have (low) polymorphisms between related and unrelated individuals and can be presented by both MHC class I and class II molecules. Alloreactivity against minor MHC encoded by Y-chromosome (H-Y-mHAg) occurs when the donor is a female and recipient is a male. Marijt et al.[46] treated three mHAg HA-1- and/or HA-2-positive patients with a relapse myeloma after alloSCT with DLI from their mHAg HA-1- and/or HA-2-negative donors. HA-1- and HA-2-specific-CD8$^+$ T cells were detectable about 5–7 weeks after DLI, and patients went into complete remission.

Vago et al. first identified the loss of HLA on leukemia cells in 5 of 17 relapsed AML/MDS patients who differed from the donor's haplotype due to acquired uniparental disomy of chromosome 6p after haplo-SCT.[156] In all cases, there were no copy-number variations. T cell subsets from mononuclear donor cells produced a robust response to the original leukemic cells. However, the same T cells no longer showed cytotoxicity, INFγ release, or proliferation in response to relapsed leukemic cells. Thus T cells from both donors and patients could no longer recognize the genomic rearranged relapsed leukemia cells, suggesting leukemic cells escaped from the selective pressure of patient-specific GVL alloreactive T cells. Villabobos et al. also identified a similar mechanism with loss of mismatched HLA from uniparental disomy in relapsed leukemia cells after haplo-SCT.[157]

Another mechanism of escape is loss of heterozygosity described by McCurdy et al. in two high-risk AML patients who relapsed after haplo-SCT using PTCy.[158] Using reverse sequence-specific oligonucleotide hybridization and melting curve analysis of the targeted alleles, loss of mismatched recipient HLA alleles on the leukemic cells were identified. Single nucleotide polymorphism array for one patient showed uniparental disomy at 6p while one patient had a deletion of chromosome 6p that encompassed the mismatched HLA locus. The latter represents a different, but similar genomic mechanism and supports that the leukemic cells may lose the mismatched HLA haplotype through multiple means, resulting in evasion of the donor immune system.

Downregulation of mismatched HLA class I antigens is another escape mechanism in haplo-SCT described by Tamaki et al.[159] Despite retention of both HLA haplotypes on the leukemic cell surface of AML patients who relapsed after transplant, there was lack of mismatched HLA-A indicated by flow cytometric analysis. The authors speculated that there might be impairment in epigenetic regulation of the gene that caused downregulation of HLA class I on unshared alleles. Most recently Christopher et al. described dysregulation of pathways involved in adaptive and innate immunity, including downregulation of MHC class II genes (HLA-DPA1, HLA-DPB1, HLA-DQB1, and HLA-DRB1) in relapsed AML following allogeneic stem cell transplant.[160] T cell exhaustion with reduced cytotoxicity from both MHC class I and II dysfunction has also been reported as an escape mechanism for patients with relapsed AML and B-ALL after HSCT.[161,162]

Strategies to Prevent Relapse

Bidirectional transplacental trafficking of maternal and fetal cells during pregnancy with development of microchimerism in both mother and fetus has been well documented. Antibodies directed against paternal HLA antigens and memory type T lymphocytes directed against paternal major and minor histocompatibility antigens from the fetus frequently circulate in multiparous women.[163,164] In theory, both maternal humoral and cellular immunity can mediate graft-versus-tumor effect if used as a donor. Indeed, Stern et al. found an improved 5-year survival in acute leukemia patients receiving maternal donor cells after TCD haplo-SCT with relapse rates lower from maternal donors than that from paternal donors.[165] Thus, when sibling, parents, or offspring are potential donors, maternal donors should be considered as priority in the haplo-SCT setting.

There is a range of possible HLA mismatch in haplo-SCT. Mismatch combination causing GVL effect may not be the same ones that cause GVHD. Studying a cohort of 4643 Japanese patients with hematologic malignancies after HLA-A, HLA-B, and HLA-DR matched-unrelated donor stem cell transplant, Kawase et al. identified four HLA-Cw and six HLA-DPB1 mismatch combinations responsible for a decreased risk of disease relapse.[166] The authors also found that amino acid substitutions ser9C-Tyr9C, Phe99C-Tyr99C, and Arg156C-Leu156C in HLA-Cw were linked to a decreased risk of relapse, although no such effect was identified in HLA-DPB1. Thus, donor selection with known HLA-Cw and HLA-DPB1 mismatches or amino acid substitutions known to decrease relapse risk should be considered when available.

The presence of KIR2DS1 on NK cells from the donor graft appears to provide protection against AML relapse, and KIR3DS1 was also associated with reduced mortality.[167] Mancusi et al. showed that the KIR ligand−mismatched donors with activating receptors KIR2DS1 and KIR3DS1 expression have a survival advantage during haplo-SCT because of a reduced infection rate and mortality.[168]

T cells that express γδ TCRs do not appear to require antigen processing and MHC presentation of peptide epitopes.[87] They do engage with MHC class Ib molecules and are believed to recognize lipid antigens. These γδ T cells are most abundant in the gut mucosa. In a long-term follow-up study of 153 acute leukemia transplant patients receiving partially mismatched and TCD grafts using either OKT3 or T10B9 anti-T cell antibodies, an increased number of γδ T cells was associated with better 5-year leukemia-free and overall survival.[169] Thus γδ T cells appear to exert protective role against leukemia relapse. Indeed, adoptive transfer of ex vivo expanded γδ T cells is now being explored for leukemia after allogeneic stem cell transplant.[170]

CONCLUSION

Haplo-SCT has evolved from an early problematic approach to now a widely adapted option for patients in need of alternative donors. With improved immune reconstitution, lower incidence of GVHD and infection, the clinical outcomes of haplo-SCT with PTCy are now comparable to that of HLA-matched donor transplants. Like HLA-matched transplant, relapse after haplo-SCT has become the major cause of transplant failure. Future studies that focus on relapse prevention and enhancement of GVL effect will likely enhance its utility.

REFERENCES

1. Cowan MJ, Wara DW, Weintrub PS, Pabst H, Ammann AJ. Haploidentical bone marrow transplantation for severe combined immunodeficiency disease using soybean agglutinin-negative, T-depleted marrow cells. *J Clin Immunol.* 1985;5:370–376.

2. Reisner Y, et al. Transplantation for severe combined immunodeficiency with HLA-A,B,D,DR incompatible parental marrow cells fractionated by soybean agglutinin and sheep red blood cells. *Blood.* 1983;61:341–348.

3. Bozdech MJ, et al. Transplantation of HLA-haploidentical T-cell-depleted marrow for leukemia: addition of cytosine arabinoside to the pretransplant conditioning prevents rejection. *Exp Hematol.* 1985;13:1201–1210.

4. Beatty PG, et al. Marrow transplantation from related donors other than HLA-identical siblings. *N Engl J Med.* 1985;313:765–771.

5. Aversa F, et al. Successful engraftment of T-cell-depleted haploidentical "three-loci" incompatible transplants in leukemia patients by addition of recombinant human granulocyte colony-stimulating factor-mobilized peripheral blood progenitor cells to bone marrow inoculum. *Blood.* 1994;84:3948–3955.

6. Handgretinger R, et al. Megadose transplantation of purified peripheral blood CD34(+) progenitor cells from HLA-mismatched parental donors in children. *Bone Marrow Transplant.* 2001;27:777–783.

7. Locatelli F, Bauquet A, Palumbo G, Moretta F, Bertaina A. Negative depletion of alpha/beta+ T cells and of CD19+ B lymphocytes: a novel frontier to optimize the effect of innate immunity in HLA-mismatched hematopoietic stem cell transplantation. *Immunol Lett.* 2013;155:21–23.

8. Bertaina A, et al. HLA-haploidentical stem cell transplantation after removal of alphabeta+ T and B cells in children with nonmalignant disorders. *Blood.* 2014;124: 822–826.

9. Martelli MF, et al. HLA-haploidentical transplantation with regulatory and conventional T-cell adoptive immunotherapy prevents acute leukemia relapse. *Blood.* 2014; 124:638–644.

10. Huang XJ, et al. Combined transplantation of G-CSF primed allogeneic bone marrow cells and peripheral blood stem cells in treatment of severe aplastic anemia. *Chin Med J.* 2004;117:604–607.

11. Huang XJ, et al. Haploidentical hematopoietic stem cell transplantation without in vitro T-cell depletion for the treatment of hematological malignancies. *Bone Marrow Transplant.* 2006;38:291–297.

12. Lv M, Chang Y, Huang X. Everyone has a donor: contribution of the Chinese experience to global practice of haploidentical hematopoietic stem cell transplantation. *Front Med.* 2018;13(1):45–56.

13. Luznik L, Jalla S, Engstrom LW, Iannone R, Fuchs EJ. Durable engraftment of major histocompatibility complex-incompatible cells after nonmyeloablative conditioning with fludarabine, low-dose total body irradiation, and posttransplantation cyclophosphamide. *Blood.* 2001;98: 3456–3464.

14. Kasamon YL, et al. Nonmyeloablative HLA-haploidentical bone marrow transplantation with high-dose posttransplantation cyclophosphamide: effect of HLA disparity on outcome. *Biol Blood Marrow Transplant.* 2010;16:482–489.

15. Luznik L, et al. HLA-haploidentical bone marrow transplantation for hematologic malignancies using nonmyeloablative conditioning and high-dose, posttransplantation cyclophosphamide. *Biol Blood Marrow Transplant.* 2008;14:641–650.

16. Ciurea SO, et al. Haploidentical transplant with posttransplant cyclophosphamide vs matched unrelated donor transplant for acute myeloid leukemia. *Blood.* 2015;126:1033–1040.

17. Kanate AS, et al. Reduced-intensity transplantation for lymphomas using haploidentical related donors vs HLA-matched unrelated donors. *Blood.* 2016;127: 938–947.

18. Ghosh N, et al. Reduced-intensity transplantation for lymphomas using haploidentical related donors versus HLA-matched sibling donors: a center for international blood and marrow transplant research analysis. *J Clin Oncol.* 2016;34:3141–3149.

19. Bashey A, et al. Comparison of outcomes of hematopoietic cell transplants from T-replete haploidentical donors using post-transplantation cyclophosphamide with 10 of 10 HLA-A, -B, -C, -DRB1, and -DQB1 allele-matched unrelated donors and HLA-identical sibling donors: a multivariable analysis including disease risk index. *Biol Blood Marrow Transplant.* 2016;22:125–133.

20. Devillier R, et al. HLA-matched sibling versus unrelated versus haploidentical related donor allogeneic hematopoietic stem cell transplantation for patients aged over 60 Years with acute myeloid leukemia: a single-center donor comparison. *Biol Blood Marrow Transplant.* 2018; 24:1449–1454.

21. Rocha V, Gluckman E, Eurocord-Netcord r, European B, Marrow Transplant g. Improving outcomes of cord blood transplantation: HLA matching, cell dose and other graft- and transplantation-related factors. *Br J Haematol.* 2009; 147:262–274.

22. Gmur JP, et al. Pure red cell aplasia of long duration complicating major ABO-incompatible bone marrow transplantation. *Blood.* 1990;75:290—295.

23. Nakamae H, et al. Cytopenias after day 28 in allogeneic hematopoietic cell transplantation: impact of recipient/ donor factors, transplant conditions and myelotoxic drugs. *Haematologica.* 2011;96:1838—1845.

24. Tsai SB, et al. Frequency and risk factors associated with cord graft failure after transplant with single-unit umbilical cord cells supplemented by haploidentical cells with reduced-intensity conditioning. *Biol Blood Marrow Transplant.* 2016;22:1065—1072.

25. Olsson R, et al. Graft failure in the modern era of allogeneic hematopoietic SCT. *Bone Marrow Transplant.* 2013; 48:537—543.

26. Petersdorf EW, et al. Major-histocompatibility-complex class I alleles and antigens in hematopoietic-cell transplantation. *N Engl J Med.* 2001;345:1794—1800.

27. Lang P, et al. Long-term outcome after haploidentical stem cell transplantation in children. *Blood Cells Mol Dis.* 2004;33:281—287.

28. Ciceri F, et al. A survey of fully haploidentical hematopoietic stem cell transplantation in adults with high-risk acute leukemia: a risk factor analysis of outcomes for patients in remission at transplantation. *Blood.* 2008;112: 3574—3581.

29. Koh LP, Rizzieri DA, Chao NJ. Allogeneic hematopoietic stem cell transplant using mismatched/haploidentical donors. *Biol Blood Marrow Transplant.* 2007;13: 1249—1267.

30. Mattsson J, Ringden O, Storb R. Graft failure after allogeneic hematopoietic cell transplantation. *Biol Blood Marrow Transplant.* 2008;14:165—170.

31. Murphy WJ, Kumar V, Bennett M. Acute rejection of murine bone marrow allografts by natural killer cells and T cells. Differences in kinetics and target antigens recognized. *J Exp Med.* 1987;166:1499—1509.

32. Raff RF, et al. Characterization of host cells involved in resistance to marrow grafts in dogs transplanted from unrelated DLA-nonidentical donors. *Blood.* 1986;68: 861—868.

33. Masouridi-Levrat S, Simonetta F, Chalandon Y. Immunological basis of bone marrow failure after allogeneic hematopoietic stem cell transplantation. *Front Immunol.* 2016;7:362.

34. Cudkowicz G, Bennett M. Peculiar immunobiology of bone marrow allografts. I. Graft rejection by irradiated responder mice. *J Exp Med.* 1971;134:83—102.

35. Murphy WJ, Kumar V, Bennett M. Rejection of bone marrow allografts by mice with severe combined immune deficiency (SCID). Evidence that natural killer cells can mediate the specificity of marrow graft rejection. *J Exp Med.* 1987;165:1212—1217.

36. Exner BG, Colson YL, Li H, Ildstad ST. In vivo depletion of host CD4+ and CD8+ cells permits engraftment of bone marrow stem cells and tolerance induction with minimal conditioning. *Surgery.* 1997;122:221—227.

37. Kernan NA, et al. Clonable T lymphocytes in T cell-depleted bone marrow transplants correlate with development of graft-v-host disease. *Blood.* 1986;68:770—773.

38. Bierer BE, et al. Regulation of cytotoxic T lymphocyte-mediated graft rejection following bone marrow transplantation. *Transplantation.* 1988;46:835—839.

39. Terenzi A, et al. Residual clonable host cell detection for predicting engraftment of T cell depleted BMTs. *Bone Marrow Transplant.* 1993;11:357—361.

40. Xu H, et al. CD8(+), alphabeta-TCR(+), and gammadelta-TCR(+) cells in the recipient hematopoietic environment mediate resistance to engraftment of allogeneic donor bone marrow. *J Immunol.* 2002;168: 1636—1643.

41. Lowin B, Hahne M, Mattmann C, Tschopp J. Cytolytic T-cell cytotoxicity is mediated through perforin and Fas lytic pathways. *Nature.* 1994;370:650—652.

42. Zimmerman Z, et al. Effector cells derived from host CD8 memory T cells mediate rapid resistance against minor histocompatibility antigen-mismatched allogeneic marrow grafts without participation of perforin, Fas ligand, and the simultaneous inhibition of 3 tumor necrosis factor family effector pathways. *Biol Blood Marrow Transplant.* 2005;11:576—586.

43. Kernan NA, Flomenberg N, Dupont B, O'Reilly RJ. Graft rejection in recipients of T-cell-depleted HLA-nonidentical marrow transplants for leukemia. Identification of host-derived antidonor allocytotoxic T lymphocytes. *Transplantation.* 1987;43:842—847.

44. Zimmerman Z, et al. Cytolytic pathways used by effector cells derived from recipient naive and memory T cells and natural killer cells in resistance to allogeneic hematopoietic cell transplantation. *Biol Blood Marrow Transplant.* 2005;11:957—971.

45. Kraus AB, et al. Early host CD8 T-cell recovery and sensitized anti-donor interleukin-2-producing and cytotoxic T-cell responses associated with marrow graft rejection following nonmyeloablative allogeneic bone marrow transplantation. *Exp Hematol.* 2003;31:609—621.

46. Marijt WA, et al. Hematopoiesis-restricted minor histocompatibility antigens HA-1- or HA-2-specific T cells can induce complete remissions of relapsed leukemia. *Proc Natl Acad Sci USA.* 2003;100:2742—2747.

47. Vogt MH, de Paus RA, Voogt PJ, Willemze R, Falkenburg JH. DFFRY codes for a new human male-specific minor transplantation antigen involved in bone marrow graft rejection. *Blood.* 2000;95:1100—1105.

48. Anasetti C, et al. Effect of HLA compatibility on engraftment of bone marrow transplants in patients with leukemia or lymphoma. *N Engl J Med.* 1989;320:197—204.

49. Flomenberg N, et al. Impact of HLA class I and class II high-resolution matching on outcomes of unrelated donor bone marrow transplantation: HLA-C mismatching is associated with a strong adverse effect on transplantation outcome. *Blood.* 2004;104:1923—1930.

50. Petersdorf EW, et al. Optimizing outcome after unrelated marrow transplantation by comprehensive matching of

HLA class I and II alleles in the donor and recipient. *Blood.* 1998;92:3515−3520.

51. Gill S, Olson JA, Negrin RS. Natural killer cells in allogeneic transplantation: effect on engraftment, graft- versus-tumor, and graft-versus-host responses. *Biol Blood Marrow Transplant.* 2009;15:765−776.

52. Long EO. Regulation of immune responses through inhibitory receptors. *Annu Rev Immunol.* 1999;17:875−904.

53. Tu MM, Mahmoud AB, Makrigiannis AP. Licensed and unlicensed NK cells: differential roles in cancer and viral control. *Front Immunol.* 2016;7:166.

54. Sun K, et al. Mouse NK cell-mediated rejection of bone marrow allografts exhibits patterns consistent with Ly49 subset licensing. *Blood.* 2012;119:1590−1598.

55. Bordignon C, et al. The role of residual host immunity in graft failures following T-cell-depleted marrow transplants for leukemia. *Ann N Y Acad Sci.* 1987;511:442−446.

56. De Santis D, et al. Natural killer cell HLA-C epitopes and killer cell immunoglobulin-like receptors both influence outcome of mismatched unrelated donor bone marrow transplants. *Tissue Antigens.* 2005;65:519−528.

57. Beelen DW, et al. Genotypic inhibitory killer immunoglobulin-like receptor ligand incompatibility enhances the long-term antileukemic effect of unmodified allogeneic hematopoietic stem cell transplantation in patients with myeloid leukemias. *Blood.* 2005;105:2594−2600.

58. Warren RP, Storb R, Weiden PL, Mickelson EM, Thomas ED. Direct and antibody-dependent cell-mediated cytotoxicity against HLA identical sibling lymphocytes. Correlation with marrow graft rejections. *Transplantation.* 1976;22:631−635.

59. Ciurea SO, et al. High risk of graft failure in patients with anti-HLA antibodies undergoing haploidentical stem-cell transplantation. *Transplantation.* 2009;88:1019−1024.

60. Ciurea SO, et al. Donor-specific anti-HLA Abs and graft failure in matched unrelated donor hematopoietic stem cell transplantation. *Blood.* 2011;118:5957−5964.

61. Morin-Papunen L, Tiilikainen A, Hartikainen-Sorri AL. Maternal HLA immunization during pregnancy: presence of anti HLA antibodies in half of multigravidous women. *Med Biol.* 1984;62:323−325.

62. Barge AJ, Johnson G, Witherspoon R, Torok-Storb B. Antibody-mediated marrow failure after allogeneic bone marrow transplantation. *Blood.* 1989;74:1477−1480.

63. Ciurea SO, et al. Complement-binding donor-specific anti-HLA antibodies and risk of primary graft failure in hematopoietic stem cell transplantation. *Biol Blood Marrow Transplant.* 2015;21:1392−1398.

64. Yoshihara S, et al. Risk and prevention of graft failure in patients with preexisting donor-specific HLA antibodies undergoing unmanipulated haploidentical SCT. *Bone Marrow Transplantation.* 2012;47:508−515.

65. Chang YJ, et al. Donor-specific anti-human leukocyte antigen antibodies were associated with primary graft failure after unmanipulated haploidentical blood and marrow transplantation: a prospective study with randomly assigned training and validation sets. *J Hematol Oncol.* 2015;8:84.

66. Ruggeri A, et al. Impact of donor-specific anti-HLA antibodies on graft failure and survival after reduced intensity conditioning-unrelated cord blood transplantation: a Eurocord, Societe Francophone d'Histocompatibilite et d'Immunogenetique (SFHI) and Societe Francaise de Greffe de Moelle et de Therapie Cellulaire (SFGM-TC) analysis. *Haematologica.* 2013;98:1154−1160.

67. Nordlander A, Mattsson J, Sundberg B, Sumitran-Holgersson S. Novel antibodies to the donor stem cell population CD34+/VEGFR-2+ are associated with rejection after hematopoietic stem cell transplantation. *Transplantation.* 2008;86:686−696.

68. Remberger M, et al. Major ABO blood group mismatch increases the risk for graft failure after unrelated donor hematopoietic stem cell transplantation. *Biol Blood Marrow Transplant.* 2007;13:675−682.

69. Taylor PA, et al. Preformed antibody, not primed T cells, is the initial and major barrier to bone marrow engraftment in allosensitized recipients. *Blood.* 2007;109:1307−1315.

70. Reisner Y, Martelli MF. Tolerance induction by 'megadose' transplants of CD34+ stem cells: a new option for leukemia patients without an HLA-matched donor. *Curr Opin Immunol.* 2000;12:536−541.

71. Pilat N, et al. Treg-therapy allows mixed chimerism and transplantation tolerance without cytoreductive conditioning. *Am J Transplant.* 2010;10:751−762.

72. Joffre O, et al. Prevention of acute and chronic allograft rejection with CD4+CD25+Foxp3+ regulatory T lymphocytes. *Nat Med.* 2008;14:88−92.

73. Steiner D, et al. Overcoming T cell-mediated rejection of bone marrow allografts by T-regulatory cells: synergism with veto cells and rapamycin. *Exp Hematol.* 2006;34:802−808.

74. Steiner D, Brunicki N, Blazar BR, Bachar-Lustig E, Reisner Y. Tolerance induction by third-party "off-the-shelf" CD4+CD25+ Treg cells. *Exp Hematol.* 2006;34:66−71.

75. Ruggeri L, et al. Effectiveness of donor natural killer cell alloreactivity in mismatched hematopoietic transplants. *Science.* 2002;295:2097−2100.

76. Ruggeri L, et al. Donor natural killer cell allorecognition of missing self in haploidentical hematopoietic transplantation for acute myeloid leukemia: challenging its predictive value. *Blood.* 2007;110:433−440.

77. Murphy WJ, Bennett M, Kumar V, Longo DL. Donor-type activated natural killer cells promote marrow engraftment and B cell development during allogeneic bone marrow transplantation. *J Immunol.* 1992;148:2953−2960.

78. Asai O, et al. Suppression of graft-versus-host disease and amplification of graft-versus-tumor effects by activated natural killer cells after allogeneic bone marrow transplantation. *J Clin Investig.* 1998;101:1835−1842.

79. Gladstone DE, Bettinotti MP. HLA donor-specific antibodies in allogeneic hematopoietic stem cell transplantation: challenges and opportunities. *Hematology Am Soc Hematol Educ Program*. 2017;2017:645–650.

80. Amrolia PJ, et al. Adoptive immunotherapy with allodepleted donor T-cells improves immune reconstitution after haploidentical stem cell transplantation. *Blood*. 2006; 108:1797–1808.

81. Korngold R, Sprent J. Lethal graft-versus-host disease after bone marrow transplantation across minor histocompatibility barriers in mice. Prevention by removing mature T cells from marrow. *J Exp Med*. 1978;148: 1687–1698.

82. Powles RL, et al. Mismatched family donors for bone-marrow transplantation as treatment for acute leukaemia. *Lancet*. 1983;1:612–615.

83. Or-Geva N, Reisner Y. The evolution of T-cell depletion in haploidentical stem-cell transplantation. *Br J Haematol*. 2016;172:667–684.

84. Vadakekolathu J, Rutella S. T-cell manipulation strategies to prevent graft-versus-host disease in haploidentical stem cell transplantation. *Biomedicines*. 2017;5.

85. Aversa F, et al. Treatment of high-risk acute leukemia with T-cell-depleted stem cells from related donors with one fully mismatched HLA haplotype. *N Engl J Med*. 1998; 339:1186–1193.

86. Aversa F, et al. Full haplotype-mismatched hematopoietic stem-cell transplantation: a phase II study in patients with acute leukemia at high risk of relapse. *J Clin Oncol*. 2005;23:3447–3454.

87. Vantourout P, Hayday A. Six-of-the-best: unique contributions of gammadelta T cells to immunology. *Nat Rev Immunol*. 2013;13:88–100.

88. Bethge WA, et al. Haploidentical allogeneic hematopoietic cell transplantation in adults using CD3/CD19 depletion and reduced intensity conditioning: an update. *Blood Cells Mol Dis*. 2008;40:13–19.

89. Kaynar L, et al. TcRalphabeta-depleted haploidentical transplantation results in adult acute leukemia patients. *Hematology*. 2017;22:136–144.

90. Wang Y, et al. Long-term follow-up of haploidentical hematopoietic stem cell transplantation without in vitro T cell depletion for the treatment of leukemia: nine years of experience at a single center. *Cancer*. 2013;119: 978–985.

91. Emadi A, Jones RJ, Brodsky RA. Cyclophosphamide and cancer: golden anniversary. *Nat Rev Clin Oncol*. 2009;6: 638–647.

92. Raiola AM, et al. Unmanipulated haploidentical bone marrow transplantation and posttransplantation cyclophosphamide for hematologic malignancies after myeloablative conditioning. *Biol Blood Marrow Transplant*. 2013;19:117–122.

93. Raj K, et al. Peripheral blood hematopoietic stem cells for transplantation of hematological diseases from related, haploidentical donors after reduced-intensity conditioning. *Biol Blood Marrow Transplant*. 2014;20: 890–895.

94. Rizzieri DA, et al. Partially matched, nonmyeloablative allogeneic transplantation: clinical outcomes and immune reconstitution. *J Clin Oncol*. 2007;25:690–697.

95. Danby R, Rocha V. Improving engraftment and immune reconstitution in umbilical cord blood transplantation. *Front Immunol*. 2014;5:68.

96. Ogonek J, et al. Immune reconstitution after allogeneic hematopoietic stem cell transplantation. *Front Immunol*. 2016;7:507.

97. van Besien K, Childs R. Haploidentical cord transplantation-The best of both worlds. *Semin Hematol*. 2016;53:257–266.

98. Jain N, et al. Immune reconstitution after combined haploidentical and umbilical cord blood transplant. *Leuk Lymphoma*. 2013;54:1242–1249.

99. van Besien K, et al. Cord blood chimerism and relapse after haplo-cord transplantation. *Leuk Lymphoma*. 2017;58: 288–297.

100. Chang YJ, Zhao XY, Huang XJ. Immune reconstitution after haploidentical hematopoietic stem cell transplantation. *Biol Blood Marrow Transplant*. 2014;20: 440–449.

101. Fry TJ, Mackall CL. Immune reconstitution following hematopoietic progenitor cell transplantation: challenges for the future. *Bone Marrow Transplantation*. 2005; 35(Suppl 1):S53–S57.

102. Yew PY, et al. Quantitative characterization of T-cell repertoire in allogeneic hematopoietic stem cell transplant recipients. *Bone Marrow Transplantation*. 2015;50: 1227–1234.

103. Hori S, Nomura T, Sakaguchi S. Control of regulatory T cell development by the transcription factor Foxp3. *Science*. 2003;299:1057–1061.

104. Cobbold SP, et al. Induction of foxP3+ regulatory T cells in the periphery of T cell receptor transgenic mice tolerized to transplants. *J Immunol*. 2004;172:6003–6010.

105. Xystrakis E, et al. Identification of a novel natural regulatory CD8 T-cell subset and analysis of its mechanism of regulation. *Blood*. 2004;104:3294–3301.

106. Robb RJ, et al. Identification and expansion of highly suppressive CD8(+)FoxP3(+) regulatory T cells after experimental allogeneic bone marrow transplantation. *Blood*. 2012;119:5898–5908.

107. Cooper MA, Fehniger TA, Caligiuri MA. The biology of human natural killer-cell subsets. *Trends Immunol*. 2001; 22:633–640.

108. Park BG, et al. Reconstitution of lymphocyte subpopulations after hematopoietic stem cell transplantation: comparison of hematologic malignancies and donor types in event-free patients. *Leuk Res*. 2015;39:1334–1341.

109. Mackall C, et al. Background to hematopoietic cell transplantation, including post transplant immune recovery. *Bone Marrow Transplant*. 2009;44:457–462.

110. Suryani S, et al. Differential expression of CD21 identifies developmentally and functionally distinct subsets of human transitional B cells. *Blood*. 2010;115:519–529.

111. Corre E, et al. Long-term immune deficiency after allogeneic stem cell transplantation: B-cell deficiency is

associated with late infections. *Haematologica.* 2010;95:
1025−1029.

112. Omazic B, Lundkvist I, Mattsson J, Permert J, Nasman-
Bjork I. Memory B lymphocytes determine repertoire oli-
goclonality early after haematopoietic stem cell
transplantation. *Clin Exp Immunol.* 2003;134:159−166.

113. Bemark M, Holmqvist J, Abrahamsson J, Mellgren K.
Translational Mini-Review Series on B cell subsets in disease. Reconstitution after haematopoietic stem cell transplantation - revelation of B cell developmental pathways
and lineage phenotypes. *Clin Exp Immunol.* 2012;167:
15−25.

114. Williams KM, Gress RE. Immune reconstitution and implications for immunotherapy following haematopoietic
stem cell transplantation. *Best Pract Res Clin Haematol.*
2008;21:579−596.

115. Roll P, et al. Effect of ATG-F on B-cell reconstitution after
hematopoietic stem cell transplantation. *Eur J Haematol.*
2015;95:514−523.

116. Petersen SL, et al. A comparison of T-, B- and NK-cell
reconstitution following conventional or nonmyeloablative conditioning and transplantation with bone marrow
or peripheral blood stem cells from human leucocyte antigen identical sibling donors. *Bone Marrow Transplant.*
2003;32:65−72.

117. Storek J, Wells D, Dawson MA, Storer B, Maloney DG.
Factors influencing B lymphopoiesis after allogeneic hematopoietic cell transplantation. *Blood.* 2001;98:
489−491.

118. Chang YJ, et al. Immune reconstitution following unmanipulated HLA-mismatched/haploidentical transplantation compared with HLA-identical sibling
transplantation. *J Clin Immunol.* 2012;32:268−280.

119. Gkazi AS, et al. Clinical T cell receptor repertoire deep
sequencing and analysis: an application to monitor immune reconstitution following cord blood
transplantation. *Front Immunol.* 2018;9:2547.

120. Oevermann L, et al. Immune reconstitution and strategies for rebuilding the immune system after haploidentical stem cell transplantation. *Ann N Y Acad Sci.* 2012;
1266:161−170.

121. Chaudhry MS, Velardi E, Malard F, van den Brink MR.
Immune reconstitution after allogeneic hematopoietic
stem cell transplantation: time to T up the thymus.
J Immunol. 2017;198:40−46.

122. Mehta RS, Rezvani K. Immune reconstitution post allogeneic transplant and the impact of immune recovery on
the risk of infection. *Virulence.* 2016;7:901−916.

123. Rutella S, Zavala F, Danese S, Kared H, Leone G. Granulocyte colony-stimulating factor: a novel mediator of
T cell tolerance. *J Immunol.* 2005;175:7085−7091.

124. Barfield RC, et al. A one-step large-scale method for T-
and B-cell depletion of mobilized PBSC for allogeneic
transplantation. *Cytotherapy.* 2004;6:1−6.

125. Chen X, et al. Rapid immune reconstitution after a
reduced-intensity conditioning regimen and a CD3-
depleted haploidentical stem cell graft for paediatric

refractory haematological malignancies. *Br J Haematol.*
2006;135:524−532.

126. Federmann B, et al. Immune reconstitution after haploidentical hematopoietic cell transplantation: impact of
reduced intensity conditioning and CD3/CD19 depleted
grafts. *Leukemia.* 2011;25:121−129.

127. Bethge WA, et al. Haploidentical allogeneic hematopoietic cell transplantation in adults with reduced-intensity
conditioning and CD3/CD19 depletion: fast engraftment
and low toxicity. *Exp Hematol.* 2006;34:1746−1752.

128. Hayday AC. Gammadelta T cells and the lymphoid stress-
surveillance response. *Immunity.* 2009;31:184−196.

129. Drobyski WR, Majewski D. Donor gamma delta T lymphocytes promote allogeneic engraftment across the major histocompatibility barrier in mice. *Blood.* 1997;89:
1100−1109.

130. Chang YJ, Huang XJ. Haploidentical SCT: the mechanisms underlying the crossing of HLA barriers. *Bone
Marrow Transplant.* 2014;49:873−879.

131. O'Donnell PV, et al. Nonmyeloablative bone marrow
transplantation from partially HLA-mismatched related
donors using posttransplantation cyclophosphamide.
Biol Blood Marrow Transplant. 2002;8:377−386.

132. Retiere C, et al. Impact on early outcomes and immune
reconstitution of high-dose post-transplant cyclophosphamide vs anti-thymocyte globulin after reduced intensity conditioning peripheral blood stem cell allogeneic
transplantation. *Oncotarget.* 2018;9:11451−11464.

133. Sun YQ, Chang YJ, Huang XJ. Update on current research
into haploidentical hematopoietic stem cell
transplantation. *Expert Rev Hematol.* 2018;11:273−284.

134. Ali MY, et al. Reassessing the definition of myeloid
engraftment after autotransplantation: it is not necessary
to see $0.5 \times 10(9)/l$ neutrophils on 3 consecutive days to
define myeloid recovery. *Bone Marrow Transplant.* 2002;
30:749−752.

135. Atilla E, Atilla PA, Bozdag SC, Demirer T. A review of infectious complications after haploidentical hematopoietic stem cell transplantations. *Infection.* 2017;45:403−411.

136. Aversa F, et al. Immunity to infections after haploidentical hematopoietic stem cell transplantation. *Mediterr J
Hematol Infect Dis.* 2016;8:e2016057.

137. Balletto E, Mikulska M. Bacterial infections in hematopoietic stem cell transplant recipients. *Mediterr J Hematol
Infect Dis.* 2015;7:e2015045.

138. Tian DM, et al. Rapid recovery of CD3+CD8+ T cells on
day 90 predicts superior survival after unmanipulated
haploidentical blood and marrow transplantation. *PLoS
One.* 2016;11:e0156777.

139. Tischer J, et al. Virus infection in HLA-haploidentical hematopoietic stem cell transplantation: incidence in the
context of immune recovery in two different transplantation settings. *Ann Hematol.* 2015;94:1677−1688.

140. Ziakas PD, Kourbeti IS, Mylonakis E. Systemic anti-
fungal prophylaxis after hematopoietic stem cell transplantation: a meta-analysis. *Clin Ther.* 2014;36:
292−306 e291.

141. Saral R, Burns WH, Laskin OL, Santos GW, Lietman PS. Acyclovir prophylaxis of herpes-simplex-virus infections. *N Engl J Med.* 1981;305:63–67.

142. Boeckh M, et al. Valganciclovir for the prevention of complications of late cytomegalovirus infection after allogeneic hematopoietic cell transplantation: a randomized trial. *Ann Intern Med.* 2015;162:1–10.

143. Chemaly RF, et al. Letermovir for cytomegalovirus prophylaxis in hematopoietic-cell transplantation. *N Engl J Med.* 2014;370:1781–1789.

144. Houghtelin A, Bollard CM. Virus-specific T cells for the immunocompromised patient. *Front Immunol.* 2017;8:1272.

145. Barrett AJ, Prockop S, Bollard CM. Virus-specific T cells: broadening applicability. *Biol Blood Marrow Transplant.* 2018;24:13–18.

146. Roddie C, Peggs KS. Immunotherapy for transplantation-associated viral infections. *J Clin Investig.* 2017;127:2513–2522.

147. Bollard CM, Heslop HE. T cells for viral infections after allogeneic hematopoietic stem cell transplant. *Blood.* 2016;127:3331–3340.

148. Themeli M, Riviere I, Sadelain M. New cell sources for T cell engineering and adoptive immunotherapy. *Cell Stem Cell.* 2015;16:357–366.

149. Solh M, et al. Post-relapse survival after haploidentical transplantation vs matched-related or matched-unrelated hematopoietic cell transplantation. *Bone Marrow Transplant.* 2016;51:949–954.

150. Farhadfar N, Hogan WJ. Overview of the progress on haploidentical hematopoietic transplantation. *World J Transplant.* 2016;6:665–674.

151. Kanda J, Chao NJ, Rizzieri DA. Haploidentical transplantation for leukemia. *Curr Oncol Rep.* 2010;12:292–301.

152. Dermime S, et al. Immune escape from a graft-versus-leukemia effect may play a role in the relapse of myeloid leukemias following allogeneic bone marrow transplantation. *Bone Marrow Transplant.* 1997;19:989–999.

153. Chewning JH, Gudme CN, Hsu KC, Selvakumar A, Dupont B. KIR2DS1-positive NK cells mediate alloresponse against the C2 HLA-KIR ligand group in vitro. *J Immunol.* 2007;179:854–868.

154. Symons HJ, et al. Improved survival with inhibitory killer immunoglobulin receptor (KIR) gene mismatches and KIR haplotype B donors after nonmyeloablative, HLA-haploidentical bone marrow transplantation. *Biol Blood Marrow Transplant.* 2010;16:533–542.

155. Goulmy E. Minor histocompatibility antigens: from transplantation problems to therapy of cancer. *Hum Immunol.* 2006;67:433–438.

156. Vago L, et al. Loss of mismatched HLA in leukemia after stem-cell transplantation. *N Engl J Med.* 2009;361:478–488.

157. Villalobos IB, et al. Relapse of leukemia with loss of mismatched HLA resulting from uniparental disomy after haploidentical hematopoietic stem cell transplantation. *Blood.* 2010;115:3158–3161.

158. McCurdy SR, et al. Loss of the mismatched human leukocyte antigen haplotype in two acute myelogenous leukemia relapses after haploidentical bone marrow transplantation with post-transplantation cyclophosphamide. *Leukemia.* 2016;30:2102–2106.

159. Tamaki H, et al. Different mechanisms causing loss of mismatched human leukocyte antigens in relapsing t(6;11)(q27;q23) acute myeloid leukemia after haploidentical transplantation. *Eur J Haematol.* 2012;89:497–500.

160. Christopher MJ, et al. Immune escape of relapsed AML cells after allogeneic transplantation. *N Engl J Med.* 2018;379:2330–2341.

161. Liu L, et al. T cell exhaustion characterized by compromised MHC class I and II restricted cytotoxic activity associates with acute B lymphoblastic leukemia relapse after allogeneic hematopoietic stem cell transplantation. *Clin Immunol.* 2018;190:32–40.

162. Kong Y, et al. PD-1(hi)TIM-3(+) T cells associate with and predict leukemia relapse in AML patients post allogeneic stem cell transplantation. *Blood Canc J.* 2015;5:e330.

163. Verdijk RM, et al. Pregnancy induces minor histocompatibility antigen-specific cytotoxic T cells: implications for stem cell transplantation and immunotherapy. *Blood.* 2004;103:1961–1964.

164. van Kampen CA, et al. Pregnancy can induce long-persisting primed CTLs specific for inherited paternal HLA antigens. *Hum Immunol.* 2001;62:201–207.

165. Stern M, et al. Survival after T cell-depleted haploidentical stem cell transplantation is improved using the mother as donor. *Blood.* 2008;112:2990–2995.

166. Kawase T, et al. HLA mismatch combinations associated with decreased risk of relapse: implications for the molecular mechanism. *Blood.* 2009;113:2851–2858.

167. Venstrom JM, et al. HLA-C-dependent prevention of leukemia relapse by donor activating KIR2DS1. *N Engl J Med.* 2012;367:805–816.

168. Mancusi A, et al. Haploidentical hematopoietic transplantation from KIR ligand-mismatched donors with activating KIRs reduces nonrelapse mortality. *Blood.* 2015;125:3173–3182.

169. Godder KT, et al. Long term disease-free survival in acute leukemia patients recovering with increased gammadelta T cells after partially mismatched related donor bone marrow transplantation. *Bone Marrow Transplant.* 2007;39:751–757.

170. Handgretinger R, Schilbach K. The potential role of gammadelta T cells after allogeneic HCT for leukemia. *Blood.* 2018;131:1063–1072.

CHAPTER 15

Therapeutic Apheresis

ROBERT A. DESIMONE, MD • SABRINA EWA RACINE-BRZOSTEK, MD, PHD • HUY P. PHAM, MD, MPH

INTRODUCTION

Apheresis describes a procedure in which whole blood is removed from a subject, separated into components (such as red blood cells [RBC], white blood cells, platelets, and plasma), and selective components are removed while the rest is reinfused back to the person with or without the use of replacement fluid(s).[1] This procedure can be used to collect blood component(s) for transfusions (donor apheresis), or it can be used as a therapeutic modality to treat diseases (therapeutic apheresis [TA]), which is the primary focus of this chapter. Common TA procedures are therapeutic plasma exchange (TPE), red blood cell exchange (RBCX) with or without isovolemic hemodilution, leukocytapheresis, thrombocytapheresis, and extracorporeal photopheresis (ECP). The common goals of these procedures are to remove the disease mediator(s) and potentially supplement missing component(s) via replacement fluid(s). Many of these procedures are performed for immune-related conditions.

McLeod's criteria are usually used to evaluate a TA consult.[2] There are three components of McLeod's criteria:[2]

(1) There must be a clear understanding of the mechanism of disease to enable a good rationale for apheresis.
(2) The abnormality that makes apheresis plausible should be able to be corrected by TA.
(3) There should be clinical evidence of outcome improvement by performing the TA procedure (and not just statistically significant results).

To assist apheresis practitioners with TA consults, the Writing Committee of the Journal of Clinical Apheresis (JCA) Special Issue 2019 of the American Society for Apheresis (ASFA) publishes Guidelines on the use of TA every 3 years since 2007.[3] The most recent version of the Guidelines will be forthcoming in 2019 (eighth edition) at the time of this writing. In this edition, a panel of 13 members from diverse backgrounds (Transfusion Medicine/Apheresis, Hematology, Nephrology, Pediatrics, and Critical Care Medicine) across the United States and Europe reviewed the medical literature for new developments in the understanding and current management/treatment of the disease as well as any changes in the evidence surrounding the use of TA as a treatment modality using a process similar to one that was employed in previous editions of the Guidelines. Finally, a total of 84 diseases and 157 indications are included in the 2019 version of the ASFA Guidelines. Of note, these are only the indications that currently have enough evidence to support (or not support) the use of TA. The Guidelines do not contain all the diseases that have been treated by TA and reported in the medical literature or the diseases that may be treated by TA. Furthermore, each disease and/or indication is also accompanied by an ASFA category (Table 15.1) and grade of recommendation (Table 15.2).

BASICS OF APPROACHING AN APHERESIS CONSULT

There are multiple ways of approaching an apheresis consult. However, many apheresis practitioners start with the ASFA Guidelines to determine if the consult's indication is legitimate. It is advisable to perform a brief literature review to ensure that there is no recent published studies since the release of the ASFA Guidelines that may have a significant impact on the apheresis indication. Furthermore, the patient's hemodynamic and cardiopulmonary status along with comorbidities and/or medications should also be taken into account when evaluating the suitability of the apheresis treatment. Finally, availability of alternative therapies that may be potentially efficacious as apheresis but with less adverse risks should be explored.

Once apheresis is determined to be indicated, the next step would be to decide what apheresis procedure

Immunologic Concepts in Transfusion Medicine. https://doi.org/10.1016/B978-0-323-67509-3.00015-9

TABLE 15.1
ASFA Category Indications.[3]

Category	Description
I	Disorders for which apheresis is accepted as first-line therapy, either as a primary standalone treatment or in conjunction with other modes of treatment
II	Disorders for which apheresis is accepted as second-line therapy, either as a standalone treatment or in conjunction with other modes of treatment
III	Optimal role of apheresis therapy is not established. Decision making should be individualized
IV	Disorders in which published evidence demonstrates or suggests apheresis to be ineffective or harmful. IRB approval is desirable if apheresis treatment is undertaken in these circumstances.

Adapted with permission from Schwartz J, Padmanabhan A, Aqui N, et al. Guidelines on the use of therapeutic apheresis in clinical practice-evidence-based approach from the writing committee of the American society for apheresis: the seventh special Issue. *J Clin Apher.* 2016;31(3):149–162.

(TPE vs. RBCX vs. ECP vs. therapeutic leukocytapheresis or thrombocytapheresis) shall be performed. Additionally, the location where apheresis is performed as well as type of access should be discussed with the requesting clinical team. The urgency of the procedure (emergent [typically perform within hours] vs. urgent [within 24 hour] vs. routine) as well as other technical information (frequency and total number of the procedures, replacement fluid, anticoagulant, necessity of blood and/or albumin prime, electrolyte repletion, etc.) needs to be evaluated.[4] Finally, especially in the scenario where TA is administered as a therapeutic trial, criteria for TA termination, preferably as objective as possible, should be discussed and agreeable before the initiation of TA with the requesting physician.

BASICS OF APHERESIS MATH

Although in most scenarios, the apheresis device can calculate the required volume of replacement fluid and if fluid priming of the device is necessary, it is essential for apheresis practitioners to understand basic principles of apheresis math to ensure a safe and effective procedure. There are many ways of estimating the blood

volume (BV) of an adult; however, the most common formula used is the Nadler's formula (shown later).[5]

- For males,

$$TBV = (0.3669 * [height\ (m)^3] \\ + (0.03219 * [weight\ (kg)] + 0.6041$$

- For females,

$$TBV = (0.3561 * [height\ (m)^3] \\ + (0.03308 * [weight\ (kg)] + 0.1833$$

Once the BV is known, plasma volume (PV) can be calculated as $PV = BV \times (1\text{-Hct})$.

Extracorporeal volume (ECV) and ERCV refer to the volume of whole blood and red blood cells (RBCs) outside of the patient's circulation at any given moment during the procedure. ECV and ERCV depend upon the apheresis procedure (or kits) as provided by the manufacturer(s). It is recommended that the patient's ECV not exceed 10%–15% of their BV, with additional concerns considered for patients with multiple comorbidities, particularly those affecting the patient's hemodynamic and cardiopulmonary status.[6] If the ECV exceeds 10%–15%, priming the apheresis kit with RBCs and/or 5% albumin is advisable to avoid procedural hypotension. Furthermore, given the potential of procedural blood volume shifts, care must be taken that the patient's intraprocedural Hct to be maintained at tolerable levels, which may vary in accordance with the patient's clinical status. Should the calculated intraprocedural Hct be less than the patient's lowest tolerable Hct, priming of the apheresis kit with RBCs is advisable. Moreover, if the patient is connected to multiple life-supporting devices, then the effective ECV and ERCV is the sum of each individual device's ECV and ERCV, respectively. When calculating either the volume ratio or the intraprocedural Hct, the effective TBV, ECV, and/or ERCV should be used.

ADVERSE EVENTS OF APHERESIS

TA is not a benign procedure. Common procedure-related complications are usually hypotension (can be related to fluid shifts during the procedure) and citrate toxicity (due to the use of citrate as an anticoagulant (which can cause metabolic alkalosis, leading to hypocalcemia and/or hypokalemia). Furthermore, if the replacement fluid is not plasma, depletion of coagulation factors can be observed in patients undergoing TPE. For example, fibrinogen is effectively removed by TPE, and it can decrease as much as ~60% after 1-plasma volume exchange. Therefore, it is important

TABLE 15.2
Grading Recommendations.[3]

Recommendation Grade	Description	Methodological Quality of Supporting Evidence	Implications
1A	Strong recommendation, high-quality evidence	RCTs without important limitations or overwhelming evidence from observational studies	Strong recommendation, can apply to most patients in most circumstances without reservation
1B	Strong recommendation, moderate-quality evidence	RCTs with important limitations or exceptional strong evidence from observational studies	Strong recommendation, can apply to most patients in most circumstances without reservation
1C	Strong recommendation, low-quality evidence	Observational studies or case series	Strong recommendation, but may change when higher quality evidence becomes available
2A	Weak recommendation, high-quality evidence	RCTs without important limitations or overwhelming evidence from observational studies	Weak recommendation, best action may differ depending on circumstances
2B	Weak recommendation, moderate-quality evidence	RCTs with important limitations or exceptional strong evidence from observational studies	Weak recommendation, best action may differ depending on circumstances
2C	Weak recommendation, low-quality evidence	Observational studies or case series	Very weak recommendation; other alternatives may be equally reasonable

Adapted with permission from Schwartz J, Padmanabhan A, Aqui N, et al. Guidelines on the use of therapeutic apheresis in clinical practice-evidence-based approach from the writing committee of the American society for apheresis: the seventh special Issue. *J Clin Apher.* 2016; 31(3):149–162.

to monitor the patient's hemostasis closely, especially when performing TPE without plasma as the replacement fluid. Other complications can be related to catheter (bleeding, thrombosis, and/or infection) or replacement fluid (allergic reaction and/or transfusion reaction if a blood component is the replacement fluid).

THERAPEUTIC PLASMA EXCHANGE

Case 1 Myasthenia Gravis: A Case for TPE With Albumin Replacement

A 73-year-old male presents to the emergency room (ER) with complaints of fever, shortness of breath, generalized weakness, difficulty speaking, and drooping eyelids. As per his family, he had been diagnosed with myasthenia gravis (MG) 9 months prior. Upon initial diagnosis, he had experienced worsening of vision in the evening hours when he read. He also had complained of fatigue on chewing and occasional difficulty swallowing. Initially, he had been treated with pyridostigmine but his symptoms returned within a few months, despite increase in dosage. He had been placed on prednisone after becoming refractory to the acetylcholinesterase (AChE) inhibitor. He recently achieved stable control of his symptoms and his prednisone dose had been tapered to the lowest effective level. He returned home from a trip with his grandchildren the day prior, during which the children fell ill with a cough and fever. His family noted that he himself woke up this morning with a fever and mild cough.

In the ER, his vital signs revealed a fever of 38°C, a respiratory rate of 16 with oxygen saturation of 95% and a pulse of 84. On physical exam, rales were heard in the right upper lung on auscultation. Bilateral ptosis was noted, and he had reduced strength in all four extremities, but had normal reflexes. Impending myasthenic crisis was suspected on account of the rapid worsening of weakness and suspicion of respiratory infection. The patient was admitted to the intensive care unit (ICU) and required intubation on arrival.

The transfusion medicine service was consulted immediately, and TPE was urgently performed.

This case demonstrates how MG may present on initial diagnosis and how rapid worsening may decompensate into a myasthenic crisis. MG is an autoimmune neurologic disease wherein autoantibodies cause functional alterations of the postsynaptic portion of the neuromuscular junction (NMJ), resulting in neuromuscular transmission impairment. Clinically, as with the patient in this case, this manifests as skeletal muscle weakness that can be generalized or localized. This weakness, usually symmetrical, may be more proximal than distal, with the classical presentation describing diplopia and ptosis. Other typical symptoms include difficulty chewing, swallowing, or slurred speech. Weakness and fatigue increase with any repetitive muscle use; as such, many complain of worsening symptoms as the day progresses into the evening.[7] The Osserman Classification allows the standardization of clinical symptoms, which aids in prognosis and therapeutic decision making. The classification divides MG into five main classes, from Class I (defined as any eye muscle weakness or possible ptosis with no other evidence of muscle weakness) up to Class V (defined as symptoms requiring intubation with or without mechanical ventilation).[8,9]

The exact mechanism leading to the autoimmunity described in MG remains unknown. However, the literature on the pathogenesis of MG keeps growing[7,9–11] and several distinct antibodies have been implicated in the disease.[12] The diagnosis of MG is confirmed by a positive test for the autoantibodies specific to MG. The three most common are autoantibodies against the acetylcholine receptor (AChR), muscle-specific kinase (MuSK) or lipoprotein receptor-related protein 4 (LRP4). A majority (70%) of patients test positive for AChR antibodies[12,13] and these antibodies bind to the extracellular domain of the AChR, impeding signal transduction. They are typically IgG1 and IgG3 subclass that activate the complement cascade and lead to further NMJ damage. Furthermore, it is believed these antibodies are capable of antigenic modulation, causing crosslinking of the receptor and subsequent receptor internalization.[12,14] Therefore, AChR antibody concentrations may not directly correlate with symptom severity, as the loss of functional AChR may lead to MG symptoms.[6]

MuSK antibodies are detected in 1%–10%[15] of MG patients and found in 30%–40% of AChR antibody-negative MG patients.[11] MuSK is a protein expressed in the postsynaptic muscle membrane and is necessary for AChR function. Different from the AChR antibody,

the MuSK antibody belongs to the IgG4 subclass and does not bind complement. This antibody does not modulate the AChR function but instead inhibits AChR clustering and impairs the end-plate alignment by binding the extracellular domain.[12] These patients have more severe weakness with marked symptoms in the facial and bulbar muscles, while limb weakness and ocular weakness are less common. MuSK antibody-positive patients may be less responsive to AChE inhibitors.

LRP4 antibodies are found in 1%–5% of MG patients[16,17] and 2%–27% of patients lacking the AChR and MuSK antibodies. These antibodies are not as well characterized but are IgG1 subclass antibodies, can disrupt LRP4 ligand binding, and can activate complement. LRP4 is a receptor for agrin and plays a role in stimulating MuSK kinase activity, thereby allowing the downstream signaling cascade for AChR clustering.[18] Most LRP4 antibody-positive patients have milder symptoms, presenting with ocular and/or mild generalized weakness, and rarely enter a myasthenic crisis.[6]

Approximately 10% of MG patients are seronegative and have no positive tests for antibodies against AChR, MuSK, or LRP4.[7] These may be patients who have low affinity or low concentrations of the AChR, MuSk, or LRP4 antibodies or have pathogenic antibodies against yet undefined antigens in the postsynaptic membrane. Repeat testing can lead to identification of a responsible antibody, and retesting is recommended 6–18 months after initial diagnosis.[12] MG-associated antibodies to other muscle antigens have been reported, including the striated muscle antigen titin, ryanodine receptor, and agrin.[19–21]

The first-line therapy for MG is an AChE inhibitor, such as pyridostigmine or neostigmine; however, MuSK-positive MG patients may have an insufficient or suboptimal response. As with the patient discussed in the case earlier, most MG patients require immunosuppressive medications. Prednisone and prednisolone are usually the glucocorticoids prescribed for initial immunomodulation, and are tapered to the lowest effective dose. Due to the heterogeneity of the disease, it is difficult to find a treatment approach ideal for all patients. As such, other steroid sparing immunosuppressants such as cyclosporine, tacrolimus, methotrexate, and rituximab have also been used.[9]

MG patients with severe MG exacerbations or those believed to have impending myasthenic crisis, as in the case earlier, require an ICU admission to allow intubation and fast acting immunosuppression. Often times, MG exacerbations or myasthenic crisis may coexist with another condition, such as severe infections. During these scenarios, intravenous immune globulin and TPE are regarded equally equivalent.[22–26] These therapies have a rapid effect and could be used in sequence if a patient responds to one therapy but not the other. Intravenous immune globulin (IVIG) may be more convenient but TPE anecdotally may have a faster effect,[27] and improvements can be seen within 24 hours. To ensure long-term improvement, TPE or IVIG is combined with higher doses of immunosuppressive drugs, as the effects of TPE or IVIG may subside within 2–4 weeks posttreatment.[3]

According to the most recent ASFA guidelines, the use of TPE is a Category I (recommendation Grade 1B) for moderate-to-severe MG.[3] TPE is used to remove the aforementioned circulating MG autoantibodies. The replacement fluid for MG is usually 5% albumin, as patients typically do not need replacement of the coagulation factors found in plasma products. Typically, depending on the clinical scenario, TPE is performed every other day for five procedures to allow IgG equilibrium between the intra- and extravascular space. TPE may also have immunomodulatory effects in MG patients, as the procedure also removes cytokines responsible for activating regulatory T lymphocytes.[28,29] MG patients have been found to have higher levels of cytokines such as IL-2, IL-4, IL-10, and IFN-γ.[30]

TPE with immunoadsorption (IA) and double filtration (DF) are two technologies being investigated to provide more selective removal of the MG antibodies. IA allows the selective removal of immunoglobulins from separated plasma through high-affinity adsorbers, columns filled with different adsorbents such as tryptophan-linked polyvinyl alcohol gel or a staphylococcal protein A, which could immobilize the pathogenic MG antibodies. DF involves the filtering of plasma through a plasma separator and then a second filter to separate albumin from larger molecules (immunoglobulins, immune complexes). These technologies allow for the return of the patient's plasma without the need for plasma or albumin supplementation, diminishing the risk of transfusion reactions.[31,32,28,33]

TPE may also be performed perioperatively for thymectomy and is a Category I (recommendation Grade 1C) by ASGA guidelines. Thymic abnormalities, usually a thymoma or thymic hyperplasia, can be associated with MG. When present, thymoma is associated with an AChR antibody-positive MG and 10% of MG cases are attributed to a thymoma. It is speculated that the thymoma cells contain muscle-specific antigens and perhaps AChR expression can be activated in thymic epithelial cells. Autoreactive T cells specific for AChR may escape the normal intrathymic surveillance and could stimulate B lymphocytes in the periphery to produce antibodies against AChR.[27] As such, thymectomy is performed for all MG patients with a thymoma or in early onset AChR MG patients. IVIG is administered or TPE is performed to minimize the risk for postthymectomy MG exacerbation.[9]

Case 2 Thrombotic Thrombocytopenia Purpura: A Case for TPE with Plasma Replacement

A 45-year-old female with no significant medical history presented to a small suburban ER with a severe headache and malaise that had worsened over the last few weeks. On the morning of presentation, she states that she had awoken with a headache that caused visual disturbances and noted her urine was a dark amber color. She noted unprovoked small bruises on her arm and a subjective fever. In the ER, she had a temperature of 38.1°C, but all other vital signs were within normal limits. On physical examination, she appeared to be lucid and oriented, however appeared pale with petechia on her upper extremities. Cardiac, pulmonary, and abdominal examination revealed no abnormalities. Laboratory results drawn and made available to the ER revealed anemia and thrombocytopenia, with a hemoglobin of 8.1 g/dL and platelet count of 15,000/μL. The peripheral blood smear was significant for "split cells" or schistocytes. The coagulation studies were within normal limits. She had several abnormalities on her comprehensive metabolic panel: lactate dehydrogenase (LDH) at 1000 IU/L, indirect bilirubin at 1.9 mg/dL, creatinine of 1.8 mg/dL. The direct Coombs test was negative. The possibility of thrombotic thrombocytopenia purpura (TTP) was high on the differential diagnosis and the patient was admitted to the hospital. She was transfused with a unit of plasma while the outside clinical apheresis service was notified for emergent TPE. ADAMTS13 levels were also ordered, and the result was pending.

TTP is a type of thrombotic microangiopathy (TMA) that is characterized by microangiopathic hemolytic anemia (MAHA), thrombocytopenia, and a severe deficiency in ADAMTS13, a von Willebrand factor (vWF) cleaving protease.[34,35] The deficiency of ADAMTS13 is severe and can be acquired (due to ADAMTS13 autoantibodies) or congenital (due to an autosomal recessive mutation in the ADAMTS13 gene on chromosome 9q34).[36] This case demonstrates the classic presentation of a patient with TTP, which is characterized by the pentad of fever, hemolytic anemia, thrombocytopenia, renal failure, and neurologic symptomology.[37,38] However, in clinical practice adhering to this pentad is considered obsolete, as less than 10% of patients present with all five symptoms.[39] In fact, if an unexplained MAHA with a thrombocytopenia is present and there is high clinical suspicion of TTP, immediate treatment is warranted before organ failure occurs.[38,40] Furthermore, it should be emphasized that these clinical features may not be specific to TTP, as TTP signs and symptoms overlap with other TMA syndromes. As further research is performed, it is becoming clear that TTP is distinguished from other TMA in that severe ADAMTS13 deficiency is the pathogenesis of TTP and it may be distinguished clinically by its mild renal involvement and more severe thrombocytopenia when compared to other TMA, such as hemolytic uremic syndrome.[41]

ADAMST13 cleaves vWF multimers and, in its absence, ultralarge multimers of vWF circulate and cause platelet adhesion. This results in thrombi within the microcirculation, consumption of platelets, ischemia within the kidneys, brain, heart, GI tract, and/or other organs. ADAMTS13 activity levels less than 5%−10% are diagnostic of TTP and the presence of anti-ADAMTS13 antibodies is suggestive of acquired TTP.[39] Several assays now exist to measure ADAMTS13 activity levels, although these assays are not always readily available,[40] as is demonstrated in our clinical case earlier.

According to the ASFA guidelines, the use of TPE is a Category I (Recommendation Grade 1A) for TTP treatment[3] and is considered a life-saving therapy, as left untreated it has a >90% overall mortality.[42] Therefore, TPE should be initiated as soon as possible. As with the MG case described previously, TPE is effective due to the removal of an autoantibody, in addition to the ultralarge vWF multimers and the associated inflammatory cytokines. However, plasma is used as the replacement fluid so as to restore the ADAMTS13 protease activity. As demonstrated in the case earlier, if TPE cannot be initiated immediately, plasma infusions may temporarily replenish ADAMTS13 levels until TPE arrangements could be made. In contrast, simple infusion of plasma, cryoprecipitate (which contains ADAMTS13), or vWF concentrate can be used to increase ADAMTS13 levels in congenital TTP, as it is the result of a constitutive deficiency of ADAMTS13 and not due to an autoantibody.[3]

TPE for acquired TTP is performed daily until the platelet count is $>150,000 \times 10^9$/L and LDH returns to normal for several days. After cessation of TPE, the patient is monitored closely for relapse and/or exacerbation. Monitoring includes daily CBC and LDH. As with MG, during an acute episode of TTP, corticosteroids are often given for initial immunomodulation.

However, these treatments do not reliably eliminate the cells that produce the inhibitory antibodies. Rituximab, an anti-CD20 monoclonal antibody, has been shown to have a high response rate in refractory patients[43] and now is often incorporated as an adjunctive agent with initial TPE. It is important to note that, in practice, there should be an 18−24 hour interval between rituximab infusion and TPE.[3] Other immunosuppression agents that may also be used as adjunctive therapy include cyclosporine, azathioprine, vincristine, and/or bortezomib.[39] Recently, caplacizumab, a nanoantibody that inhibits the interaction between vWF and platelets, is approved for the treatment of TTP. However, currently it is unclear how this medication will be incorporated into the TTP treatment algorithm.[44]

Case 3 Donor-Specific Antibodies in Kidney Transplant Recipients: A Case of Possible Unforeseen Immunological Driven Effects of TPE.

A 35-year-old female is undergoing evaluation for a second kidney transplant after graft failure within 2 years of her first transplant due to noncompliance with immunosuppressive therapy. Before the first ABO-compatible transplant, she had been on several years of hemodialysis due to diabetic nephropathy that resulted in end-stage renal disease. Her calculated panel-reactive antibody (cPRA) using microarray single antigen beads is 99%, which includes multiple class II HLA antibodies. She had no potential living donors and despite being placed on the deceased donor list for 3 years, was unsuccessful for a match. Recently, a living donor becomes available in a paired exchange pool, but she needs to undergo desensitization to minimize the risk of rejection.

Kidney transplants in recipients possessing antibodies against mismatched donor HLA antigens are at high risk for antibody-mediated rejection (AMR). The HLA antigen system is broken into two broad categories based on their expression on cell membranes—Class I and Class II. Class I consists of the HLA-A, -B, and -C antigens and are found on all nucleated cells; whereas, Class II consists of HLA-DR, -DQ, and -DP antigens and are expressed only by antigen-presenting cells (APC).[45]

Preformed HLA antibodies could develop from previous exposure to foreign HLA antigens during transfusion, pregnancy, or previous transplantation. Preformed antibodies can cause hyperacute rejection. After the initial production of antibodies from the first HLA antigen exposure, a period of latency may occur, only to be reactivated upon reexposure. This reactivation is T-cell mediated, requiring the stimulation of APC, and results in complement activation and cytotoxic destruction of the graft vessel endothelium and nephron tubules.[46]

Several tests have been developed to access the recipients pretransplant risk of rejection and to detect HLA antibodies. The complement-dependent cytotoxicity (CDC) crossmatch evaluates for the presence of preformed antibodies.[47] A positive CDC crossmatch predicts the risk of hyperacute rejection and its utilization in excluding poor recipient-donor matches reduces hyperacute rejection. However, this test is not highly sensitive and does not detect all clinically relevant antibodies.[48] Recently, more sensitive assays involving ELISA, flow cytometry, and Luminex platforms have been used to detect donor-specific HLA antibodies (DSA) and are included in the recipient's organ waiting list profile to allow better matching and exclusion of unacceptable HLA antigen mismatches.[48] The cPRA[49] has been developed to estimate the likelihood of finding an acceptable donor by utilizing the HLA frequency data from the donor population. It is defined as the percentage of donors expected to have HLA antigens *unacceptable* for a candidate. Therefore, in the case example earlier, a cPRA of 99% predicts that a donor would negative crossmatch with a recipient at probability of 1%.

To expand the donor pool for patients with poor cPRA, immunologically incompatible living-donor renal transplantation may be performed after the reduction of DSA. When compared to patients remaining on dialysis while awaiting an HLA compatible organ, incompatible live-donor transplantation after desensitization provided a significant survival benefit for patients with HLA sensitization. Impressively, 8 years posttransplant the survival advantage was more than double.[50]

The desensitization protocol is a multipart and intricate regimen combining the use of immunosuppressive therapies, TPE and in some cases splenectomy to lower the levels of preformed antibodies.[51] The DSA levels are rechecked after desensitization and changes to the HLA antibody levels are modified in the donor-recipient profile. As such, the ASFA guidelines state that the use of TPE is a Category I (Recommendation Grade 1B) for the desensitization of kidney recipients undergoing a living donor transplant. TPE may be performed daily or every other day pretransplant until the crossmatch is negative. It could continue postoperatively or if AMR occurs.[3]

TPE has the same ASFA category I (Recommendation Grade 1B) for renal AMR. It could be performed daily or every other day for ∼5−6 procedures.[3] As with the use of TPE in the aforementioned desensitization protocols, its utility in AMR is the removal of DSA, which cause injury to the renal graft. IVIG may also be administered after TPE sessions to possibly neutralize the DSA and inhibit complement binding and activation. Rituximab also has played a role in AMR therapy by depleting B lymphocytes and in effect reducing the pool of antibody-producing plasma cells. Other therapies used include bortezomib and antithymocyte globulin, which induce plasma cell and B-lymphocyte apoptosis.[52]

A curious phenomenon of antibody rebound post-TPE has been described,[53,54] and may explain the variability of DSA removal by TPE. Theoretically, TPE removes all circulating immunoglobulins without regard for specificity. However, it had been observed that post-TPE there would be a greater reduction of HLA Class II DSA compared to Class I.[53,55,56] Yamada et al.[53] propose four possible mechanisms that may account for this rebound phenomenon. The first possible cause may be the activation of naïve cells by the TPE process itself. During the transplant process, there is a high level of active donor antigens present and these TPE-activated naïve cells become sensitized to these higher levels of existing antigens on the transplanted kidney. This leads to the production of de novo DSAs. A second mechanism describes memory B lymphocytes also possibly becoming activated by the TPE process, resulting in the increased production of some but not other DSAs. Yamada et al. cite work by Paglieroni et al. wherein B-lymphocytes were more activated 7−9 days after TPE.[57]

An intriguing third possible explanation suggests a decrease in negative feedback on the DSA-producing B cells when DSA levels decrease post-TPE—ultimately resulting in an increase of DSA production. Additionally, as many kidney transplant patients receive multipart-regimented therapies combining the use of various immunosuppressive therapies, the use of therapies such as IVIG would further the decrease in the initial DSA production.[58,59] Ultimately, this allows for a greater net result of DSA production after the effects of IVIG have diminished. Finally, a fourth explanation focuses less on the effects of TPE and the possible absorption of DSA early in AMR by the healthy transplanted kidney tissue. The DSA levels remain low but as the AMR progresses, the increase in tissue damage releases the previously bound antibodies into the circulation.[53]

This case demonstrates that the effects of TPE may go beyond the simple bulk removal of plasma that contains the pathologic antibodies, immune complexes, and cytokines.[60,61] TPE also can play immunomodulatory roles. For instance, it can shift the T-helper cell (Th1/Th2) balance toward Th2. It has also been reported to suppress the production of proinflammatory cytokines such as IFN-γ and IL-2.[62,63]

EXTRACORPOREAL PHOTOPHERESIS
Overview of Procedure
ECP is an immunomodulatory procedure. During ECP, a small percentage of the patient's circulating mononuclear cells (MNCs) are collected utilizing a centrifuge bowl, including pathogenic or autoreactive T-lymphocytes, and undergo ex vivo incubation with a psoralen compound and subsequent exposure to ultraviolet A (UVA) light. The treated cells are then reinfused into the patient.[64] Approved by the United States Food and Drug Administration in 1988 for the treatment of cutaneous T-cell lymphoma (CTCL), ECP is categorized by ASFA as a primary, first-line adjunctive treatment or supportive therapy for CTCL. ASFA also acknowledges ECP as a second-line therapy, either as a standalone treatment or in conjunction with other therapies, for cellular/recurrent rejection and rejection prophylaxis in cardiac transplants as well as acute and chronic graft-versus-host disease (GVHD).[3]

ECP is commonly performed using the UVAR XTS or CELLEX automated photopheresis systems (Therakos Inc., Exton, PA). Heparin or acid-citrate dextrose can be used as anticoagulants for either system, although both systems are only officially approved for use with heparin. For the UVAR XTS, which is a discontinuous flow, single-needle procedure, 125 or 225 mL of whole blood is collected into a centrifuge bowl; the buffy coat is collected and the remaining blood components are returned to the patient. Following collection, the MNC suspension is incubated with methoxypsoralen and pumped through a photoactivation chamber for exposure to UVA light, after which it is reinfused to the patient. The general procedure for the CELLEX is similar to the UVAR XTS, however, the CELLEX can achieve continuous flow using double-needle modes. ECP can also be performed in an off-line fashion using two devices with a standard cell separator for MNC collection followed by UVA irradiation as is the practice in several centers in Europe.

Case 4 Acute Graft-Versus-Host Disease
A 45-year-old male with acute myeloid leukemia went into chronic remission status-post allogeneic, HLA-matched hematopoietic stem-cell transplant (HSCT); however, the patient was diagnosed with stage 4 acute graft-versus-host disease (aGVHD) of the skin and rectum on day +55. The aGVHD was resistant to steroids, infliximab, and basiliximab. He underwent ECP with dramatic improvement in symptoms, and now receives two treatments every other week as an outpatient.

GVHD following HSCT is associated with significant morbidity and mortality. Steroids are first-line management, and immunosuppressive agents such as infliximab, rituximab, and alemtuzumab are second-line.[65,66] Immunosuppression carries significant risks, including infection, reduced graft-versus-leukemia effect, and secondary malignancies.[67] Because this patient was resistant to steroids and multiple second-line therapies, he was started on ECP twice a week until improvement of his symptoms. The ideal schedule and duration of ECP for management of GVHD has not been definitively established, and there is great variation in practice. Typically, most practitioners will start with single-day treatments 2−3 times per week, sometimes as consecutive days but others will utilize 1−2 day breaks in between treatments. Treatment is continued until clinical improvement, followed by progressive tapering. To date, clinical trials comparing different ECP treatment schedules for the treatment of GVHD have not been conducted.

ECP's mechanism of action in GVHD has not been fully elucidated, but it has been proposed to result in a shift from an inflammatory (T_h1) state to a tolerance (T_h2) state; thus, inducing tolerance of donor T lymphocytes to host antigens. A typical ECP treatment results in reinfusion of approximately 5×10^6 MNCs; during their photoactivation, monofunctional, and bifunctional DNA adducts form, leading to MNC apoptosis within 24−48 hour. The apoptotic MNCs are engulfed by APCs, and their antigens are presented in the context of major histocompatibility complex I and II.[68,69] The downstream effects described in both GVHD and cardiac transplant patients include reduced proinflammatory cytokines (IL-2, TNF-α, IFN-γ) and increased antiinflammatory cytokines (TGF-β) through arginine metabolism pathways, as well as increased populations of regulatory T cells.[70,71] The emergence of regulatory T-cell populations during ECP treatments has been correlated with clinical response.[72] Other proposed mechanisms of action in GVHD include expansion of memory CD8+ T cells[73] and differentiation of monocytes to immature dendritic cells, which then may acquire the ability to secrete IL-10.[74,75] In addition, decreased lymphocytes have been correlated with ECP response in chronic GVHD, highlighting dysregulation of B lymphocytes as a potential contributing factor.[76]

Case 5 Cutaneous T-Cell Lymphoma

A 67-year-old female presents with extensive (75% body surface area involvement) with CTCL. She underwent ECP with dramatic improvement in skin symptoms after a few treatments.

In a seminal clinical trial, ECP showed improvement in symptoms in 27 of 37 (73%) patients receiving treatments.[77] There is a conundrum when considering the clinical effects of ECP. On the one hand, it has the ability to immunize against CTCL antigens as an immunostimulator; whereas, on the other hand, in GVHD and organ transplant rejection it has the ability to induce tolerance and act as an immunomodulator. No other therapy is used for both tolerance and immunity. Because dendritic cells are positioned in both antigen-specific T-cell immunity and tolerance, a central role for them has been suggested. In contrast, in GVHD and organ transplant rejection, ECP has been shown to reduce proinflammatory cytokines and increase T regulatory cells; in CTCL, the same therapy has been shown to reduce T regulatory cells, increase proinflammatory cytokines, and thus lead to an effector T-cell response. The presence of necrotic cells leads to a mature dendritic cell phenotype with an increase in expression of costimulatory ligands and a downstream effector T-cell response; whereas, the presence of apoptotic cells leads to an immature dendritic cell phenotype with a reduced expression of costimulatory ligands and a regulatory T-cell response.[78]

ECP has been shown to have a direct impact on the development of a dendritic cell phenotype from processed monocytes. For example, ECP has been shown to increase coexpression of HLA-DR and cytoplasmic CD83 in monocytes, the coexpression of which suggests the development of a dendritic cell phenotype. In addition, ECP has been shown to upregulate 12 critical genes involving in dendritic cell biology in monocytes following processing.[79]

CONCLUSIONS

As discussed, apheresis is not a benign procedure. The ASFA Guidelines on the use of therapeutic apheresis assist apheresis practitioners in understanding the medical indications and the technical information of the apheresis procedure. If appropriately utilized, therapeutic apheresis can be a powerful treatment modality for many autoimmune conditions as outlined earlier.

CONFLICTS OF INTEREST

HPP is a speaker and consultant for Alexion Pharmaceuticals. RD and SER do not have any conflict of interest to report.

REFERENCES

1. Pham HP, Schwartz J. How to approach an apheresis consultation using the American Society for Apheresis guidelines for therapeutic apheresis procedures. *ISBT Sci Ser.* 2015;10(S1):79−88.
2. McLeod BC. An approach to evidence-based therapeutic apheresis. *J Clin Apher.* 2002;17(3):124−132.
3. Schwartz J, Padmanabhan A, Aqui N, et al. Guidelines on the use of therapeutic apheresis in clinical practice-evidence-based approach from the writing committee of the American society for apheresis: the seventh special Issue. *J Clin Apher.* 2016;31(3):149−162.
4. Russi G, Marson P. Urgent plasma exchange: how, where and when. *Blood Transfus.* 2011;9(4):356−361.
5. Nadler SB, Hidalgo JH, Bloch T. Prediction of blood volume in normal human adults. *Surgery.* 1962;51(2):224−232.
6. Pham HP, Schwartz J. How we approach a patient with symptoms of leukostasis requiring emergent leukocytapheresis. *Transfusion.* 2015;55(10):2306−2311. quiz 2305.
7. Gilhus NE. Myasthenia gravis. *N Engl J Med.* 2016;375(26):2570−2581.
8. Jaretzki 3rd A, Barohn RJ, Ernstoff RM, et al. Myasthenia gravis: recommendations for clinical research standards. Task force of the medical scientific advisory board of the myasthenia gravis foundation of America. *Neurology.* 2000;55(1):16−23.
9. Sanders DB, Wolfe GI, Benatar M, et al. International consensus guidance for management of myasthenia gravis: executive summary. *Neurology.* 2016;87(4):419−425.
10. Mantegazza R, Bernasconi P, Cavalcante P. Myasthenia gravis: from autoantibodies to therapy. *Curr Opin Neurol.* 2018;31(5):517−525.
11. Evoli A. Myasthenia gravis: new developments in research and treatment. *Curr Opin Neurol.* 2017;30(5):464−470.
12. Gilhus NE, Skeie GO, Romi F, Lazaridis K, Zisimopoulou P, Tzartos S. Myasthenia gravis - autoantibody characteristics and their implications for therapy. *Nat Rev Neurol.* 2016;12(5):259−268.
13. Peeler CE, De Lott LB, Nagia L, Lemos J, Eggenberger ER, Cornblath WT. Clinical utility of acetylcholine receptor antibody testing in ocular myasthenia gravis. *JAMA Neurol.* 2015;72(10):1170−1174.
14. Meriggioli MN, Sanders DB. Muscle autoantibodies in myasthenia gravis: beyond diagnosis? *Expert Rev Clin Immunol.* 2012;8(5):427−438.

15. Guptill JT, Sanders DB, Evoli A. Anti-MuSK antibody myasthenia gravis: clinical findings and response to treatment in two large cohorts. *Muscle Nerve.* 2011;44(1):36–40.

16. Zisimopoulou P, Evangelakou P, Tzartos J, et al. A comprehensive analysis of the epidemiology and clinical characteristics of anti-LRP4 in myasthenia gravis. *J Autoimmun.* 2014;52:139–145.

17. Pevzner A, Schoser B, Peters K, et al. Anti-LRP4 autoantibodies in AChR- and MuSK-antibody-negative myasthenia gravis. *J Neurol.* 2012;259(3):427–435.

18. Kim N, Stiegler AL, Cameron TO, et al. Lrp4 is a receptor for Agrin and forms a complex with MuSK. *Cell.* 2008; 135(2):334–342.

19. Skeie GO, Mygland A, Aarli JA, Gilhus NE. Titin antibodies in patients with late onset myasthenia gravis: clinical correlations. *Autoimmunity.* 1995;20(2):99–104.

20. Mygland A, Aarli JA, Matre R, Gilhus NE. Ryanodine receptor antibodies related to severity of thymoma associated myasthenia gravis. *J Neurol Neurosurg Psychiatry.* 1994; 57(7):843–846.

21. Gasperi C, Melms A, Schoser B, et al. Anti-agrin autoantibodies in myasthenia gravis. *Neurology.* 2014;82(22): 1976–1983.

22. Barth D, Nabavi Nouri M, Ng E, Nwe P, Bril V. Comparison of IVIg and PLEX in patients with myasthenia gravis. *Neurology.* 2011;76(23):2017–2023.

23. Qureshi AI, Choudhry MA, Akbar MS, et al. Plasma exchange versus intravenous immunoglobulin treatment in myasthenic crisis. *Neurology.* 1999;52(3):629–632.

24. Gajdos P, Chevret S, Toyka KV. Intravenous immunoglobulin for myasthenia gravis. *Cochrane Database Syst Rev.* 2012;12:CD002277.

25. Ortiz-Salas P, Velez-Van-Meerbeke A, Galvis-Gomez CA, Rodriguez QJ. Human immunoglobulin versus plasmapheresis in guillain-barre syndrome and myasthenia gravis: a meta-analysis. *J Clin Neuromuscul Dis.* 2016; 18(1):1–11.

26. Gajdos P, Chevret S, Toyka K. Plasma exchange for myasthenia gravis. *Cochrane Database Syst Rev.* 2002;4: CD002275.

27. Gilhus NE, Verschuuren JJ. Myasthenia gravis: subgroup classification and therapeutic strategies. *Lancet Neurol.* 2015;14(10):1023–1036.

28. Zhang L, Liu J, Wang H, et al. Double filtration plasmapheresis benefits myasthenia gravis patients through an immunomodulatory action. *J Clin Neurosci.* 2014;21(9): 1570–1574.

29. Zhang Y, Wang HB, Chi LJ, Wang WZ. The role of FoxP3+CD4+CD25hi Tregs in the pathogenesis of myasthenia gravis. *Immunol Lett.* 2009;122(1):52–57.

30. Yeh JH, Wang SH, Chien PJ, Shih CM, Chiu HC. Changes in serum cytokine levels during plasmapheresis in patients with myasthenia gravis. *Eur J Neurol.* 2009;16(12): 1318–1322.

31. Grob D, Simpson D, Mitsumoto H, et al. Treatment of myasthenia gravis by immunoadsorption of plasma. *Neurology.* 1995;45(2):338–344.

32. Yeh JH, Chiu HC. Comparison between double-filtration plasmapheresis and immunoadsorption plasmapheresis in the treatment of patients with myasthenia gravis. *J Neurol.* 2000;247(7):510–513.

33. Haas M, Mayr N, Zeitlhofer J, Goldammer A, Derfler K. Long-term treatment of myasthenia gravis with immunoadsorption. *J Clin Apher.* 2002;17(2):84–87.

34. Furlan M, Robles R, Galbusera M, et al. von Willebrand factor-cleaving protease in thrombotic thrombocytopenic purpura and the hemolytic-uremic syndrome. *N Engl J Med.* 1998;339(22):1578–1584.

35. Tsai HM, Lian EC. Antibodies to von Willebrand factor-cleaving protease in acute thrombotic thrombocytopenic purpura. *N Engl J Med.* 1998;339(22):1585–1594.

36. Krogh AS, Waage A, Quist-Paulsen P. Congenital thrombotic thrombocytopenic purpura. *Tidsskr Nor Laegeforen.* 2016;136(17):1452–1457.

37. George JN, Nester CM. Syndromes of thrombotic microangiopathy. *N Engl J Med.* 2014;371(7):654–666.

38. Coppo P, Cuker A, George JN. Thrombotic thrombocytopenic purpura: toward targeted therapy and precision medicine. *Res Pract Thromb Haemost.* 2019;3(1):26–37.

39. Joly BS, Coppo P, Veyradier A. Thrombotic thrombocytopenic purpura. *Blood.* 2017;129(21):2836–2846.

40. Sadler JE, Moake JL, Miyata T, George JN. Recent advances in thrombotic thrombocytopenic purpura. *Hematology Am Soc Hematol Educ Program.* 2004:407–423.

41. Winters JL. Plasma exchange in thrombotic microangiopathies (TMAs) other than thrombotic thrombocytopenic purpura (TTP). *Hematology Am Soc Hematol Educ Program.* 2017;2017(1):632–638.

42. Rock GA, Shumak KH, Buskard NA, et al. Comparison of plasma exchange with plasma infusion in the treatment of thrombotic thrombocytopenic purpura. Canadian Apheresis Study Group. *N Engl J Med.* 1991;325(6): 393–397.

43. Scully M, McDonald V, Cavenagh J, et al. A phase 2 study of the safety and efficacy of rituximab with plasma exchange in acute acquired thrombotic thrombocytopenic purpura. *Blood.* 2011;118(7):1746–1753.

44. Peyvandi F, Scully M, Kremer Hovinga JA, et al. Caplacizumab for acquired thrombotic thrombocytopenic purpura. *N Engl J Med.* 2016;374(6):511–522.

45. Robson KJ, Ooi JD, Holdsworth SR, Rossjohn J, Kitching AR. HLA and kidney disease: from associations to mechanisms. *Nat Rev Nephrol.* 2018;14(10): 636–655.

46. Nishio-Lucar A, Balogun RA, Sanoff S. Therapeutic apheresis in kidney transplantation: a review of renal transplant immunobiology and current interventions with apheresis medicine. *J Clin Apher.* 2013;28(1):56–63.

47. Patel R, Terasaki PI. Significance of the positive crossmatch test in kidney transplantation. *N Engl J Med.* 1969; 280(14):735–739.

48. Susal C, Dohler B, Ruhenstroth A, et al. Donor-specific antibodies require preactivated immune system to harm renal transplant. *EBioMedicine.* 2016;9:366–371.

49. Cecka JM. Calculated PRA (CPRA): the new measure of sensitization for transplant candidates. *Am J Transplant.* 2010;10(1):26–29.
50. Montgomery RA, Lonze BE, King KE, et al. Desensitization in HLA-incompatible kidney recipients and survival. *N Engl J Med.* 2011;365(4):318–326.
51. Keith DS, Vranic GM. Approach to the highly sensitized kidney transplant candidate. *Clin J Am Soc Nephrol.* 2016; 11(4):684–693.
52. Zhang R. Donor-specific antibodies in kidney transplant recipients. *Clin J Am Soc Nephrol.* 2018;13(1):182–192.
53. Yamada C, Ramon DS, Cascalho M, et al. Efficacy of plasmapheresis on donor-specific antibody reduction by HLA specificity in post-kidney transplant recipients. *Transfusion.* 2015;55(4):727–735. quiz 726.
54. Dau PC. Increased antibody production in peripheral blood mononuclear cells after plasma exchange therapy in multiple sclerosis. *J Neuroimmunol.* 1995;62(2): 197–200.
55. Zachary AA, Montgomery RA, Ratner LE, et al. Specific and durable elimination of antibody to donor HLA antigens in renal-transplant patients. *Transplantation.* 2003;76(10): 1519–1525.
56. Zachary AA, Montgomery RA, Leffell MS. Factors associated with and predictive of persistence of donor-specific antibody after treatment with plasmapheresis and intravenous immunoglobulin. *Hum Immunol.* 2005;66(4): 364–370.
57. Paglieroni T, Caggiano V, MacKenzie MR. Effects of plasmapheresis on peripheral blood mononuclear cell populations from patients with macroglobulinemia. *J Clin Apher.* 1987;3(4):202–208.
58. Mayer L, Stohl W, Cunningham-Rundles C. Feedback inhibition of B cell differentiation by monomeric immunoglobulin. *Int Rev Immunol.* 1989;5(2):189–195.
59. Tawfik DS, Cowan KR, Walsh AM, Hamilton WS, Goldman FD. Exogenous immunoglobulin downregulates T-cell receptor signaling and cytokine production. *Pediatr Allergy Immunol.* 2012;23(1):88–95.
60. Winters JL. Plasma exchange: concepts, mechanisms, and an overview of the American Society for Apheresis guidelines. *Hematology Am Soc Hematol Educ Program.* 2012;2012:7–12.
61. Reeves HM, Winters JL. The mechanisms of action of plasma exchange. *Br J Haematol.* 2014;164(3):342–351.
62. Goto H, Matsuo H, Nakane S, et al. Plasmapheresis affects T helper type-1/T helper type-2 balance of circulating peripheral lymphocytes. *Ther Apher.* 2001;5(6):494–496.
63. Shariatmadar S, Nassiri M, Vincek V. Effect of plasma exchange on cytokines measured by multianalyte bead array in thrombotic thrombocytopenic purpura. *Am J Hematol.* 2005;79(2):83–88.
64. Zic JA, Miller JL, Stricklin GP, King Jr LE. The North American experience with photopheresis. *Ther Apher.* 1999;3(1): 50–62.
65. Dignan FL, Clark A, Amrolia P, et al. Diagnosis and management of acute graft-versus-host disease. *Br J Haematol.* 2012;158(1):30–45.
66. Jacobsohn DA. Optimal management of chronic graft-versus-host disease in children. *Br J Haematol.* 2010; 150(3):278–292.
67. Inamoto Y, Flowers ME, Lee SJ, et al. Influence of immunosuppressive treatment on risk of recurrent malignancy after allogeneic hematopoietic cell transplantation. *Blood.* 2011; 118(2):456–463.
68. Voll RE, Herrmann M, Roth EA, Stach C, Kalden JR, Girkontaite I. Immunosuppressive effects of apoptotic cells. *Nature.* 1997;390(6658):350–351.
69. Gallucci S, Lolkema M, Matzinger P. Natural adjuvants: endogenous activators of dendritic cells. *Nat Med.* 1999; 5(11):1249–1255.
70. Peritt D. Potential mechanisms of photopheresis in hematopoietic stem cell transplantation. *Biol Blood Marrow Transplant.* 2006;12(1 Suppl 2):7–12.
71. George JF, Gooden CW, Guo L, Kirklin JK. Role for CD4(+)CD25(+) T cells in inhibition of graft rejection by extracorporeal photopheresis. *J Heart Lung Transplant.* 2008;27(6):616–622.
72. Di Biaso I, Di Maio L, Bugarin C, et al. Regulatory T cells and extracorporeal photochemotherapy: correlation with clinical response and decreased frequency of proinflammatory T cells. *Transplantation.* 2009;87(9):1422–1425.
73. Yamashita K, Horwitz ME, Kwatemaa A, et al. Unique abnormalities of CD4(+) and CD8(+) central memory cells associated with chronic graft-versus-host disease improve after extracorporeal photopheresis. *Biol Blood Marrow Transplant.* 2006;12(1 Suppl 2):22–30.
74. Spisek R, Gasova Z, Bartunkova J. Maturation state of dendritic cells during the extracorporeal photopheresis and its relevance for the treatment of chronic graft-versus-host disease. *Transfusion.* 2006;46(1):55–65.
75. Rutella S, Danese S, Leone G. Tolerogenic dendritic cells: cytokine modulation comes of age. *Blood.* 2006;108(5): 1435–1440.
76. Kuzmina Z, Greinix HT, Knobler R, et al. Proportions of immature CD19+CD21- B lymphocytes predict the response to extracorporeal photopheresis in patients with chronic graft-versus-host disease. *Blood.* 2009; 114(3):744–746.
77. Edelson R, Berger C, Gasparro F, et al. Treatment of cutaneous T-cell lymphoma by extracorporeal photochemotherapy. Preliminary results. *N Engl J Med.* 1987;316(6): 297–303.
78. Adamski J, Kinard T, Ipe T, Cooling L. Extracorporeal photopheresis for the treatment of autoimmune diseases. *Transfus Apher Sci.* 2015;52(2):171–182.
79. Berger C, Hoffmann K, Vasquez JG, et al. Rapid generation of maturationally synchronized human dendritic cells: contribution to the clinical efficacy of extracorporeal photochemotherapy. *Blood.* 2010;116(23):4838–4847.

CHAPTER 16

Passive Monoclonal and Polyclonal Antibody Therapies

J. PETER R. PELLETIER, MD, FCAP, FASCP • FAISAL MUKHTAR, MBBS, MD, FCAP, FASCP

PASSIVE POLYCLONAL ANTIBODIES THERAPY

Passive Polyclonal Antibody Treatment Overview

Polyclonal immunoglobulins have been in use since the 19th century to protect against infectious agents, toxins, and disease conditions such as those with an autoimmune etiology. These immunoglobulin preparations are made from pools of selected human donors or animals with high titers of antibodies against viruses and toxins. These antibody treatments provide passive transfer of high titer antibodies that either reduces risk or reduces severity of infection. They are used to prevent hemolytic disease of the newborn and modify inflammatory reactions. Earlier drugs were very nonselective and patients frequently succumbed to infection due to suppression of both antibody-mediated (humoral) and cell-mediated arms of the immune system. Today, the principal approach is to alter lymphocyte function using drugs or antibodies against immune proteins. However, with the advent of human organ and tissue transplantation (e.g., kidney, heart, bone marrow, and/or peripheral blood stem cells) as treatment options, these polyclonal antibody therapies in combination with other treatment regimens are being used to lower the ability of the body's immune system to reject these transplants. However, their use is not without risk, as complications include development of immune complexes and severe allergic reactions. A summary of these polyclonal antibody therapies may be found in Table 16.2.

Immunosuppressive Agents: Disease Modifying

Antithymocyte globulin (rabbit)/thymoglobulin; antithymocyte globulin (equine)/Atgam

Description. Rabbit antithymocyte globulin (rATG) and equine antithymocyte globulin (eATG) are purified, pasteurized preparation of lymphocyte depleting polyclonal gamma immunoglobulin (IgG) raised against human thymus lymphocytes in rabbits and horses, respectively. They are used in prevention and/or treatment of renal transplant rejection worldwide.[1–7]

History of antibody use. rATG induction in combination with immunosuppressive therapy is more effective in preventing episodes of acute renal graft rejection in adult renal transplant recipients, in recurrent episodes of acute rejection,[8,9] and those acute rejections that are not responsive to high-dose corticosteroid therapy than other monoclonal antibody preparations.[10,11] rATG recipients had a lower incidence of biopsy-confirmed acute rejection episodes,[12] greater event-free survival up to 10 years posttransplantation, and greater graft survival up to 5 years posttransplantation.[13]

Mechanisms of action. The exact mechanism of these polyclonal antibodies has not been fully understood.[3,4,14–20] However, being polyclonal, they display specificity toward a wide variety of surface antigens (Ags) expressed on T and B-lymphocytes, dendritic cells, natural killer (NK) cells, and endothelial cells. However, T-cell depletion is considered to play a key role by modulating the expression of lymphocyte surface antigens involved in a wide variety of functions such as T-cell activation to endothelial adherence, activation of certain transcription factors, and interference with numerous immune cell processes, such as cytokine production, chemotaxis, endocytosis, cell stimulation, and proliferation.[14–20]

In vitro studies indicate that binding of eATG to cells is generally nonspecific; the drug binds to visceral tissues, including thymus and testis cell membranes and nuclear and cytoplasmic components of tissues such as tonsil, kidney, and liver,[21] and is extensively bound to bone marrow cells,[22] and to other peripheral blood cells besides lymphocytes.[21]

Diseases treated. As mentioned earlier, both antithymocyte globulins are used for treatment and prevention

Immunologic Concepts in Transfusion Medicine. https://doi.org/10.1016/B978-0-323-67509-3.00016-0

of acute renal allograft rejection.[2–8] More rATG recipients have been reported to achieve the endpoint of successful response (return of serum creatinine levels to baseline by end of treatment or within 14 days of treatment initiation). However, among those who achieved a successful response, fewer episodes of recurrent rejection occurred with rATG within 90 days of treatment cessation.[2] eATG is also used for treating moderate-to-severe aplastic anemia in patients who are unsuitable for bone marrow transplantation.[3,23,24]

Adverse effects. The most common adverse effects are fever, thrombocytopenia, leukopenia, gastrointestinal disorders, and/or concurrent infection.[1,2] Cytomegalovirus (CMV) infection was generally higher with rATG except in high-risk patients.[1,25] eATG therapy may result in reactivation of or infection with CMV, herpes simplex virus,[25] or Epstein–Barr virus.[26] The incidence of malignancies is generally lower with rATG therapy.[27] This product is made of equine and human blood components, so it may carry a risk of transmitting infectious agents such as viruses, and theoretically, the Creutzfeldt–Jakob disease (CJD) agent.

Update. There has been recent evidence that the addition of human anti-T-lymphocyte globulin (ATLG) plus cyclosporine and methotrexate to standard graft-versus-host disease (GVHD) prophylaxis is preferred over standard GVHD prophylaxis alone because it improves the probability of survival without relapse and of chronic GVHD after myeloablative peripheral blood stem-cell transplantation from a human leukocyte antigen (HLA)-identical sibling donor for patients with acute leukemia in remission. Additionally, this therapy provides better quality of life and shorter immunosuppressive treatment compared to standard GVHD prophylaxis without ATLG.[22]

Antitoxin and Immune Globulins: Disease Modifying
Tetanus immune globulin/Baytet/Hypertet
Description. Tetanus immune globulin (TIG) is a specific solvent-detergent-treated plasma-derived product obtained from donors immunized with tetanus toxoid. TIG contains tetanus antitoxin that provides temporary passive immunity to individuals who have low or no immunity to the toxin produced by *Clostridium tetani*.[28,29]

Mechanisms of action. TIG contains tetanus antitoxin antibodies, which neutralize the free form of the powerful exotoxin produced by *Clostridium tetani*.[28,30]

TIG can only neutralize unbound exotoxin; it does not affect toxin already bound to nerve endings.[31]

Diseases treated. TIG is used to provide passive immunity to tetanus as part of a postexposure prophylaxis regimen following an injury in patients whose immunization is incomplete or uncertain or if it has been more than 10 years since last dose of tetanus toxoid.[1,3–9]

Adverse reaction. Slight soreness at injection site, mild fever, and rarely sensitization to repeated injections of human immune globulin has been reported.[28]

Antitoxin and Immune Globulins: Disease Modifying
Cytomegalovirus immune Globulin/Cytogam
Description. Cytomegalovirus immune globulin IV (CMV-IG) is a purified immune globulin (hyperimmune globulin) that contains immunoglobulin G (IgG) derived from pooled adult human plasma selected for high titers of anti-CMV antibodies.[32]

Mechanisms of action. CMV-IG provides relatively high concentration of antibodies directed against CMV. It provides prophylaxis against CMV infection or disease in immunocompromised individuals.[32–43] Results from in vitro studies and mice indicate that anti-CMV antibodies can neutralize the pathogenic properties of CMV.[42–44] As CMV usually targets a population of bone marrow-derived myeloid lineage progenitor cells, antibody-neutralization of the virus alone may not be enough to prevent or make active disease less severe in already CMV-infected individuals.[42,44–47]

Disease treated. CMV-IG provides passive immunity to individuals who are at risk for primary CMV infection/disease, or secondary CMV disease (reactivation of CMV).[41,42,44–46,48–51] It is also prescribed for the prophylaxis of CMV disease associated with transplantation of kidney, lung, liver, pancreas, and heart. With the exception of CMV-seronegative recipients of kidneys from CMV-seropositive donors, CMV-IG prophylaxis should be considered in conjunction with ganciclovir.

Adverse reactions. Most frequent adverse reactions reported are flushing, chills, muscle cramps, back pain, fever, nausea, vomiting, arthralgia, and wheezing.[32,34–36] There is a slight risk of hemolysis, as intravenous immunoglobulin (IVIG) products can contain blood group antibodies, which may act as a hemolysin and induce in vivo coating of red blood cells with immunoglobulin, causing a positive direct antiglobulin reaction. Transfusion-related acute lung injury (noncardiogenic pulmonary edema) and thrombotic events have been reported in patients receiving IVIG preparations.[32]

Similar to all other products made from human plasma, this CMV-IG also carries the possibility for transmission of blood-borne viral agents and the CJD agent. However, this IVIG is treated with a solvent detergent viral inactivation procedure to inactivate a wide spectrum of lipid-enveloped viruses, including HIV-1, HIV-2, Hepatitis B, and Hepatitis C.

Antivenin [latrodectus mactans]/black widow spider antivenin—antivenin Micrurus fulvius/eastern and Texas coral snake antivenin—crotalidae polyvalent immune Fab/Crofab

Description. These antivenins are sterile, nonpyrogenic, purified, and lyophilized preparation of specific venom-neutralizing serum globulins obtained from the blood serum of healthy horses exposed to the venom of black widow spiders and eastern coral snake (*Micrurus fulvius*) venom, respectively.[52–55] In contrast, crofab is an antivenin made up of ovine Fab (monovalent) immunoglobulin fragments obtained from blood of healthy sheep immunized with North American Crotalinae subfamily of venomous snakes that includes rattlesnakes, copperheads, cottonmouth, or water moccasins.[56]

Mechanisms of action. Mode of action of these antivenins is unknown.[52] However, they probably act by neutralizing venom of black widow spiders and coral snakes.[54] Crofab is a venom-specific Fab fragment of IgG that works by binding and neutralizing venom toxins, facilitating their redistribution away from target tissues and their elimination from the body.[56]

Disease treated. These antivenins are indicated for patients with symptoms due to bites by black widow spider (*Latrodectus mactans*)[52] and bites of two genera of coral snakes, that is, Micrurus (including the eastern and Texas varieties) and Micruroides (the Sonoran or Arizona variety), found in southeastern Arizona and southwestern New Mexico.[52,57–59] Antivenin *Micrurus fulvius* (equine origin) is indicated only for treatment and management of adult and pediatric patients exposed to North American crotalid envenomation.[54]

Adverse effects. Immediate systemic reactions (allergic reactions or anaphylaxis) and death can occur in patients sensitive to antivenin from horse serum.[52,60]

Most common adverse reactions to crofab are urticaria, rash, nausea, pruritus, and back pain.[61,62]

High antibody titer influenza fresh frozen plasma

Description. Use of convalescent (persons who have recovered from a particular infection) donor plasma with high hemagglutination inhibition titer against certain influenza strains has been recommended as a primary therapy for severe respiratory infectious diseases including influenza, severe acute respiratory syndrome, and Middle East respiratory syndrome.[63]

History of antibody use. A meta-analysis of previous cohort studies during the 1918 influenza pandemic showed a case-fatality rate of 16% among subjects treated with plasma, serum, or whole blood compared to 37% among controls. Similarly, in 2009, a cohort study using convalescent plasma for the treatment of pandemic H1N1 influenza resulted in a mortality of 20% in the treatment group versus 54% in the control group.[64]

Mechanisms of action. Antiinfluenza convalescent plasma decreases the rate of viral shedding measured by neutralizing antibody titer and hemagglutination inhibition.[65] Both preexisting immunity (previous infections and vaccinations) as well as any immune response occurring after illness onset makes this mechanism of action more complex.

Disease classifications treated. Influenza, severe acute respiratory syndrome, and Middle East respiratory syndrome.[63]

Adverse effects. Convalescent plasma seems safe. The serious adverse events reported are related to the underlying influenza, its complications, preexisting comorbidities, and not due to the convalescent plasma usage.

High antibody titer ebola fresh frozen plasma

Description. Antibodies to the Ebola virus (EV) in whole blood or plasma from convalescent donors may be effective in the treatment of EV infection.

History of antibody use. The World Health Organization (WHO) has stated that convalescent blood or plasma is an option in the treatment of Ebola.[66] In 1999, transfusion of locally collected convalescent blood helped to decrease Ebola mortality.[67] Therefore,

WHO has recommended the collection of convalescent plasma to treat patients with Ebola virus infection.

Mechanisms of action. This fresh frozen plasma (FFP) has high titers of antibodies directed against Ebola virus.[68]

Adverse effects. Convalescent plasma seems safe with few adverse effects.[69,70]

Digoxin immune Fab/DigiFab; Digibind

Description. Digoxin immune Fab is a sterile, purified, lyophilized monovalent preparation of bovine immunoglobulin Fab fragments that binds to digoxin. These Fab fragments are obtained from the blood of healthy sheep immunized with a digoxin derivative, digoxindicarboxymethoxylamine, a digoxin analogue that contains the functionally essential cyclopentaperhydrophenanthrene: lactone ring moiety coupled to keyhole limpet hemocyanin. The final product is prepared by taking the immunoglobulin fraction of the ovine serum, digesting it with papain, and isolating the digoxin-specific Fab fragments by affinity chromatography.[71-79]

Mechanisms of action. DigiFab or Digibind have antigen-binding fragments that bind to free digoxin molecules that results in an equilibrium shift away from binding to receptors, thereby reversing the cardiotoxic effects of the glycoside.[71,72,75,76,78,80-87] Subsequently, Fab-digoxin complexes are cleared by the kidney and reticuloendothelial system. Due to papain treatment, the Fab fragments lack the antigenic determinants of the Fc fragment resulting in reduced immunogenicity to patients as opposed to intact immunoglobulin products.[71,72,75,76,78,79,84,88,89]

Diseases treated. Digoxin immune Fab is indicated for patients with either life-threatening or potentially life-threatening digoxin toxicity or overdose.[71,79,90-95] Data from clinical trials have showed that both DigiFab and Digibind reduce levels of free digoxin in the serum to below the limit of assay quantitation for several hours after Fab administration.

Adverse reactions. Digoxin immune Fab (ovine) generally is well tolerated following intravenous (IV) administration.[71-73,76,78] Hypokalemia may occur, sometimes developing rapidly in patients receiving digoxin immune Fab (ovine).[71,72,79,96,97] DigiFab should not be administered to patients with a known history of hypersensitivity to papaya or papain unless the benefits outweigh the risks.

Immune Globulins: Antiinfective
Hepatitis B immune globulin/HepaGam B/nabi-HB/BayHepB/HyperHEP B S/D

Description. Hepatitis B immune globulin (HBIG) is a specific immune globulin (hyperimmune globulin) that contains antibody to hepatitis B surface antigen (anti-HBs) prepared from plasma of healthy donors with high titer (>1:100,000) of anti-HBs antibody. It provides temporary passive immunity against hepatitis B virus (HBV).[98-104]

HepaGam-B is a solvent/detergent-treated sterile solution of purified gamma globulin containing antibody to HBs antigen that contains high titers of anti-HBs from plasma donated by healthy screened donors. Both HBIG and HepaGam-B are manufactured by a solvent/detergent (S/D) treatment procedure that is effective in inactivating lipid-enveloped viruses such as hepatitis B virus, hepatitis C virus, and human immunodeficiency virus type 1 and type 2. However, S/D is less effective against nonlipid-enveloped viruses such as hepatitis A virus and parvovirus B-19.[100,101,104]

Mechanisms of action. It provides passive immunization for individuals exposed to the hepatitis B virus by binding to the surface antigen and reducing rate of hepatitis B infection.

Diseases treated. HBIG provides passive prophylactic immunity to HBV infection for prevention of perinatal HBV infection in neonates born to HBs antigen-positive (HBsAg-positive) mothers,[100-106] for postexposure prophylaxis in susceptible individuals exposed to HBV or HBsAg-positive materials (e.g., blood, plasma, serum),[100-104,107-109] sexual exposure to HBsAg-positive persons, for household exposure to persons with acute HBV infection, and for prevention of HBV recurrence in liver transplant recipients who are HBsAg-positive (HepaGam-B only).[104,110-117] HBIG is not indicated for treatment of active hepatitis B infection and is ineffective in the treatment of chronic active hepatitis B infection.[105]

Adverse reactions. The local adverse reactions that may occur at the site of injection after intramuscular (IM) administration are pain, tenderness, swelling, and erythema.[100,101,109] The systemic effects that may occur after IM administration are urticaria, angioedema, nausea, vomiting, myalgia, headache, flu- or cold-like symptoms, lightheadedness, and malaise have been reported.[100,101,104]

Varicella zoster immune globulin/VariZIG

Summary. Varicella zoster immune globulin (VZIG) is a specific immune globulin (hyperimmune globulin). VZIG is prepared from plasma of donors selected for high titers of antibodies to varicella zoster virus (anti-VZV) and used to provide temporary passive immunity against VZV.[118-120]

Mechanisms of action. VZIG acts by neutralizing varicella zoster virus via high titers of IgG antibodies present in the plasma used.

Diseases treated. VZIG is used for postexposure prophylaxis of varicella (chickenpox) in individuals who do not have evidence of varicella immunity and are at high risk for severe varicella infection and its complications. These high risk individuals include immunocompromised patients such as neonates whose mothers have signs and symptoms of varicella around the time of delivery (i.e., 5 days before to 2 days after), premature infants born at ≥28 weeks of gestation who are exposed during the neonatal period and whose mothers do not have evidence of immunity, premature infants born at <28 weeks of gestation or who weigh ≤1000 g at birth and were exposed during the neonatal period regardless of their mothers' evidence of immunity status, and finally pregnant women.[118,119,121,122]

VZIG is now recommended for outbreak control and postexposure treatment, and the vaccine is available to children with humoral immunodeficiencies and selected children with HIV infection.[122] Use of VZIG for postexposure prophylaxis in pregnant women exposed to VZV may prevent or reduce severity of varicella in the woman but does not prevent fetal infection.[119,121]

VZIG is not indicated for individuals who previously received age-appropriate varicella vaccination and subsequently became immunocompromised because of disease or immunosuppressive therapy later in life. Bone marrow transplant recipients should be considered susceptible to varicella regardless of previous history of varicella or varicella vaccination in themselves or their donors. However, those who develop varicella or herpes zoster after transplantation should be considered immune to varicella.[119]

Adverse reactions. The most common adverse effects reported with VZIG in clinical trials in pregnant women, infants, and immunocompromised adults and children were injection site pain, headache, chills, fatigue, rash,

and nausea. Severe hypersensitivity reactions may occur following administration of VZIG.[118]

Rimabotulinumtoxin B/Myobloc

Summary. Rimabotulinumtoxin B, a type B botulinum toxin produced by fermentation of the bacterium *Clostridium botulinum* type B (Bean strain), is a neuromuscular blocking agent (neurotoxin) and inhibitor of acetylcholine release at motor nerve terminals.[123-126]

Mechanisms of action. Rimabotulinumtoxin B and other botulinum toxin serotypes act by inhibiting acetylcholine release at the neuromuscular junction via a three-step process, that is, toxin binding, toxin internalization, and inhibition of acetylcholine release into the neuromuscular junction leading to chemical denervation and flaccid paralysis.[123,124,126,127]

Diseases treated. Rimabotulinumtoxin B is used for management of adults with cervical dystonia (also called as spasmodic torticollis) to reduce severity of abnormal head positioning and neck pain through reduction of undesired or excessive contraction of striated or smooth (involuntary) muscle.[128-131]

Adverse reactions. The most common adverse effects reported with Botulinum toxin are dry mouth, dysphagia, dyspepsia, and injection site pain.[123,132-134] Serious hypersensitivity reactions have been rarely reported with onabotulinumtoxin A.[127]

Botulism immune globulin/BabyBIG

Summary. Botulism immune globulin IV (BIG-IV) is a specific immune globulin (hyperimmune globulin) that is prepared from plasma of adult volunteer donors immunized with pentavalent botulinum toxoid, which neutralizes free botulinum toxin types A and B. It is one of the most poisonous substances known and exists in seven antigenic variants (types A to G).[120,121,135]

Mechanisms of action. BIG-IV is a human-derived antitoxin that neutralizes botulinum toxin. BIG-IV has a half-life of approximately 28 days in vivo and large capacity to neutralize the toxin.[135]

Disease treated. Infant botulism occurs when young infants ingest spores of *Clostridium botulinum* that then germinate, colonize the GI tract, and produce botulinum toxin. This neurotoxin causes generalized weakness and loss of muscle tone. A single infusion will neutralize the toxin for at least 6 months and toxins type A or B that may be absorbed from the colon of an infant younger than 1 year old.[121,135−139]

Adverse effect. Mild, transient, blush-like erythematous rash on the face or trunk occurred in 9% −14% of infants receiving BIG-IV in clinical studies.[135,140]

Rabies immune globulin/bayrab/HyperRAB, imogam Rabies, KedRAB
Description. Rabies immune globulin (RIG) is a sterile solution of specific IgG that contains antibody to rabies antigen. It is used to provide temporary passive immunity to rabies infection as part of a postexposure prophylaxis regimen in unvaccinated individuals exposed to the disease or virus.[141−144]

Mechanisms of action. RIG is a human-derived antitoxin that neutralizes rabies virus so that virus spread is reduced and its infective or pathogenic properties are inhibited. Specific rabies antibodies present in RIG neutralizes rabies. It should be used in conjunction with rabies vaccine and can be administered through the seventh day after the first dose of vaccine is given. RIG provides immediate, temporary rabies virus-neutralizing antibodies until the patient responds to active immunization and produces virus-neutralizing antibodies.[121,141−144]

Diseases treated. Given to all persons suspected of exposure to rabies with one exception, those who have been previously immunized with rabies vaccine and have a confirmed adequate rabies antibody titer should receive only vaccine.

Adverse reactions. Most common local adverse effects include tenderness, pain, muscle soreness, or stiffness that may occur at the site of injection. Low-grade fever, headache, and malaise may also occur.[141−143]

Immune Globulins: Immunomodulation
Rho(D) immune globulin/WinRho; RhoGam; Rhophylac, MicRhoGAM, BatRhoD, HyperRho
Summary. Rho(D) immune globulin (RhIG) consists of anti-Rho(D) IgG antibodies to the red blood cell Rho(D) antigen. RhIG is prepared from human pools of plasma of Rho(D)-negative donors immunized with Rho(D)-positive red blood cells after cold alcohol fractionation, and subsequent purification and infectious disease reduction technologies.[145−150]

Mechanisms of action. The exact mechanism of action of Rho(D) immune globulin in the suppression of formation of anti-Rho(D) is not fully known.

In the treatment of preventing D alloimmunization, RhIG binds to Rho(D) antigen that entered the maternal circulation during fetal−maternal hemorrhage (FMH) involving an Rho(D)-positive fetus or transfusion with Rho(D)-positive blood, preventing stimulation of the mother's primary immune response to Rho(D) antigen. Therefore, by preventing the active production of anti-Rho (D) by the mother, the risk of hemolytic disease of the fetus and newborn in future pregnancies is decreased.[145−149]

In the treatment of idiopathic thrombocytopenic purpura (ITP), administration of Rho(D) immune globulin to Rho(D)-positive individuals is believed to cause transient mononuclear macrophage Fc receptor (FcR) blockade by complexes within the reticuloendothelial system, particularly the spleen, which spares the patient's IgG-coated platelets. This FcR blockade and decreased Fc-mediated phagocytosis of antibody-coated platelets result in increases of platelet counts in ITP patients.[145,149,151−156]

Diseases treated. Prevent D alloimmunization in D-negative women of childbearing potential if the neonate is D+, weak-D positive, or D untested, and following perinatal events associated with FMH such as abortion, ectopic pregnancy, amniocentesis, chorionic villus sampling, external cephalic version, abdominal trauma, and antepartum hemorrhage. It is also used to prevent D alloimmunization in D-negative individuals who receive D+ blood components such as whole blood-derived platelets, apheresis platelets, and/or granulocytes. Similarly, it is used for the treatment of ITP in D+ patients who had not undergone splenectomy.[145−147,149,151−153,157−164] Some preparations of Rho(D) immune globulin may be administered IM or IV (Rhophylac, WinRho SDF), whereas others are labeled for IM use only (MICRhoGAM, RhoGAM, HyperRHO S/D Full Dose, HyperRHO S/D Mini-Dose).[145−147,149,165] When used for ITP treatment, RhIG must be administered IV.[145,149]

Adverse reactions. Generally, mild with the most common being headache, fever, chills, pain at the injection site and, rarely, hypersensitivity reactions. Some degree of hemolysis is inevitable, but this is predictable and transient.[146,147]

Immunoglobulin (generic)/bbrands: Bivigam, Carimune, Cuvitru, Flebogamma, Gammagard, GamaSTAN, Gammaked, Gammaplex, Gamunex-C, Hizentra, Hyqvia, Octagam Privigen

Summary. Immune globulin IM (IMIG), immune globulin IV (IVIG), and immune globulin subcutaneous are sterile, nonpyrogenic preparations of globulins containing many antibodies normally present in adult human blood. Immune globulins (IG) are collected either by whole blood donations as recovered plasma (20%), or by apheresis as source plasma (80%). IVIG is a highly purified product consisting mostly of IgG with a half-life of 21–28 days.

Hyperimmune globulin (Hyper-Ig) products are manufactured from donors with high Ig titers with specificity to antigenic determinant(s) of interest. High titers of these donors can be achieved by natural immunity, prophylactic immunizations, or through targeted immunizations. Hyper-Ig products should contain at least fivefold-increased titers compared to standard preparations of IVIG.

IVIG production is regulated by the IUIS/WHO (International Union of Immunological Societies/World Health Organization), which require the following:

- Source material must be plasma obtained from a minimum pool of 10,000 donors;
- Product must be free of prekallikrein activator, kinins, plasmin, preservatives, or other potentially harmful contaminants;
- IgA content and IgG aggregate levels need to be as low as possible;
- Product must contain at least 90% intact IgG;
- IgG should maintain opsonin activity, complement binding, and other biological activities;
- IgG subclasses should be present in similar proportions to those in normal pooled plasma;
- Antibody levels against at least two species of bacteria (or toxins) and two viruses should be determined;
- Product must demonstrate at least 0.1 international units of hepatitis B antibody per mL, and hepatitis A radioimmunoassay titer of at least 1:1000;
- Manufacturer should specify the contents of the final product, including the diluent and other additives, and any chemical modification of IgG.[166–172]

Mechanisms of action. The mechanisms of Ig-induced immunomodulation are incompletely understood but include macrophage Fc receptor blockage by immune complexes formed between IVIG and native antibodies, modulation of complement, suppression of antibody production, suppression of inflammatory cytokines and chemokines, and/or antiidiotypic regulation of autoreactive B-lymphocytes or antibodies.

As IVIG contains a diverse group of antibody specificities, which protects recipients against multiple infections by eliminating opsonized infectious organisms via antibody-dependent cell-mediated cytotoxicity or by complement activation. This is followed by lysis and/or neutralization of soluble infectious proteins by immune complex formation and elimination through the RES.[166,170,173–175]

Diseases treated. IVIG is indicated for the treatment of primary immune deficiency, secondary immune deficiency, ITP, Kawasaki disease, and congenital hypogammaglobulinemia. Currently, there is an extensive list of diseases for which IVIG could be used. It also has immunomodulatory properties resulting in an increasing list of both FDA-approved and nonapproved indications.

IMIG is used to provide passive immunity to hepatitis A virus infection for preexposure or postexposure prophylaxis in susceptible individuals who are at risk of or have been exposed to the virus. IMIG and IVIG are used to prevent or modify symptoms of measles (rubeola) in susceptible individuals exposed to the disease <6 days. IVIG is used for replacement therapy to promote passive immunity in patients with primary humoral immunodeficiency who are unable to produce sufficient amounts of IgG antibodies and in the management of ITP to increase platelet counts, to prevent and/or control bleeding, or to allow these patients to undergo surgery.

IVIG is used for prevention of bacterial infections in patients with hypogammaglobulinemia and/or recurrent bacterial infections associated with B-cell Chronic Lymphocytic Leukemia. IVIG is used in conjunction with aspirin therapy for initial treatment of the acute phase of Kawasaki disease. IVIG is also used to treat chronic inflammatory demyelinating polyneuropathy to improve neuromuscular disability and impairment, and for maintenance therapy to prevent relapse. Furthermore, IVIG is used for maintenance treatment to improve muscle strength and disability in adults with multifocal motor neuropathy.[166–201]

Adverse reactions. Approximately 2%–10% of infusions are associated with adverse reactions that include those at the infusion site (erythema, pain, swelling, pruritus, heat), phlebitis, eczema, fever, chills, myalgias, malaise, flushing, rash, diaphoresis, pruritus, bronchospasm, chest pain, back pain, extremity pain, dizziness, blood pressure changes, nausea, vomiting, and headache.[167,170,172,177–179,181–183]

PASSIVE MONOCLONAL ANTIBODY TREATMENT

In the late 20th century (~1986), monoclonal antibodies were developed. The first monoclonal antibodies (Mabs) were of xenographic source and were wrought with problems of immunogenicity. These early Mabs did not gain favor until chimerization took pace in the mid-1990s, and in 1998 two Mabs were approved to treat one respiratory syncytial virus and the other certain breast cancers. Further development to humanize and then generate fully human Mab led to an evolution of therapies utilizing these agents. Mabs are being researched or approved to treat a multitude of diseases that include oncologic, inflammatory, autoimmune, cardiovascular, respiratory, neurologic, allergic, benign hematologic, infectious, orthopedic, coagulopathic, and metabolic indications and to decrease disease morbidity (diminution of pain), modify disease progression (i.e., macular degeneration, diabetes), and potentially alter anatomic development. In this section of the chapter, we will review the history of use of these passive monospecific antibody therapies, their mechanism of action, pharmacologic-therapeutic classification, particular medical indication, adverse reactions, and potential future use of these medications.[201]

Mechanism of action

Depending on the antigenic target of these antibodies multiple events are set into action. Immunologic changes occur as the specific antigens are presented more efficiently to effector cells. Some of these actions create decreased inflammatory and allergic responses, while other effects generate antibody-dependent cytotoxicity (ADCC) and complement-dependent cytotoxicity (CDC). Other actions can block receptor interaction with ligands by either binding with ligands or their cognate receptors (i.e., allow activation of NK cells). Interactions may also directly cause initiation of programmed cell death (apoptosis), cessation of growth/replication/proliferation, or lead to changes in metabolism. Moreover, there are also antibodies against infectious agents to prevent cell adhesion for entry, spread, replication, and contagion. Antibodies may also be directed against toxins leading to various methods of inactivation.[201]

Adverse reactions

Depending on their mode of action, Mabs are associated with a myriad of side effects. They can be associated with immunogenicity that can cause a decrease in their effectiveness. Antineoplastic antibodies can be associated with tumor lysis syndrome. Similarly, reactivation of underlying infections can occur leading to progressive multifocal leukoencephalopathy, HBV, fungal, parasitic, or tuberculosis infections. Other adverse reactions include but are not limited to initiation of autoimmune disorders, increased risk for malignancy, cardiac arrhythmia, angina/ischemia, cytopenias, hemorrhage, and allergic reactions including anaphylaxis, embryo–fetal toxicity (if can cross placental barrier), and even death.

TYPES OF ILLNESS TREATED
Oncology

Malignancies can be caused by infectious agents, toxins, or genetic mutations with changes in control of growth, proliferation, or programmed cell death. Historically these have been treated with a variety of radiation therapies to eradicate malignant cells or with chemotherapeutic agents to enhance maturity, decrease proliferation, or cause destruction of cancer cells. In some cases intense high-dose chemotherapy is used to cause cancer remission with stem cell transplants for subsequent rescue. Passive antibody therapy may replace or be additive to other pharmacology therapies and increase chances for complete remission, prolong disease-free survival, and overall survival.

B-cell chronic lymphocytic leukemia

Rituximab (Rituxan) is a chimeric murine/human Mab (IgG1κ) that binds to CD20 (human B-lymphocyte-restricted differentiation antigen, Bp35 {controlling differentiation and possible calcium ion channel}). Its mechanism of action is not entirely clear and may involve CDC and ADCC. Many studies have shown this antibody to have an additive benefit to standard chemotherapy alone. This antibody has been approved by the FDA to treat chronic lymphocytic leukemia (CLL) since 1997. Nowadays, this medication is often combined with ibritumomab in treating CLL (to be discussed with non-Hodgkin's lymphoma).[202,203]

Alemtuzumab (Campath) binds to CD52 and is a humanized rat Mab (IgG1κ) binding to receptors on both T and B cells as well as macrophages, NK cells, and neutrophils, leading to CDC and ADCC. The resultant cytopenias lead to a severe immunocompromised state. Alemtuzumab was FDA approved as a single agent in the treatment of B-cell CLL in 2001.[204]

Ofatumumab (Ocrevus) is a human Mab (IgG1κ) with CDC that binds to CD20 near the cellular membrane. In phase II studies, this agent had 86% objective response rate (ORR) when used alone and with CHOP therapy had 100% ORR and 62% complete remission (CR); whereas, in phase III trials, this Mab showed ORR of 10% after rituximab relapse. This medication was approved by the FDA to treat CLL in 2009.[205]

Monalizumab is a humanized Mab (IgG4κ) that binds to CD94/NKG2A (an inhibitory signal receptor transmitter) on NK cells. Monalizumab demonstrated blockade of NKG2A/HLA-E and restores the ability of NK cells to lyse B cells in vitro. In addition, this Mab was shown to be of benefit in murine models. Ongoing phase I/II studies will be completed in 2019.[206]

Otlertuzumab is a humanized Mab fragment (IgG Fab') with specificity to CD37 that induces both ADCC and caspase-independent apoptosis. In a phase II study both better progression-free survival (PFS) and ORR were observed when used with bendamustine compared to bendamustine used alone.[207]

Urelumab is a human Mab (IgG4κ) with specificity to CD134 (an immune checkpoint inhibitor). This antibody has completed safety phase I dosing trials. Higher doses lead to significant hepatotoxicity. Safe dosing is now established in clinical phase II studies to be completed in 2020.[208,209]

Ulocuplumab is a human Mab with specificity to CD184 (CXCR4). *In vitro* studies showed apoptotic effects via production of oxygen species that was not associated with better caspase activation than AMD3100. Phase I studies were completed in 2014, no manuscripts were found for review. This medication is presently in phase II trials against acute myelocytic leukemia (AML) to be completed in 2021.[210,211]

Other monoclonal antibodies not demonstrating benefit in clinical trials for CLL include apolizumab, dacetuzumab, and gomiliximab (aka lumiliximab)[212–215]

Acute myelocytic leukemia

AML is the leading cause of leukemic mortality in the United States (US). Over the last 10 years therapy has not changed significantly for this disease. Novel therapies have been developed in the last decade, some showing temporal success and some showing a brighter tomorrow.[216]

AMG330 is a bispecific T-cell engager (BiTE) antibody with specificity for CD3 and CD33. This Mab is currently in clinical trials to be completed in 2020 for treatment of AML. A BiTE antibody stimulates ADCC (via T cells) in the presence of antigenic targets on cells of interest. In vitro studies have shown effective lysis of

AML cells, while in animal studies it has demonstrated significant decrease in tumor burden.[217]

IMGN632 is an anti-CD123 antibody complexed to a DNA mono-alkylating agent. In vitro studies showed it had more potency against AML cells than to normal myeloid progenitor cells. In animal models there was an excellent response rate against tumor cells. Ongoing clinical trials will be completed in 2021.[216]

Talacotuzumab is a humanized monoclonal antibody (IgG1-2κ) with specificity to interleukin (IL)-3 receptor subunit-α (CD123, a growth and differentiating receptor). This antibody induces ADCC both in vitro and in animal models. Phase III clinical trials were reportedly completed in 2018; published results are forthcoming.[218]

Samalizumab is a humanized Mab (IgG2/IgG4κ) with specificity to CD200 (OX-2membrane glycoprotein) is in phase II trials to be completed in 2021.[219]

Ficlatuzumab is a humanized Mab (IgG1κ) in a phase I trial to treat refractory/relapsing AML to be completed in 2020.[220]

Other Mab not demonstrating benefit in clinical trials or withdrawn following postmarketing for AML include gemtuzumab ozogamicin (FDA approved 2000 withdrawn 2010 secondary to venoocclusive disease) and lintuzumab (*no* added benefit over standard chemotherapy).[221–223]

Multiple Myeloma

Daratumumab (Darzalex) is a human Mab (IgG1κ) with specificity to CD38 (functions reportedly include receptor-mediated adhesion and signaling events, as well as important bifunctional ectoenzymatic activities that contribute to intracellular calcium mobilization. This Mab mechanism of action is thought to induce CDC, ADCC, antibody-dependent cellular phagocytosis, and apoptosis. This medication is used to treat refractory and recurrent multiple myeloma.[224,225]

Silutuximab (Sylvant) is a chimeric Mab (IgG1κ) with specificity to IL-6. This medication was FDA approved in 2014 for multicentric Castleman's disease (MCD) with HIV negative and HHV-8 negative. There are ongoing studies in phase II clinical trials to be completed in 2019.[226,227]

B-cell acute lymphoblastic leukemia (B-cell ALL)

Blinatumomab (Blincyto) is a mouse double heavy-chain fragment (Murine {scFv - kappa − heavy} − {scFv - heavy − kappa}) with specificity for CD19 and CD3 known as a BiTE. This Mab's mode of action is by directing CD3$^+$ effector memory T cells to CD19$^+$ target cells leading to T-cell activation and B-cell apoptosis. This biologic is used to treat relapsed/refractory cell ALL. In phase III trials event-free survival almost tripled and duration of remission almost doubled.[228–230]

Hodgkin's lymphoma

Hodgkin's lymphoma is a rare malignancy affecting young adults with a peak incidence in patients >55 years old. Up to 40% of these patients can develop relapsing disease. Brentuximab vedotin (Adcentrix) is a chimeric humanized Mab drug conjugate (Mab + linker + payload {IgG1κ +protease cleavage linker + monomethyl auristatin E [MMAE]}) with specificity to CD30 (a cell membrane protein of the tumor necrosis factor receptor superfamily member 8. MMAE is a microtubule-disrupting agent. The combination of this a Mab and drug conjugate disrupts the intracellular microtubule network causing cell cycle arrest at G2/M stage and apoptosis. This medication has a 43% PFS at 30 months.[231]

Mab to look out for in the future include Camidanlumab tesirine (ADCT-301) a human Mab (IgG1κ). This Mab has specificity to CD25 (a IL-2 receptor alpha subunit) with a drug conjugate. The drug is released intracellularly and causes DNA interstrand crosslinks. This Mab is in phase I studies to be completed in 2019 for Hodgkin's and non-Hodgkin's T- and B-cell lymphomas. In addition, there are clinical phase I studies against multiple solid tumors to be completed in 2021.[232,233]

Agents abandoned or not found to be beneficial include apolizumab, denintuzumab mafodotin (HBU-12), iratumumab (MDX060), and lucatumumab (HCD122).[212,234,235]

Anaplastic large cell lymphoma

Brentuximab vedotin (Adcentrix) is an FDA-approved medication for patients with refractory or relapsed anaplastic large cell lymphoma who achieved CR. This Mab had 79% OS and 57% PFS at 5 years, with median response duration not reached at time of publication.[236]

Breast Cancer

Atezolizumab (Tecentriq) is an FcγR binding–deficient, fully humanized Mab (IgG1κ). This Mab binds to programmed death ligand I (PD-L1) to prevent interaction with receptors PD-1 and B7.1 (a costimulatory cell-surface protein), reversing T-cell suppression. Activation of B7.1 can potentially stimulate long-term responses through development of new immunity via priming and activation of T cells in lymph nodes. A lack of FcγR binding decreases ADCC of the T cells enabling more tumor-specific T cell to remain active. This medication was approved by the FDA in 2019 to treat triple negative (estrogen receptor, progesterone receptor, human epidermal growth factor receptor-2) unresectable or metastatic breast cancers.[237,238]

Colorectal Cancer

Bevacizumab (Avastin) is a humanized Mab (IgG1κ) with specificity to vascular endothelial growth factor-a (VEGF-A) that acts as an inhibitor of angiogenesis. It was FDA approved for treatment of colorectal cancer and has recently been approved for multiple other cancers including ovarian, fallopian cancers, renal cell carcinoma, and recurrent glioblastoma multiforme (GBM).[239,240]

Urothelial Carcinoma

Atezolizumab (Tecentriq) is FDA approved as a single agent in urothelial carcinoma and for patients with disease progression despite other chemotherapy treatment.[241,242]

Nonsmall cell lung cancer

Atezolizumab (Tecentriq) is FDA approved as a single agent for nonsmall cell lung cancer (NSCLC).

Bevacizumab (Avastin) is FDA approved for treatment of locally advanced, recurrent or metastatic, nonsquamous NSCLC.

Nivolumab (Opdivo) is an FDA-approved human Mab (IgG4κ) immunoglobulin and blocks PD-1 preventing interaction PD-1 and its ligands PD-L1 and PD-L2. It is used to treat RCC, NSCLC, Hodgkin's lymphoma, melanoma, small cell lung cancer, colorectal cancer, and squamous cell carcinoma of the head and neck. In phase III clinical trials, nivolumab performed better than docetaxel in the treatment of NSCLC.[243–245]

Ovarian/cervical fallopian cancer

Bevacizumab (Avastin) is FDA approved for treatment of locally advanced, recurrent or metastatic, ovarian, cervical, and fallopian cancers after treatment with chemotherapy regimens and surgery.[246]

Merkel Cell Carcinoma

Merkel cell carcinoma is a rare aggressive cutaneous malignancy caused by infection with polyoma virus and exposure to ultraviolet radiation. This cancer was classically treated with chemotherapeutic agents leading to rare durable responses. Avelumab (Bavencio) is a fully human Mab (IgG1λ) with specificity to PD-L1. This Mab was approved by the FDA for treatment of Merkel cell carcinoma in 2017. Treatment with this Mab increases response rates to about 50% and extended durable response times approximately five times.[247,248] This Mab is in clinical trial to treat other solid tumors including but not limited to hepatocellular, ovarian, esophagogastric, colorectal NSCLC, testicular, urothelial, and adrenocortical carcinomas.[249]

Neuroblastoma

Neuroblastoma is an aggressive tumor of children with a 5-year survival of about 50%. Treatment classically is high-dose intensive chemotherapy, myeloablative chemotherapy with stem cell rescue, and/or irradiation therapy. Dinutuximab (Unituxin) is a chimeric Mab (IgG1κ) with specificity to GD2 ganglioside that has mechanisms of action via CDC and ADCC. This Mab is used in patients who have had at least a partial response to classic therapy.[250,251]

Glioblastoma Multiforme

GBM is the most common malignant primary brain tumor in adults. This disease remains incurable.

Bevacizumab (Avastin) is FDA approved for treatment of recurrent GBM as salvage therapy. This medication with chemotherapy increases overall survival by 4 months but as a single agent is not effective.[252]

Relatlimab (BMS-986,016) is a human Mab (IgG4κ) with specificity to lymphocyte activation gene 3 (LAG3, CD223) and is in phase I clinical trials to be completed in 2020 for treatment of GBM.[253]

Tanibirumab (aka Olinvacimab, TTAC-0001) is a human Mab (IgG1) with specificity to vascular endothelial growth factor receptor-2 (VEFR-2) and is in phase II studies to treat GBM to be completed in 2020.[254−256]

Malignant Ascites

Catumaxomab (Removab) is a trifunctional rat/murine hybrid antibody (IgG2a/IgG2b). Catumaxomab consists of one "half" (one heavy chain and one light chain) of an antiepithelial cell adhesion molecule (anti-EpCAM) antibody and one-half of an anti-CD3 antibody, so that each molecule of catumaxomab can bind both EpCAM and CD3. In addition, the Fc-region can bind to an Fc receptor on accessory cells such as other antibodies, which has led to calling the drug a trifunctional antibody. This antibody's mechanism of action is through ADCC. It is approved for use in Europe for malignant ascites from ovarian, gastric, colon, pancreatic, breast, and endometrial carcinoma and is a pending review for approval by the FDA.[257−260]

Cutaneous squamous cell carcinoma

Cemiplimab (Libtayo) is a human Mab (IgG4) for treatment of cutaneous squamous cell carcinoma (CSCC) that is metastatic or locally advanced and not amenable to surgery. CSCC is second only to basal cell carcinoma as the most common skin cancer. Surgical intervention is not possible in 5% of patients. This Mab offers a treatment with less morbidity than palliative radiation or surgery, and gives an ORR in 50% of these otherwise untreatable patients. There are many additional phase II studies involving this Mab to be completed from 2020 to 23.[261,262]

AUTOIMMUNE/INFLAMMATORY DISEASES

Inflammatory Bowel Disease

Inflammatory bowel disease (IBD) pathophysiology remains unknown but may have genetic, infectious, autoimmune origins including cell-mediated immunity. These diseases may be classified as ulcerative colitis (UC), isolated to the colon, or Crohn's disease primarily found in the colon but may involve the entire gastrointestinal tract. With long-standing active disease, malignancy is much more frequent in UC than in Crohn's disease. Mild UC is treated with antiinflammatory agents such as sulfasalazine and glucocorticosteroids. For more severe disease, high-dose steroids may be used to maintain disease quiescent and low-dose steroids to keep disease in remission. Low-dose chemotherapeutic agent or immunosuppressive agent may also be added if dose of corticosteroids is too high to maintain remission. Surgery may be necessary to control disease. For Crohn's disease, medical therapy is usually less successful in managing the disease and surgery may be necessary but is not curative as in UC. For both of these disease processes, passive antibody therapy may offer not only control of disease but possible complete remission from mucosal damage.[263,264]

Adalimumab (two formulations: Humira and Amjevita) is a recombinant human Mab (IgG1) with specificity to tumor necrosis factor alpha (TNF-α). Both forms are FDA approved to treat Crohn's disease as well as multiple types of rheumatoid arthritis. In Crohn's disease, this medication decreases signs and symptoms of disease and is able to induce clinical remissions.[265,266]

Certolizumab (Cimzia) is a recombinant humanized m fragment with TNF-α as target. It is FDA approved for both Crohn's disease and Rheumatoid arthritis.[267−269]

Vedolizumab (Entyvio) is a humanized Mab (IgG1κ) that has selectivity for integrin α4β7 and is FDA approved for treatment of Crohn's disease. This

Mab mode of action is to selectively block trafficking of memory T cells into inflamed gut tissue by inhibiting α4β7-mucosal addressin cell adhesion molecule-1 (MAd-CAM-1) interaction with intestinal vasculature. This medication has shown a good safety profile with no cases of promyelocytic leukemia (PML), no increased risk of infections, malignancies compared with classically treated IBD, and low incidence of infusion-related reactions. This medication is also FDA approved for UC.[270,271]

Infliximab (Remicade, Inflectra, Remsira) is a chimeric Mab (IgG1κ) with specificity to TNF-α and is FDA approved for IBD and multiple inflammatory arthritic diseases. This medication allows for steroid-free remission within months of starting therapy.[272]

Natalizumab (Tysabri) is a humanized Mab (IgG2κ) with selectivity to CD62L (L selectin α4 subunit of α4β1 and α4β7 integrins of leukocytes, not neutrophils, VLA-4). This Mab is FDA approved for Crohn's disease and multiple sclerosis. This medications is effective in induction of clinical remission in moderate-to-severe Crohn's disease. This medication does have the risk of PML.[273,274]

Other Mab being studied for Crohn's disease but not yet approved by the FDA include Ustekinumab, brazikumab, etrolizumab, risankizumab, and ontamalimab. In contrast, Mabs studied but not beneficial for Crohn's disease include andecaliximab, eldelumab, and fontolizumab. Refer to Table 16.1.

Ulcerative Colitis
Mabs being studied for UC but not yet approved by the FDA include bimekizumab, etrolizumab, golimumab, mirikizumab, ravagalimab, sacituzumab govitecan, ontamalimab, and vatelizumab. Refer to Table 16.1.

Autoimmune Diseases
Autoimmune diseases affect many organs and tissues including liver, gall bladder, pancreas (β islet cells in diabetes mellitus), nerve junctions (myasthenia gravis), thyroid, bone and joints, blood vessels, and multiorgan systems, systemic lupus erythematosus (SLE). Autoimmune arthritis is of multiple types including psoriatic, sclerosis, rheumatoid arthritis (RA), and SLE. Many of these diseases are mediated by antibody or cellular autoimmunity but ultimately appear to be secondary to an underlying abnormality in T-cell immune-regulatory control. These disease processes are historically controlled with antiinflammatory agents, immunosuppressive/immunomodulatory agents, or low-dose chemotherapy. Those with resultant hormone deficiencies are supplemented with hormones depleted by the disease process. It is hoped that passive antibody therapy will mitigate the sequelae of these inflammatory processes.

Plaque psoriasis/psoriatic arthritis
Psoriasis affects 2%–3% of the world population and is an inflammatory skin disease. Brodalumab (Siliz) is a human Mab (IgG2κ) with specificity to IL-17 receptor A (IL-17RA). It is FDA approved for treatment of plaque psoriasis, and its mechanism of action is by inhibiting IL-17A, IL-17F, IL-17C, IL-25, and IL-17A/F heterodimer cytokine-induced responses including release of proinflammatory cytokines. When compared to ustekinumab, response rates nearly doubled with brodalumab in phase II and phase III trials during induction and maintenance therapies.[275,276]

Other therapies currently also approved or being studied for treatment of this disease include bermekimab (MABp1,T2-18C3, CA-18C3, Xilonix), bimekizumab, briakinumab, certolizumab pegol (Cimzia), etanercept (Enbrel), infliximab (Remicade, Inflectra, Remsima), itolizumab (Alzumab), adalimumab (Humira, Amjevita), ustekinumab (Stelara), secukinumab (AIN457, Cosentyx), guselkumab (Tremfya), tildrakizumab (MK-3222, SCH-900,222, Ilumya, Ilumetri), risankizumab (ABBV-066, BI-655,066), mirikizumab (LY3074828), namilumab (MT203), netakimab, and vunakizumab. Refer to Table 16.1.

Withdrawn from market or ineffective for treating psoriasis include efalizumab (Raptiva), fezakinumab, bleselumab, and teplizumab (MGA031, PRV-031, hOKT3g1(Ala-Ala)) Refer to Table 16.1.

Systemic juvenile idiopathic arthritis
Abatacept (Orencia) is a recombinant soluble fusion protein of the extracellular domain of human cytotoxic T-lymphocyte-associated antigen 4 (CTLA-4) linked to the modified Fc portion of human IgG1. Its mechanism of action is as selective costimulation modulator as it inhibits T lymphocyte activation by binding to CD80 and CD86, thereby blocking interaction with CD28. This interaction provides a costimulatory signal necessary for full activation of T lymphocytes. This medication is FDA approved for both juvenile idiopathic arthritis (JIA) and adult RA.[277–279]

Rheumatoid Arthritis
Certolizumab pegol alone or with methotrexate improves quality of life in RA and may cause disease remission and reduce joint damage.[280]

TABLE 16.1
Summary of Monoclonal Antibody Therapies.

Generic Drug Name	Brand Name	Type of Antibody	AHFS Classification	Dosage Form(s)	Target
8H9		Iodine 124 monoclonal antibody (Murine)	Antineoplastic Neuroblastoma, sarcoma, metastatic brain cancers Another study Sloan Kettering using I^{331} version phase I good results	Intravenous	B7–H3
Abagovomab		Monoclonal antibody (Murine) An antiidiotypic mAb that mimics ovarian cancer CA125 protein	Antineoplastic Phase II study for ovarian cancer Phase III good immune response but no increase RFS or OS no benefit	Subcutaneous	CA-125
Abatacept	Orencia FDA 2005 EU 2010	Recombinant soluble fusion protein of the extracellular domain of human cytotoxic T-lymphocyte-associated antigen 4 (CTLA-4) linked to the modified Fc portion of human immunoglobulin G1 (IgG1).	Disease modifying Rheumatoid arthritis Juvenile and adult psoriatic arthritis (phase III)	Subcutaneous or intravenous	Selective costimulation modulator, inhibits T cell (T lymphocyte) activation by binding to CD80 and CD86, thereby blocking interaction with CD28. This interaction provides a costimulatory signal necessary for full activation of T lymphocytes.
Abciximab c7Ec Fab	ReoPro FDA 1994 EU 1995 (country-specific approval)	Human-murine chimera Recombinant mono clonal IgG1 Fab	Procedure modification High-risk coronary intervention Platelet aggregation inhibitor	Intravenous	Platelet glycoprotein IIb/IIIa receptor (CD41 7E3)/Intergrin α-IIb
Abituzumab DI17E6 EMD525797		Humanized mono clonal antibody IgG2κ	Antineoplastic Colorectal cancer phase I 2013, phase II 2015 primary endpoint PFS not met Sclerosing interstitial lung disease phase II terminated 2018 slow enrollment Prostate phase IIno significant increase PFS	Intravenous	CD51 (?integrin alpha V)

Continued

TABLE 16.1
Summary of Monoclonal Antibody Therapies.—cont'd

Generic Drug Name	Brand Name	Type of Antibody	AHFS Classification	Dosage Form(s)	Target
Abrilumab AMG 181			Phase II study discontinued development (2016)		Integrin α-4 β-7
Actoxumab		Human monoclonal antibody	Disease modifying *Clostridium difficile* Phase I and II anti-CDTB1 much better		*Clostridium difficile* toxin A
Adalimumab	Humira FDA 2002 EU 2003 Amjevita FDA 2016 EU 2017	Recombinant human IgG1 monoclonal antibody	Disease modifying Humira **Rheumatoid arthritis; juvenile idiopathic arthritis; psoriatic arthritis; ankylosing spondylitis; Crohn's disease, plaque psoriasis** Amjevita Arthritis; juvenile rheumatoid arthritis; psoriatic arthritis; rheumatoid colitis; ulcerative Crohn's disease; psoriasis; spondylitis; ankylosing Possibly hemolytic disease of newborn	Injection subcutaneous	TNF-α
Adecatumumab MT-201		Recombinant human monoclonal antibody IgG1κ	Antineoplastic Breast phase Ib+, colorectal and prostate Phase II completed Phase III soon?	Intravenous	EpCAM (CD326) epithelial cell adhesion molecule
Aducanumab		Human monoclonal antibody IgG1	Disease modifying Alzheimer's disease Phase III x 2 ongoing started 2015	Intravenous	Beta-amyloid (N-terminus 3–6) soluble oligomers and insoluble fibrils
Afasevikumab		Human monoclonal antibody IgG1κ	Disease modifying Multiple sclerosis Phase I completed Nothing in pubmed	Subcutaneous	IL17A and IL17F
Afelimomab		Murine F(ab') Antibody Fab' fragment IgG3κ	Disease modifying Sepsis Phase III trial marginal benefit abandoned		TNF-α

Name	Trade name/Approval	Type	Indication/Status	Route	Target
Alacizumab pegol		Humanized monoclonal antibody F(ab')₂	Limited information on development; Cancer		VEGFR2
Alemtuzumab LDP-03 Campath-1H	Lemtrada FDA 2014 EU 2013 MS Campath FDA 2001 EU 2001 CLL	Humanized rat monoclonal antibody IgG1κ	Antineoplastic **B-Cell CLL**, CTCL, T cell lymphoma Disease modifying **Multiple sclerosis** (phase III) Not effective for kidney transplant conditioning or rejection prevention	Intravenous	CD52
Alirocumab	Praluent FDA 2015 EU 2015	Human monoclonal antibody IgG1	Disease modifying Decrease cholesterol Phase III	Subcutaneous	Proprotein convertase subtilisin kexin type 9 (PCSK9)
Altumomab pentetate In[98]	Hybri-ceaker	Murine monoclonal antibody IgG1	Diagnostic purpose radiology colorectal cancer (diagnosis)		CEA
ALX-0171		Trimeric nanobody	Antiinfectious RSV phase II 2020	Inhalation	RSVF
Amatuximab MORAb-009		Chimeric murine–human monoclonal antibody IgG1κ	Antineoplastic Ovarian cancer Phase II Now research on using to treat mesotheliomas Phase I/II Pancreatic cancer	Intravenous	Mesothelin Prohibits binding of MSLN with antigen CA125/MUC16
AMG330		Bispecific T-cell engager (BiTE)	Antineoplastic AML phase I AML 2020	Intravenous	CD33 and CD3
Anatumomab mafenatox		Murine monoclonal fragment Fab	Antineoplastic Nonsmall cell lung carcinoma		Tumor-associated glycoprotein 72 (TAG-72)
Andecaliximab GS 5745		Chimeric monoclonal antibody IgG4κ	Antineoplastic gastric cancer phase I, II, III ongoing or gastroesophageal junction adenocarcinoma phase III ongoing Crohn phase II no response, UC	Intravenous	Gelatinase B is a matrix metalloproteinase-9 (MMP-9)
Anetumab ravtansine In[98]		Human monoclonal antibody IgG1λ	Antineoplastic ovarian phase II, lung, pancreatic phase I, breast now research on using to treat mesotheliomas Phase II Cervical cancer ?preclinical		Mesothelin Prohibits binding of MSLN with antigen CA125/MUC16

Continued

TABLE 16.1
Summary of Monoclonal Antibody Therapies.—cont'd

Generic Drug Name	Brand Name	Type of Antibody	AHFS Classification	Dosage Form(s)	Target
Anifrolumab		Human monoclonal antibody IgG1κ	Disease modifying Systemic lupus erythematosus phase I and IIb 2018	Intravenous	Interferon α/β receptor
Anrukinzumab (=IMA-638)		Humanized monoclonal antibody IgG1κ	Disease modifying Asthma phase II ?results UC phase II no benefit		IL-13
Apolizumab		Humanized monoclonal antibody	Antineoplastic non-Hodgkin's lymphoma abandoned 2009 toxic effects 2009 CLL phase I/II		HLA-DRβ
Arcitumomab	CEA-Scan FDA 1996 EU 1996 Withdrawn EU market 2005	Murine monoclonal antibody IgG1 Fab'	Diagnostic imaging Gastrointestinal cancers Colorectal cancers		CEA
Ascrinvacumab		Human monoclonal antibody	Antineoplastic mesothelioma Nothing in pub med or web search		Activin receptor-like kinase 1
Aselizumab		Humanized monoclonal antibody	Disease modifying Severe injured patients phase II 2004, no benefit		L-selectin (CD62L)
Atezolizumab MPDL3280A	Tecentriq FDA 2016	Fc engineered, humanized monoclonal antibody IgG1κ	Antineoplastic agent, treat metastatic **urothelial carcinoma, non-small cell lung cancer** Phase III Bladder/urothelial cancer phase I Breast cancer phase Ib **triple marker neg breast cancer**	Intravenous	Binds to PD-L1 and blocks interactions with the PD-1 and B7.1 receptors FDA-approved atezolizumab (TECENTRIQ, Genentech, Inc.), in combination with bevacizumab, paclitaxel, and carboplatin for the first-line treatment of patients with metastatic nonsquamous, nonsmall cell lung cancer (NSq NSCLC) with no EGFR or ALK genomic tumor aberrations

Name	Approval	Antibody type	Use / Notes	Route	Target
Atidortoxumab		Human monoclonal antibody IgG1κ	Limited information on use and development	Negative search PubMed-internet	*Staph aureus* alpha toxin
Atinumab		Human monoclonal antibody IgG4κ	Disease modifying Acute spinal cord injury		RTN4
Atorolimumab	Developed??	Human monoclonal antibody IgG3	Disease modifying hemolytic disease of the newborn		Rhesus factor
Avelumab	Bavencio FDA 2017	Human monoclonal antibody IgG1λ	Antineoplastic Cancers, ovarian, gastric, nonsmall cell lung (NSCLC), metastatic, solid tumors phase II Studies completed metastatic **Merkel cell carcinoma**	Intravenous	PD-L1
Azintuxizumab vedotin		Chimeric/humanized monoclonal antibody IgG1	Antineoplastic Nothing in PubMed		CD319
BAN-2401		Humanized monoclonal antibody IgG1	Disease modifying Alzheimer A phase IIb study ongoing started 2013	Intravenous	Soluble Aβ amyloid protofibrils
Bapineuzumab		Humanized IgG1 monoclonal antibody	Disease modifying Alzheimer's disease Phase III no more studies discontinued research 2012 ARIA-E, amyloid-related imaging abnormalities—edema	Intravenous	Beta amyloid Fibrillary and soluble β amyloid
Basiliximab	Simulect FDA 1998 EU 1998	Chimeric monoclonal antibody IgG1κ	Immunosuppressive agents **Prophylaxis of acute rejection in allogeneic renal transplantation**	Intravenous	CD25 (α chain of IL-2 receptor)
Bavituximab		Chimeric monoclonal antibody IgG1κ IgG3 (SUNRISE trial)	Cancer, viral infections (Hep C) phase III NSCLC failed to improve survival Sunrise trial stopped Feb 2016, phase II/III breast cancer, phase II pancreatic cancer, phase I/II trial hepatocellular carcinoma, phase I malignant melanoma + rectal cancer good response rectal; not for prostate cancer, phase II hepatitis C not resulted?		Phosphatidylserine

Continued

TABLE 16.1
Summary of Monoclonal Antibody Therapies.—cont'd

Generic Drug Name	Brand Name	Type of Antibody	AHFS Classification	Dosage Form(s)	Target
BAY-103356 CDP 571	Humicade Senlizumab	Humanized monoclonal antibody IgG4κ	For research only Phase II 1995		TNF α
BCD-100		Human monoclonal antibody	Antineoplastic Phase II/III melanoma NCT03269565 (complete Dec 2019)	Intravenous	Programmed cell death-1 (PD1)
Bectumomab	LymphoScan	Fab'-IgG2κ	Antineoplastic Non-Hodgkin's lymphoma (detection)		CD22
Begelomab	Begedina	Murine IgG2b	Disease modifying GvHD phase II/III		DPP4 binds CD26 on T lymphocytes
Belantamab mafodotin		Humanized monoclonal antibodymab	Antineoplastic	No studies or info on clinical trial, PubMed, FDA substance	BCMA
Belatacept	Nulojix FDA 2011	Soluble fusion Protein consisting of the modified extracellular domain of CTLA-4 fused to Fc domain of a recombinant human monoclonal antibody IgG1	Immunosuppressive agents **Prophylaxis renal transplant rejection in adults** Phase III FDA approved	Intravenous	Selectively inhibits T-cell activation through costimulation blockade binds to both CD80 and CD86 blocking CD28
Belimumab	Benlysta FDA 2011 EU 2011 LymphoStat-B	Human monoclonal antibody IgG1λ	Disease modifying Kidney transplant phase II Treat **SLE** (testing phase III for renal involvement) Phase II Rheum arthritis failure Phase II Srogren ± GVHD ongoing	Intravenous Subcutaneous	B-cell activating factor (BAFF), B-lymphocyte stimulator
Bemarituzumab		Humanized monoclonal antibody	Antineoplastic		FGFR2
Benralizumab	Fasenra FDA 2017 EU 2017	Humanized monoclonal antibody IgG1κ	Disease-Modifying Asthma phase III completed **Severe asthma eosinophilic subtype**	Subcutaneous	Interleukin-5 (IL-5α) receptor alpha subunit-directed cytolytic (CD125)

Name	Brand/Status	Antibody type	Indication/use	Route	Target
Berlimatoxumab		Human monoclonal antibody	Staph aureus bicomponent leukocidin		No studies clinical, no find creative, zero pub med
Bermekimab MABp1 T2-18C3 CA-18C3	Xilonix	Human monoclonal antibody IgG1κ	Disease modifying psoriasis phase III x2 2020 Ank spond II 2022 Psor arth II 2020 III 2020	Subcutaneous Intravenous	IL17A
Bersanlimab		Human monoclonal antibody			ICAM-1
Bertilimumab	CAT-214	Human monoclonal antibody IgG4κ	Disease modifying Severe allergic disorders phase II atopic dermititis Ongoing studies bullous pemphigoid and ulcerative colitis phase II	Intravenous	CCL11 (eotaxin-1)
Besilesomab	Scintimun EU 2010 Not FDA approved	Murine monoclonal antibody IgG1κ	Diagnostic use Inflammatory lesions and metastases (detection)		CEA-CAM8-related antigen
Bevacizumab	Avastin FDA 2004 EU 2005	Humanized monoclonal antibody IgG1κ BiTE	Antineoplastic agent Antiangiogenesis inhibitor **Colorectal cancer 2004, NSCLC 2006, RCC 2009,** GBM phase III, **ovarian cancer, metastatic cervical cancer, fallopian** 2014 Breast cancer (FDA removed approval for breast cancer 2010) **Recurrent glioblastoma multiform Nonsquamous nonsmall cell lung cancer**	Intravenous solution or ophthalmic injection May not be so good for GBM or ovarian	VEGF-A anti-angiogenesis inhibitor
Bezlotoxumab	Zinplava FDA 2016 EU 2017	Human monoclonal antibody IgG1	Disease modifying phase III studies done MODIFY I and II Modify III ongoing Pseudomembranous colitis	Intravenous	*Clostridium difficile* colitis anti-B toxin

Continued

TABLE 16.1
Summary of Monoclonal Antibody Therapies.—cont'd

Generic Drug Name	Brand Name	Type of Antibody	AHFS Classification	Dosage Form(s)	Target
Biciromab	FibriScint	Murine monoclonal fragment Fab' IgG1κ	Detect cardiovascular thromboembolism (diagnosis)		Fibrin II, beta chain
Bimagrumab BYM338		Human monoclonal antibody IgG1λ	Disease modifying Myostatin inhibitor DM II decrease BMI phase II Sporadic inclusion body myositis phase III not meet endpoint Treat sarcopenia in older adults phase II	Intravenous	Activin A receptor type IIB (ACVR2B)
Bimekizumab		Humanized monoclonal antibody IgG1κ	Disease modifying Ankylosing spondylitis (2018 II, 2022 II, +), plaque psoriasis (2021 III, 2020 III, 2019 III, +), psoriatic arthritis (2020), RA (2017 II), UC phase II	Subcutaneous	IL 17A and IL 17F
Bivatuzumab mertansine		Humanized monoclonal antibody IgG1	Antineoplastic squamous cell carcinoma, breast phase I fail x2, head/neck or esophagus phase I fail, toxicity		CD44 v6
Bleselumab		Human monoclonal antibody IgG4κ	Disease modifying organ transplant rejection phase II 2020 to prevent FSGS in kidney transplant patients Phase II psoriasis- medication tolerated with minimal reaction, no benefit to disease process	Intravenous	CD40
Blinatumomab	Blincyto FDA 2014 EU 2015	Murine(scFv - kappa - heavy) - (scFv - heavy - kappa) BiTE	Antineoplastic Ph chrom neg pre-B ALL (CD19+) phase II **B-cell precursor acute lymphoblastic leukemia (ALL) initial or relapsed/ refractory**	Intravenous	Bispecific T-cell engager monoclonal antibody construct that directs CD-3 positive effector memory T cells to CD19-positive target cells
Blontuvetmab	Blontress	Canine monoclonal antibody IgG2 κ/λ	Veterinary treat canine B-cell lymphoma		CD20

Name	Approval/Status	Antibody type	Indication/Status	Route	Target
Blosozumab		Humanized IgG4κ	Disease modifying Osteoporosis 3 phase I and one phase 2 injection site reaction and antibodies to antibody	Intravenous Subcutaneous	SOST Antisclerostin
Bococizumab RN316 PF-04950615		Humanized IgG2κ	Disease modifying Dyslipidemia Phase III 2019 Discontinued secondary to antidrug antibodies, no primary endpoint achieved	Subcutaneous intravenous	Neural apoptosis-regulated proteinase 1 PCSK9 (proprotein convertase subtilisin/kexin type 9, neural apoptosis-regulated convertase 1, NARC1, NARC-1, proproteine convertase 9, PC9)
Brazikumab		Human monoclonal antibody IgG2λ	Disease modifying Ulcerative colitis phase II 2021 Phase I/II completed Crohn. Phase III ongoing	Subcutaneous	IL23
Brentuximab vedotin	Adcetris FDA 2013 Breakthrough therapy status by FDA 2018	Chimeric humanized monoclonal antibody IgG1κ	Antineoplastic **Hodgkin lymphoma** **Anaplastic large-cell lymphoma**	Intravenous	CD30 (TNFRSF8) an antibody-drug conjugate (ADC) 3 parts: anti-CD30 (cAC10, a cell membrane protein of the tumor necrosis factor receptor), a microtubule disrupting agent monomethyl auristatin E (MMAE) and a protease-cleavable linker that attaches MMAE covalently to cAC10. The combination disrupts the intracellular microtubule network causing cell-cycle arrest and apoptotic cellular death
Briakinumab		Human monoclonal antibody	Disease modifying psoriasis, Drug development stopped for psoriasis, phase IIb study in Crohn's	Intravenous	IL-12, IL-23
Brodalumab AMG827	Siliz FDA 2016	Human monoclonal antibody IgG2κ	Disease modifying **Plaque psoriasis** Completed phase III	Subcutaneous	Receptor IL-17RA

Continued

TABLE 16.1
Summary of Monoclonal Antibody Therapies.—cont'd

Generic Drug Name	Brand Name	Type of Antibody	AHFS Classification	Dosage Form(s)	Target
Brolucizumab RTH258 ESBA1008	FDA review 2018	Humanized single chain antibody fragment (scFv κ)	Disease modifying Wet or age-related macular degeneration phase III to be completed Sept 2018, 2020 HAWK (NCT02307682) and HARRIER (NCT02434328) phase III trials good results	Intravitreal https://www.novartis.com/news/media-releases/new-novartis-phase-iii-data-brolucizumab-demonstrate-reliability-12-week-treatment-interval	VEGFA
Brontictuzumab		Humanized IgG2λ	Antineoplastic Phase I Colorectal Lymphoid Adenoid cystic Solid tumors	Intravenous	Notch 1
Burosumab KRN23	Crysvita FDA 2018	Human monoclonal antibody IgG1κ	Disease modifying X-linked hypophosphatemia Phase III completed	Subcutaneous https://www.creativebiolabs.net/burosumab-overview.htm	FGF 23 phosphaturic hormone fibroblast growth factor 23
Cabiralizumab		Humanized monoclonal antibody IgG4κ	Antineoplastic metastatic pancreatic cancer phase II 2020 Many other cancers phase I	Intravenous	CSF1R
Camidanlumab tesirine ADCT-21		Human monoclonal antibody	Antineoplastic B-cell Hodgkin's lymphoma, non-Hodgkin lymphoma, acute lymphoblastic leukemia, acute myeloid leukemia 2018 phase I Advanced solid tumors with literature evidence of CD25(+) treg content Head and neck Nonsmall cell lung Gastric, esophageal, Pancreas, bladder, Renal cell, melanoma, Triple-negative breast, ovarian phase I 2021	Intravenous	CD25

Name	Trade name/Approval	Type	Indication	Route	Target
Sinilimab Camrelizumab IBI308	China pending approval	Humanized monoclonal antibody IgG4κ	Antineoplastic Phase III nasopharyngeal cancer 2021 Phase III esophageal cancer 2021		Programmed cell death 1 (PDCD1)
Canakinumab ACZ885	Ilaris FDA 2009 EU 2009	Human monoclonal antibody IgG1κ	Disease modifying **Cryopyrin-associated periodic syndromes Including familial cold auto-inflammatory syndrome and Muckle—Wells syndrome; tumor necrosis factor receptor-associated periodic syndrome (TRAPS); hyperimmunoglobulin D syndrome (HIDS)/ mevalonate kinase deficiency (MKD) and familial Mediterranean fever (FMF) Systemic Juvenile idiopathic arthritis** Treat Juvenile idiopathic arthritis phase III NSCLC 2025 phase III CVD rejected by FDA Behcet	Subcutaneous	IL-1β
Cantuzumab mertansine		Humanized monoclonal antibody IgG1κ	Antineoplastic Colorectal cancer phase I 2007	Intravenous	Mucin CanAg
Cantuzumab ravtansine		Humanized monoclonal antibody IgG1κ	Antineoplastic Cancers		MUC1
Caplacizumab-yhdp	Cablivi (Nanobody program) FDA 2019 EU 2018	Humanized single variable domain antibody (bivalent nanobody)	Disease modifying Inhibits interaction vWF and platelets Treat acquired TTP Phase III Hercules study completed	Intravenous Subcutaneous	VWF

Continued

TABLE 16.1
Summary of Monoclonal Antibody Therapies.—cont'd

Generic Drug Name	Brand Name	Type of Antibody	AHFS Classification	Dosage Form(s)	Target
Capromab pendetide	Prostascint FDA 1996	Murine monoclonal antibody	Diagnostic imaging Prostatic carcinoma cells detection	Intravenous	Tumor surface antigen PSMA
Carlumab		Human monoclonal antibody IgG1κ	Antineoplastic Prostate phase II no long term benefit Pulm fibrosis phase II no benefit	Intravenous	hMCAF/MCP-1 (human macrophage/monocyte chemotactic protein-1)
Carotuximab TRC105		Chimeric monoclonal antibody IgG1κ	Antineoplastic angiosarcoma Hepatocellular car phase I/II 2020 Glioblastoma multi-phase II 2014 terminated poor accrual ?results Angiosarcoma phase III 2019 TAPPAS trial Prostate ca phase II 2021 NSCLC phase I 2019	Intravenous	Endoglin (CD105)
Catumaxomab	Removab FDA approved pend 2017) EU approved 2009	Removab: A trifunctional rat/murine hybrid antibody IgG2a/IgG2b	Antineoplastic Removab Ovarian cancer phase II, malignant ascites phase II, gastric cancer phase II (ovarian, gastric, colon, pancreatic, breast, endometrial) Proxinium Head and neck cancer	Intraperitoneal	EpCAM, CD3 Catumaxomab consists of one "half" (one heavy chain and one light chain) of an anti-EpCAM antibody and one half of an anti-CD3 antibody, so that each molecule of catumaxomab can bind both EpCAM and CD3. In addition, the Fc-region can bind to an Fc receptor on accessory cells like other antibodies, which has led to calling the drug a trifunctional antibody.
cBR96-doxorubicin immuno-conjugate aka SGN-15		Humanized monoclonal antibody IgG1κ	Antineoplastic Cancer Sponsorship ceased 2005		

Name	Trade name / FDA	Type	Indication	Route	Target
Cedelizumab	CIMZIA	Humanized monoclonal antibody IgG4κ	Prevent organ transplant rejection	Intravenous	CD4
Cemiplimab	Libtayo FDA 2018	Human monoclonal antibody IgG4	Antineoplastic Nonsmall cell lung cancer (NSCLC) phase I 2021, phase II 2022 × 3 III 2022 × 3 Oropharynx phase II 2022 Multiple myeloma phase II 2022 Ovarian ca phase II 2022 Head neck squamous cell carcinoma phase II 2020 **Cutaneous squamous cell** Glioblastoma multiforme phase II 2021 Lung ca phase II 2022 Cervical cancer phase III 2023	Intravenous	Programmed cell death receptor PCDC1
Cergutuzumab amunaleukin Aka RO6895882, CEA-IL2v		Humanized monoclonal antibody	Antineoplastic phase I Dec 2018	Intravenous	IL2
Certolizumab pegol CDP870	Cimzia FDA 2008 EU 2009	Recombinant, humanized antibody Fab' fragment	Disease-Modifying **Crohns** **Rheumatoid arthritis** (phase IIIs completed) Psoriatic arthritis phase III Ankylosing spondylitis	Subcutaneous	Tumor necrosis factor α blocker
Cetrelimab	Relatimab	Human monoclonal antibody IgG4κ	Antineoplastic	Nothing on PubMed or creative lab Substance is registered with FDA	Programmed cell death 1
Cetuximab IMC-225	Leukeran Erbitux FDA 2004 EU 2004	Recombinant chimeric monoclonal antibody IgG1κ	Antineoplastic agent **Metastatic colorectal cancer** and head and neck cancer NSCLC	Intravenous solution	EGFR
Citatuzumab bogatox		Humanized Fab IgG1κ	Antineoplastic ovarian cancer and other solid tumors	Study phase I terminated 2008	EpCAM

Continued

TABLE 16.1
Summary of Monoclonal Antibody Therapies.—cont'd

Generic Drug Name	Brand Name	Type of Antibody	AHFS Classification	Dosage Form(s)	Target
Cixutumumab		Human monoclonal antibody IgG1κ	Antineoplastic Solid tumors Sarcoma phase II Esophageal cancer phase II Rhabdomyosarcoma phase II no benefit Liver cancer phase I Low antitumor effect Pancreas no benefit 2012	Intravenous	IGF-1 receptor (CD221)
Clazakizumab ALD–518		Humanized monoclonal antibody	Disease modifying rheumatoid arthritis phase II 2015 × 3 Crohn disease phase II 2013 Highly sensitized renal transplant candidates phase II 2020 Treat post-tx rejection kidney phase II 2020 Antibody-mediated rejection phase III 2027	Subcutaneous	IL6
Clenoliximab		Chimeric monoclonal antibody	Disease modifying Rheum Arth No study since 2003		CD4
Clivatuzumab tetraxetan (90)Y-clivatuzumab tetraxetan	hPAM4-Cide	Humanized monoclonal antibody IgG1κ	Antineoplastic Pancreatic cancer Phase III 2017 PANCRIT-1 study. Study terminated no increase improvement of overall survival		MUC1
Codrituzumab		Humanized monoclonal antibody IgG1κ	Antineoplastic HCC Phase Ib no response Phase II no response		Glypican 3
Cofetuzumab pelidotin		Humanized monoclonal antibody IgG1κ	Antineoplastic	Nothing on PubMed or creative lab Substance is not registered with FDA	Protein tyrosine kinase 7 (PTK7)

Name	Status	Type	Indication	Route	Target
Coltuximab ravtansine SAR3419		Chimeric monoclonal antibody IgG1 conjugated to DM4 (N2'-(4-((3-carboxypropyl)dithio)-4-methyl-1-oxopentyl)-N2'-deacetylmaytansine)	Antineoplastic Relapse/refractory ALL phase II 2015 low clinical response Phase II moderate response		CD19
Conatumumab AMG655		Human monoclonal antibody IgG1κ	Antineoplastic Phase II 2019: Advanced solid tumors Carcinoid Colorectal cancer Locally advanced Lymphoma Metastatic cancer Nonsmall cell lung cancer Sarcoma Solid tumors Colon cancer phase Ib/II no benefit	Intravenous	TRAIL–R2
Concizumab		Humanized IgG4κ	Disease modifying Hemophilia A and B phase II 2020	Subcutaneous	Kunitz-type protease inhibitor 2 domain of tissue factor pathway inhibitor (TFPI)
Cosfroviximab ZMapp		Chimeric monoclonal antibody IgG1κ Triple monoclonal antibody cocktail	Disease modifying Ebola virus Ongoing studies show benefit but not enough enrolled to power study		Ebola virus glycoprotein
Crenezumab RG7412 MABT5102A		Humanized monoclonal antibody IgG4	Disease modifying Alzheimer's disease phase III study ongoing prodromal/mild AD 2021 Phase III 2022	Intravenous	1-40-β-amyloid
Crizanlizumab SelG1	FDA review possible 2019	Humanized monoclonal antibody IgG2κ	Disease modifying Sickle cell disease phase II 2022 children Phase II adults decrease pain crisis	Intravenous	P Selectin
Crotedumab		Human monoclonal antibody IgG4κ	Disease modifying DM type II	No results	GCGR

Continued

TABLE 16.1
Summary of Monoclonal Antibody Therapies.—cont'd

Generic Drug Name	Brand Name	Type of Antibody	AHFS Classification	Dosage Form(s)	Target
Cusatuzumab ARGX-110		Humanized monoclonal antibody IgG1	Antineoplastic Phase I completed safe Phase I/II CTCL dec 2018 Nasopharyngeal carcinoma 2018	Intravenous	CD70
Dacetuzumab HU-S2C6 ASKP1240 SGN-40		Humanized monoclonal antibody IgG1	Antineoplastic Hematologic cancers Multiple myeloma phase I 2007 Large B-cell lymphoma phase II 2009 enrollment stopped no benefit CLL phase II 2006 NHL phase I Renal transplant (CIRRUS I) phase II 2022 SLE nephritis phase II 2020	Intravenous	CD40
Daclizumab	Zenapax Zinbryta FDA 1997 EU 1999 Zenapax withdrawn from market Apr 2009 for commercial reasons Zinbryta withdrawal 2018 secondary to risk/benefit profile	Humanized monoclonal antibody IgG1κ	Disease modifying Prevention of organ transplant rejections Phase IV kidney transplants, multiple sclerosis phase III 2018 pulled from market secondary inflammatory brain disorders Biogen Heart transplant phase IV 108 studies Zanapax discontinued from market by Roche (basiliximab replace)		CD25 (α chain of IL-2 receptor)
Dalotuzumab		Humanized monoclonal antibody IgG1κ	Antineoplastic Phase I multiple Phase II breast no improvement × 2 Phase III colon no improvement Ped solid phase I	Intravenous	IGF-1 receptor (CD221)

Name	Antibody type	Indication / trials	Route	Target / mechanism
Dapirolizumab pegol	Humanized monoclonal antibody IgG1κ	SLE phase II Nov 2018 Phase I safe	Intravenous	CD154 (CD40L)
Daratumumab Darzalex FDA 2015 EU 2016	Human IgG1κ	Antineoplastic agent **Multiple myeloma relapse/refractory** Phase III completed	Intravenous solution	CD38 Induces CDC, ADCC, ADCP, and apoptosis
Dectrekumab QAX576	Human monoclonal antibody IgG1κ	Cancers, asthma phase II, idiopathic pulmonary fibrosis, eosinophilic Esophagitis phase II some benefit but primary endpoint not achieved, Keloids, Crohn's disease phase II trials 2013	Nothing on PubMed Substance is registered with FDA, creative lab	IL-13
Demcizumab	Humanized monoclonal antibody IgG2κ	Antineoplastic NSCLC phase II 2018 Phase I safety established with 50% tumor regression response	Intravenous	Delta-like ligand 4DLL4 DLL4 and Notch1, signaling stimulated by DLL4 plays a role in development of blood vessels throughout life
Denintuzumab mafodotin HBU-12 SGN-CD19A	Humanized monoclonal antibody IgG1κ Antibody-drug conjugate (ADC) composed of a humanized anti-CD19 monoclonal antibody conjugated to the microtubule-disrupting agent monomethyl auristatin F (MMAF)	Antineoplastic LBCL phase II terminated study by company Acute lymphoblastic leukemia and B-cell non-Hodgkin lymphoma Phase I 2017 Phase II 2018 terminated by sponsor	Intravenous	CD19
Denosumab AMG162 Prolia FDA 2010 EU 2010 Xgeva FDA 2011 EU 2011	Human monoclonal antibody IgG2	Disease modifying Osteoporosis FREEDOM trial, bone metastases, etc. 186 studies Phase III completed Melanoma phase II 2022 Bone giant cell tumor phase II 2025	Subcutaneous	Receptor activator of nuclear factor kappa-B ligand (RANKL) Xgeva: Prevention of skeletal-related events (SREs) in adults with bone metastases from breast and castration-resistant prostate cancer. Prolia: Osteoporosis

Continued

TABLE 16.1
Summary of Monoclonal Antibody Therapies.—cont'd

Generic Drug Name	Brand Name	Type of Antibody	AHFS Classification	Dosage Form(s)	Target
Depatuxizumab mafodotin ABT 414		Chimeric humanized monoclonal antibody IgG1κ CONJUGATED TO AURISTATIN F	Glioblastoma Phase III Nov 2019 Children phase III 2020	Intravenous	EGFR
Derlotuximab biotin Iodine (131 I) derlotuximab biotin		Chimeric monoclonal antibody IgG1κ	Immunoassays Potential for glioblastoma multiforme		Histone complex
Detumomab		Murine monoclonal antibody IgG1	Antineoplastic B-lymphoma cell	Nothing on PubMed or clinical trials Substance is not registered with FDA, is on creative lab	CD3E
Dezamizumab GSK-2398852		Humanized monoclonal antibody IgG1κ	Disease modifying Treat amyloidosis Transthyretin cardiomyopathy amyloidosis (ATTR-CM), suspended pending data review Aug 2018 phase I x 4	Intravenous	Serum amyloid P component
Dinutuximab APN311	Unituxin FDA 2015 EU 2015 then withdrawn EU	Chimeric monoclonal antibody IgG1κ	Antineoplastic Neuroblastoma phase I 2022 SCLC phase III Nov 2019 Osteosarcoma phase II Dec 2018 **Neuroblastoma** phase II 2020	Intravenous	GD2 ganglioside
Diridavumab CR6261		Human monoclonal antibody IgG1λ	Disease modifying Infectious disease/influenza A Very good response in animal study mice Phase II 2019	Intravenous	Influenza A hemagglutinin
Domagrozumab PF-06252616		Humanized monoclonal antibody IgG1κ	Disease modifying Duchenne muscular dystrophy phase II 2018 Phase I completed		GDF-8

Drug	Status/Brand	Antibody type	Clinical	Route	Target
Dorlimomab aritox		F(ab')₂	Murine	Nothing on PubMed or clinical trials Substance is not registered with FDA, or creative lab	Programmed cell death protein-1 (CD279) PCDP1
Dostarlimab TSR042 WBP285	FDA review pending 2019	Humanized monoclonal antibody IgG4κ	Antineoplastic Solid tumor Phase I, II, III studies ongoing Ovarian CA (first study) phase III 2023		
Drozitumab PRO95780 rhuMAB DR5		Human monoclonal antibody IgG1λ	Antineoplastic Colorectal cancer Ib 2012 Preclinical rhabdomyosarcoma 2018 Chondrosarcoma not efficacious NHL results?	Intravenous	Death receptor 5 (DR5)
Duligotuzumab MEHD7945A		Human monoclonal antibody IgG1κ	Antineoplastic squamous head and neck phase II no benefit Colon ca phase II no benefit		Anti-EGFR × Anti-HER3 bispecific antibody
Dupilumab	Dupixent FDA 2017	Human monoclonal antibody IgG4	Disease modifying asthma, **atopic dermatitis** Ongoing studies	Subcutaneous	IL4
Durvalumab	Imfinzi FDA 2017	Human monoclonal antibody IgG1κ	Antineoplastic agent Treat NSCLC stage III phase I, urothelial carcinoma	Intravenous	PD-L1 (CD274) and CD80—inhibit binding of programmed death ligand 1 to PD-1 and CD80 allowing T cell to recognize and kill tumor cells
Dusigitumab MEDI 573		Human monoclonal antibody IgG2λ	Antineoplastic Breast cancer phase II results? HCC phase II results?	Intravenous	ILGF2
Duvortuxizumab MGD011		Chimeric/humanized monoclonal antibody	Antineoplastic B-cell malignancy Phase I/II Jul 2018/2020	Intravenous	CD19, CD3E
Ecromeximab KW2871		Chimeric monoclonal antibody IgG1κ	Antineoplastic Metastatic melanoma Phase I/II clinical activity limited	Intravenous	GD3 ganglioside

Continued

TABLE 16.1
Summary of Monoclonal Antibody Therapies.—cont'd

Generic Drug Name	Brand Name	Type of Antibody	AHFS Classification	Dosage Form(s)	Target
Eculizumab	Soliris PNH FDA 2007 EU 2007 aHUS, and myasthenia gravis FDA 2018 EU 2018 Japan 2018	Humanized monoclonal antibody IgG1/4	Immuno-regulation **Paroxysmal nocturnal hemoglobinuria (PNH), atypical hemolytic uremic syndrome (HUS) Generalized myasthenia gravis (MG)** Phase II CAD	Intravenous	C5
Edobacomab E5		Murine monoclonal antibody	No improved survival		Endotoxin
Edrecolomab	Panorex	Murine monoclonal antibody IgG2κ	Antineoplastic Colorectal carcinoma phase III 2003 no improvement	Intravenous	Glycoprotein EpCAM/17-1A
Efalizumab	Raptiva FDA 2003 EU 2004 Withdrawn both markets 2009	Recombinant humanized monoclonal antibody IgG1κ	Disease modifying (2003 approved) psoriasis	Subcutaneous Voluntary withdrawal 2009	Human CD11a Increase risk progressive multifocal leukoencephalopathy (PML)
Efungumab MYC123	Mycograb Mycograb C28Y	Human scFv	Antiinfectious agent Invasive Candida infection	Intravenous	Heat shock protein 90 (Hsp90)
Eldelumab Mdx 1100		Human monoclonal antibody IgG1κ	Crohn's disease phase IIa no significant response, ulcerative colitis phase IIb prim endpoint not achieved Rheum arthritis phase II	Intravenous	Interferon γ-induced protein CXCL 10
Elezanumab PR-1432051 ABT-555		Human monoclonal antibody IgG1λ	Spinal cord injury and multiple sclerosis phase II 2021	Intravenous	REPULSIVE GUIDANCE MOLECULE FAMILY MEMBER A (RGMA)
Elgemtumab LJM716		Human IgG1κ	Antineoplastic Breast gastric phase I	Intravenous	ERBB3 (HER3)
Elotuzumab PDL063	Empliciti FDA 2015 EU 2016	Human IgG1κ	Antineoplastic Multiple myeloma Phase III completed and ongoing	Intravenous	SLAMF7

Elsilimomab B-E8	Humanized monoclonal antibody IgG1	Antineoplastic multiple myeloma Not effective in mice		IL-6
Emactuzumab RG7155	Humanized monoclonal antibody IgG1	ANTINEOPLASTIC Phase I 2019 solid tumors Phase II 2025 REDIRECT study ovarian, fallopian tube cancer Pancreatic phase II 2020		HUMAN MACROPHAGE COLONY-STIMULATING FACTOR RECEPTOR (CSF1R, CD115)
Emapalumab NI-0501 Gamifant FDA 2018 EU pending	Human monoclonal antibody IgG1λ	Hemophagocytic lymphohistiocytosis Phase III 2021	Intravenous	Interferon γ
Emibetuzumab LA480 LY2875358	Humanized monoclonal antibody IgG4κ Bivalent antibody	Antineoplastic NSCLC phase II 2020 Advanced cancer Gastric safe ?effective adenocarcinoma Gastroesophageal junction adenocarcinoma Hepatocellular cancer Renal cell carcinoma Nonsmall cell lung cancer phase II Jan 2018 Phase I safe with tumor response	Intravenous	Hepatocyte growth factor receptor (HHGFR) and MET signaling
Emicizumab ACE910 Hemlibra FDA 2018	Humanized monoclonal antibody IgG4κ Bispecific	Disease modifying Hemophilia A phase III 2020 With or without inhibitors	Subcutaneous	Activated F9, F10
Enapotamab vedotin	Human monoclonal antibody IgG1κ	Antineoplastic	Nothing on PubMed or clinical trials Substance is not registered with FDA, or creative lab	Human growth factor receptor AXL
Enavatuzumab PDL192	Humanized monoclonal antibody IgG1κ	Antineoplastic Phase I 2011 No responses and liver pancreatic toxicity	Intravenous	TWEAK receptor
Enfortumab vedotin FDA review pending 2019	Human monoclonal antibody	Antineoplastic bladder cancer phase I Phase II ongoing		Nectin-4 Anti-Nectin-4 Monoclonal antibody attached to a microtubule-disrupting agent, monomethyl auristatin E (MMAE)

Continued

TABLE 16.1
Summary of Monoclonal Antibody Therapies.—cont'd

Generic Drug Name	Brand Name	Type of Antibody	AHFS Classification	Dosage Form(s)	Target
Enlimomab pegol		Murine monoclonal antibodyIgG2a	Disease modifying Stroke	Nothing on PubMed or clinical trials Substance is not registered with FDA	ICAM-1 (CD54)
Enoblituzumab MGA 271		Humanized monoclonal antibody IgG1κ	Antineoplastic Phase I 2022 children Neuroblastoma Rhabdomyosarcoma Osteosarcoma Ewing sarcoma Wilms tumor Desmoplastic small round cell tumor Phase I melanoma, NSCLC 2018 Phase II prostate 2021		CD276 (B7–H3)
Enokizumab MEDI528		Humanized monoclonal antibody IgG1κ	Asthma phase II No improvement	Intravenous	IL9
Enoticumab REGN421		Human monoclonal antibody IgG1κ	Antineoplastic Phase 1 2014 ovarian cancer +		Delta-like canonical notch ligand 4 (DLL4)
Ensituximab NEO-201 NPC-1C		Chimeric monoclonal antibody IgG1κ	Antineoplastic Phase II pancreatic and colorectal cancer 2017	Intravenous	5AC
Enterecept RHU-TNFR:FC	Enbril FDA 2003	1-235-Tumor necrosis factor receptor fusion protein attached to recombinant human IgG1 Fc fragment	Disease modifying Antirheumatic drug Not effective for inflammatory bowel disease	Subcutaneous	TNFα
Epitumomab cituxetan AS-1402 HuHMFG-1	Sontuzumab	Humanized monoclonal antibody IgG1	Antineoplastic Breast cancer phase II 2012 no benefit		Episialin MS4A1 (membrane-spanning 4-domains subfamily A member 1, CD20 (HMFG-1)
Epratuzumab HLL2 AMG412		Humanized monoclonal antibody IgG1κ ADCC/CDC	Antineoplastic B-ALL phase III ongoing 2018 Disease modifying SLE phase III no improvement	Intravenous	CD22

Name	Brand/Status	Type	Indication/Phase	Route/Notes	Target
Eptinezumab ALD403	FDA review possible 2019	Monoclonal antibody IgG1κ	Disease modifying Migraine phase III		Calcitonin gene-related peptide
Erenumab	Aimovig FDA May 2018	Human monoclonal antibody IgG2λ	Disease modifying Migraine phase III		Calcitonin gene-related peptide (CGRP)
Erlizumab Rhumab CD18		Humanized IgG1 F(ab')$_2$ fragment	Antineoplastic (lab tests) Immunosuppressive drug phase I study cough up blood and phase II did not meet goals Heart attack, stroke, traumatic shock ??no successful CD18 drug to date	LGL type leukemia	ITGB2 (CD18) and LFA-1 block growth factor of blood vessels stop lymphocytes from moving into inflamed tissue
Ertumaxomab	Rexomun	Rat/murine hybrid triomab, murine IgG2a HET2 target, RAT IgG2bλ CD3 target	Antineoplastic Breast Gastric, esophageal Phase II studies terminated company to focus on other plans not safety concerns concentrate on catumaxomab Phase I found safe 2016	Intravenous	HER2/neu, CD3
Etaracizumab or etaratuzumab MEDI-522	Abegrin Vitaxin	Humanized monoclonal antibody IgG2κ	Antineoplastic Melanoma phase II 2010 not beneficial, prostate cancer, ovarian cancer small and large bowel cancer phase I and II completed results unreported 2017	Intravenous	Integrin αvβ3
Etigilimab		Humanized monoclonal antibody IgG1κ		Nothing on pubmed or clinical trials Substance is registered with FDA, or is not in creative lab	TIGIT T-cell immunoreceptor with Ig and ITIM domains
Etrolizumab PRO145223 RHUMAB BETA7		Humanized monoclonal antibody IgG1κ	Disease modifying Inflammatory bowel disease UC phase III 2020 × 4/2023/2024/2025 Crohn phase III 2021	Subcutaneous	Integrin β7 Inhibits binding of αEβ7 to E-cadherin
Evinacumab REGN1500		Human monoclonal antibody IgG4κ	Disease modifying Dyslipidemia Phase II 2020 Phase III 2020/2022		Angiopoietin 3

Continued

TABLE 16.1
Summary of Monoclonal Antibody Therapies.—cont'd

Generic Drug Name	Brand Name	Type of Antibody	AHFS Classification	Dosage Form(s)	Target
Evolocumab	Repatha FDA 2015 EU 2015	Human monoclonal antibody IgG2λ	Disease modifying hypercholesterolemia Completed phase III Heterozygous familial hypercholesterolemia, CVD	Subcutaneous	Proprotein convertase subtilisin kexin type 9 (PCSK9)
Exbivirumab		Humanized monoclonal antibody IgG1λ	Disease modifying prevent disease Hep B	Oral therapy Abstract of randomized study of 50 patients	Hepatitis B surface antigen
Fanolesomab RB5-IGM	NeutroSpec	Murine monoclonal antibody	Diagnostic imaging Appendicitis (diagnosis only)		CD15
Faralimomab		Murine monoclonal antibody IgG1		Nothing on PubMed or clinical trials Substance is not registered with FDA, or is not in creative lab	Interferon receptor
Faricimab RG7716 RO6867461		Humanized monoclonal antibody IgG1mab	Disease modifying angiogenesis, ocular vascular diseases STAIRWAY, BOULEVARD, RHINE, Yosemite phase II and III studies phase III 2022 for diabetes maculae edema AMD LUCERNE phase III 2022 TENAYA phase III 2022	Intravitreous	ANTIVASCULAR ENDOTHELIAL GROWTH FACTOR/ ANTIANGIOPOIETIN 2 BISPECIFIC ANTIBODY (VEGF-A and Ang-2)
Farletuzumab MORAB-003		Humanized monoclonal antibody IgG1κ	Antineoplastic Ovarian cancer phase III subgroup may benefit	Intravenous	Folate receptor 1
Fasinumab REGN475 SAR164877 MT5547		Human monoclonal antibody IgG4κ	Disease modifying acute sciatic pain phase III Knee arthritis pain phase III 2021	Subcutaneous (auto injector)	Human nerve growth factor (HNGF)
FBTA05 Bi20	Lymphomun	Rat IgG2b (CD3)/murine IgG2a (CD20) hybrid trifunct	Antineoplastic Chronic lymphocytic leukemia trial terminated recruitment too slow	Intravenous?	CD20/CD3

Felvizumab	Humanized monoclonal antibody IgG1κ	Antiinfectious agent Respiratory syncytial virus infection	Nothing on PubMed or clinical trials Substance is not registered with FDA, but is in creative lab	Respiratory syncytial virus
Fezakinumab	Human monoclonal antibody IgG1λ	Disease modifying Rheumatoid arthritis, psoriasis (not good for) Atopic dermatitis phase IIb good results	Intravenous	IL-22
Fibatuzumab Ifabotuzumab	Humanized monoclonal antibody IgG1κ	Disease modifying Myelodysplastic syndrome Research in Australia for GBM phase I		Ephrin receptor A3
Ficlatuzumab SCH 900105 AV 299	Humanized monoclonal antibody IgG1κ	Antineoplastic Head and neck cancer phase I 2020 Pancreatic phase I 2023 NSCLC phase I/II 2013 AML phase I 2020	Intravenous	Hepatocyte growth factor (HGF) hepapoietin A
Figitumumab CP751871	Human monoclonal antibody IgG2κ Ceased development in 2011 by pfizer	Antineoplastic Adrenocortical carcinoma, nonsmall cell lung carcinoma etc. ?additional benefit in phase I		Insulin-like growth factor receptor IGF-1 receptor (CD221)
Firivumab	Human monoclonal antibody IgG1κ	Disease modifying Influenza A virus hemagglutinin	Nothing on PubMed or clinical trials Substance is registered with FDA, and is in creative lab	INFLUENZA A VIRUS HEMAGGLUTININ HA
Flanvotumab IMC20D7S	Human monoclonal antibody IgG1κ	Antineoplastic Melanoma phase I 2012	Intravenous No published data	TYRP1 (glycoprotein 75)
Fletikumab	Human monoclonal antibody IgG4	Disease modifying Rheumatoid arthritis phase IIa good, phase IIb no results		IL 20
Flotetuzumab MGD006 S80880	Humanized di-scFv dual affinity retargeting (DART) to CD123 and CD3	Antineoplastic Hematologic malignancies (ALL, NHL) Phase II not yet recruiting 2018	Intravenous?	IL 3 receptor

Continued

TABLE 16.1
Summary of Monoclonal Antibody Therapies.—cont'd

Generic Drug Name	Brand Name	Type of Antibody	AHFS Classification	Dosage Form(s)	Target
Fontolizumab	HuZAF	Humanized monoclonal antibody IgG	Disease modifying Treat Crohn's clinical development stopped despite some benefit phase II ustekinumab is better		IFN-γ
FOR46		Antibody drug conjugate	Antineoplastic Phase I for multiple myeloma failed remission or relapse Phase I prostate cancer	Intravenous	CD46
Foralumab		Human monoclonal antibody IgG1κ	Disease modifying NASH phase II 2019	Oral	CD3 epsilon
Foravirumab		Human monoclonal antibody IgG1κ	Disease modifying rabies (prophylaxis)	Nothing in pub med or clinical trials	Rabies virus glycoprotein
Fremanezumab LBR-101 RN307	Ajovy FDA 2018	Humanized monoclonal antibody IgG2κ	Disease modifying migraine and cluster headache phase III 2019	Subcutaneous	α-Calcitonin gene-related peptide
Fresolimumab		Humanized monoclonal antibody IgG4	Disease modifying Idiopathic pulmonary fibrosis (IPF), scleroderma, focal segmental glomerulosclerosis (phase 2), cancer (kidney cancer and melanoma)	Need larger study for FSGS Good response scleroderma https://newdrugapprovals.org/2016/01/30/fresolimumab/	TGF β 1
Frovocimab LY3015014		Humanized monoclonal antibody IgG4κ	Disease modifying hypercholesterolemia Completed phase II trials 2014 good response and safe	Subcutaneous	PROPROTEIN CONVERTASE SUBTILISIN KEXIN 9 (PCSK9)
Frunevetmab https://en.wikipedia.org/wiki/List_of_therapeutic_monoclonal_antibodies - cite_note-WHOList 116-17 NV-02		Veterinary monoclonal antibody IgG1κ	Veterinary		Feline muscle nerve growth factor

Name	Type	Indication/Status	Route	Target
Fulranumab AMG403	Human monoclonal antibody IgG2κ	Disease modifying Pain osteoarthritis pain phase III 2017	Subcutaneous	Nerve growth factor
Galcanezumab LY2951742 Emgality FDA 2018	Humanized monoclonal antibody IgG4κ	Disease modifying Migraine Phase III completed Cluster HA phase III 2020	Subcutaneous	Calcitonin gene-related polypeptides (CGRPs) α and β
Galiximab IDEC-114	Chimeric monoclonal antibody IgG1λ ADCC/CDC	Antineoplastic lymphoma phase II 2015 minimal response ORR 10.3%	Intravenous	CD80
Gancotamab MM-302	Human cFv Single chain fragment	Antineoplastic Breast cancer phase I–III	Intravenous	HER2/neu
Ganitumab AMG479	Human monoclonal antibody IgG1κ	Antineoplastic Pancreatic phase III—no increase benefit Phase III for rhabdomyosarcoma and Ewings 2021 Not beneficial in NSCLC	Intravenous	IGF-1 receptor (CD221)
Gantenerumab R04909832 R1450	Human monoclonal antibody IgG1κ	Disease modifying Alzheimers Phase III stopped for potential futility additional studies at higher dosing (DIAN in a phase II/III trial in individuals at risk For and with early-stage autosomal-dominant AD phase III 2021	Subcutaneous	Beta amyloid
Gatipotuzumab PankoMab-GEX	Humanized monoclonal antibody IgG1κ	Antineoplastic Ovarian, non-small cell lung cancer (NSCLC), colorectal cancer (CRC), breast cancer (BC), gynecological cancers (GYN) phase I used for diag/prog now	Intravenous	Musculus, antimucin (MUC1)
Gavilimomab ABX-CBL	Murine monoclonal antibody IgM	Disease modifying Graft versus host disease phase III completed 2005 less effective than antithymocyte antibody		CD147 (basigin)

Continued

TABLE 16.1
Summary of Monoclonal Antibody Therapies.—cont'd

Generic Drug Name	Brand Name	Type of Antibody	AHFS Classification	Dosage Form(s)	Target
Gedivumab RG7745 RO6876802		Human monoclonal antibody IgG1κ	Disease modifying Influenza virus A	No studies PubMed/clinical trials	Influenza virus hemagglutinin HA
Gemtuzumab ozogamicin	Mylotarg AML FDA 2000 Voluntary withdrawal 2010 VOD now black box warning Returned to market with FDA approval 2017	Humanized monoclonal antibody IgG4/toxin conjugate	Antineoplastic Acute myelogenous leukemia Many ongoing and completed studies	Intravenous	CD33
Gevokizumab XOMA 052		Humanized monoclonal antibody IgG2κ	Disease modifying DM phase II (late stage) no results Other dz too 24 studies behcet uveitis failed primary end point phase III (Eyeguard _B) 2015	Subcutaneous	IL-1β
Gilvetmab PD1		Veterinary monoclonal antibody IgG2κ	Antineoplastic	No studies clinical trial, pub med	*CANIS FAMILIARIS* PROGRAMMED CELL DEATH PROTEIN 1 (PCDC1)
Gimsilumab MORAb-022		Human monoclonal antibody IgG1	Disease modifying Rheumatoid arthritis Asthma Phase I poster presentation of safety results good 2016	Intravenous	HUMAN GRANULOCYTE-MACROPHAGE COLONY-STIMULATING FACTOR (CSF2)
Girentuximab WX-G250 CG250	Rencarex Reductane	Chimeric monoclonal antibodyIgG1κ Radioactive labeled ab	Antineoplastic Clear cell renal cell carcinoma for treatment and imaging	Intravenous	Carbonic anhydrase 9 (CA-IX)
Glemba-tumumab vedotin CR011		Human monoclonal antibody IgG2κ Antibody drug complex	Antineoplastic Melanoma phase II, breast cancer	Intravenous	**Human glycoprotein NMB extracellular domain** (GPNMB)
Golimumab CNTO 148	Simponi FDA 2009 EU 2009	Human monoclonal antibody IgG1κ	Disease modifying **Rheumatoid arthritis, psoriatic arthritis**, juvenile rheum arth, **ankylosing spondylitis** many studies, UC, DM1 phase I (2020, 2021)	Subcutaneous, intravenous	TNF-α

Drug	Status	Antibody type	Indication	Route	Target
Gomiliximab IDEC-152 Lumiliximab ST-152		Chimeric monoclonal antibody IgG1κ ADCC/CDC	Allergic asthma ? Antineoplastic CLL Phase I, phase 2/3 2014 Failed efficacy		CD23 (IgE receptor)
Gosuranemab BIIB092 IPN-007	FDA orphan drug status	Humanized monoclonal antibody IgG4κ	Progressive supranuclear palsy Phase I 2020 Alzheimer 2021	Intravenous	τ protein
Guselkumab CNTO 1959	Tremfya FDA ?	Human monoclonal antibody IgG1λ	Disease modifying Psoriasis Adenomatous polyposis	Subcutaneous	IL23A
Hu3F8		Humanized monoclonal antibody IgG3	Antineoplastic Phase I For neuroblastoma mod tox and substantial effect on tumor Phase II ongoing	Intravenous	GD2 ganglioside
Ianalumab		Human monoclonal antibody IgG1κ	Immunomodulation Autoimmune hepatitis		Human cytokine receptor BAFF-R
Ibalizumab	Trogarzo FDA/EU approved	Humanized monoclonal antibody IgG4	Disease modifying anti-HIV Phase III		CD4
Ibritumomab tiuxetan IDEC-129 IDEC-IN2B8 IDEC-Y2B8	Zevalin FDA 2002 EU 2004	Murine monoclonal antibody IgG1κ YT[77] or In[98] bound	Antineoplastic **Follicular non-Hodgkin's lymphoma, B-cell NHL,** multiple myeloma conditioning for BMT, B-cell DLCL, mantle cell Many studies		CD20 (human B-lymphocyte-restricted differentiation antigen, Bp35)
Icrucumab IMC 18F1		Human monoclonal antibody IgG1κ	Antineoplastic No benefit breast phase II No benefit colon phase II No benefit urothelial phase II	Intravenous	Vascular endothelial growth factor receptor (VEGFR-1)
Idarucizumab	Praxbind FDA 2015 EU 2015	Humanized monoclonal antibody Fab fragment	Antidotes Drug reversal agent Reversal of anticoagulant effects of dabigatran Phase III trial RE-VERSE AD	Intravenous	Dabigatran etexilate

Continued

TABLE 16.1
Summary of Monoclonal Antibody Therapies.—cont'd

Generic Drug Name	Brand Name	Type of Antibody	AHFS Classification	Dosage Form(s)	Target
Igovomab	Indimacis-125	Murine F(ab')$_2$	Diagnostic imaging Ovarian cancer (diagnosis)		
Iladatuzumab vedotin RG7986		Humanized monoclonal antibody IgG1κ	Antineoplastic	Nothing in PubMed or clinical trials	Human gene B29 protein (CD97B)
Imalumab BAX69		Human monoclonal antibody IgG1κ	Antineoplastic	Intraperitoneal infusion, intravenous	Macrophage migration inhibitory factor (MIF)
Imaprelimab		Humanized IgG1κ	Antineoplastic	Nothing in PubMed or clinical trials	Melanoma cell adhesion molecule (MCAM)
Imciromab pentetate	Myoscint FDA approved 1996 Withdrawn from market	Murine monoclonal antibody fragment Fab IgG2aκ	Diagnostic Cardiac imaging		Cardiac myosin
Imgatuzumab RG7160 RO5083945 GA201 HUMA-B		Humanized monoclonal antibody IgG1κ	Antineoplastic Colorectal 2013 Head and neck 2017 NSCLC 2017		Epidermal growth factor receptor (EGFR, HER1)
IMGN632		Monoclonal antibody with antibody drug conjugate	Antineoplastic AML, ALL phase I 2021 NCT03386513	Intravenous	CD123
Inclacumab RG1512 RO4905417		Human monoclonal antibody IgG4κ	Disease modifying Cardiovascular disease phase II	Intravenous	Selectin P
Indatuiximab ravtansine		Chimeric monoclonal antibody IgG4κ	Antineoplastic Preclinical breast cancer		CD138 (syndecan-1) SDC1
Indusatumab vedotin TAK-264 MLN0264		Human monoclonal antibody IgG1κ conjugated via a mc-val-cit-PABC linker to monomethyl auristatin E {MMAE (5F9-mc-val-cit-PABC-MMAE)}	Antineoplastic Gastrointestinal, pancreatic, gastroesophageal Safe phase I, phase II pancreatic min response, three studies terminated by company business	Intravenous	Guanylate cyclase C (GUCY2C)

Inebilizumab MEDI-551		Humanized monoclonal antibody IgG2κ ADCC	Antineoplastic Refractory DLBCL phase II 2016 Disease modifying systemic sclerosis, multiple sclerosis Neuromyelitis optica	Intravenous	CD19
Infliximab	Remicade FDA 1998 EU 1999 Inflectra FDA 2016 EU 2013 Remsima EU 2013	Human-murine chimera IgG1κ Human constant, murine variable region	Disease modifying Remicade Crohn's disease; ulcerative colitis; rheumatoid arthritis; ankylosing spondylitis; psoriatic arthrits; plaque psoriasis Inflectra Spondylitis; ankylosing; arthritis; rheumatoid colitis; ulcerative arthritis; psoriatic Crohn's disease; psoriasis Remsima Spondylitis; ankylosing arthritis; rheumatoid colitis; ulcerative Crohn's disease; arthritis; psoriatic psoriasis	Intravenous solution	TNF-α
Inolimomab		Murine monoclonal antibody	Disease modifying GVHD phase III No better than ATG in 3 studies Abandoned not in 2017 Cochrane review		CD25 (α chain of IL-2 receptor)
Inotuzumab ozogamicin G544	Besponsa FDA 2017	Humanized monoclonal antibody IgG4κ ADCC/ CDC	Antineoplastic ALL phase II 2023 Multiple other studies	Intravenous	CD22
Intetumumab CNTO095		Human monoclonal antibody IgG1κ	Antineoplastic Solid tumors (prostate cancer, melanoma) Melanoma phase II possible benefit 2011 Prostate cancer no additional benefit 2013 phase II	Intravenous	CD51
Ipilimumab	Yervoy FDA 2011 EU 2011	Human monoclonal antibody IgG1κ	Antineoplastic agent Bladder carcinoma (trials ongoing) Melanoma		

Continued

TABLE 16.1
Summary of Monoclonal Antibody Therapies.—cont'd

Generic Drug Name	Brand Name	Type of Antibody	AHFS Classification	Dosage Form(s)	Target
Ipilimumab MDX010 MDX101 BMS-734016	Yervoy FDA 2011 melanoma Metastatic renal cancer/colorectal cancer 2018	Human monoclonal antibody IgG1κ	Antineoplastic **Melanoma (checkmate 067) Renal cell carcinoma (checkmate 214) Colorectal cancer** Pancreatic?	Intravenous	CD152 cytotoxic T-lymphocyte-associated antigen 4 (CTLA-4) and blocks interaction with its ligands CD80/CD86
Iratumumab MDX060		Human monoclonal antibody IgG1κ	Antineoplastic Hodgkin's lymphoma phase II completed Clinical research discontinued 2009	Intravenous	CD30 (tumor necrosis factor receptor superfamily, Member 8; TNFRSF8) aka Ki-1 Ag
Isatuximab SAR650984	FDA review possible 2019	Chimeric monoclonal antibody IgG1κ	Antineoplastic multiple myeloma Phase I 2019 Phase II 2022 Phase III 2025	Intravenous	CD 38
Iscalimab CFZ533		Human monoclonal antibody IgG1κ	Disease modifying Potential treat autoimmune disease Lupus nephritis phase II 2020 Myasthenia gravis GVHD Kidney transplant 2022 phase II Preclinicals	Intravenous	CD40
Istiratumab MM-005 MM-141		Human monoclonal antibody IgG1	Antineoplastic Advanced solid tumors Pancreatic cancer phase II 2018		Insulin-like growth factor I receptor/neuregulin receptor HER3 (IGF1R, CD221)
Itolizumab	Alzumab FDA	Humanized monoclonal antibody IgG1κ	Disease modifying Psoriasis GVHS phase II 2022		CD6
Ixekizumab	Taltz	Humanized monoclonal antibody	Disease modifying Phase III radiographic axial spondyloarthritis Psoriatic arthritis	Subcutaneous	IL 17A

Name	Construction	Indication / Notes	Route	Target
Keliximab Became clenoliximab IgG4	Chimeric monoclonal antibody IgG1λ	Disease modifying Chronic asthma Rheumatoid arthritis		CD4
Labetuzumab CEA-Cide hMN14	Humanized monoclonal antibody IgG1	Antineoplastic Colorectal cancer Gastrointestinal phase II 2021 imagin Phase II completed therapy 2003	Intravenous	CEA
Lacnotuzumab MCS110	Humanized monoclonal antibody IgG1κ	Antineoplastic Breast, pigmented villonodular synovitis (PVNS) Squam ESOP phase II 2024 Gastric 2019		CSF1, MCSF
Ladiratuzumab vedotin	Humanized monoclonal antibody IgG1κ Antibody drug conjugate	Antineoplastic Phase I triple-negative breast cancer 2017 ongoing study		LIV-1
Lampalizumab RG7417	Humanized monoclonal fragment IgG1κ	Disease modifying Geographic atrophy secondary to age-related macular degeneration phase III Jan 2018 ineffective	Intravitreous	Complement factor D (CFD)
Lanadelumab Takhzyro FDA 2018 SHP643 DX-2930	Human monoclonal antibody IgG1κ	Disease modifying Angioedema phase III 2019	Subcutaneous	Kallikrein (KLKB1)
Landogrozumab LY2495655	Humanized monoclonal antibody IgG4κ	Disease modifying Muscle wasting disorders, i.e., after hip surgery phase II Pancreatic cancer phase II no benefit cancer, some muscle improvement but primary objective not met	Intravenous Subcutaneous	Human growth differentiating factor 8 (GDF-8) aka myostatin (MSTN)
Laprituximab emtansine IMGN289	Chimeric monoclonal antibody	No trials or PubMed or creative lab only in FDA registry ?new		EGFR
Larcaviximab ZMAPP	Chimeric monoclonal antibody IgG1κ	Disease modifying Ebola virus	No studies clinical trial or PubMed	Ebolavirus glycoprotein

Continued

TABLE 16.1
Summary of Monoclonal Antibody Therapies.—cont'd

Generic Drug Name	Brand Name	Type of Antibody	AHFS Classification	Dosage Form(s)	Target
Lebrikizumab MILR1444A TNX-650 RG-3637 PRO301444		Humanized monoclonal antibody IgG4κ	Disease modifying Asthma phase III Atopic dermatitis HL phase II 2007	Subcutaneous injection	Interleukin-13 (IL-13)
Lemalesomab		Murine monoclonal antibody IgG1κ	Diagnostic agent		NCA-90 (granulocyte antigen)
Lendalizumab Olendalizumab ALXN-1007		Humanized monoclonal antibody IgGκ	Disease modifying Antiphospholipid syndrome GI GVHD	Intravenous	Anticomplement 5A
Lenvervimab		Humanized IgG1κ	Disease modifying Hepatitis B	No studies in clinical trials or PubMed	Hepatitis B surface antigen
Lenzilumab KB-003		Human monoclonal antibody	Antineoplastic chronic myelomonocytic leukemia and juvenile myelomonocytic leukemia phase I	Intravenous	GRANULOCYTEMACROPHAGE COLONY-STIMULATING FACTOR (GM-CSF)
Lerdelimumab CAT-152	Trabio	Human monoclonal antibody IgG4	Disease modifying Phase I studies ?Cancer and fibrosis Trials stopped for fibrosis after glaucoma surgery		Transforming growth factor β 2
Leronlimab PRO-140	FDA review 2018	Humanized IgG4κ	Disease modifying HIV phase III ongoing no results published good results phase II	Subcutaneous	Chemokine receptor 5 (CCR5)
Lesofavumab RG70026		Human monoclonal antibody IgG1κ	Disease modifying Influenza A	No studies clinical trials or PubMed	Hemagglutinin HA
Letolizumab		Humanized synthetic light chain variable region (scFv)	Disease modifying inflammatory diseases	No studies clinical trials or PubMed or creative labs	TRAP
Lexatumumab HGS1018 HGS-ETR2		Human monoclonal antibody IgG1λ	Antineoplastic Breast Pancreatic	Intravenous	Tumor necrosis factor receptor superfamily member 10B/death receptor 5 (TRAIL–R2)

Name		Antibody type	Indication/Status	Route/Study	Target
Libivirumab		Humanized monoclonal antibody IgG1κ	Antiinfectious Prevent disease Hep B	Oral therapy Abstract of randomized study of 50 patients	Hepatitis B surface antigen
Lifastuzumab vedotin DBNIB0600A		Humanized monoclonal antibody	Antineoplastic Ovarian cancer Phase 2	Intravenous	Phosphate-sodium cotransporter
Ligelizumab QGE031		Humanized monoclonal antibody IgG1κ	Disease modifying SSevere asthma and chronic spontaneous urticaria phase II and III ongoing trial 2021	Subcutaneous	Immunoglobulin E (IGHE)
Lilotomab satetraxetan	Betalutin	Murine monoclonal antibody IgG1	Antineoplastic NHL 2020/phase II 2025 Diffuse Ig B-cell lymphoma 2019		CD37
Lintuzumab SGN33		Humanized monoclonal antibody IgG1κ	Antineoplastic AMLphase I/II 2022 Mult myeloma phase I 2020 Myelodysplastic phae II 2011	Intravenous	CD33
Lirilumab IPH2102		Human monoclonal antibody IgG4	Antineoplastic Solid and hematological cancers No good aml, squam cell head neck no good, bladder cancer ongoing? May benefit MDS	Intravenous	Killer cell immunoglobulin like (KIR2D) Block the interaction between KIR2DL-1,-2,-3 inhibitory receptors and their ligands
Lodelcizumab LFU720		Humanized monoclonal antibody IgG1κ	Disease modifying Hypercholesterolemia	Unknown studies in clinical trials and PubMed	Proprotein convertase subtilisin/kexin type 9 (PCSK9)
Lokivetmab	Cytopoint FDA approved for dogs only	Canis monoclonal antibody IgG2κ	Disease modifying Veterinary Clinical signs of atopic dermatitis in dogs		Canis lupus familiaris IL31
Loncastuximab tesirine ADCT-402		Chimeric monoclonal antibody IgG1κ	Antineoplastic Diffuse large B-cell lymphoma phase II 2020	Intravenous	CD19
Lorvotuzumab mertansine BB-10901 IMGN901		Humanized monoclonal antibody IgG1κ	Antineoplastic SCLC Ovarian AML phase II Wilm, rhabdomyosarcoma, Neuroblast, MPNST, Synovial sarcoma 2018 phase II	Intravenous	CD56

Continued

TABLE 16.1
Summary of Monoclonal Antibody Therapies.—cont'd

Generic Drug Name	Brand Name	Type of Antibody	AHFS Classification	Dosage Form(s)	Target
Losatuxizumab vedotin ABBV-221		Chimeric/humanized monoclonal antibody IgG1	Antineoplastic		Epidermal growth factor (EGRF, ERBB1 HER1)
Lucatumumab HCD122	Discontinued development by Novartis 2013	Human monoclonal antibody IgG1κ	Antineoplastic; Multiple myeloma, non-Hodgkin's lymphoma, Hodgkin's lymphoma	Intravenous	CD40
Lulizumab pegol		Humanized monoclonal antibody	Disease modifying; SLE; Phase I safe; Phase II no response	Intravenous; Subcutaneous	CD28
Lumretuzumab RG7116 RO5479599		Humanized monoclonal antibody IgG1κ	Antineoplastic	Intravenous	CD28; receptor for tyrosine-protein kinase(erbB-3, HER3)
Lupartumab amadotin BAY-1129980		Human monoclonal antibody IgG	Antineoplastic; Phase I terminated Why?	Intravenous	GPI- anchored cell surface-associated protein C4.4A (LYPD3)
Lutikizumab ABT981		Humanized monoclonal antibody	Disease modifying; Osteoarthritis; Phase IIa no effect	Subcutaneous	Interleukin 1 alpha/interleukin 1 beta
Mapatumumab HGS1012		Human monoclonal antibody IgG4λ	Antineoplastic; Hepatocellular no benefit; Multiple myeloma; Cervical cancer; NSCLC no benefit; NHL; Bladder cancer may be beneficial		Tumor necrosis factor receptor superfamily member 10A; cytokine receptor DR4 (death receptor 4 tumor necrosis receptor apoptosis-induced ligand (TRAIL-R1)
Margetuximab MGAH22		Chimeric/Humanized monoclonal antibody IgG1κ	Antineoplastic; Breast cancer; Gastric cancer/GEC phase Ib/II trial	Intravenous	erbB2/HER2
Marstacimab PF-06741086		Human monoclonal antibody IgG1λ	Disease modifying; Bleeding with hemophilia phase II 2020	Subcutaneous	Tissue pathway factor inhibitor (TFPI)

Name	Brand/Approval	Type	Indication/Status	Route	Target
Maslimomab		Murine monoclonal antibody	Immunosuppressive Unknown no studies and not listed in creative lab or FDA		T-cell receptor
Matuzumab EMD 72000		Humanized monoclonal antibody IgG1κ	Antineoplastic Colorectal, lung and stomach cancer weakly beneficial	Intravenous	Epidermal growth factor receptor (EGFR)
Mavrilimumab CAM3001		Human monoclonal antibody IgG4λ	Disease modifying rheumatoid arthritis phase IIb good	Subcutaneous	GMCSF receptor α-chain
MEDI565 MT111 AMG211		Fab IgG1 BiTE	Antineoplastic Gastrointestinal adenocarcinoma phase I 2018	Intravenous	CD3 and CEA
Mepolizumab SB-240563	Bosatria Nucala FDA 2015 EU 2015	Human monoclonal IgG1κ	Disease modifying No benefit in eosinophilic esophagitis Beneficial allergic **severe asthma**	Subcutaneous	Interleukin-5 (IL-5) antagonist
Metelimumab CAT 192		Humanized monoclonal antibody IgG4	Disease modifying Scleroderma	Dropped from further development	TGF β 1
Milatuzumab HLL1 IMMU-115		Humanized monoclonal antibody IgG1κ	Antineoplastic Multiple myeloma Lupus Leukemia	Intravenous	CD74
Minretumomab MOAB CC49		Murine monoclonal antibody IgG1	Diagnostic Tumor detection/diagnostic/prognostic Failed phase I clinical trials		Tumor-associated glycoprotein 72 (TAG-72)
Mirikizumab LY3074828		Humanized monoclonal antibody	Disease modifying Psoriasis phase III 2020 UC phase III 2023 LUCENT 1 2021 phase III LUCENT 2 2022	Intravenous	IL23A
Mirvetuximab soravtansine M9346A IMGN853		Chimeric monoclonal antibody IgG1	Antineoplastic Ovarian phase III 2019 Breast ca phase II 2020	Intravenous	Folate receptor alpha
Mitumomab BEC-2		Murine monoclonal antibody	Antineoplastic SCLC phase III no benefit 2005	Subcutaneous	GD3 ganglioside
Modotuximab 1024 DS Zatuximab Futuximab SYM004		Chimeric monoclonal antibody IgG1κ	Antineoplastic Antineoplastic Colorectal Phase 2019 Phase III 2025	Subcutaneous	EGFR extracellular domain III/HER1

Continued

TABLE 16.1
Summary of Monoclonal Antibody Therapies.—cont'd

Generic Drug Name	Brand Name	Type of Antibody	AHFS Classification	Dosage Form(s)	Target
Mogamulizumab AMG761 KM8761	Poteligeo FDA 2018	Humanized monoclonal antibody IgG1κ	Antineoplastic Adult T-cell leukemia/lymphoma Solid tumors Many studies ongoing	Intravenous	CC chemokine receptor CCR4
MOR202 MOR03087		Human monoclonal antibody IgG1	Antineoplastic multiple myeloma phase I 2018	Intravenous	CD38
Monalizumab NN8765 IPH2201		Humanized monoclonal antibody IgG4κ	Disease modifying Rheumatoid arthritis, antineoplastic gynecologic malignancies, and other cancers phase II 2021 NSCLC phase II 2022 s/p stem cell transplant phase I 2020 CLL phase II 2019	Intravenous	Killer cell lectin-like receptor subfamily C member1 (NKG2A, CD159A, CD94) that recognize nonclassical HLA (i.e., HLA-E)
Morolimumab		Human monoclonal antibody IgG1	?Diagnostic	No studies in pub med, creative lab or FDA substance	Rhesus factor
Mosunetuzumab RG7828 BTCT4465A		Humanized monoclonal antibody IgG1κ bispecific	Antineoplastic NHL phase II 2023 DLBCL phase II 2023	Intravenous Subcutaneous	CD3E, MS4A1, CD20
Motavizumab MEDI-524	Numax FDA not approved 2010 Older drug just as effective with less side effects	Humanized monoclonal antibody IgG1κ	Disease modifying Respiratory syncytial virus phase III completed Safety concerns hives and allergic reactions	Intramuscular	Respiratory syncytial virus glycoprotein F
Moxetumomab pasudotox	Lumoxiti FDA 2018	Recombinant immunotoxin comprised of a variable fragment (Fv) of a Murine IgG4 anti-CD22 monoclonal antibody Fused to a truncated fragment of Pseudomonas exotoxin A	Antineoplastic Hairy cell leukemia Phase I ALL peds	Intravenous	CD22

Name	Antibody type	Indication	Route	Target
Muromonab-CD3 Muromab Aka teplizimab/ MGA031 — Orthoclone OKT3 FDA 1986 EU 1986 (country specific approval)	Humanized monoclonal antibody IgG2aκ	Disease modifying Prevention of kidney transplant rejection Many trials GVHD, NASH and T2DM, giant cell myocarditis AbATE	Intravenous Oral	CD3
Nacolomab tafenatox	Murine monoclonal fragment Fab	Antineoplastic ?Colorectal cancer	No studies in clinical trial or PubMed	C242 antigen
Namilumab MT203	Human monoclonal antibody IgG1κ	Disease modifying Ank spond psoriasis, RA phase II	Subcutaneous	Colony-stimulating factor 2 (CSF2)
Naptumomab estafenatox TTS-CD3 ANYARA ABR-217620	Murine monoclonl antibody fragment Fab	Antineoplastic Nonsmall cell lung carcinoma, renal cell carcinoma phase III completed primary endpoint not achieved	Intravenous	Tumor-associated antigen 5T4
Naratuximab emtansine IMGN529	Chimeric monoclonal antibody IgG1κ	Antineoplastic B-Cell lymphoma NHL	Intravenous	Tetraspanin-26 (CD37)
Narnatumab IMC-RON-8 Ron8	Human monoclonal antibody IgG1κ	Antineoplastic Solid tumors phase I	Intravenous	Human cell surface receptor RON (CD 135) macrophage-stimulating 1 receptor
Natalizumab Antegran Antegren — Tysabri FDA 2004 EU 2006	Humanized monoclonal antibody IgG4κ	Disease modifying **Relapsing multiple sclerosis, Crohn's disease**	Intravenous	L selectin (CD62L) α4-subunit of α4β1 and α4β7 integrins of leukocytes (except neutrophils) (VLA-4)
Navicixizumab OMP 305B83	Humanized/chimeric monoclonal antibody IgG2κ	Antineoplastic Phase I study colorectal gyn tumors	Intravenous	Delta-like 4 (DLL4) Vascular endothelial growth factor A (VEGF-A)
Navivumab CT-P27	Human monoclonal antibody IgG1κ	Disease modifying Influenza A	No studies PubMed	Influenza A virus hemagglutinin HA
Naxitamab HU3F8	Humanized monoclonal antibody IgG3	Antineoplastic High-risk neuroblastoma and refractory osteomedullary disease study 2023	?Intravenous	c-Met Ganglioside anti-GD2
Nebacumab	Humanized monoclonal antibody IgM	Withdrawn for safety, Efficacy and commercial reasons		Endotoxin

Continued

TABLE 16.1
Summary of Monoclonal Antibody Therapies.—cont'd

Generic Drug Name	Brand Name	Type of Antibody	AHFS Classification	Dosage Form(s)	Target
Necitumumab IMC-11F8	Portrazza FDA 2015 EU 2016	Human monoclonal antibody IgG1κ	Antineoplastic Nonsmall cell lung carcinoma	Intravenous	EGFR
Nemolizumab CIM331 CD14152		Humanized monoclonal antibody IgG2κ	Disease modifying Eczema phase I and II	Subcutaneous	Interleukin-31 receptor A (IL31RA)
NEOD001 Birtamimab ELT1-01 HU2A4		Humanized monoclonal antibody IgG1κ	Disease modifying Primary systemic amyloidosis lack clinical benefit	Intravenous	Amyloid A protein/ amyloid light chain
Nesvacumab REGN910 SAR307746		Human monoclonal antibody IgG1κ	Antineoplastic Solid tumors not as beneficial as other agents in breast cancer Disease modifying Macular degeneration	Intravenous	Angiopoietin 2
Netakimab		Chimeric monoclonal antibody	Disease modifying Psoriasis PLANETA study (Russia, future EU and China)		Interleukin 17A
Nimotuzumab	Theracim Theraloc	Humanized monoclonal antibodyIgG1κ	Antineoplastic Squamous cell carcinoma, head and neck cancer, nasopharyngeal cancer, glioma	Intravenous	EGFR
Nirsevimab MEDI8897		Human monoclonal antibody IgG1κ	Disease modifying Respiratory syncytial virus phase II 2018	Intramuscular	Respiratory syncytial virus fusion protein (RSVFR)

Generic name	Brand/Approval	Antibody type	Indication	Route	Target/Mechanism
Nivolumab	Opdivo FDA 2015 EU 2015	Human monoclonal antibody IgG4κ immunoglobulin	Antineoplastic agent Programmed death receptor-1 (PD-1) blocking antibody **NSCLC**, bladder cancer, **renal cell cancer phase III 2021 Hodgkin lymphoma Melanoma Small cell lung cancer Squamous carcinoma head and neck Colorectal cancer** GBM no added benefit 2017	Intravenous	Blocks the interaction between PD-1 and its ligands, PD-L1 and PD-L2
Nofetumomab merpentan	Verluma FDA 1996 No longer marketed in USA	Murine monoclonal fragment IgG2bκ Fab	Antitumor Cancer diagnostic imaging SCLC		Membrane-spanning 4-domains, subfamily A, member 1
Obiltoxaximab ETI-204	Anthim FDA 2016	Chimeric monoclonal antibody IgG1κ	Disease modifying Bacillus anthracis anthrax phase IV 2021	Intravenous Intramuscular	*Bacillus anthracis* spores PA component of *B. anthracis* toxin
Obinutuzumab GA101HUMAB RG7159 RO5072759 Afutuzumab	Gazyvaro FDA 2013	Humanized monoclonal antibody IgG1κ	Antineoplastic lymphoma phase II (MCL, DLBCL) **Chronic lymphocytic leukemia** Phase II 2021	Intravenous	CD20 Induces B-cell apoptosis
Ocaratuzumab LY2469298 AME-133V		Humanized monoclonal antibody IgG1κ	Antineoplastic NHL Pemphigus phase III	Intravenous	CD20
Ocrelizumab	Ocrevus FDA 2017	Humanized monoclonal antibody IgG1κ	Disease modifying Multiple sclerosis	Intravenous	CD20
Odulimomab		Murine monoclonal antibody	Disease modifying Transplant rejection Only studied in mice		Lymphocyte function-associated antigen-1 (LFA-1 (CD11a))
Ofatumumab	Arzerra FDA 2009 EU 2010	Human monoclonal antibody IgG1κ Complement-dependent cytotoxicity (CDC)	Antineoplastic **CLL** Phase III 10% ORR after ritux Phase II as first line 86% ORR With CHOP 100% ORR with 62% CR	Intravenous	CD20
Olaratumab IMC3G3	Lartruvo FDA 2016 EU 2016	Human monoclonal antibody IgG1κ	Antineoplastic **Sarcoma** phase II 2023 Ovarian not beneficial	Intravenous	Platelet derived growth factor receptor alpha (PDGF-R α)

Continued

TABLE 16.1
Summary of Monoclonal Antibody Therapies.—cont'd

Generic Drug Name	Brand Name	Type of Antibody	AHFS Classification	Dosage Form(s)	Target
Oleclumab MEDI9447		Human monoclonal antibody IgG1λ	Antineoplastic pancreatic phase II 2021 Colorectal cancer Bladder cancer phase I 2020 Breast cancer phase II 2022 NSCLC phase II 2022	Intravenous?	5'-nucleotidase CD73
Olokizumab		Humanized monoclonal antibody IgG4κ	Disease modifying rheumatoid arthritis Phase I 2014 phase IIb mod results		IL6
Omalizumab IGE25 RG3648	Xolair	Humanized monoclonal antibody IgG1κ	Disease modifying allergic asthma Urticaria	Subcutaneous	IgE Fc region
Omburtamab		Murine monoclonal antibody IgG1κ	Antineoplastic Neuroblastoma Phase III 2022	Intracerebroventricular treatment	CD276
OMS721		Human monoclonal antibody	Disease modifying Atypical hemolytic uremic syndrome phase III 2020 Lupus nephritis phase II 2018	Intravenous	Mannan-binding lectin-associated serine protease-2 (MASP-2)
Onartuzumab PRO143966 RO5490258 METMAB		Humanized monoclonal antibody IgG	Antineoplastic	Intravenous	Human scatter factor receptor kinase
Ontuxizumab MORAB-004		Chimeric/humanized monoclonal antibody	Antineoplastic No clinical response	Intravenous	Endosialin tumor endothelial marker-1 (TEM1)
Onvatilimab		Human monoclonal antibody IgG1κ		Nothing in PubMed	Vista (V-domain immunoglobulin suppression of T activation (VSIR)
Opicinumab BIIB033		Human monoclonal antibody IgG1	Disease modifying multiple sclerosis Phase II 2020		Leucine-rich repeat and immunoglobulin domain containing neurite outgrowth inhibitor receptor interacting protein-1 (LINGO-1) LINGO-1

Name	Type	Indication/Status	Route	Target
Oportuzumab monatox VB4-845 Vicinium Proxinium FDA 2005 EU 2005 Additional approval pending 2019	Humanized monoclonal antibody fragment scFv	Antineoplastic Bladder phase III **Head and neck cancer**	Intravescical	Epithelial cell adhesion molecule (EPCAM) and tumor-associated calcium signal transducer 1 (TACSTD1) and pseudomonas exotoxin A immunotoxin fusion protein (anti-EPCAM antibody fragment-Pseudomonas exotoxin fusion protein)
Oregovomab MAB-B43.13 OvaRex	Murine monoclonal antibody IgG1κ Antidiopathic antibody to ovarian antigen CA-125	Antineoplastic Ovarian cancer Not effective in achieving increase RFS or OS Ovarian phase I 2021 Phase II 2019	Subcutaneous Intravenous	CA-125
Orticumab RG7418	Human monoclonal antibody fragment Fab	Disease modifying Antinflammatory		Oxidized low-density lipoprotein oxLDL
Otelixizumab	Chimeric humanized monoclonal antibody IgG1	Disease modifying Diabetes mellitus type 1 TTEDD phase II DEFEND-1 phase III failed DEFEND-2 phase III- no real benefit	Subcutaneous	CD3
Otilimab MOR103 GSK3196165	Human monoclonal antibody IgG1λ	Disease modifying Osteoarthritis, rheumatoid arthritis phase II 2012 Multiple sclerosis phase II 2014	Intravenous	Granulocyte-macrophage colony-stimulating factor (GMCSF)
Otlertuzumab TRU-016	Humanized monoclonal antibody IgG fragment	Antineoplastic CLL phase I and II 2014 and 2019	Intravenous	CD37
Oxelumab OX40L R4930 HUMAB OX40L	Human monoclonal antibody IgG1κ	Disease modifying Asthma mainly preclinical mice Many clinical studies ongoing leukemia and asthma	Intravenous	OX-40 (CD252)
Ozanezumab GSK1223249	Humanized IgG1	Disease modifying ALS phase II 2015 ALS no good	Intravenous	Neurite outgrowth inhibitor (NOGO-A)

Continued

TABLE 16.1
Summary of Monoclonal Antibody Therapies.—cont'd

Generic Drug Name	Brand Name	Type of Antibody	AHFS Classification	Dosage Form(s)	Target
Ozoralizumab ATN 103		Humanized monoclonal antibody	Disease modifying Rheumatoid arthritis phase II 2012	Subcutaneous	TNF-α
Pagibaximab		Chimeric monoclonal antibody	Disease modifying Staph sepsis low birth weight infants Phase II/III studies 2010	Intravenous	Lipoteichoic acid
Palivizumab	Synagis, Abbosynagis FDA 1998 EU 1999	Humanized monoclonal antibody IgG1κ	Disease modifying RSV many phase III studies	Intramuscular	F protein of respiratory syncytial virus
Pamrevlumab FG-3019		Human monoclonal antibody IgG1κ	Disease modifying Idiopathic pulmonary fibrosis (IPF), Antineoplastic Pancreatic cancer Muscular dystrophy phase II 2021 Diabetes nephropathy		Connective tissue growth factor (CTGF) Insulin-like growth factor binding protein 8 (IGFBP-8)
Panitumumab ABENIX ABX-EGFhttps://en.wikipedia.org/wiki/List_of_therapeutic_monoclonal_antibodies - cite-note-WHOList91-38	Vectibix FDA 2006 EU 2007	Human monoclonal antibody IgG2κ	Antineoplastic **Metastatic colorectal cancer**	Intravenous	EGFR/erbB-1/HER1
PankoMab-GEX Gatipotuzumab		Humanized monoclonal antibody IgG1κ	Antineoplastic Phase IIb 2017 Phase I solid tumors 2019	Intravenous	Tumor-specific glycosylation of MUC1
Panobacumab Aerumab 11 AR-101 KBPA-101		Human monoclonal antibody	Antimicrobial *Pseudomonas aeruginosa* infection	Intravenous	*Pseudomonas aeruginosa* serotype O11

Name	Type	Status	Route	Target
Parsatuzumab MEGF0444A RG-7414	Human monoclonal antibody IgG1κ	Antineoplastic Colorectal cancer phase II 2014 no benefit		Epidermal growth factor-like domain 7 (EGFL7)
Pascolizumab	Humanized monoclonal antibody	Disease modifying Not effective trials aborted		IL-4
Pasotuxizumab	Chimeric/humanized monoclonal antibody fragment	Antineoplastic	No studies	Folate hydrolase/prostate-specific membrane antigen (PSMA)
Pateclizumab RG7415 PRO283698 MLTA3698A	Humanized monoclonal antibody IgG1κ	Disease modifying rheumatoid arthritis Phase II not as efficacious as adalimumab but had response	Subcutaneous	Lymphotoxin-α
Patritumab AMG888 U3-1287	Human monoclonal antibody IgG1κ	Antineoplastic May not be beneficial head/neck NSCLC CT site		ErbB3 (HER3)
Spartalizumab *PDR001* FDA review possible 2019	Humanized monoclonal antibody	Antineoplastic Breast cancer phase II 2021 NSCLC 2021 Melanoma phase II 2022 Phase III 2020	Intravenous	PD1, PDCD1, CD279
Pembrolizumab MK-3475 Keytruda FDA 2014 EU 2015 FDA 2018 for metastatic Merkel cell carcinoma, HCC, NSCLC	Humanized monoclonal antibody IgG4κ	Antineoplastic Squamous carcinoma trachea, **NSCLC**, urothelial (HCC phase II) Melanoma cHL, LgB cell lymph Gastric cancer **Cervical cancer** Hepatocellular **carcinoma**	Intravenous Trials for multiple myeloma discontinued by FDA	PD-1
Pemtumomab HMFG1 antibody labeled with 90Yttrium Theragyn	Murine monoclonal antibody	Antineoplastic Phase III Europe 2009/US 2013 no benefit after 3.5 years follow-up		MUC1/human milk fat globule antigen 1 (HMFG1)
Perakizumab	Humanized monoclonal antibody IgG1κ	Disease modifying psoriatic arthritis Phase I discontinued		IL 17A

Continued

TABLE 16.1
Summary of Monoclonal Antibody Therapies.—cont'd

Generic Drug Name	Brand Name	Type of Antibody	AHFS Classification	Dosage Form(s)	Target
Pertuzumab	Perjeta FDA2012 EU 2013 Omnitarg	Humanized monoclonal antibody IgG1	Antineoplastic agent HER2-positive metastatic **breast cancer** Gastric/breast cancer Phase III gastric	Intravenous	Extracellular dimerization domain (subdomain II) of the human epidermal growth factor receptor 2 protein (HER2/neu)
Pexelizumab		Humanized scFv	Disease modifying acute myocardial infarctions	APEX-AMI trial negative results PRIMO-CABG I and II trials no significant benefit	C5
Pidilizumab CT-011		Humanized monoclonal antibody IgG1κ	Antineoplastic Mult myeloma DLBCL Pontine glioma Pancreas Melenaoma HCC Antinfection	Intravenous	PD-1
Pinatuzumab vedotin		Humanized monoclonal antibody ADC consisting of the microtubule-disrupting agent, monomethyl auristatin E (MMAE), conjugated to an anti-CD22 mAbvia the protease-cleavable peptide linker maleimidocaproylvaline-citrulline(vc)-p-aminobenzoyloxycarbonyl	Antineoplastic B-cell NHL phase I study good response Phase II completion 2019	Intravenous	CD22
Pintumomab		Murine monoclonal antibody	Not therapeutic Diagnostic imaging adenocarcinoma antigen		Adenocarcinoma (imaging)
Placulumab		Human monoclonal antibody V-kappaJ2 FC	Disease modifying pain and inflammatory diseases Development discontinued 2012		Human TNF

Name	Type	Indication/Status	Route	Target
Plozalizumab MLN1202 HU1D9	Humanized monoclonal antibody IgG1κ	Disease modifying Diabetic nephropathy and arteriovenous graft patency RA no benefit	Intravenous	CC chemokine receptor 2 (CCR2)
Pogalizumab MOXR0916 RO7021608 Vonlerolizumab	Humanized monoclonal antibody IgG1κ	Antineoplastic Solid tumors phase I 2019 may be safe but may not be effective No formal manuscripts yet	Intravenous	Tumor necrosis factor receptor superfamily member 4 (ACT35, OX40, CD134)
Polatuzumab vedotin FCU2711 RO5541077-000	Humanized monoclonal antibody IgG1κ	Antineoplastic NHL phase II 2019 DLBCL phase III 2023	Intravenous	CD79B
Ponezumab RN1219 PF-04360365	Humanized monoclonal antibody IgG2	Disease modifying Alzheimer's disease Safe but no clinical efficacy 2013	Intravenous	Human beta-40-amyloid Aβ40
Porgaviximab C2G4	Chimeric monoclonal IgG1κ	Antiinfectious Ebola virus disease	No known ongoing studies	Zaire ebolavirus glycoprotein
Prasinezumab PRX002 RG7935 RO7046015	Humanized monoclonal antibody IgG1κ	Disease modifying Parkinson's disease Phase II 2021	Intravenous	Anti-alpha-synuclein (NACP)
Prezalizumab AMG-557 MEDI5872	Humanized monoclonal antibody IgG2	Disease modifying SLE phase II 2018 Sjogren's	Subcutaneous	B7-related protein inducible T-cell costimulator ligand (ICOSL)
Priliximab cMT 412 CEN 000029	Chimeric monoclonal antibody	Disease modifying Crohn's disease, multiple sclerosis	IN FDA no known studies	CD4
Pritoxaximab	Chimeric monoclonal antibody IgG1κ	Antiinfectious		E. coli shiga toxin type-1
Pritumumab	Human monoclonal antibody IgG1κ	Antineoplastic Brain cancer Phase II studies in Japan, could not find literature reportedly increase survivability 10 fold		Vimentin

Continued

TABLE 16.1
Summary of Monoclonal Antibody Therapies.—cont'd

Generic Drug Name	Brand Name	Type of Antibody	AHFS Classification	Dosage Form(s)	Target
Quilizumab MEMP1972A RG-7449 Anti-M1		Humanized monoclonal antibody IgG1κ	Disease modifying Asthma phase II 2014 no great benefit Urticaria phase II 2014 no great benefit Allergic rhinitis	Subcutaneous Intravenous	M1 prime segment of membrane bound IgE (IGHE)
Racotumomab	Vaxira	Murine monoclonal antibody IgG1κ	Antineoplastic Nonsmall cell lung cancer phase III 2016 cimavax better (recombinant EGF injection) 2 more months survival over placebo Neuroblastoma phase II 2020	Intradermal Subcutaneous	N-glycolylneuraminic acid gangliosides (NGNA ganglioside)
Radretumab F16SIP L19SIP radiolabeled with j331		Human monoclonal antibody Imaging study PET	Antineoplastic Lymphoma brain mets 2012 phae I Stage III NSclC		Fibronectin extra domain-B
Rafivirumab CR57		Human monoclonal antibody IgG1λ Used in cocktail and with vaccination	Antiinfectious Rabies (prophylaxis)	No known studies	Rabies virus glycoprotein
Ralpancizumab RN317 PF-05335810		Humanized monoclonal antibody IgG2κ	Disease modifying Dyslipidemia phase I 2017		PCSK9 (proprotein convertase subtilisin/ kexin type 9, neural apoptosis-regulated convertase 1, NARC1, NARC-1, proprotein convertase 9, PC9)
Ramucirumab LY3009806 IMC-1121B	Cyramza FDA 2014 EU 2014	Human monoclonal antibody IgG1κ	Antineoplastic Urothelial phase III done **Adenocarcinoma stomach and GE junction phase II 2023** Colorectal cancer NSCLC HCC phase III 2017 no additional benefit	Intravenous	VEGFR2

Name	Trade name / Approval	Antibody type	Route	Indication / Status	Target
Ranevetmab NV-01		Veterinary monoclonal antibody IgG1κ canine		Disease modifying Osteoarthritis in dogs	Nerve growth factor-β (NGF-β)
Ranibizumab RBZ RG-3645 RHuFAb	Lucentis FDA 2006 EU 2007	Humanized monoclonal fragment IgG1κ Fab	Intravitreal	Disease modifying **Macular degeneration** (wet form) post market studies phase II	Vascular endothelial growth factor A (VEGF-A)
Ravagalimab PR-1629977 ABBV-323		Humanized monoclonal antibody IgG1κ	Intravenous Subcutaneous	Disease modifying UC phase II 2023	CD40
Ravulizumab ALXN1210	Ultomiris FDA 2019 EU pending	Humanized monoclonal antibody IgG2/IgG4κ	Intravenous	Disease modifying Paroxysmal nocturnal hemoglobinuria (PNH) Phase III 2021 similar to eculizumab, atypical hemolytic uremic syndrome phase III 2021	Complement C5 (C5)
Raxibacumab	ABthrax FDA 2012	Human monoclonal antibody IgG1λ	Intravenous	Antiinfectious Treat inhalation anthrax	*Bacillus anthracis* protective antigen
Refanezumab GSK249320		Humanized monoclonal antibody IgG1κ	Intravenous	Disease modifying recovery of motor function after stroke Phase II completed 2011 no benefit	Myelin-associated glycoprotein
Regavirumab MCA C23 TI-23		Human monoclonal antibody		Antiinfectious Cytomegalovirus glycoprotein B ONLY STUDIES IN RATS 1994	Cytomegalovirus infection
Relatlimab BMS-986016		Human monoclonal antibody IgG4κ	Intravenous	Antineoplastic Melanoma phase II 2022 Colon cancer phase II 2022 Chordoma phase II 2020 Cannot find manuscripts but company website phase II good results Glioblastoma phase I 2020	Lymphocyte activation gene 3 (LAG3) CD223
Remtolumab ABT-122		Human monoclonal antibody	Subcutaneous	Disease modifying RA Phase II 2016 no increased benefit over adalimumab	Interleukin 17 alpha, TNF-α

Continued

TABLE 16.1
Summary of Monoclonal Antibody Therapies.—cont'd

Generic Drug Name	Brand Name	Type of Antibody	AHFS Classification	Dosage Form(s)	Target
Reslizumab DCP 835 Scheme 55700 CEP-38072	Cinqair FDA 2016 EU 2016	Humanized monoclonal antibody IgG4κ	Disease modifying Inflammations of the airways asthma completed and ongoing, skin and gastrointestinal tract, polyarteritis stage II 2018 Rhino sinusitis 2020	Intravenous Subcutaneous	IL-5
Rilotumumab AMG-102		Human monoclonal antibody IgG2κ	Antineoplastic Gastric completed phase III 2015 not effective NSCLC phase II 2014 no benefit Glioma phase II no response	Intravenous	Hepatocyte growth factor (HGF)
Rinucumab REGN2176		Human monoclonal antibody IgG4κ	Disease modifying neovascular age-related macular degeneration phase II 2014	Intravitreal	Platelet-derived growth factor receptor beta
Risankizumab ABBV-066 BI-655066	FDA/EU pending approval	Humanized monoclonal antibody IgG1κ	Disease modifying Crohn's disease phase II good, phase III ongoing psoriasis phase II response better than ustekinumab, psoriatic arthritis, and asthma	Subcutaneous	IL23A
Rituximab GP2013 IDEC-102 RG-105	MabThera, Rituxan FDA 1997 EU 1998	Chimeric monoclonal antibody IgG1κ	Antineoplastic Non-Hodgkin lymphomas, chronic lymphocytic leukemias, some autoimmune disorders, i.e., rheumatoid arthritis, >2K studies ongoing	Subcutaneous	CD20
Rivabazumab pegol		Humanized monoclonal antibody fragment Fab' IgG1κ	Antiinfectious	No studies found	*Pseudomonas aeruginosa* type III secretion system
Rmab	Rabishield Made in India	Human monoclonal antibody	Antiinfectious Postexposure prophylaxis of rabies		Rabies virus G glycoprotein

Name/codes	Status/brand	Type	Indication	Route	Target
Robatumumab 19D12 SCH 717454 MK-7454 P04722		Human monoclonal antibody IgG1κ	Antineoplastic Colorectal phase II 2009 little benefit Ewings no response 2016	Intravenous	Insulin-like growth factor I (IGF-1 receptor) (CD221)
Roledumab		Human monoclonal antibody IgG1κ	Immunomodulation Rh disease Phase III 2017	Intravenous	RHD
Romilkimab SAR156597 HUBTI3_2_1		Humanized chimeric monoclonal antibody IgG4 bispecific	Disease modifying Systemic sclerosis phase II 2019 Pulm fibrosis phase II 2017 no benefit	Subcutaneous	Interleukin 13 and IL4
Romosozumab	Evenity FDA pending EU pending Japan 2018	Humanized monoclonal antibody IgG2κ	Disease modifying Postmenopausal osteoporosis phase III study FRAME Men phase III BRIDGE phase III	Intravenous	Sclerostin/scleroscin SOST
Rontalizumab rhuMAb IFNalpha		Humanized monoclonal antibody	Disease modifying Systemic lupus erythematosus phase II 2013 end points not met	Subcutaneous	IFN-α
Rosmantuzumab OMP-131R10		Humanized monoclonal antibody IgG1κ	Antineoplastic Colorectal cancer phase I 2018	Intravenous	Root plate-specific spondin r-spondin-3 WNT? (wingless/integrated)
Rovalpituzumab tesirine SC0002 SC16LD6.5 ABBV-181		Humanized monoclonal antibody IgG1κ	Antineoplastic Small cell lung cancer phase I 2018 Phase II 2024	Intravenous	Delta-like ligand-3 (DLL3)
Rovelizumab Hu23F2G	LeukArrest	Humanized monoclonal antibody IgG1κ	Disease modifying Hemorrhagic shock, MI stroke phase III goals not met 2000		CD11, CD18
Rozanolixizumab UCB7665		Chimeric/humanized monoclonal antibody IgG4κ	Thrombocytopenia ITP phase II 2019 Myasthenia gravis phase II 2018	Subcutaneous Intravenous	Neonatal Fc receptor (FCGRT)

Continued

TABLE 16.1
Summary of Monoclonal Antibody Therapies.—cont'd

Generic Drug Name	Brand Name	Type of Antibody	AHFS Classification	Dosage Form(s)	Target
Ruplizumab	Antova	Humanized monoclonal antibody	Disease modifying lupus and lupus nephritis not effective Life-threatening thromboembolism	BioDrugs. 2004; 18(2): 95–102. Costimulation blockade in the treatment of rheumatic diseases	CD154 (CD40L)
Sacituzumab govitecan IMMU-132	FDA/EU pending approval	Humanized monoclonal antibody IgG1κ	Antineoplastic agent Prostate cancer phase II 2021 Urothelial phase II 2020 Trip neg breast ca phase III 2020 NSCLC SCLC UC	Intravenous	Tumor-associated calcium signal transducer 2 (TROP-2) inhibits topoisomerase I
Samalizumab ALXN6000 BAML–16–001–S1		Humanized monoclonal antibody IgG2/G4κ	Antineoplastic CLL MM phase I 2010 (terminated by sponsor) AML phase II 2021	Intravenous	OX-2 membrane glycoprotein (CD200)
Samrotamab vedotin		Chimeric/humanized monoclonal antibody IgG1κ	Antineoplastic	No studies found	Leucine-rich repeat-containing protein 15 (LRRC15)
Sarilumab REGN88 SAR153191	Kevzara FDA?EU/Japan under review approved in Canada	Human monoclonal antibody IgG1κ	Disease modifying rheumatoid arthritis phase III 2015/2020/2027(preg exposure), ankylosing spondylitis Juvenile idiopathic arthritis phase II 2022	Subcutaneous	IL6
Satralizumab SA237 Sapelizumab	FDA review possible 2019	Humanized monoclonal antibody IgG2κ	Disease modifying Neuromyelitis optica phase III 2019/2020	Subcutaneous?	IL6 receptor
Satumomab pendetide	OncoScint CR103 FDA 1992	Murine monoclonal antibody IgGκ fragment Fab'	Diagnostic imaging Detection colorectal and ovarian cancer	Intravenous	Tumor-associated glycoprotein (TAG-72)
Secukinumab AIN457	Cosentyx FDA 2015 EU 2015	Human monoclonal antibody IgG1κ	Disease modifying Uveitis, rheumatoid arthritis psoriasis phase II 2019 over 100 other studies **arthritis; psoriatic psoriasis; spondylitis; ankylosing**	Subcutaneous	IL 17A

Name/Code	Antibody type	Indication/Phase	Route	Target
Selicrelumab CP 870.893 RG7876 RO-7009789	Human monoclonal antibody IgG2κ	Antineoplastic Solid tumors phase I 2020 Pancreatic cancer phase II 2020 Colon cancer phase II 2021 Mesothelioma phase ib 2015	Subcutaneous Intravenous	Tumor necrosis factor receptor superfamily member 5 (CD40)
Seribantumab MM121 SAR256212	Human monoclonal antibody IgG2λ	Antineoplastic Breast phase II 2020 Ovarian phase I 2014	Intravenous	Receptor tyrosine-protein kinase erbB-3 (HER3)
Setoxaximab	Chimeric monoclonal antibody IgG1κ	Antiinfection E. coli	No known studies or clinical use	E. coli shiga toxin type-2
Setrusumab BPS804 MOR05813	Human monoclonal antibody IgG2	Disease modifying Osteogenesis imperfecta phase II 2020	Intravenous	Sclerostin (SOST)
Sevirumab MSL-109		Antiinfectious CMV retinitis early termination trial secondary to safety Phase II 2003		Cytomegalovirus infection
SHP647 Ontamalimab PF-00547659	Human monoclonalantibodyIgG2κ	Disease modifying Crohn's/UC phase III 2020–2025 × 7 Phase II study 2007 better response in UC than in Crohn (?more time needed to evaluate clinical significance	Subcutaneous	Mucosal addressin cell adhesion molecule (MADCAM)
Sibrotuzumab BIBH1 F19	Humanized monoclonal antibody IgG1κ	Antineoplastic Colorectal cancer phase II 2003 failed Lung cancer2001	Intravenous	FAP
Sifalimumab MDX-1103 MEDI-545 CP145	Humanized monoclonal antibody IgG1κ	Disease modifying SLE phase II 2015 dermatomyositis, polymyositis	Intravenous Subcutaneous	IFN-α
Siltuximab CLLB8 CNTO-328 Sylvant FDA 2014 EU 2014	Chimeric monoclonal antibody IgG1κ	Antineoplastic Multiple myeloma phase II 2019 DM type I phase I 2017 Schizophrenia adjunct 2020 phase II **Multicentric Castleman's disease (MCD) with HIV negative and HHV-8 negative**	Intravenous	IL-6

Continued

TABLE 16.1
Summary of Monoclonal Antibody Therapies.—cont'd

Generic Drug Name	Brand Name	Type of Antibody	AHFS Classification	Dosage Form(s)	Target
Simtuzumab AB0024 GS-6624		Humanized monoclonal antibody IgG4κ	Disease modifying Hepatic fibrosis Phase II 2016 no benefit Pulm fibroses phase II 2017 no benefit Myelo fibr 2017 phase II	Subcutaneous Intravenous	Lysyl oxidase homolog 2 (LOXL2)
Siplizumab MEDI-507		Humanized monoclonal antibody IgG1κ	Antineoplastic		CD2 T Or NK cells
Sirtratumab vedotin		Human monoclonal antibody	Antineoplastic	Nothing in PubMed or clinical trials	SLITRK6
Sirukumab		Human monoclonal antibody IgG1κ	Disease modifying Rheumatoid arthritis Phase III done good results	Subcutaneous	IL-6
Sofituzumab vedotin		Humanized monoclonal antibody	Antineoplastic Ovarian pancreatic Phase I (2014)		CA-125
Solanezumab LY2062430		Humanized monoclonal antibody IgG1	Disease modifying Alzheimer's Phase III study discontinued no effect In preclinical trial for secondary prevention 2022 Hereditary AD phase III 2021	Intravenous	Beta amyloid
Solitomab MT110-011 AMG110		Murine monoclonal antibody bispecific T-cell engager (BiTE)	Antineoplastic Gastrointestinal, lung, and other cancers Phase I 2015	Intravenous	Epithelial cell adhesion molecule (EpCAM) CD3
Sonepcizumab LT1009	iSONEP	Humanized monoclonal antibody	Disease modifying Choroidal and retinal neovascularization phase II 2015 not so good Antineoplastic phase II renal cancer 2017 potential	Intravenous Intravitreous	Sphingosine-1-phosphate (S1P)
Stamulumab		Humanized monoclonal antibody	Disease modifying muscular dystrophy Animal studies, minimal efficacy Phase I/II studies ongoing (no improvement)	Intravenous	Myostatin

Name		Antibody type	Clinical	Route	Target
Sulesomab IMMU-MN3	LeukoScan EU 1997	Murine monoclonal IgG1 fragment Fab'	Diagnostic Osteomyelitis (imaging)		NCA-90 (granulocyte antigen)
Suptavumab REGN2222 SAR438584		Human monoclonal antibody IgG1κ	Antiinfectious Medically attended lower respiratory disease phase III 2017 not meet primary endpoint Another study no data yet at 30 mg/kg dose	Intramuscular	Resp sync virus fusion protein (RSVFR)
Sutimilimab BIVV009		Chimeric/humanized monoclonal antibody IgG4κ	Disease modifying cold agglutinin disease phase III 2020	Intravenous	Complement C1s (C1s)
Suvizumab KD-247		Humanized monoclonal antibody IgG1κ	Antiinfectious HIV Phase I KD-247 2007	Intravenous	Human immunodeficiency virus glycoprotein 120 third variable loop
Suvratoxumab MEDI4893		Human monoclonal antibody IgG1κ	Disease modifying Nosocomial pneumonia phase II 2018	Intravenous	Staphylococcus aureus alpha toxin
Tabalumab LY2127399		Human monoclonal lantibodyIgG4κ	Antineoplastic Rheum arthr phase III 2013 no signif response SLE phase III 2015 endpoints not met Mult myelo phase I 2014 may not treat but be prognostic	Subcutaneous	Cytokine B-cell activating factor (BAFF)
Tacatuzumab tetraxetan HAFP-31	AFP-Cide	Humanized monoclonal antibody yttrium[77]	Antineoplastic	No studies in clinical trial or PubMed	Alpha-fetoprotein
Tadocizumab C4G1 YM337		Humanized monoclonal antibody fragment IgG1κ Fab'	Disease modifying Percutaneous coronary intervention phase I 1999 ?not further developed		Integrin αIIbβ3
Talacotuzumab CSL362 JNJ-56022473		Humanized monoclonal antibody IgG1-2κ	Antineoplastic AML phase III 2018 MDS phase II 2019 SLE 2019 phase I	Intravenous	Interleukin 3 receptor subunit-α (IL3Rα, CD123)
Talizumab C21/AL-90 TNX-901		Humanized monoclonal antibody IgG1κ	Disease modifying Peanut allergy Allergic reaction Phase II 2003 good results legal issues shelved the drug	Subcutaneous	IgE

Continued

TABLE 16.1
Summary of Monoclonal Antibody Therapies.—cont'd

Generic Drug Name	Brand Name	Type of Antibody	AHFS Classification	Dosage Form(s)	Target
Tamtuvetmab AT-005	Tactress	Canine monoclonal antibody IgG2λ			CD52
Tanezumab RN624 PF-4383119	FDA review possible 2019	Humanized monoclonal antibody IgG2	Disease modifying Pain Osteoarthritis Back pain Metastatic cancer pain Phase II ~2008		Nerve growth factor (NGF)
Tanibirumab Olinvacimab TTAC-0001		Human monoclonal antibody IgG1	Disease modifying Antineoplastic Phase I glioblastoma 2020 Breast cancer phase I 2020 AMD murine no human studies found	Intravenous	VEFR-2
Taplitumomab paptox		Murine monoclonal antibody IgG1κ	Antineoplastic	No studies pub med or clinical trials	CD19
Tarextumab OMP-59R5		Human monoclonal antibody IgG2	Antineoplastic Phase II trial NSCLC no benefit 2017 Pancreatic phase II 2017	Intravenous	Notch2/3, Notch receptor
Tavolimab MEDI0562		Chimeric/humanized monoclonal antibody IgG1κ	Antineoplastic Head and neck phase I 2024 Ovarian cancer phase II 2023		Tumor necrosis factor receptor superfamily member 4 (TNFRS4) OX40L receptor (CD134)
Technetium (99 mTc) acritumomab		Rabbit monoclonal IgG	Not for use in humans-research purpose only		CEA
Technicium (99 mTc) Fanolesomab	NeutroSpec FDA2004	Murine monoclonal IgM radiolabeled	Disease modifying osteomyelitis Sales and marketing suspended (2005) **Diagnostic scans for acute appendicitis**	Intravenous	CD15
Tefibazumab INH–H2002	Aurexis	Humanized monoclonal antibody IgG1κ	Antiinfectious Staphylococcus aureus infection Phase II 2006	Intravenous	Clumping factor A

Name	Type	Indication/Phase	Status/Other	Route	Target
Telimomab aritox (TAB-885)	Recombinant murine monoclonal antibody Fab with ricin	Antineoplastic T Cell lymphoma/leukemia		No studies in pub med or clinical trials	CD5
Telisotuzumab vedotin ABT-700	Humanized monoclonal antibody IgG1κ	Antineoplastic Phase I 2017 SCLC phase II 2022 NSCLC phase II 2021		Intravenous	Hepatocyte growth factor receptor HGFR
Tenatumomab	Murine monoclonal antibody IgG2b	Antineoplastic Phase I 2017 Phase II brain tumors 2010		Intravenous	P24821, tenascin C
Teneliximab	Chimeric monoclonal antibody IgG1	Not in clinical trials 2009			CD40 (TNF receptor superfamily member 5)
Teplizumab MGA031 PRV-031 hOKT3g1(Ala-Ala)	Humanized monoclonal antibody IgG1κ	Disease modifying type I DM phase II completion AbATE trial 2019 Psoriasis phase I and II completed 2010 study stopped secondary to injection reaction severe allergy		Intravenous Subcutaneous	CD3
Tepoditamab	Human monoclonal antibody IgG1κ bispecific	Antineoplastic		No studies on PubMed or clinical trials	c-type dendritic cell-associated lectin 2 (CLEC-2A, MCLA-117) and CD3
Teprotumumab RV001 R-1507 RO4858696 HZN-001	Human monoclonal antibody	Disease modifying Thyroid eye disease phase II 2017 Graves phase III 2020	FDA review possible 2019	Intravenous	Insulin-like growth factor receptor type I (IGF-1 receptor) (CD221)
Tesidolumab LFG316 NOV-4	Human monoclonal antibody	Phase I 2017 PNH phase II 2020 AMD phase II 2015 not beneficial		Intravenous Intravitreous	C5
Tetulomab tetraxetan LU-177	Humanized monoclonal antibody	Antineoplastic Animal studies 2013	Betalutin	Subcutaneous	CD37
Tezepelumab MEDI9929 AMG-157	Human monoclonal antibody IgG2λ	Disease modifying Asthma, atopic dermatitis Phase II 2017		Subcutaneous	Thymic stromal lymphopoietin (TSLP)

Continued

TABLE 16.1
Summary of Monoclonal Antibody Therapies.—cont'd

Generic Drug Name	Brand Name	Type of Antibody	AHFS Classification	Dosage Form(s)	Target
Theralizumab TGN1412 TAB08		Humanized monoclonal antibody	Antineoplastic Solid tumors phase I 2020 Disease modifying Rheum arth, SLE phase II	Intravenous	CD28 History of cytokine storm at higher doses 2006
Tibulizumab LY3090106		Humanized monoclonal antibody bispecific tetravalent	Disease modifying Autoimmune disorder Phase I 2020	Subcutaneous Intravenous No manuscripts found specific to this antibody	Human B-cell activating factor of the tumor necrosis factor family interleukin 17 (BAFF)
Tigatuzumab CS-1008 TRA-8		Humanized monoclonal antibody IgG1κ	Antineoplastic Colon phase II 2011no added benefit Colon phase I 2013 NSCLC phase II 2011 no benefit Pancreatic phase II 2008 benefit TN breast canc 2015 phase II no added benefit		Cytokine receptor DR5 (death receptor 5) TRAIL–R2
Tildrakizumab MK-3222 SCH-900222	Ilumya Ilumetri FDA 2018	Humanized monoclonal antibody IgG1κ	Immunologically mediated inflammatory disorders Mod/severe psoriasis phase III 2018-20	Subcutaneous	IL23
Timigutuzumab		Humanized monoclonal antibody IgG1κ	Antineoplastic	No studies in clinical trial or PubMed	erbB2/HER2
Timolumab BTT-1023		Human monoclonal antibody	Disease modifying Scler cholang phase II 2019	Intravenous	AOC3
Tiragotumab MTIG-7192A RG6058 RO7092284		Human monoclonal antibody IgG1κ	Antineoplastic Phase I 2020 NSCLC phase II 2021 HL phase II 2019	Intravenous Nothing published yet	T-cell IG and immune-receptor tyrosine-based inhibitory motif (TIGIT)
Tislelizumab	China pending approval	Humanized monoclonal antibody	Antineoplastic NSCLC phase III 2020 Gastric phase III 2022 Esophageal cancer phase III 2021 NHL phase II 2020	Intravenous Nothing published yet 2019	PCDC1, CD279

			Indication	Route	Target
Tisotumab vedotin		Human monoclonal antibody IgG1κ	Antineoplastic Ovary cancer Cervix cancer Endometrium cancer Bladder cancer Prostate cancer Esophagus cancer Lung cancer, NSCLC Squamous cell carcinoma of the head and neck Pancreatic phase II 2022/3	Intravenous	Coagulation factor III
Tocilizumab MRA R-1569 RG-1569 RHPM-1 RO-4877533 Atlizumab	Actemra, RoActemra FDA 2010 EU 2009	Humanized monoclonal antibody IgG1κ	Disease modifying **rheumatoid arthritis** >100 studies Behcet syndrome	Intravenous Subcutaneous	IL-6 receptor
Tomuzotuxi-mabfibri		Humanized monoclonal antibody IgG1κ	Antineoplastic Phase I 2019		EGFR, HER1
Toralizumab E-6040 IDEC-131		Humanized monoclonal antibody IgG1κ	Disease modifying rheumatoid arthritis, lupus nephritis etc. Phase II trials failed with TE		CD154 (CD40L)
Tosatoxumab		Human monoclonal antibody IgG1λ	Antiinfectious	No studies PubMed or Clin trials	*Staphylococcus aureus* α-hemolysin
Tositumomab and iodine 131 Tositumomab	Bexxar FDA 2003	Murine monoclonal antibody IgG2aλ	Antineoplastic Follicular lymphoma (**NHL**) >100 studies	Intravenous	CD20
Tovetumab MEDI-575		Human monoclonal antibody IgG2κ	Antineoplastic Phase I/II 2012 Glioblastoma limited clin activity	Intravenous	Platelet-derived growth factor receptor α (CD140a)
Tralokinumab CAT-354		Human monoclonal antibody IgG4	Disease modifying asthma phase IIb +/−, atopic dermatitis phase II 2016	Intravenous Subcutaneous	IL-13

Continued

TABLE 16.1
Summary of Monoclonal Antibody Therapies.—cont'd

Generic Drug Name	Brand Name	Type of Antibody	AHFS Classification	Dosage Form(s)	Target
Trastuzumab 4D5v8 R-597 SYD977	Herceptin FDA 1998 EU 2000 Herceptin Hylecta FDA 2019 — trastuzumab/ hyaluronidase Herzuma 2018	Humanized monoclonal antibody IgG1κ	Antineoplastic **Breast cancer Gastric and gastro-esophageal junction cancer** HER2-positive phase III	Subcutaneous Intravenous	HER2/neu
Trastuzumab Deruxtecan DS-8201	Hercion FDA breakthrough therapy	Antibody drug conjugate humanized antibody IgG1κ with topoisomerase I inhibitor (DXd)	Antineoplastic breast cancer phase I study breast, gastric, colorectal, salivary, and nonsmall cell lung cancer participated in part 2 2020 phase II DESTINY-Breast01		HER2
Trastuzumab emtansine RG-3502 PRO132365	Kadcyla FDA2013 EU 2013	Humanized monoclonal antibody IgG1κ as ADC	Antineoplastic **Breast cancer**	Intravenous	HER2/neu
TRBS07	Ektomab	3funct	Antineoplastic Melanoma	GD2 ganglioside	Tribbles-related protein (TRB) family members are the mammalian orthologs of Drosophila tribbles. Tribbles was originally identified as a cell cycle regulator during Drosophila development. Tribbles genes are evolutionary conserved, and three TRB genes (TRB1, TRB2 and TRB3) have been identified in mammals. TRBs are considered pseudokinases because they lack an ATP binding site or one of the

conserved catalytic motifs essential for kinase activity. Instead, TRBs play important roles in various cellular processes as scaffolds or adaptors to promote the degradation of target proteins and to regulate several key signaling pathways. Recent research has focused on the role of TRBs in tumorigenesis and neoplastic progression. In this review, we focus on the physiological roles of TRB family members in tumorigenesis through the regulation of the ubiquitin-proteasome system and discuss TRBs as biomarkers or potential therapeutic targets in cancer

Name		Type	Target	Indication	Route
Tregalizumab BT-061		Humanized monoclonal antibody IgG1κ	CD4	Disease modifying Rheumatoid arthritis Phase IIb no benefit	Subcutaneous
Tremelimumab (aka ticilimumab)	*CP-675,206	Human monoclonal antibody IgG2	CTLA4 (cytotoxic T lymphocyte-associated antigen 4, CD152)	Antineoplastic agent NSCLC, small cell lung cancer, urethelial cancer phase II 2020, head and neck cancer and colon phase I 2021 Mesothelial phase IIb DETERMINE not beneficial >100 studies	
Trevogrumab REGN1033 SAR391786		Human monoclonal antibody IgG4κ	Myostatin, growth differentiation factor 8 (GDF8)	Disease modifying Muscle atrophy due to orthopedic disuse and sarcopenia phase II 2020	
TRL3d3 3D3		IgG	Ati-G protein antibody (RSVGV)	Studies only in mice to this point	

Continued

TABLE 16.1
Summary of Monoclonal Antibody Therapies.—cont'd

Generic Drug Name	Brand Name	Type of Antibody	AHFS Classification	Dosage Form(s)	Target
Tucotuzumab celmoleukin EMD-273066 HUKS-IL2		Humanized monoclonal antibody IgG1	Antineoplastic Ovarian phase II 2008 Lung, kidney, bladder phase I 2000 no benefit	Intravenous	Interleukin2 (EpCAM)
Tuvirumab		Humanized monoclonal antibody	Antiinfectious Not effective in achieving primary efficacy as assessed by neutralization of circulating HBsAg	Intravenous	Hepatitis B virus surface antigen
Ublituximab TG-1101	FDA review pending 2019	Chimeric monoclonal antibodyIgG1κ	Antineoplastic Chronic lymphocytic leukemia, follicular cell lymphoma phase II 2020 Disease modifying Multiple sclerosis phase II 2019, phase III 2021 Awaiting result looks good prelim	Intravenous	CD20 MS4A1
Ulocuplumab		Human monoclonal antibody IgG4	Antineoplastic CLL phase I 2014 Phase I/II Waldenstrom macroglobulinemia 2025 Phase I/II AML 2021	Intravenous	CXCR4 (CD184)
Urelumab BMS-663513		Human monoclonal antibody IgG4κ	Antineoplastic CLL phase II 2020 Solid tumors phase II 2023	Intravenous	Human receptor 4-1BB (CD137)
Urtoxazumab TMA-15		Humanized monoclonal antibody IgG1κ	Disease modifying EHEC animal studies	Intravenous	*Escherichia coli* (EHEC) shiga toxin 2
Ustekinumab	Stelara FDA 2009 EU 2009	Human monoclonal antibody IgG1κ	Disease modifying Crohn disease **Plaque psoriasis** Psoriatic arthritis	Subcutaneous Intravenous	p40 subunit of interleukin 12 (IL-12p40), IL-23
Utomilumab PF-05082566		Human monoclonal antibody IgG2	Antineoplastic Diffuse large B-cell lymphoma Phase I 2021 phase II 2020 Breast phase II 2025	Intravenous	4-1BB (CD137)

Name	Brand/Approval	Antibody type	Indication/Phase	Route	Target/Mechanism
Vadastuximab talirine H2H12EC		Chimeric monoclonal antibody IgG1κ	Antineoplastic Acute myeloid leukemia phase II 2017 phase III 2017 MDS phase II 2017	Intravenous	CD33
Vanalimab Mitazalimab		Humanized monoclonal antibody IgG1λ	Antineoplastic?	No studies clinical trial or PubMed	Immune checkpoint receptor, tumor necrosis receptor family CD40, (TNFRSF5)
Vandortuzumab vedotin		Humanized monoclonal antibody	Antineoplastic Prostate cancer		STEAP1
Vantictumab OMP-18R5		Human monoclonal antibody IgG2mab	Antineoplastic NSCLC, breast phase I 2017	Intravenous	Frizzled receptor
Vanucizumab RG-7221 RO5520985		Humanized monoclonal antibody IgG1κ bispecific ANG-2/VEGF-Amab	Antineoplastic Phase I 2018	Intravenous	Angiopoietin 2/vascular endothelial growth factor A
Vapaliximab BTT-1002 HUVAP		Chimeric monoclonal antibody IgG2κ		No studies in PubMed or clinical trials	Vascular adhesion protein AOC3 (VAP-1)
Varisacumab GNR-011 R-84		Human monoclonal antibody IgG1κ		No studies in PubMed or clinical trials	VEGF-A
Varlilumab CDX-1127		Human monoclonal antibody IgG1κ	Antineoplastic Solid tumors and hematologic malignancies Phase I 2017, phase II 2019/20 Melanoma phase II 2018/21	Intravenous	CD27
Vatelizumab GBR500 SAR339658		Humanized monoclonal antibody IgG4	Disease modifying UC phase II 2016 MS phase II 2016 withdrawn lack of efficacy		A2β1 integrin I domain ITGA2 (CD49b)
Vedolizumab LDP02 MLN02	Entyvio FDA 2014 EU 2014	Humanized monoclonal antibody IgG1κ	Disease modifying **Crohn disease** **Ulcerative colitis** In CD resolution extraintestinal manifestations	Intravenous	Integrin α4β7 Selectively blocks trafficking of Memory T cells to inflamed gut tissue by inhibiting a4b7-mucosal addressin cell adhesion molecule-1 (MAd-CAM-1) interaction

Continued

TABLE 16.1
Summary of Monoclonal Antibody Therapies.—cont'd

Generic Drug Name	Brand Name	Type of Antibody	AHFS Classification	Dosage Form(s)	Target
Veltuzumab IMMU-106 HA20		Humanized monoclonal antibody IgG1κ	Antineoplastic Non-Hodgkin's lymphoma phase II 2013 ITP phase II 2016	Subcutaneous	CD20
Vepalimomab		Murine monoclonal antibody			AOC3 (vascular adhesion protein-1)
Vesencumab MNRP1685A		Human monoclonal antibody IgG1mab	Antineoplastic Solid malignancies Phase I 2011 proteinuria		Neuropilin1 (NRP1)
Visilizumab	Nuvion	Humanized monoclonal antibody IgG2	Disease modifying Prevent GVHD Not effective in UC		CD3
Vobarilizumab		Humanize monoclonal scFv	Disease modifying inflammatory autoimmune diseases	Nothing in PubMed	IL6R
Volociximab M200		Chimeric monoclonal antibody IgG4κ	Antineoplastic Solid tumors NSCLC phase I/II 2010 Disease modifying phase I AMD terminated no results		Integrin α5β1
Vopratelimab JTX-2011		Humanized monoclonal antibody IgG1κ	Antineoplastic Solid tumors phase II 2022	Intravenous	Inducible T-cell costimulator (ICOS)
Vorsetuzumab mafodotin H1F6 SGN-70		Humanized monoclonal antibody	Antineoplastic Phase I 2017	Intravenous	CD70
Votumumab	HumaSPECT Diagnostic EU 1998 Withdrawn from market 2003	Human monoclonal antibody	Diagnostic Human colon cancer imaging		Tumor antigen Cytokeratin tumor-associated antigen (CTAA16.88)

Name	Status/Trade	Antibody type	Indication/Phase	Route	Target
Vunakizumab SHR-1314		Humanized monoclonal antibody IgG1	Disease modifying Psoriasis phase II 2019	Subcutaneous Nothing published	Interleukin 17 alpha
Xentuzumab BI-836845		Humanized monoclonal antibody	Antineoplastic Breast, prostate, solid phase I 2019	Intravenous No clinical studies published	Insulin-like growth factor (IGF1, IGF2)
XMAB-5574 Tafasitamab MOR00208	FDA review possible 2019	Humanized monoclonal immunoglobulin fragment κ Fc	Antineoplastic Diffuse large B-cell lymphoma phase II 2015/18/19/22 phase III 2022	Intravenous	CD19
Zalutumumab 2F8 HUMAX-EGFR	HuMax-EGFr Suspended for commercialization	Human monoclonal antibody	Antineoplastic Squamous cell carcinoma of the head and neck phase II 2011 phase III 2016	Intravenous	EGFR
Zanolimumab	HuMax-CD4 (trade name)	Humanized monoclonal antibody IgG1κ	Antineoplastic CTCL Phase II good results Phase III suspended by company?	Intravenous	CD4
Zenocutuzumab		Humanized monoclonal antibody IgG1 bispecific epidermal growth factor receptors her2,her3	Antineoplastic		ERBB3, HER3
Ziralimumab		Human monoclonal antibody IgM	Disease modifying immunosuppressive	No studies clinical trials or PubMed	CD147 (basigin)
Zolbetuximab IMAB362 Claudiximab		Chimeric monoclonal antibody IgG1κ ADCC enhance antibody	Antineoplastic gastric cancer phase I, IIb Phase III 2023 Gastrointestinal adenocarcinomas and pancreatic tumor	Intravenous	Claudin protein (CLDN18.2)
Zolimomab aritox H65-RTA ZX-CD5	Orthozyme CD 5 plus	Human monoclonal antibody IgG1	Disease modifying	Not effective in preventing GVHD 1994	CD5

Auristatins are water-soluble dolastatin analogs of dolastatin 10. Dolastatin 10 belongs to dolastatin family and it can powerfully bind to tubulin, thus inhibiting polymerization mediated through the binding to the vinca alkaloid-binding domain, and causes cell to accumulate in metaphase arrest.

Ankylosing Spondylitis

Certolizumab pegolis is also approved for use with ankylosing spondylitis.

Systemic Lupus Erythematosus

Belimumab (Benlysta) is a human Mab (IgG1λ) that binds to B-cell activating factor and acts as a B-lymphocyte stimulator-specific inhibitor. It was approved by the FDA in 2011 for treatment of adult patients with active, autoantibody-positive SLE receiving standard therapy. This medication also decreases episodic frequency of lupus nephritis.[281–283]

Cardiovascular Disease

Despite marked improvement in survival from cardiovascular disease, this illness remains the number one cause of mortality in the US. This process causes injury to the endothelium of blood vessels of the heart secondary to toxins, accumulation of cholesterol, or chronic low-grade inflammation. Treatment has been preventive, primarily during actual injury or following injury. Therapies involve changes in behavior (diet, exercise, and cessation of tobacco use), pharmacologic to control contributing underlying illness (hypercholesterolemia, hypertension, diabetes type I and II), to diminish injury through thrombolytics, stents, vasodilators, supplemental oxygen, or to control sequelae of infarctions (cardiac dysfunction/failure). Passive antibody therapies are being tried to decrease the effects of some of the contributing factors of atherosclerotic plaque formation.

Abciximab (ReoPro) is a chimeric recombinant monoclonal fragment (IgG1 Fab') with specificity to platelet glycoprotein IIb/IIIa receptor (CD41 7E3)/Intergrin α-IIb that prevents platelets from binding to fibrinogen. This Mab also prevents coagulation factor XIII from binding to platelets allowing stabilization of clots and are more easily lysed. The Fc portion of the antibody is removed to decrease thrombocytopenias. This antibody is used during high-risk coronary intervention to prevent clot formation and cardiac ischemia.[284]

Alirocumab (Praluent) is a human Mab (IgG1) with specificity to proprotein convertase subtilisin/kexin type 9. This medication is used to control cholesterol levels in patients at high risk for cardiovascular events and in patients with familial hypercholesterolemia who are not controlled by other agents.[285–287]

Evolocumab (Repatha) is a human Mab (IgG2λ) FDA approved for the treatment of hypercholesterolemia in patients with familial hypercholesterolemia or history of cardiovascular disease. This Mab has specificity to PCSK9. This medication reduced low-density lipoprotein (LDL) and cholesterol levels by 60% even after statin therapy. Hazard ratios for primary and secondary endpoints were less than one ($\sim 0.80{-}0.85$) with fewer cardiovascular-related death or infarction and stroke.[288,289]

Under future watch is frovocimab (LY3015014) a humanized Mab (IgG4κ) with specificity to PCSK9 that completed phase I and II trials. There was up to 50% reduction in LDL cholesterol levels. Phase III studies have yet to be performed.[290]

An additional antibody is lodelcizumab a humanized Mab (IgG1κ); however, no studies were found in clinicaltrials.gov or in Pubmed searches.

Bococizumab is a humanized Mab (IgG2κ) that was in phase III trial, which was discontinued secondary to primary endpoints not being achieved.[291]

NEUROLOGIC DISEASES

Besides autoimmune and malignant diseases of the neurologic system, there are also diseases of the central nervous system classified as degenerative. Such diseases include supranuclear palsy (SNP), Alzheimer's, and Parkinson's. Alzheimer's is likely the most common cause of dementia first described in 1907. This disease may be depicted as presenile or senile dementia and progresses at a similar rate no matter age of onset. This disease has a genetic predisposition causing it to occur in younger age groups. Histological changes include diffuse plaques (containing amyloid), neurofibrillary plaques, and neuronal loss especially in the hippocampus and temporal regions. Medical management may reverse some of the symptoms but does not prevent disease progression. Parkinson's is a mainly sporadic degenerative disease with a gradual progressive course mainly affecting motor function more than memory. It was first described in 1817. This is a disease of the substantia nigra characterized by loss of melanin containing nerve cells and eosinophilic intracytoplasmic inclusions. Aside from emotional support and physical therapy, medical therapy is used to decrease tremors including anticholinergic drugs for tremors at onset, beta blockers for intention tremors, and levodopa for postural imbalance and akinesia. Deep brain stimulation is also used to treat symptoms later on as disease progresses. SNP starts in the same age range as Parkinson's (middle to later in life) that was first described in 1963 with disturbances in gait and balance secondary to rigidity of trunk muscles. Loss of neurons and gliosis is seen in the midbrain. Medical treatment is relatively unsuccessful. Multiple sclerosis is a demyelinating disease most often seen in young adults. The clinical manifestations are diverse and the progression can be chronic, acute, or remitting and relapsing. Medications and therapeutic plasma exchange have been used to treat this debilitating disease with limited efficacy. Clinical trials are ongoing looking at Mab therapies for treatment of these four neurologic degenerative diseases.

Multiple Sclerosis

Alemtuzumab (Lemtrada) is a humanized Mab (IgG1κ) targeting CD52 that depletes lymphocytes (B and T cell) as reported earlier and is FDA approved for treatment of acute relapsing and remitting multiple sclerosis.[292]

Ocrelizumab (Ocrevus) is a humanized Mab (IgG1κ) with specificity to CD20 (a B-cell membrane protein). In phase II trials, there were decreases in brain lesions on imaging, and decrease rate of disability decline in primary progressive multiple sclerosis.[293]

Natalizumab (Tysabri) is a monoclonal IgG4κ humanized antibody with specificity to cell adhesion molecule (CD62L) that is FDA approved for relapsing multiple sclerosis.[294,295]

The mabs to watch out for in the future and are in clinical trials include anifrolumab a human monoclonal antibody in phase I trials; elezanumab is a human Mab (IgG1λ) with specificity to repulsive guidance molecule family member-A that is in phase II trials to be completed 2021; and finally inebilizumab (MEDI-551) is a humanized monoclonal antibody (IgG2κ) with specificity to CD19 (a B-cell lymphocyte protein). This Mab mechanism of action is via ADCC and has completed phase I trials with good safety profile and response in decreasing lesions seen on contrast enhanced magnetic resonance imaging. Otilimabis (MOR103) is a human Mab (IgG1λ) completing phase I studies with good safety profile that targets granulocyte-macrophage colony-stimulating factor. Ublituximab is in phase II clinical studies to be completed in 2019, and phase III studies are scheduled to be completed in 2021. This Mab is a chimeric Mab (IgG1κ) with specificity to CD20 MS2A1.[296–300]

Additional Mab have serious adverse effects such as daclizumab a humanized monoclonal (IgG1κ) with specificity to (CD25 {IL-2Rα}); or are ineffective as is opicinumab a human Mab IgG1 with specificity to Leucine-rich repeat and immunoglobulin domain containing neurite outgrowth inhibitor receptor interacting protein-1 which in a phase II trial was no more beneficial than placebo in treating optic neuritis in multiple sclerosis patients.[301,302]

Alzheimer's Disease

Aducanumab is a human Mab IgG1 with specificity to β-amyloid (N-terminus 3−6) soluble oligomers and insoluble fibers. Phase III clinical trials are ongoing since 2015.

BAN-2401 is a humanized Mab IgG1 with specificity to β-amyloid fibrillary and soluble β amyloid and is in phase IIb clinical studies since 2013.

Gosuranemab (BIIB092, IPN-007) is a humanized Mab IgG4κ with specificity to the tau protein and is in clinical trials to treat Alzheimer's disease scheduled to be completed in 2021. Gosuranemab is also in phase I studies to treat progressive suranuclear palsy and will be completed in 2020.

Crenezumab (RG7412, MABT5102A) is a humanized Mab IgG4 with specificity to 1−40 β-amyloid and is on phase III studies scheduled to be completed in 2021 and 2022.

Gantenerumab (RO4909832, R1450) is a human Mab IgG1κ with targets β-amyloid. This Mab on initial phase III studies was found to be ineffective. Ongoing phase II/III trials are currently in place at higher dosing in a clinical population of people with autosomal dominant form of Alzheimer's disease.

Solanezumab (LY2062430) is a humanized Mab IgG1 with specificity to beta amyloid. Initial phase III trials discontinued for lack of efficacy in preventing Alzheimer's disease. Ongoing phase III trials are now in place for secondary prevention of this disease and will be completed in 2021 and 2022.

Mab antibodies studied and were ineffective include bapineuzumab, gantenerumab (RO4909832, R1450), and ponezumab (RN1219, PF-04,360,365).

Parkinson's Disease

Prasinezumab (PRX002, RG7935, RO7046015) is a humanized Mab IgG1κ with specificity to α-synuclein. This Mab is in phase II clinical trials to treat Parkinson's and will be completed in 2021.

ALLERGIC DISEASES

Allergic reactions develop because of immunologic stimulation of IgE antibodies followed by their interaction with allergens and mast cells. Effects can be local (dermatitis) or systemic (respiratory, cardiovascular, and gastrointestinal). Treatment is either avoidance of the allergens or supportive therapy in acute allergic reactions including pharmacologic treatment with type 1 and 2 histamine blockers, glucocorticosteroids, and if life-threatening epinephrine. Passive antibody therapies are being studied and approved to curtail severe reactions.

Asthma

Asthma affects 24 million individuals in the US, and up to 10% of asthma patients have severe disease that may be uncontrolled despite high doses of standard-of-care asthma medications requiring additional use of chronic oral corticosteroids. Benralizumab (Fensenra) is a humanized Mab (IgG1κ) with specificity to CD125 (IL-5Rα). This Mab is approved to treat severe asthma of the eosinophilic subtype in ages 12 and older. Its mechanism of action is to decrease the number of eosinophils via ADCC. Basophils are also depleted.[303]

Atopic Dermatitis

Dupilumab (Dupixent) is a human monoclonal gG4 antibody with specificity to interleukin-4 receptor subunit-alpha (IL-4Rα) that is approved to treat severe atopic dermatitis in adults.[304]

COAGULOPATHY AND OTHER BENIGN HEMATOLOGIC DISEASES

Coagulopathies are usually either autoimmune or genetic. In factor VIII deficiency, recombinant factor VIII is used to replace lack of this protein. However, patients may develop antibodies to factor VIII leading to high titers of inhibitors. Furthermore, patients without deficiency may also develop autoantibodies to factor VIII de novo leading to coagulopathies. Other factor combinations as well as recombinant active factors have been created to overcome these inhibitory antibodies. Mabs with bispecific binding are also being researched as another avenue for treatment.

ITP can lead to critical low platelet levels increasing risk for severe bleeding. ITP can occur in both adult and pediatric settings as it is considered an autoimmune disease. Typically, this is treated with steroids and IVIG. In addition, as mentioned earlier, RhD⁺ patients have benefitted from polyclonal medications directed against the D antigen. Recently, Mab to treat this disease have been developed and will be discussed next.

Thrombotic thrombocytopenic purpura (TTP) is a blood disorder that does not lead to bleeding but to development of diffuse thrombi in small blood vessels. More often, this disorder is secondary to an autoimmune inhibitory antibody to the disintegrin and metalloproteinase with thrombospondin type 1 motif member-13 (ADAMTS-13), known as acquired TTP. Inhibiting this zinc containing metalloprotease leads to lack of cleavage of large multimers of von Willebrand Factor (vWF). The large vWF multimers then more easily bind to platelets resulting in platelet clots in small blood vessels. More rarely, this disorder is secondary to an inherited deficiency of ADAMTS-13. This patient population with congenital deficiency is managed with transfusion of FFP to replace the deficient enzyme. Acquired TTP is typically treated with therapeutic plasma exchange (TPE). This treatment modality removes the inhibitory antibody and ultralarge vWF multimers. Similarly, TPE will replete the missing enzyme. Immunosuppressive agents may be added if only TPE is not effective. A Mab preventing interaction of vWF and platelets was recently approved for use in treating this disorder.[305,306] Caplacizumab-yhdp (Cablivi) is a humanized single-variable-domain immunoglobulin (Nanobody) that inhibits the interaction between ultralarge vWF multimers and platelets and is directed against vWF. It induces a faster response to therapy with TPE and decreases relapse with continued use during TPE. This medication is then used post-TPE treatment until immunological evidence of disease is controlled to prevent relapse.[305,307,308] This medication was FDA approved for use in TTP in 2019.

Atypical hemolytic uremic syndrome (aHUS) is a disorder of the complement system due to uncontrolled activation. This disorder presents with thrombocytopenia, thrombi, and renal dysfunction. Historically, this illness was treated with TPE; however, end-stage renal failure occurred in 30% of patients and about 65% mortality in subsequent relapses with increasing incidence of renal failure. There are now two monoclonal antibodies approved for the treatment of aHUS. Refer to Table 16.1.

Sickle Pain Crisis

In sickle cell disease, one of the frequent complications is pain crises. This is usually treated with analgesics, oxygen, hydration, and transfusions (simple or exchange). Monoclonal antibodies are being developed to treat pain crises in sickle cell patients in both adult and pediatric populations. Crizanlizumab is a humanized Mab (IgG2κ) with specificity to selectin P. One phase II trial was completed in 2016 and three additional phase II studies will be completed between 2021 and 27 to treat vasoocclusive pain crisis. This medication may be under FDA review as early as 2019.[309,310]

INFECTIONS

Antimicrobials have historically been developed against a variety of viral, bacterial, fungal, and parasitic infections. These pharmaceuticals target differences from human cells of these particular organisms such as cell wall or membrane structure, genetic make-up, transcription/translation of genetic material, or metabolic pathways.

Often organisms develop resistance to entire categories of these medications. Earlier in the chapter, passive polyclonal antibodies were discussed in the treatment of some of these infectious agents and we will now discuss research in monoclonal therapies to pathogenic microorganisms.

Clostridium difficile

Enterocolitis from *Clostridium difficile* is a community or hospital acquired infection increasing morbidity and mortality in those that acquire it. Treatment is supportive or with fecal transplants or antibiotics. Bezlotoxumab (Zinplava) is a human Mab (IgG1) with specificity to *Clostridium difficile*'s B toxin. It is used to treat pseudomembranous colitis and prevent *C. difficile* reinfection.[311,312]

Actoxumab, a monoclonal antibody against *C. difficile* toxin A, has shown not to be clinically significant.

Respiratory Syncytial Virus

Respiratory syncytial virus (RSV) infects almost all children by 2 years old and poses extra risk in preterm infants. Supportive therapy, RSV-IG or IVIG, and antiviral therapy have been used to mitigate the sequela of this infection with optimal response yet to be seen. No vaccines have yet to be developed for this infection. Recently, monoclonal antibodies have been FDA approved or are undergoing pre/clinical trials to treat this infectious process and include palivizumab, Nirsevimab (MEDI8897), TRL3d3 (3D3), and ALX-0171.[313,314]

Not beneficial or safe in use for RSV: motavizumab, Suptavumab (REGN2222, SAR438584).

Influenza virus

Influenza is a worldwide respiratory infectious problem with cyclic epidemics yearly. Supportive therapy, yearly vaccinations, and antivirals are used to decrease the morbidity and mortality caused by this sometimes virulent pathogen. Both polyclonal and monoclonal therapies are being evaluated to better treat these infections. Mabs in pre/clinical trials include diridavumab (CR6262), firivumab, gedivumab (RG7745, RO6876802), lesofavumab (RG70026), and Navivumab (CT-P27).

Rabies

Rabies is a devastating viral infection with swift mortality if not treated quickly after initial exposure. Vaccines usually react too slowly and have to be combined with polyclonal IVIG infusions. Monoclonal therapy was previously studied but usually the virus mutates quickly and the infection is not controlled. More recently, in clinical trials, cocktails of Mabs are being tried to more closely mimic the benefits of polyclonal therapies. These Mabs include foravirumab, rafivirumab (CR57), and Rmab.

Hepatitis B virus

HBV is one of if not the most common infections in the world. Even though antivirals are available and effective, only recently they have they been widely used in the infant population and not just "high"-risk individuals. Mabs to treat this infection that are being investigated include libivirumab. Mab that is not found to be effective is tuvirumab.

Ebola

Ebola is a relatively rare but devastating hemorrhagic infection. Most care is supportive with various studies being performed to prevent/mitigate this disease. Vaccines are under development as well as passive polyclonal therapies. Mab therapies being developed or studied include porgaviximab (C2G4), cosfroviximab, and larcaviximab.

For these and other bacterial, fungal, and viral antiinfectious agents, information may be found in Table 16.1.

IMMUNOMODULATION

In solid organ transplants, cellular or humoral immunity can develop against the transplant leading to acute or chronic rejection. An additional complication with these and stem cell transplants is severe GVHD. In the past, these transplant complications were treated with high-dose glucocorticosteroids, immunosuppressive medication, chemotherapeutic agents, IVIG, or T-cell lymphocytic specific immunoglobulins. Recently, Mabs have been added to this armamentarium to better control these adverse reactions to transplantations.

Basiliximab (Simulect) is a chimeric Mab (IgG1κ) with specificity to CD25 IL-2α. The only FDA-approved indication for this medication is prophylaxis of acute rejection in renal transplant patients. There are multiple ongoing studies of this biological for other organ transplants including liver, lung, and heart as well as for inflammatory/immunologic diseases such as GVHD following stem cell transplantation, ulcerative colitis, and uveitis.[315–319]

Belatacept (Nulojix) is a soluble fusion protein consisting of the modified extracellular domain of CTLA-4 fused to the Fc domain of a recombinant human Mab

IgG1. This Mab selectively inhibits T-cell activation through costimulation blockade binding to both CD80 and CD86 while blocking CD28 via tighter binding than its parent antibody abatacept. Refer to Table 16.1.

METABOLIC SYNDROMES

Hypercholesterolemia is associated with increased risk for cardiovascular disease/atherosclerosis secondary to inherited or dietary etiologies. Diet and exercise are used to treat mild forms of these disorders. Medications such as nicotinic acid, fibrates, bile acid binding resins, and 3-hydroxy-3-methyl-glutaryl-coenzyme A reductase inhibitors are used for more severe forms of these disorders. Phase III studies have been completed with monoclonal antibodies for patients' refractory to the previously mentioned forms of therapy.

Hypophosphatemia

Burosumab (KRN23, Crysvita) is a human Mab IgG1κ with specificity to phosphaturic hormone fibroblast growth factor 23 (FGF 23). This hormone is a regulator of phosphate and vitamin D homeostasis. FGF23 inhibits the enzyme CYP27B1 and stimulates CYP24A1, thereby reducing circulating levels of 1,25-dihydroxyvitamin D (1,25(OH)2D), the active metabolite of vitamin D. This medication is FDA approved for the treatment of X-linked hypophosphatemic rickets.[320,321]

Osteoporosis

Denosumab (Prolia) is an FDA-approved human Mab (IgG2) that is a receptor activator of nuclear factor κB ligand that inhibits development and activity of osteoclasts. As Prolia, this medication is used to prevent or treat osteoporosis in women.[322-324] This medication under the trade name Xgeva is also used to prevent skeletal-related events in adults with bone metastasis from breast, prostate cancers, and multiple myeloma.[325,326]

ENDOCRINE DISORDERS

Diabetes may be classified as primary or secondary. In this chapter, we will be mainly interested in both insulin-dependent (Type I) and insulin-independent types (Type II). Type I diabetes mellitus is generally secondary to loss of β cells in the islets of Langerhans and subsequent loss of insulin production. Type II typically is secondary to decreased sensitivity to the effects of insulin. In type I, insulin is replaced exogenously depending on glucose levels. In type II, medications are given to stimulate islet cells to produce more insulin. Mabs are being developed to potentially mitigate the autoimmune process leading to Type I diabetes mellitus or the sequela of renal failure often seen with this disease. For type II, Mabs are being investigated to potentially decrease body mass index and thus decrease disease severity. Refer to Table 16.1.

OTHER CLINICAL DISORDERS

Age-related macular degeneration (AMD) is the leading irreversible cause of visual loss affecting the elderly. Two forms include a dry form with deposits in the macula or a wet form involving abnormal growth of blood vessels. The wet form, even though less frequent, is associated with more severe visual acuity loss. Antiangiogenesic drugs or laser treatments are used to slow the progression or even partially reverse visual loss. Some trials have been completed while others are ongoing using Mab to treat the wet form of AMD. Brolucizumab was found as good as if not better than aflibercept in a phase III clinical trial.[327]

Cryopyrin-associated periodic syndromes (including familial cold auto-inflammatory syndrome and Muckle-Wells syndrome); tumor necrosis factor receptor-associated periodic syndrome (TRAPS); hyperimmunoglobulin D Syndrome (HIDS)/mevalonate kinase deficiency and familial Mediterranean fever (FMF) may also respond to canakinumab.[328]

POTENTIAL FUTURE USES OF MONOCLONAL ANTIBODIES AND THEIR TARGETS

Passive antibody therapy continues to be useful clinically whether polyclonal or monoclonal therapy is implemented. Increased utilization of the classic polyclonal antibody preparations continue especially in the realm of infections. In the past 3 years, monoclonal therapy has evolved and revolutionized treatment in many areas. As targets are identified to modify disease pathology no matter its genre we continue to get a better handle on morbidity and mortality. We are learning that not only is the target important put the portion of the target mediating the effect we intend to modify is also important. Importantly, modification of antibodies to be more compatible with the immune system while decreasing rapidity of clearance also allows for more consistent therapy. There are also many targets yet to be discovered or only now being developed as in the canonical wingless/integrated (WNT) signaling. This receptor family is important in a multitude of diseases not limited to: hereditary colorectal cancer,

TABLE 16.2
Summary of Polyclonal Antibody Therapies.

Generic Drug Name	Brand Name	Additional Brand Names	AHFS Classification	Dosage Form(s)	Restricted Medication
Antithymocyte globulin (equine)	Atgam		Immunosuppressive agent	Intravenous solution	
Antithymocyte globulin (rabbit)	Thymoglobulin		Immunosuppressive agent	Intravenous solution	
Antivenin *Latrodectus mactans*	Black widow Antivenin		Serums	Intravenous solution	
Antivenin micrurus	Eastern and Texas coral Snake Antivenin		Serums	Intravenous solution	
Botulism immune globulin	BabyBIG				
Crotalidae polyvalent immune Fab	Crofab		Serums	Intravenous solution	
Cytomegalovirus immune globulin	Cytogam		Serums	Intravenous solution	Yes
Digoxin immune Fab	Digibind		Serums	Intravenous solution	
Hepatitis B immune globulin	Hepagam-B		Serums	Intramuscular solution, Intravenous solution	
Hepatitis B immune globulin	BayHepB	HepaGam B, Hyper Hep B, Nabi-HB			
High antibody titer Ebola FFP					
High antibody titer influenza FFP					

Continued

TABLE 16.2
Summary of Polyclonal Antibody Therapies.—cont'd

Generic Drug Name	Brand Name	Additional Brand Names	AHFS Classification	Dosage Form(s)	Restricted Medication
Immunoglobulin (generic)	Gamunex	Vivaglobin, Cuvitru, Privigen, gammagard, octagam, gamunex, hizentra, Bivigam, Carimune, Flebogamma, Gamastan, Gamimune, Gammaplex, gammar, Panglobulin, Panzyga, Sandoglobulin		Intravenous, Subcutaneous	Treat XLA, CVID, Hyper IgM syndromes, Wiskott Aldrich syndrome
Rabies immune globulin	Bayrab	HyperRAB, Imogam rabies, KedRAB			
Respiratory syncytial virus immune globulin	RespiGam				
Rho (D) immune globulin	WhinRho RhoGam	Rhophylac, MicRhoGAM, BatRhoD, HyperRho	Serums	Intravenous, intramuscular solutions	
Rimabotulinumtoxin B	Myobloc		Other Miscellaneous Therapeutic agents	Injection solution	Yes
Rozrolimupab			Anti-RhD Prevent isoimmunization ITP		
Tetanus immune globulin	Baytet	Hypertet			
Varicella zoster immune globulin	VariZIG				

Searched sites for table information. Monoclonal. https://www.fda.gov/Drugs/InformationOnDrugs/ApprovedDrugs/ucm279174.htm. https://fdasis.nlm.nih.gov/srs/. https://clinicaltrials. gov/ct2/. https://www.ncbi.nlm.nih.gov/pubmed/. https://chem.nlm.nih.gov/chemidplus/rn. https://druginfo.nlm.nih.gov/drugportal/. https://www.creativebiolabs.net/.

various types of sporadic cancers, intellectual disability syndrome, Alzheimer's disease, bipolar disorder, bone diseases, and vascular diseases. One monoclonal antibody rosmantuzumab (OMP-131R10), a humanized Mab (IgG1κ), is in phase I trials to treat colorectal cancer.[329,330] Other disease processes have yet to find their optimal therapy (Alzheimer's) or are advancing to fuller therapeutic benefit. The future is wide open for this newer class of pharmaceuticals as they continue to develop to full fruition.

REFERENCES

1. Sangstat Medical Corporation. *Thymoglobulin; (Antithymocyte Globulin [rabbit]) Prescribing Information*. Menlo Park, CA. December 1998.
2. Ormrod D, Jarvis B. Antithymocyte globulin (rabbit): a review of the use of Thymoglobulin in the prevention and treatment of acute renal allograft rejection. *BioDrugs*. 2000;14:255−273.
3. Kalamazoo, MI. *Pharmacia. Atgam Prescribing Information*. June 2000.
4. The Upjohn Company. *Drug Reference: Atgam*. Kalamazoo, MI. November 1981.
5. Cosimi AB. The clinical value of antilymphocyte antibodies. *Transplant Proc*. 1981;13:462−468.
6. Cosimi AB. The clinical usefulness of antilymphocyte antibodies. *Transplant Proc*. 1983;15:583−589.
7. Cho SI, Bradley JW, Carpenter CB, et al. Antithymocyte globulin, pretransplant blood transfusion, and tissue typing in cadaver kidney transplantation. *Am J Surg*. 1983;145:464−471.
8. Nelson PW, Cosimi AB, Delmonico FL, et al. Antithymocyte globulin as the primary treatment for renal allograft rejection. *Transplantation*. 1983;36:587−589.
9. Nowygrod R, Appel G, Hardy MA. Use of ATG for reversal of acute allograft rejection. *Transplant Proc*. 1981;13:469−472.
10. Hardy MA, Nowygrod R, Elberg A, et al. Use of ATG in treatment of steroid-resistant rejection. *Transplantation*. 1980;29:162−164.
11. Simonian SJ, Lyons P, Chvala R, et al. Reversal of acute cadaveric renal allograft rejection with added ATG treatment. *Transplant Proc*. 1983;15:604−607.
12. Gaber AO, First MR, Tesi RJ, et al. Results of the double-blind, randomized, multicenter, phase III clinical trial of Thymoglobulin versus Atgam in the treatment of acute graft rejection episodes after renal transplantation. *Transplantation*. 1998;66:29−37.
13. Brennan DC, Flavin K, Lowell JA, et al. A randomized, double-blinded comparison of Thymoglobulin versus Atgam for induction immunosuppressive therapy in adult renal transplant recipients. *Transplantation*. 1999; 67:1011−1018.
14. Lance EM. Mode of action of antilymphocyte serum. *Fed Proc*. 1970;29:209−211.
15. Martin WJ, Miller JFAP. Site of action of antilymphocyte globulin. *Lancet*. 1967;2:1285−1287.
16. Levey RH, Medawar PB. Nature and mode of action of antilymphocytic antiserum. *Proc Natl Acad Sci USA*. 1966;56:1130−1137.
17. Wohlman MH, Toledo-Pereyra LH, Zeichner WD. The immunosuppressive properties of antilymphocyte serum preparations: a current review. *Dial Transplant*. 1981;10: 19−28.
18. Zimmerman B, Tsui F. Immunosuppressive antilymphocyte serum: different subpopulations of T lymphocytes are influenced at different doses of antilymphocyte serum. *Transplantation*. 1979;28:323−328.
19. Bach JF. Mechanism and significance of rosette inhibition by antilymphocyte serum. In: Bach JF, Dormont J, Eyquem A, et al., eds. *International Symposium on Antilymphocyte Serum; Symposium Series on Immunobiology Standardization*. Vol. 16. New York: S Karger; 1970:189−198.
20. Pirofsky B, Beaulieu R, Bardana EJ, et al. Antithymocyte antiserum effects in man. *Am J Med*. 1974;56:290−296.
21. Greco B, Bielory L, Stephany D, et al. Antithymocyte globulin reacts with many normal human cell types. *Blood*. 1983;62:1047−1054.
22. Bonifazi F, Solano C, Wolschke C et al. GVHD prophylaxis plus ATLG after myeloablative allogeneic haemopoietic peripheral blood stem-cell transplantation from HLA-identical siblings in patients with acute leukaemia in remission: final results of quality of life and long-term outcome analysis of a phase 3 randomised study. The Lancet. Hematology, ISSN: 2352-3026, Vol: 6, Issue: 2, Page: e89-e99. https://doi.org/10.1016/S2352-3026(18)30214-X
23. Champlin RE. Treatment of aplastic anemia, pp. 480−483. In: Gale RP, moderator. Aplastic anemia: biology and treatment *Ann Intern Med*. 1981;95: 477−494.
24. Champlin R, Ho W, Gale RP. Antithymocyte globulin treatment in patients with aplastic anemia. *N Engl J Med*. 1983;308:113−118.
25. Cheeseman SH, Rubin RH, Stewart JA, et al. Controlled clinical trial of prophylactic human-leukocyte interferon in renal transplantation: effects on cytomegalovirus and herpes simplex virus infections. *N Engl J Med*. 1979; 300:1345−1349.
26. Cheeseman SH, Henle W, Rubin RH, et al. Epstein-Barr virus infection in renal transplant recipients: effects of antithymocyte globulin and interferon. *Ann Intern Med*. 1980;93(Part 1):39−42.
27. Diethelm AG, Aldrete JS, Shaw JF, et al. Clinical evaluation of equine antithymocyte globulin in recipients of renal allografts: analysis of survival, renal function, rejection, histocompatibility, and complications. *Ann Surg*. 1974;180:20−28.
28. Talecris Biotherapeutics. *HyperTET S/D (Tetanus Immune Globulin [human]) Solvent/detergent Treated Prescribing Information*. NC: Research Triangle Park; May 2008.
29. Centers for Disease Control and Prevention. General recommendations on immunization: recommendations of

the advisory committee on immunization practices (ACIP). *MMWR Recomm Rep (Morb Mortal Wkly Rep)*. 2006;55(RR-15):1−48.

30. Murphy TV, Slade BA, Broder KR, et al. Prevention of pertussis, tetanus, and diphtheria among pregnant and postpartum women and their infants recommendations of the Advisory Committee on Immunization Practices (ACIP). *MMWR Recomm Rep (Morb Mortal Wkly Rep)*. 2008;57:1−51.

31. Centers for Disease Control and Prevention. *Epidemiology and Prevention of Vaccine-Preventable Diseases*. 11th ed. Washington, DC: Public Health Foundation; 2009.

32. CSL Behring. *CytoGam (Cytomegalovirus Immune Globulin Intravenous [human][CMV-IG]) Liquid Formulation Solvent Detergent Treated Prescribing Information*. Kankakee, IL. November 2010.

33. Snydman DR, McIver J, Leszczynski J, et al. A pilot trial of a novel cytomegalovirus immune globulin in renal transplant recipients. *Transplantation*. 1984;38:553−557.

34. Snydman DR, Werner BG, Heinze-Lacey B, et al. Use of cytomegalovirus immune globulin to prevent cytomegalovirus disease in renal-transplant recipients. *N Engl J Med*. 1987;317:1049−1054.

35. Snydman DR. Prevention of cytomegalovirus-associated diseases with immunoglobulin. *Transplant Proc*. 1991;23(Suppl 3):131−135.

36. Snydman DR, Werner BG, Tilney NL, et al. Final analysis of primary cytomegalovirus disease prevention in renal transplant recipients with a cytomegalovirus-immune globulin: comparison of the randomized and open-label trials. *Transplant Proc*. 1991;23:1357−1360.

37. Werner BG, Snydman DR, Freeman R, et al. Cytomegalovirus immune globulin for the prevention of primary CMV disease in renal transplant patients: analysis of usage under treatment IND status. *Transplant Proc*. 1993;25:1441−1443.

38. Ho M. Cytomegalovirus. In: Mandell GL, Bennett JE, Dolin R, eds. *Mandell, Douglas and Bennett's Principles and Practice of Infectious Diseases*. 4th ed. New York: Churchill Livingstone; 1995:1351−1364.

39. Dickinson BI, Gora-Harper ML, McCraney SA, et al. Studies evaluating high-dose acyclovir, intravenous immune globulin, and cytomegalovirus hyperimmunoglobulin for prophylaxis against cytomegalovirus in kidney transplant recipients. *Ann Pharmacother*. 1996;30: 1452−1464.

40. Snydman DR. Cytomegalovirus immunoglobulins in the prevention and treatment of cytomegalovirus disease. *Clin Infect Dis*. 1990;12(Suppl 7):S839−S848.

41. Patel R, Snydman DR, Rubin RH, et al. Cytomegalovirus prophylaxis in solid organ transplant recipients. *Transplantation*. 1996;61:1279−1289.

42. Meyers JD. Prevention of cytomegalovirus infection after marrow transplantation. *Rev Infect Dis*. 1989;11(Suppl 7):S1691−S1705 ([PubMed]).

43. Winston DJ, Ho WG, Champlin RE. Cytomegalovirus infections after allogeneic bone marrow transplantation. *Clin Infect Dis*. 1990;12(Suppl 7):S776−S787.

44. Valantine HA. Prevention and treatment of cytomegalovirus disease in thoracic organ transplant patients: evidence for a beneficial effect of hyperimmune globulin. *Transplant Proc*. 1995;27(Suppl 1):49−57.

45. Grundy JE. Virologic and pathogenetic aspects of cytomegalovirus infection. *Clin Infect Dis*. 1990;12(Suppl 7):S711−S719.

46. Bass EB, Powe NR, Goodman SN, et al. Efficacy of immune globulin in preventing complications of bone marrow transplantation: a meta-analysis. *Bone Marrow Transplant*. 1993;12:273−282.

47. Taylor-Wiedeman J, Sissons JG, Borysiewicz LK, Sinclair JH. Monocytes are a major site of persistence of human cytomegalovirus in peripheral blood mononuclear cells. *J Gen Virol*. 1991;72:2059−2064.

48. Tsinontides AC, Bechtel TP. Cytomegalovirus prophylaxis and treatment following bone marrow transplantation. *Ann Pharmacother*. 1996;30:1277−1290.

49. Zamora MR, Fullerton DA, Campbell DN, et al. Use of cytomegalovirus (CMV) hyperimmune globulin for prevention of CMV disease in CMV-seropositive lung transplant recipients. *Transplant Proc*. 1994;26(Suppl 1): 49−51.

50. Snydman DR, Werner BG, Dougherty NN, et al. A further analysis of the use of cytomegalovirus immune globulin in orthotopic liver transplant patients at risk for primary infection. *Transplant Proc*. 1994;26(Suppl 1):23−27.

51. Aguado JM, Gomez-Sanchez MA, Lumbreras C, et al. Prospective randomized trial of efficacy of ganciclovir versus that of anti-cytomegalovirus (CMV) immunoglobulin to prevent CMV-seropositive heart transplant recipients treated with OKT3. *Antimicrob Agents Chemother*. 1995; 39:1643−1645.

52. Merck & Co. *Inc. Antivenin (Latrodectus Mactans) (Black Widow Spider Antivenin) Equine Origin Prescribing Information*. Whitehouse Station, NJ. February 2014.

53. Clark RF, Wethern-Kestner S, Vance MV, et al. Clinical presentation and treatment of black widow spider envenomation: a review of 163 cases. *Ann Emerg Med*. 1992;21: 782−787.

54. Wyeth Laboratories Inc. *Antivenin (Micrurus fulvius) (Equine Origin) (North American Coral Snake Antivenin) Prescribing Information*. Marietta, PA. August 2001.

55. *The United States Pharmacopeia, 25th Rev, and the National Formulary*. 20th ed. Rockville, MD: The United States Pharmacopeial Convention, Inc; 2002:158.

56. Protherics Inc Crofab. *(Crotalidae Polyvalent Immune Fab [ovine]) Prescribing Information*. Brentwood, TN. 2010 Sep.

57. Parrish HM. Bites by coral snakes: report of 11 representative cases. *Am J Med Sci*. 1967;253:561.

58. Identification and distribution of North American venomous snakes. In: Russell FE, ed. *Snake Venom Poisoning*. Philadelphia: JB Lippincott Company; 1980: 45−86.

59. Roze JA. New world coral snakes (Elapidae): a taxonomic and biologic summary. *Mem Inst Butantan, Sao Paulo*. 1982;46:305−338.

60. Anon. Treatment of snakebite in the USA. *Med Lett Drugs Ther.* 1982;24:87–89.

61. Clark RF, McKinney PE, Chase PB, et al. Immediate and delayed allergic reactions to Crotalidae polyvalent immune Fab (ovine) antivenom. *Ann Emerg Med.* 2002;39:671–676.

62. Lavonas EJ, Ruha AM, Banner W, et al. Unified treatment algorithm for the management of crotaline snakebite in the United States: results of an evidence-informed consensus workshop. *BMC Emerg Med.* 2011;11:2.

63. England PH. MERS-CoV: clinical decision making support for treatment. https://www.gov.uk/government/publications/mers-covclinical-decision-making-support-for-treatment (accessed Nov 8, 2016).

64. Luke TC, Kilbane EM, Jackson JL, Hoffman SL. Meta-analysis: convalescent blood products for Spanish influenza pneumonia: a future H5N1 treatment? *Ann Intern Med.* 2006;145:599–609.

65. Hung IF, To KK, lee CK, et al. Convalescent plasma treatment reduced mortality in patients with severe pandemic influenza A (H1N1) 2009 virus infection. *Clin Infect Dis.* 2011;52:447–456.

66. Gulland A. First Ebola treatment is approved by WHO. *BMJ.* 2014;349:g5539.

67. Mupapa K, Massamba M, Kibadi K, et al. Treatment of Ebola hemorrhagic fever with blood transfusions from convalescent patients. International Scientific and Technical Committee. *J Infect Dis.* 1999;179:S18–S23.

68. Klein HG. Should blood be an essential medicine? *N Engl J Med.* 2013;368:199–201.

69. Ala F, Allain JP, Bates I, et al. External financial aid to blood transfusion services in sub-Saharan Africa: a need for reflection. *PLoS Med.* 2012;9:e1001309.

70. Burnouf T, Emmanuel J, Mbanya D, et al. Ebola: a call for blood transfusion strategy in sub-Saharan Africa. *Lancet.* 2014;384:1347–1348.

71. *GlaxoSmithKline. Digibind (Digoxin Immune Fab [ovine]) Prescribing Information.* NC: Research Triangle Park; September 2003.

72. Smith TW, Haber E, Yeatman L, et al. Reversal of advanced digoxin intoxication with Fab fragments of digoxin-specific antibodies. *N Engl J Med.* 1976;294:797–800.

73. Smith TW, Butler VP, Haber E, et al. Treatment of life-threatening digitalis intoxication with digoxin-specific Fab antibody fragments. *N Engl J Med.* 1982;307:1357–1362.

74. Cole PL, Smith TW. Use of digoxin-specific Fab fragments in the treatment of digitalis intoxication. *Drug Intell Clin Pharm.* 1986;20:267–270.

75. Smith TW, Butler VP, Haber E. Cardiac glycoside-specific antibodies in the treatment of digitalis intoxication. In: Haber E, Krause RM, eds. *Antibodies in Human Diagnosis and Therapy.* New York: Raven Press; 1977:365–389.

76. Wenger TL, Butler VP, Haber E, et al. Treatment of 63 severely digitalis-toxic patients with digoxin-specific antibody fragments. *J Am Coll Cardiol.* 1985;5:118–123A.

77. Larbig D, Raff U, Haasis R. Reversal of digitalis effects by specific antibodies. *Pharmacology.* 1979;18:1–8.

78. Smolarz A, Roesch E, Lenz E, et al. Digoxin specific antibody (Fab) fragments in 34 cases of severe digitalis intoxication. *J Toxicol Clin Toxicol.* 1985;23:327–340.

79. Protherics Inc. *Digifab (Digoxin Immune Fab [ovine]) Prescribing Information.* Brentwood, TN. September 2010.

80. Smith TW. Use of antibodies in the study of the mechanism of action of digitalis. *Ann N Y Acad Sci.* 1974;242:731–736.

81. Watson JF, Butler VP. Biologic activity of digoxin-specific antisera. *J Clin Investig.* 1972;51:638–648 ([PubMed]).

82. Butler VP. Antibodies as specific antagonists of toxins, drugs, and hormones. *Pharmacol Rev.* 1982;34:109–114.

83. Gardner JD, Kiino DR, Swartz TJ, et al. Effects of digoxin-specific antibodies on accumulation and binding of digoxin by human erythrocytes. *J Clin Investig.* 1973;52:1820–1833.

84. Sullivan JB. Immunotherapy in the poisoned patient. *Med Toxicol.* 1986;1:47–60.

85. Boucher BA, Lalonde RL. Digoxin-specific antibody fragments for the treatment of digoxin intoxication. *Clin Pharm.* 1986;5:826–827.

86. Schmidt DH, Butler VP. Reversal of digoxin toxicity with specific antibodies. *J Clin Investig.* 1971;50:1738–1744.

87. Butler VP, Schmidt DH, Smith TW, et al. Effects of sheep digoxin-specific antibodies and their Fab fragments on digoxin pharmacokinetics in dogs. *J Clin Investig.* 1977;59:345–349.

88. Curd JG, Smith TW, Jaton JC, et al. The isolation of digoxin-specific antibody and its use in reversing the effects of digoxin. *Proc Natl Acad Sci USA.* 1971;68:2401–2406.

89. Nisonoff A. Enzymatic digestion of rabbit gamma globulin and antibody and chromatography of digestion products. *Methods Med Res.* 1964;10:134–141.

90. Lapostolle F, Borron SW, Verdier C, et al. Digoxin-specific Fab fragments as single first-line therapy in digitalis poisoning. *Crit Care Med.* 2008;36:3014–3018.

91. Eyal D, Molczan KA, Carroll LS. Digoxin toxicity: pediatric survival after asystolic arrest. *Clin Toxicol.* 2005;43:51–54.

92. Bateman DN. Digoxin-specific antibody fragments: how much and when? *Toxicol Rev.* 2004;23:135–143.

93. Schaeffer TH, Mlynarchek SL, Stanford CF, et al. Treatment of chronically digoxin-poisoned patients with a newer digoxin immune fab–a retrospective study. *J Am Osteopath Assoc.* 2010;110:587–592.

94. Ip D, Syed H, Cohen M. Digoxin specific antibody fragments (Digibind) in digoxin toxicity. *BMJ.* 2009;339:b2884.

95. Flanagan RJ, Jones AL. Fab antibody fragments: some applications in clinical toxicology. *Drug Saf.* 2004;27:1115–1133.

96. Ware JA, Young JB, Luchi RJ, et al. Treatment of severe digoxin toxicity with digoxin-specific antibodies: a case report. *Tex Med.* 1983;79:57–59.

97. Nicholls DP, Murtagh JG, Holt DW. Use of amiodarone and digoxin specific Fab antibodies in digoxin overdosage. *Br Heart J.* 1985;53:462−464.

98. Centers for Disease Control and Prevention. General recommendations on immunization: recommendations of the advisory committee on immunization practices (ACIP). *MMWR Recomm Rep (Morb Mortal Wkly Rep).* 2006;55(RR-15):1−47.

99. American Academy of Pediatrics. *2006 Red Book: Report of the Committee on Infectious Diseases.* 27th ed. Elk Grove Village, IL: American Academy of Pediatrics; 2006.

100. Talecris. *HyperHEP B S/D (Hepatitis B Immune Globulin [human] Solvent/detergent Treated) Prescribing Information.* June 2007.

101. Nabi. *Nabi-HB (Hepatitis B Immune Globulin [human] Solvent/detergent Treated and Filtered) Prescribing Information.* Boca Raton, FL. June 2003.

102. Centers for Disease Control and Prevention. A comprehensive immunization strategy to eliminate transmission of hepatitis B virus infection in the United States. Recommendations of the Advisory Committee on Immunization Practices (ACIP). Part I: immunization of infants, children, and adolescents. *MMWR Recomm Rep (Morb Mortal Wkly Rep).* 2005;54(RR-16):1−33.

103. Centers for Disease Control and Prevention. A comprehensive immunization strategy to eliminate transmission of hepatitis B virus infection in the United States. Recommendations of the Advisory Committee on Immunization Practices (ACIP). Part II: immunization in adults. *MMWR Recomm Rep (Morb Mortal Wkly Rep).* 2006;55(RR-16):1−33.

104. Apotex. *HepaGam B (Hepatitis B Immune Globulin Intravenous [human]) Prescribing Information.* Weston, FL. April 2007.

105. American Academy of Pediatrics. *2006 Red Book: Report of the Committee on Infectious Diseases.* 27th ed. Elk Grove Village, IL: American Academy of Pediatrics; 2006.

106. Centers for Disease Control and Prevention. Recommended immunization schedules for persons 0 through 18 years−United States, 2009. *MMWR Morb Mortal Wkly Rep.* 2009;57. Q1-4.

107. Centers for Disease Control Immunization Practices Advisory Committee (ACIP). Protection against viral hepatitis: recommendations of the immunization practices advisory committee (ACIP). *MMWR Recomm Rep (Morb Mortal Wkly Rep).* 1990;39(RR-2):1−26.

108. Centers for Disease Control and Prevention. Sexually transmitted diseases treatment guidelines. *MMWR Recomm Rep (Morb Mortal Wkly Rep).* 2006;55(RR-11):1−94.

109. Centers for Disease Control and Prevention. Updated US Public Health Service guidelines for the management of occupational exposures to HBV, HCV, and HIV and recommendations for postexposure prophylaxis. *MMWR Morb Mortal Wkly Rep.* 2001;50(No. RR-11):1−51.

110. Coffin CS, Terrault NA. Management of hepatitis B in liver transplant recipients. *J Viral Hepat.* 2007;14(Suppl1):37−44.

111. Yilmaz N, Shiffman ML, Stravitz RT, et al. Prophylaxis against recurrence of hepatitis B virus after liver transplantation: a retrospective analysis spanning 20 years. *Liver Int.* 2008;28:72−78.

112. Gish RG, McCashland T. Hepatitis B in liver transplant recipients. *Liver Transplant.* 2006;12:S54−S64.

113. Anderson RD, Chinnakotla S, Guo L, et al. Intramuscular hepatitis B immunoglobulin (HBIG) and nucleosides for prevention of recurrent hepatitis B following liver transplantation: comparison with other HBIG regimens. *Clin Transplant.* 2007;21:510−517.

114. Gane EJ, Angus PW, Strasser S, et al. Lamivudine plus low-dose hepatitis B immunoglobulin to prevent recurrent hepatitis B following liver transplantation. *Gastroenterology.* 2007;132:931−937.

115. Nath DS, Kalis A, Nelson S, et al. Hepatitis B prophylaxis post-liver transplant without maintenance hepatitis B immunoglobulin therapy. *Clin Transplant.* 2006;20:206−210.

116. Eisenbach C, Sauer P, Mehrabi A, et al. Prevention of hepatitis B virus recurrence after liver transplantation. *Clin Transplant.* 2006;20(Suppl):111−116.

117. Zheng S, Chen Y, Liang T, et al. Prevention of hepatitis B recurrence after liver transplantation using lamivudine or lamivudine combined with hepatitis B immunoglobulin prophylaxis. *Liver Transplant.* 2006;12:253−258.

118. Cangene Corporation. *Varizig Varicella Zoster Immune Globulin (Human) Lyophilized Powder for Solution for Injection for Intramuscular Administration Only Prescribing Information.* Winnipeg, Canada. December 2012.

119. Centers for Disease Control and Prevention. Prevention of varicella: recommendations of the advisory committee on immunization practices (ACIP). *MMWR Recomm Rep (Morb Mortal Wkly Rep).* 2007;56(RR-4):1−40.

120. National Center for Immunization and Respiratory Diseases. General recommendations on immunization — recommendations of the advisory committee on immunization practices (ACIP). *MMWR Recomm Rep (Morb Mortal Wkly Rep).* 2011;60:1−64.

121. American Academy of Pediatrics. *Red Book: 2009 Report of the Committee on Infectious Diseases.* 28th ed. Elk Grove Village, IL: American Academy of Pediatrics; 2009.

122. Centers for Disease Control and Prevention (CDC). FDA approval of an extended period for administering VariZIG for postexposure prophylaxis of varicella. *MMWR Morb Mortal Wkly Rep.* 2012;61:212.

123. Solstice Neurosciences. *Myobloc (rimabotulinumtoxinB) Injection Prescribing Information.* South San Francisco, CA. May 2010.

124. Brashear A, Lew MF, Dykstra DD, et al. Safety and efficacy of NeuroBloc (botulinum toxin type B) in type A-responsive cervical dystonia. *Neurology.* 1999;53:1439−1446.

125. Terranova W, Breman JG, Locey RP, et al. Botulism type B: epidemiologic aspects of an extensive outbreak. *Am J Epidemiol.* 1978;108:150−156.

126. Cheng CM, Chen JS, Patel RP. Unlabeled uses of botulinum toxins: a review, part 1. *Am J Health Syst Pharm.* 2006;63:145−152.

127. Allergan. *Botox (onabotulinumtoxinA) for Injection Prescribing Information.* Irvine, CA. September 2013.

128. Bell MS, Vermeulen LC, Sperling KB. Pharmacotherapy with botulinum toxin: harnessing nature's most potent neurotoxin. *Pharmacotherapy.* 2000;20:1079−1091.

129. Tsui JK. Botulinum toxin as a therapeutic agent. *Pharmacol Ther.* 1996;72:13−24.

130. Moore AP. Botulinum toxin A (BoNT-A) for spasticity in adults. What is the evidence? *Eur J Neurol.* 2002;9(Suppl 1):42−47.

131. Corry IS, Cosgrove AP, Duffy CM, et al. Botulinum toxin A compared with stretching casts in the treatment of spastic equinus: a randomised prospective trial. *J Pediatr Orthop.* 1998;18:304−311.

132. Figgit DP, Noble S. Botulinum toxin B: a review of its therapeutic potential in the management of cervical dystonia. *Drugs.* 2002;62:705−722.

133. Lew MF, Adornato BT, Duane DD, et al. Botulinum toxin type B: a double-blind, placebo-controlled, safety and efficacy study in cervical dystonia. *Neurology.* 1997;49:701−707.

134. Anon. Botulinum toxin for cervical dystonia. *Med Lett Drugs Ther.* 2001;43:63−64.

135. California Department of Public Health. *BabyBIG (Botulism Immune Globulin Intravenous [human]) Prescribing Information.* Richmond, CA. January 2012.

136. Arnon SS. Creation and development of the public service orphan drug Human Botulism Immune Globulin. *Pediatrics.* 2007;119:785−789 ([PubMed]).

137. Infant Botulism Treatment and Prevention Program. Division of Communicable Disease Control, California Department of Health Services. From IBTPP website. Accessed 2012 Mar 26. [Web].

138. Underwood K, Rubin S, Deakers T, et al. Infant botulism: a 30-year experience spanning the introduction of botulism immune globulin intravenous in the intensive care unit at Childrens Hospital Los Angeles. *Pediatrics.* 2007; 120:e1380−e1385 ([PubMed]).

139. Arnon SS. Infant botulism. In: Feigin RD, Cherry JD, Demmler-Harrison GJ, et al., eds. *Feigin: Feigin and Cherry's Textbook of Pediatric Infectious Diseases.* 6th ed. Philadelphia, PA: Saunders Elsevier; 2009.

140. Arnon SS, Schechter R, Maslanka SE, et al. Human botulism immune globulin for the treatment of infant botulism. *N Engl J Med.* 2006;354:462−471.

141. Talecris Biotherapeutics, Inc. *HyperRAB S/D (Rabies Immune Globulin [human] Solvent/detergent Treated) Prescribing Information.* NC: Research Triangle Park; March 2008.

142. Sanofi Pasteur. *Imogam Rabies-HT (Rabies Immune Globulin [human] USP, Heat Treated) Prescribing Information.* Swiftwater, PA. December 2005.

143. Centers for Disease Control and Prevention. Human rabies prevention—United States, 2008. Recommendations of the advisory committee on immunization practices. *MMWR Recomm Rep (Morb Mortal Wkly Rep).* 2008;57(RR-3):1−27.

144. Centers for Disease Control and Prevention. Use of a reduced (4-dose) vaccine schedule for postexposure prophylaxis to prevent human rabies. Recommendations of the Advisory Committee on Immunization Practices. *MMWR Recomm Rep (Morb Mortal Wkly Rep).* 2010;59(RR-2):1−9.

145. Cangene bioPharma. *WinRho SDF (Rho [D] Immune Globulin Intravenous [human]) Prescribing Information.* Baltimore, MD. December 2010.

146. Grifols Therapeutics. *HyperRHO S/D Mini-Dose (Rho [D] Immune Globulin [human]) Prescribing Information.* NC: Research Triangle Park; September 2012.

147. Ortho-Clinical Diagnostics. *Rho-GAM (Rho [D] Immune Globulin [human]) Ultra-filtered PLUS and MICRhoGAM (Rho [D] Immune Globulin [human]) Ultra-filtered PLUS Prescribing Information.* NJ: Raritan; November 2012.

148. The United States pharmacopeia. *23rd Rev, and the National Formulary.* 18th ed. Rockville, MD: The United States Pharmacopeial Convention, Inc; 1995:350.

149. CSL Behring. *Rhophylac (Rho [D] Immune Globulin Intravenous [human]) Prescribing Information.* IL: Kankakee; October 2012.

150. Kumar S. Universal RDH genotyping in fetuses. *BMJ.* 2008;336:783.

151. Bussel JB, Graziano JN, Kimberly RP, et al. Intravenous anti-D treatment of immune thrombocytopenic purpura: analysis of efficacy, toxicity, and mechanism of effect. *Blood.* 1991;77:1884−1893.

152. Becker T, Küenzlen E, Salama A, et al. Treatment of childhood idiopathic thrombocytopenic purpura with Rhesus antibodies (anti-D). *Eur J Pediatr.* 1986;145:166−169.

153. Andrew M, Blanchette VS, Adams M, et al. A multicenter study of the treatment of childhood chronic idiopathic thrombocytopenic purpura with anti-D. *J Pediatr.* 1992; 120:522−527.

154. Scaradavou A, Woo B, Woloski BMR, et al. Intravenous anti-D treatment of immune thrombocytopenic 20. Ballow M. Mechanisms of action of intravenous immunoglobulin therapy and potential use in autoimmune connective tissue diseases. *Cancer.* 1991;68:1430−1436.

155. Ballow M. Mechanisms of action of intravenous immunoglobulin therapy and potential use in autoimmune connective tissue diseases. *Cancer.* 1991;68:1430−1436.

156. Kniker WT. Immunosuppressive agents, γ-globulin, immunomodulation, immunization, and aphresis. *J Allergy Clin Immunol.* 1989;84:1104−1107.

157. Blanchette V, Imbach P, Andrew M, et al. Randomised trial of intravenous immunoglobulin G, intravenous anti-D, and oral prednisone in childhood acute immune thrombocytopenic purpura. *Lancet.* 1994;344:703−707.

158. Berchtold P, McMillan R. Therapy of chronic idiopathic thrombocytopenic purpura in adults. *Blood.* 1989;74:2309−2317.

159. Rodeghiero F, Schiavotto C, Castaman G, et al. A follow-up study of 49 adult patients with idiopathic thrombocytopenic purpura treated with high-dose immunoglobulins and anti-D immunoglobulins. *Haematologica.* 1992; 77:248−252.

160. Stasi R, Stipa E, Masi M, et al. Long-term observation of 208 adults with chronic idiopathic thrombocytopenic purpura. *Am J Med.* 1995;98:436–442.

161. Landonio G, Galli M, Nosari A, et al. HIV-related severe thrombocytopenia in intravenous drug-users: prevalence, response to therapy in a medium-term follow-up, and pathogenetic evaluation. *AIDS.* 1990;4:29–34.

162. Hoffman DM, Caruso RF, Mirando T. Human immunodeficiency virus-associated thrombocytopenia. *Dicp Ann Pharmacother.* 1989:157–160.

163. Food and Drug Administration. FDA Application: Search Orphan Drug Designations and Approvals. Silver Spring, MD. From FDA website (http://www.accessdata.fda.gov/scripts/opdlisting/oopd/index.cfm). Accessed 2013 Jul 2.

164. Oksenhendler E, Bierling P, Brossard Y, et al. Anti-RH immunoglobulin therapy for human immunodeficiency virus-related immune thrombocytopenic purpura. *Blood.* 1988;71:1499–1502.

165. Okwundu CI, Afolabi BB. Intramuscular versus intravenous anti-D for preventing Rhesus alloimmunization during pregnancy. *Cochrane Database Syst Rev.* 2013;1: CD007885.

166. CSL Behring. *Carimune NF, Nanofiltered (Immune Globulin Intravenous [human] Lyophilized for Solution) Prescribing Information.* IL: Kankakee; November 2016.

167. Baxalta US Inc. *Gammagard S/D (Immune Globulin Intravenous [human] IgA Less than or Equal to 2.2 mcg/mL in a 5% Solution) Prescribing Information.* Westlake Village, CA. September 2016.

168. Grifols USA. *GamaSTAN S/D (Immune Globulin IM [human]) Prescribing Information.* NC: Research Triangle Park; June 2017.

169. Octapharma USA. *Octagam (Immune Globulin Intravenous [human] 5% Liquid) Prescribing Information.* Hoboken, NJ. August 2015.

170. Grifols Therapeutics Inc. *Gamunex-C (Immune Globulin Intravenous [human] 10% Caprylate/chromatography Purified) Prescribing Information.* NC: Research Triangle Park; September 2016.

171. Baxalta US Inc. *Gammagard S/D (Immune Globulin Intravenous [human] IgA Less than 1 mcg/mL in a 5% Solution) Prescribing Information.* Westlake Village, CA. September 2016.

172. CSL Behring. *Privigen (Immune Globulin Intravenous [human] 10% Liquid) Prescribing Information.* Kankakee, IL. October 2016.

173. American Academy of Pediatrics. *Red Book: 2015 Report of the Committee on Infectious Diseases.* 30th ed. Elk Grove Village, IL: American Academy of Pediatrics; 2015.

174. NIH Consensus Development Conference. Intravenous immunoglobulin: prevention and treatment of disease. *J Am Med Assoc.* 1990;264:3189–3193.

175. Hughes RA, Donofrio P, Bril V, et al. Intravenous immune globulin (10% caprylate-chromatography purified) for the treatment of chronic inflammatory demyelinating polyradiculoneuropathy (ICE study): a randomised placebo-controlled trial. *Lancet Neurol.* 2008;7:136–144.

176. CSL Behring. *Hizentra (Immune Globulin Subcutaneous [human] 20% Liquid) Prescribing Information.* Kankakee, IL. October 2016.

177. Bio Products Laboratory (distributed by BPL Inc). *Gammaplex (Immune Globulin Intravenous [human] 5% Liquid for Intravenous Use) Prescribing Information.* Hertfordshire, UK. September 2015.

178. Biotest Pharmaceuticals. *Bivigam (Immune Globulin Intravenous [human] 10% Liquid) Prescribing Information.* Boca Raton, FL. April 2014.

179. Grifols USA. *Flebogamma 10% DIF (Immune Globulin Intravenous [human] Solution for Intravenous Administration) Prescribing Information.* Los Angeles, CA. January 2016.

180. Octapharma USA. *Octagam (Immune Globulin Intravenous [human] 10% Liquid) Prescribing Information.* Hoboken, NJ. November 2015.

181. Baxalta US Inc. *Hyqvia (Immune Globulin [human] 10% with Recombinant Human Hyaluronidase Solution for Subcutaneous Administration) Prescribing Information.* Westlake Village, CA. April 2016.

182. Baxalta US Inc. *Cuvitru (Immune Globulin Subcutaneous [human] 20% Solution) Prescribing Information.* Westlake Village, CA. September 2016.

183. Kedrion Biopharma. *Gammaked (Immune Globulin Intravenous [human] 10% Caprylate/chromatography Purified) Prescribing Information.* Fort Lee, NJ. September 2016.

184. Advisory Committee on Immunization Practices (ACIP), Fiore AE, Wasley A, et al. Prevention of hepatitis A through active or passive immunization: recommendations of the advisory committee on immunization practices (ACIP). *MMWR Recomm Rep (Morb Mortal Wkly Rep).* 2006;55(RR-7):1–23.

185. Centers for Disease Control and Prevention. Update: prevention of hepatitis A after exposure to hepatitis A virus and in international travelers. Updated recommendations of the advisory committee on immunization practices (ACIP). *MMWR Morb Mortal Wkly Rep.* 2007;56: 1080–1084.

186. Nelson NP. Updated dosing instructions for immune globulin (human) GamaSTAN S/D for hepatitis a virus prophylaxis. *MMWR Morb Mortal Wkly Rep.* 2017;66: 959–960.

187. Centers for Disease Control and Prevention. *CDC Health Information for International Travel.* Atlanta, GA: US Department of Health and Human Services; 2018 (Updates may be available at: CDC website).

188. McLean HQ, Fiebelkorn AP, Temte JL, et al. Prevention of measles, rubella, congenital rubella syndrome, and mumps, 2013: summary recommendations of the Advisory Committee on Immunization Practices (ACIP). *MMWR Recomm Rep (Morb Mortal Wkly Rep).* 2013; 62(RR-04):1–34.

189. Gardulf A, Nocolay U, Asensio O, et al. Rapid subcutaneous IgG replacement therapy is effective and safe in children and adults with primary immunodeficiencies-a prospective, multi-national study. *J Clin Immunol.* 2006; 26:177–185.

190. Nicolay U, Kiessling P, Berger M, et al. Health-related quality of life and treatment satisfaction in north american patients with primary immunedeficiency diseases receiving subcutaneous IgG self-infusions at home. *J Clin Immunol.* 2006;26:65–72.

191. Gaspar J, Berritsen B, Jones A. Immunoglobulin replacement treatment by rapid subcutaneous infusion. *BMJ.* 1998;79:48–51.

192. Grifols USA. *Flebogamma 5% DIF (Immune Globulin Intravenous [human] Solution for Intravenous Administration) Prescribing Information.* Los Angeles, CA. April 2015.

193. Kurtsberg J, Friedman HS, Chaffee S, et al. Efficacy of intravenous gamma globulin in autoimmune-mediated pediatric blood dyscrasias. *Am J Med.* 1987;83(Suppl 4A):4–9.

194. Lusher JM, Warrier I. Use of intravenous gamma globulin in children and adolescents with idiopathic thrombocytopenic purpura and other immune thrombocytopenias. *Am J Med.* 1987;83(Suppl 4A):10–16.

195. Berkman SA, Lee ML, Gale RP. Clinical uses of intravenous immunoglobulins. *Ann Intern Med.* 1990;112:278–292.

196. Cooperative Group for the Study of Immunoglobulin in Chronic Lymphocytic Leukemia. Intravenous immunoglobulin for the prevention of infection in chronic lymphocytic leukemia. *N Engl J Med.* 1988;319:902–907.

197. Knapp MJ, Colburn PA. Clinical uses of intravenous immune globulin. *Clin Pharm.* 1990;9:509–529.

198. Newburger JW, Takahashi M, Burns JC, et al. The treatment of Kawasaki syndrome with intravenous gamma globulin. *N Engl J Med.* 1986;315:341–347.

199. Nagashima M, Matsushima M, Matsuoka H, et al. High-dose gammaglobulin therapy for Kawasaki disease. *J Pediatr.* 1987;110:710–712.

200. Newburger JW, Takahashi M, Gerber MA, et al. Diagnosis, treatment, and long-term management of Kawasaki disease: a statement for health professionals from the committee on rheumatic fever, endocarditis and Kawasaki disease, council on cardiovascular disease in the young, American heart association. *Circulation.* 2004;110:2747–2771.

201. Singh S, Tank NK, Dwiwedi P, Charan J, et al. Monoclonal antibodies: a review. *Curr Clin Pharmacol.* 2018;13:85–99. https://doi.org/10.2174/1574884712666170809124728. PMID:28799485.

202. HIGHLIGHTS OF PRESCRIBING INFORMATION: RITUXAN HYCELA (rituximab and hyaluronidase human) injection, for subcutaneous use Initial U.S. Approval: 2017. Revised 6/2017. Available at: https://www.accessdata.fda.gov/drugsatfda_docs/label/2017/761064s000lbl.pdf.

203. Salles G, Barrett M, Robin Foà R, et al. Rituximab in B-cell hematologic malignancies: a review of 20 Years of clinical experience. *Adv Ther.* 2017;34:2232–2273. https://doi.org/10.1007/s12325-017-0612-x. PMID: 28983798.

204. Qi J, Chen S, Chiorazzi N, Rader C. An IgG1-like bispecific antibody targeting CD52 and CD20 for the treatment of B-cell malignancies. *Methods.* 2019;154:70–76.

Available online 24 August 2018 at https://DOI.org/10.1016/j.ymeth.2018.08.008.

205. Zhang B. Mini-review: ofatumumab. *mAbs.* 2009;1(4):326–331. Previously published online as a mAbs E-publication: http://www.landesbioscience.com/journals/mabs/article/8895.

206. McWilliams EM, Meleb JM, Cheney C, et al. Therapeutic CD94/NKG2A blockade improves natural killer cell dysfunction in chronic lymphocytic leukemia. *OncoImmunology.* 2016;5(10):e1226720 (9 pages) Accepted 16 August 2016. Available at: https://doi.org/10.1080/2162402X.2016.1226720.

207. Robak T, Hellmann A, Kloczko J, et al. Randomized phase 2 study of otlertuzumab and bendamustine versus bendamustine in patients with relapsed chronic lymphocytic leukaemia. *Br J Haematol.* 2017;176:618–628. https://doi.org/10.1111/bjh.14464. PMID: 24843434.

208. Segal NH, Logan TF, Hodi S, et al. Results from an integrated safety analysis of urelumab, an agonist anti-CD137 monoclonal antibody. *Clin Cancer Res.* 2017;23(8):1929–1936. Published OnlineFirst October 18, 2016. Available at: http://clincancerres.aacrjournals.org/content/23/8/1929.

209. NIH: National Library of Medicine at Clinicaltrials.gov Clinical trial; Urelumab (CD137 mAb) with rituximab for relapsed, refractory or high-risk untreated chronic lymphocytic leukemia (CLL) patients. Available at: https://clinicaltrials.gov/ct2/show/NCT02420938?term=urelumab&rank=1.

210. Kashyap MK, Kumar D, Jones H, et al. Ulocuplumab (BMS-936564/MDX1338): a fully human anti-CXCR4 antibody induces cell death in chronic lymphocytic leukemia mediated through a reactive oxygen species-dependent pathway. *Oncotarget.* January 19, 2016;7(3):2809–2822. https://doi.org/10.18632/oncotarget.6465. Published online 2015 Dec 4. PMID:26646452.

211. First in Human Study to Determine the Safety, Tolerability and Preliminary Efficacy of an Anti-CXCR4 Antibody in Subjects With Acute Myelogenous Leukemia and Selected B-cell Cancers. Available at: https://clinicaltrials.gov/ct2/show/NCT01120457?term=ulocuplumab&rank=5.

212. Lin TS, Stock W, Xu H, et al. A phase I/II dose escalation study of apolizumab (Hu1D10) using a stepped-up dosing schedule in patients with chronic lymphocytic leukemia and acute leukemia. *Leuk Lymphoma.* 2009;50(12):1958–1963. https://doi.org/10.3109/10428190903186486. PMID: 19860603.

213. de Vos S, Forero-Torres A, Ansell SM, et al. A phase II study of dacetuzumab (SGN-40) in patients with relapsed diffuse large B-cell lymphoma (DLBCL) and correlative analyses of patient-specific factors. *J Hematol Oncol.* 2014;7:44. https://doi.org/10.1186/1756-8722-7-44. PMID:24919462.

214. Fayad L, Ansell SM, Advani R, et al. Dacetuzumab plus rituximab, ifosfamide, carboplatin and etoposide as salvage therapy for patients with diffuse large B-cell lymphoma relapsing after rituximab, cyclophosphamide,

doxorubicin, vincristine and prednisolone: a randomized, double-blind, placebo-controlled phase 2b trial. *Leuk Lymphoma.* 2015;56(9):2569–2578. https://doi.org/10.3109/10428194.2015.1007504. PMID: 25651427.

215. Awan FT, Hillmen P, Hellmann A, et al. A randomized, open-label, multicentre, phase 2/3 study to evaluate the safety and efficacy of lumiliximab in combination with fludarabine, cyclophosphamide and rituximab versus fludarabine, cyclophosphamide and rituximab alone in subjects with relapsed chronic lymphocytic leukaemia. *Br J Haematol.* 2014;167:466–477. https://doi.org/10.1111/bjh.13061. PMID:25130401.

216. Kovtun Y, Jones GE, Adams S, et al. A CD123-targeting antibody-drug conjugate, IMGN632, designed to eradicate AML while sparing normal bone marrow cells. *Blood Adv.* April 24, 2018;2(8):848–858. https://doi.org/10.1182/bloodadvances.2018017517. PMID:29661755.

217. Aigner M, Feulner J, Schaffer S, et al. T lymphocytes can be effectively recruited for ex vivo and in vivo lysis of AML blasts by a novel CD33/CD3-bispecific BiTE antibody construct. *Leukemia.* April 2013;27(5):1107–1115. https://doi.org/10.1038/leu.2012.341. Epub 2012 Nov 26. PMID:23178753.

218. Xie LH, Biondo M, Busfield SJ, et al. CD123 target validation and preclinical evaluation of ADCC activity of anti-CD123 antibody CSL362 in combination with NKs from AML patients in remission. *Blood Canc J.* 2017;7:e567. https://doi.org/10.1038/bcj.2017.52. published online 2 June 2017. PMID:28574487. Available at: https://www.ncbi.nlm.nih.gov/pmc/articles/PMC5520399/.

219. NIH: National Library of Medicine at Clinicaltrials.gov Clinical trial; Study of Biomarker-Based Treatment of Acute Myeloid Leukemia. Available at: https://clinicaltrials.gov/ct2/show/NCT03013998?term=samalizumab&rank=3.

220. NIH: National Library of Medicine at Clinicaltrials.gov Clinical trial; Ficlatuzumab With High Dose Cytarabine in Relapsed and Refractory AML available at: https://clinicaltrials.gov/ct2/show/NCT02109627?term=Ficlatuzumab&rank=3.

221. Egan PC, Reagan JL. The return of gemtuzumab ozogamicin: a humanized anti-CD33 monoclonal antibody–drug conjugate for the treatment of newly diagnosed acute myeloid leukemia. *OncoTargets Ther.* 2018;11:8265–8272. https://doi.org/10.2147/OTT.S150807. eCollection 2018. PMID:30538495.

222. Feldman EJ, Brandwein J, Stone R, et al. Phase III randomized multicenter study of a humanized anti-CD33 monoclonal antibody, Lintuzumab, in combination with chemotherapy, versus chemotherapy alone in patients with refractory or first-relapsed acute myeloid leukemia. *J Clin Oncol.* June 20, 2005;23(18):4110–4116. https://doi.org/10.1200/JCO.2005.09.133. PMID: 15961759.

223. Sekeres MA, Lancet JE, Wood BL, et al. Randomized, phase IIb study of low-dose cytarabine and lintuzumab versus low-dose cytarabine and placebo in older adults with untreated acute myeloid leukemia. *Haematologica.*

January 2013;98(1):119–128. https://doi.org/10.3324/haematol.2012.066613. Epub 2012 Jul 16. PMID: 22801961.

224. de Weers M, Tai YT, van der Veer MS, et al. Daratumumab, a novel therapeutic human CD38 monoclonal antibody, induces killing of multiple myeloma and other hematological tumors. *J Immunol.* 2011;186(3):1840–1848. https://doi.org/10.4049/jimmunol.1003032. Epub 2010 Dec 27. PMID:21187443. Available at: http://www.jimmunol.org/content/186/3/1840.

225. HIGHLIGHTS OF PRESCRIBING INFORMATION DARZALEX (daratumumab) injection. Revised 11/2016 Available at: https://www.accessdata.fda.gov/drugsatfda_docs/label/2016/761036s004lbl.pdf.

226. Shah JJ, Feng L, Thomas SK, et al. Siltuximab (CNTO 328) with lenalidomide, bortezomib and dexamethasone in newly-diagnosed, previously untreated multiple myeloma: an open-label phase I trial. *Blood Canc J.* 2016;6:e396. https://doi.org/10.1038/bcj.2016.4. published online 12 February 2016. PMID:26871714.

227. CENTER FOR DRUG EVALUATION AND RESEARCH; Approval Package for: APPLICATION NUMBER: 125496Orig1s000 Trade Name: Sylvant, Generic Name: siltuximab, Sponsor: Janssen Biotech, Inc, Approval Date: April 23, 2014. Available at: https://www.accessdata.fda.gov/drugsatfda_docs/nda/2014/125496Orig1s000Approv.pdf.

228. Le Jeune C, Thomas X. Potential for bispecific T-cell engagers: role of blinatumomab in acute lymphoblastic leukemia. *Drug Des Dev Ther.* February 18, 2016;10:757–765. https://doi.org/10.2147/DDDT.S83848. eCollection 2016. PMID:26937176.

229. Kantarjian H, Stein A, Gökbuget N, et al. Blinatumomab versus chemotherapy for advanced acute lymphoblastic leukemia. *N Engl J Med.* March 02, 2017;376(9):836–847. https://doi.org/10.1056/NEJMoa1609783. PMID: 28249141.

230. HIGHLIGHTS OF PRESCRIBING INFORMATION; BLINCYTO (blinatumomab) for injection, for intravenous use; Initial U.S. Approval: 2014 Revised 7/2017 https://www.accessdata.fda.gov/drugsatfda_docs/label/2017/125557s008lbl.pdf.

231. Scott LJ. Brentuximab vedotin: a review in CD30-positive Hodgkin lymphoma. *Drugs.* 2017;77:435–445. https://doi.org/10.1007/s40265-017-0705-5. Published online: 11 February 2017. PMID:28190142.

232. Flynn MJ, Zammarchi F, Tyrer PC, et al. ADCT-301, a pyrrolobenzodiazepine (PBD) dimer–containing antibody–drug conjugate (ADC) Targeting CD25-expressing hematological malignancies. *Mol Cancer Ther.* November 2016;15(11):2709–2721. Epub 2016 Aug 17. PMID:27535974.

233. Study of ADCT-301 in Patients With Relapsed or Refractory Hodgkin and Non-Hodgkin Lymphoma. Available at: https://clinicaltrials.gov/ct2/show/NCT02432235?term=Camidanlumab+tesirine&rank=3.

234. Ansell SM, Horwitz SM, Engert A, et al. Phase I/II study of an anti-CD30 monoclonal antibody (MDX-060) in

Hodgkin's Lymphoma and anaplastic large-cell lymphoma. *J Clin Oncol.* 2007;25:2764—2769. https://doi.org/10.1200/JCO.2006.07.8972. PMID:17515574.

235. Fanale M, Assouline S, Kuruvilla J, et al. Phase IA/II, multicentre, open-label study of the CD40 antagonistic monoclonal antibody lucatumumab in adult patients with advanced non-Hodgkin or Hodgkin lymphoma. *Br J Haematol.* January 2014;164(2):258—265. https://doi.org/10.1111/bjh.12630. PMID: 24219359.

236. Pro B, Advani R, Brice P, et al. Five-year results of brentuximab vedotin in patients with relapsed or refractory systemic anaplastic large cell lymphoma. *Blood.* July 26, 2018;132(4):458—459. https://doi.org/10.1182/blood-2018-05-853192. PMID:30049735.

237. Schmid P, Adams S, Rugo HS, et al. Atezolizumab and Nab-paclitaxel in advanced triple-negative breast cancer. *N Engl J Med.* 2018;379:2108—2121. https://doi.org/10.1056/NEJMoa1809615. Available at: https://www.nejm.org/doi/full/10.1056/NEJMoa1809615.

238. Adams S, Diamond JR, Hamilton E, et al. Atezolizumab Plus nab-Paclitaxel in the treatment of metastatic triple-negative breast cancer with 2-year survival follow-up a phase 1b clinical trial. *JAMA Oncol.* October 19, 2018. https://doi.org/10.1001/jamaoncol.2018.5152 [Epub ahead of print]. PMID:30347025.

239. Cremolini C, Loupakis F, Antoniotti C, et al. FOLFOXIRI plus bevacizumab versus FOLFIRI plus bevacizumab as first-line treatment of patients with metastatic colorectal cancer: updated overall survival and molecular subgroup analyses of the open-label, phase 3 TRIBE study. *Lancet Oncol.* 2015;16:1306—1315. Available at: https://doi.org/10.1016/S1470-2045(15)00122-9.

240. HIGHLIGHTS OF PRESCRIBING INFORMATION; AVASTIN (bevacizumab) injection, for intravenous use; Initial U.S. Approval: 2004 Revised 12/2017; Available at: https://www.accessdata.fda.gov/drugsatfda_docs/label/2017/125085s319lbl.pdf.

241. Inman BA, Longo TA, Ramalingam S, et al. Atezolizumab: a PD-L1—blocking antibody for bladder cancer. *Clin Cancer Res.* 2017;23:1886—1890. https://doi.org/10.1158/1078-0432.CCR-16-1417. Published OnlineFirst November 30, 2016. PMID:27903674.

242. Petrylak DP, Powles T, Bellmunt J, et al. Atezolizumab (MPDL3280A) monotherapy for patients with metastatic urothelial cancer long-term outcomes from a phase 1 study. *JAMA Oncol.* April 1, 2018;4(4):537—544. https://doi.org/10.1001/jamaoncol.2017.5440. PMID: 29423515.

243. Horn L, Spigel DR, Vokes EE, et al. Nivolumab versus docetaxel in previously treated patients with advanced non-small-cell lung cancer: two-year outcomes from two randomized, open-label, phase III trials (CheckMate 017 and CheckMate 057). *J Clin Oncol.* 2017;35:3924—3933. Available at: DOI: https://doi.org/10.1200/JCO.2017.74.3062.

244. Hodi FS, Chiarion-Sileni V, Gonzalez R, et al. Nivolumab plus ipilimumab or nivolumab alone versus ipilimumab alone in advanced melanoma (CheckMate 067): 4-year outcomes of a multicentre, randomised, phase 3 trial. *Lancet Oncol.* 2018;19(11):1480—1492. https://doi.org/10.1016/S1470-2045(18)30700-9. Epub 2018 Oct 22. PMID:30361170.

245. Cella D, Grünwald V, Escudier B, et al. Patient-reported outcomes of patients with advanced renal cell carcinoma treated with nivolumab plus ipilimumab versus sunitinib (CheckMate 214): a randomised, phase 3 trial. *Lancet Oncol.* February 2019;20(2):297—310. https://doi.org/10.1016/S1470-2045(18)30778-2. Epub 2019 Jan 15. PMID:30658932.

246. Coleman RL, Brady MF, Herzog TJ, et al. Bevacizumab and paclitaxel—carboplatin chemotherapy and secondary cytoreduction in recurrent, platinum-sensitive ovarian cancer (NRG Oncology/Gynecologic Oncology Group study GOG-0213): a multicentre, open-label, randomised, phase 3 trial. *Lancet Oncol.* June 2017;18(6): 779—791. https://doi.org/10.1016/S1470-2045(17)30279-6. Epub 2017 Apr 21. PMID:28438473.

247. Kaufman HL, Russell J, Hamid O, et al. Avelumab in patients with chemotherapy-refractory metastatic Merkel cell carcinoma: a multicentre, single-group, open-label, phase 2 trial. *Lancet Oncol.* October 2016;17(10): 1374—1385. https://doi.org/10.1016/S1470-2045(16)30364-3. Epub 2016 Sep 1. PMID:27592805.

248. HIGHLIGHTS OF PRESCRIBING INFORMATION; BAVENCIO (avelumab) injection, for intravenous use Initial U.S. Approval: 2017. Revised 3/2017; Available at:: https://www.accessdata.fda.gov/drugsatfda_docs/label/2017/761049s000lbl.pdf.

249. NIH: National Library of Medicine at Clinicaltrials.gov for 175 Studies found for: Avelumab; Also searched for MSB0010718C and Bavencio. See search details available at: https://clinicaltrials.gov/ct2/results?cond=&term=Avelumab&cntry=&state=&city=&dist=.

250. Ploessl C, Pan A, Maples KT, et al. Dinutuximab: an anti-GD2 monoclonal antibody for high-risk neuroblastoma. *Ann Pharmacother.* May 2016;50(5):416—422. https://doi.org/10.1177/1060028016632013. Epub 2016 Feb 25. PMID:26917818.

251. Dhillon S. Dinutuximab: first global approval. *Drugs.* May 2015;75(8):923—927. https://doi.org/10.1007/s40265-015-0399-5. PMID:25940913.

252. Diaz RJ, Ali S, Qadir MG, et al. The role of bevacizumab in the treatment of glioblastoma. *J Neuro Oncol.* July 2017; 133(3):455—467. https://doi.org/10.1007/s11060-017-2477-x. Epub 2017 May 19. PMID:28527008.

253. NIH: National Library of Medicine at Clinicaltrials.gov Clinical trial; Anti-LAG-3 Alone & in Combination w/Nivolumab Treating Patients w/Recurrent GBM (Anti-CD137 Arm Closed 10/16/18) Available at: https://www.clinicaltrials.gov/ct2/show/NCT02658981?term=BMS-986016&rank=7.

254. Lee SJ, Lee SY, Lee WS, et al. Phase I trial and pharmacokinetic study of tanibirumab, a fully human monoclonal antibody to vascular endothelial growth factor receptor 2, in patients with refractory solid tumors. *Investig New Drugs.* December 2017;35(6):782—790. https://doi.org/

10.1007/s10637-017-0463-y. Epub 2017 Apr 8. PMID: 28391576.

255. NIH: National Library of Medicine at Clinicaltrials.gov Clinical trial; Trial to Evaluate the Safety of TTAC-0001(Tanibirumab) in Recurrent Glioblastoma. Available at: https://www.clinicaltrials.gov/ct2/show/NCT03033524?term=tanibirumab&rank=2.

256. NIH: National Library of Medicine at Clinicaltrials.gov Clinical trial; TTAC-0001 Phase II Trial With Recurrent Glioblastoma Progressed on Bevacizumab. Available at: https://www.clinicaltrials.gov/ct2/show/NCT03856099?term=ttac-0001&rank=1.

257. Seimetz D, Lindhofer H, Bokemeyer C. Development and approval of the trifunctional antibody catumaxomab (anti-EpCAM anti-CD3) as a targeted cancer immunotherapy. *Cancer Treat Rev.* October 2010;36(6): 458–467. https://doi.org/10.1016/j.ctrv.2010.03.001. Epub 2010 Mar 27. Review. PMID:20347527.

258. Seimetz D. Novel monoclonal antibodies for cancer treatment: the trifunctional antibody catumaxomab (Removab). *J Cancer.* 2011;2:309–316. Epub 2011 May 25. PMID:21716847.

259. Fossati M, Buzzonetti A, Monego G, et al. Immunological changes in the ascites of cancer patients after intraperitoneal administration of the bispecific antibody catumaxomab (anti-EpCAM × anti-CD3). *Gynecol Oncol.* August 2015;138(2):343–351. https://doi.org/10.1016/j.ygyno.2015.06.003. Epub 2015 Jun 3. PMID:26049121.

260. Removab Catumaxomab Product Monograph from Fresnius Biotech. Available at: https://hemonc.org/docs/packageinsert/catumaxomab.pdf.

261. HIGHLIGHTS OF PRESCRIBING INFORMATION: LIBTAYO (cemiplimab-rwlc) injection, for intravenous use Initial U.S. Approval: 09/2018 Last Revised 9/2018 Available at: https://www.accessdata.fda.gov/drugsatfda_docs/label/2018/761097s000lbl.pdf.

262. Migden MR, Rischin D, Schmults CD, et al. PD-1 blockade with cemiplimab in advanced cutaneous squamous-cell carcinoma. *N Engl J Med.* July 26, 2018;379(4):341–351. https://doi.org/10.1056/NEJMoa1805131. Epub 2018 Jun 4. PMID:29863979.

263. Lee MJ, Parker CE, Taylor SR, et al. Efficacy of medical therapies for fistulizing Crohn's disease: systematic review and meta-analysis. *Clin Gastroenterol Hepatol.* 2018; 16:1879–1892. Available at: https://doi.org/10.1016/j.cgh.2018.01.030.

264. Trigo-Vicente C, Gimeno-Ballester V, García-López S, et al. Systematic review and network meta-analysis of treatment for moderate-to-severe ulcerative colitis. *Int J Clin Pharm.* 2018;40:1411–1419. Available at: https://doi.org/10.1007/s11096-018-0743-4.

265. HIGHLIGHTS OF PRESCRIBING INFORMATION: HUMIRA (adalimumab) injection, for subcutaneous use. Initial U.S. Approval: 2002 Revised 1/2019. Available at: https://www.rxabbvie.com/pdf/humira.pdf.

266. Hanauer SB, Sandborn WJ, Rutgeerts P, et al. Human anti−tumor necrosis factor monoclonal antibody (adalimumab) in Crohn's disease: the CLASSIC-I trial.

Gastroenterology. February 2006;130(2):323–333. PMID: 16472588.

267. Lee SD, Rubin DT, Sandborn WJ, et al. Reinduction with certolizumab pegol in patients with Crohn's disease experiencing disease exacerbation: 7-year Data from the PRECiSE 4 study. *Inflamm Bowel Dis.* August 2016;22(8):1870–1880. https://doi.org/10.1097/MIB.0000000000000805. PMID:27400222.

268. Winter TA, Wright J, Ghosh S, et al. Intravenous CDP870, a PEGylated Fab' fragment of a humanized antitumour necrosis factor antibody, in patients with moderate-to-severe Crohn's disease: an exploratory study. *Aliment Pharmacol Ther.* December 2004;20(11−12):1337–1346. PMID:15606396.

269. Sandborn WJ, Lee SD, Randall C, et al. Long-term safety and efficacy of certolizumab pegol in the treatment of Crohn's disease: 7-year results from the PRECiSE 3 study. *Aliment Pharmacol Ther.* October 2014;40(8): 903–916. https://doi.org/10.1111/apt.12930. Epub 2014 Aug 22. PMID:25146586.

270. Colombel JF, Sands BE, Rutgeerts P, et al. The safety of vedolizumab for ulcerative colitis and Crohn's disease. *Gut.* May 2017;66(5):839–851. https://doi.org/10.1136/gutjnl-2015-311079. Epub 2016 Feb 18. PMID:26893500.

271. Rosario M, Dirks NL, Milch C, et al. A review of the clinical pharmacokinetics, pharmacodynamics, and immunogenicity of vedolizumab. *Clin Pharmacokinet.* November 2017;56(11):1287–1301. https://doi.org/10.1007/s40262-017-0546-0. Review. PMID:28523450.

272. Inokuchi T, Takahashi S, Hiraoka S. Long-term outcomes of patients with Crohn's disease who received infliximab or adalimumab as the first-line biologics. *J Gastroenterol Hepatol.* February 6, 2019. https://doi.org/10.1111/jgh.14624 [Epub ahead of print]. PMID:30724387.

273. Nelson SML, Nguyen TM, McDonald JWD, et al. Natalizumab for induction of remission in Crohn's disease (Review). *Cochrane Database Syst Rev.* 2018;(8):CD006097. https://doi.org/10.1002/14651858.CD006097.pub3. PMID:30068022.

274. HIGHLIGHTS OF PRESCRIBING INFORMATION: TYSABRI (natalizumab) injection, for intravenous use Initial U.S. Approval: 2004 Revised 4/2018. Available at: https://www.tysabri.com/content/dam/commercial/multiple-sclerosis/tysabri/pat/en_us/pdfs/tysabri-prescribing_information.pdf.

275. Lebwohl M, Strober B, Menter A, et al. Phase 3 studies comparing brodalumab with ustekinumab in psoriasis. *N Engl J Med.* October 2015;373(14):1318–1328. https://doi.org/10.1056/NEJMoa1503824. PMID: 26422722.

276. HIGHLIGHTS OF PRESCRIBING INFORMATION: SILIQ (brodalumab) injection, for subcutaneous use. Initial U.S. Approval: 2017 Revised 2/2017. Available at: https://www.accessdata.fda.gov/drugsatfda_docs/label/2017/761032lbl.pdf.

277. Blair HA, Deeks ED. Abatacept: a review in rheumatoid arthritis. *Drugs.* July 2017;77(11):1221–1233. https://

doi.org/10.1007/s40265-017-0775-4. Review. PMID: 28608166.

278. Goldzweig O, Hashkes PJ. Abatacept in the treatment of polyarticular JIA: development, clinical utility, and place in therapy. *Drug Des Dev Ther*. January 26, 2011;5: 61–70. https://doi.org/10.2147/DDDT.S16489. PMID: 21340039.

279. HIGHLIGHTS OF PRESCRIBING INFORMATION: ORENCIA (abatacept) for injection for intravenous use injection, for subcutaneous use. Initial U.S. Approval: 2005 Revised 12/2013. Available at: https://www.accessdata.fda.gov/drugsatfda_docs/label/2013/125118s171lbl.pdf.

280. Ruiz Garcia V, Burls A, Cabello JB, et al. Certolizumab pegol (CDP870) for rheumatoid arthritis in adults (Review). *Cochrane Database Syst Rev*. 2017;(9): CD007649. https://doi.org/10.1002/14651858.CD007649.pub4. PMID:28884785.

281. Navarra SV, Guzmán RM, Gallacher AE, et al. Efficacy and safety of belimumab in patients with active systemic lupus erythematosus: a randomised, placebo-controlled, phase 3 trial. *Lancet*. 2011;377:721–731. https://doi.org/10.1016/S0140-6736(10)61354-2. Epub 2011 Feb 4. PMID:21296403.

282. Chao YS, Adcock L. *CADTH RAPID RESPONSE REPORT: Belimumab Treatment for Adults with Systemic Lupus Erythematosus: A Review of Clinical Effectiveness, Cost-Effectiveness, and Guidelines*. Ottawa: CADTH; May 2018 (CADTH rapid response report: summary with critical appraisal). Publication Date: May 23, 2018. Available at: https://www.cadth.ca/sites/default/files/pdf/htis/2018/RC0989%20Benlysta%20for%20Lupus%20Final.pdf.

283. Sciascia S, Radin M, Yazdany J, et al. Efficacy of belimumab on renal outcomes in patients with systemic lupus erythematosus: a systematic review. *Autoimmun Rev*. March 2017;16 3:287–293. https://doi.org/10.1016/j.autrev.2017.01.010. Epub 2017 Jan 29. PMID: 28147262.

284. Usta C, Turgut NT, Bedel A. How abciximab might be clinically useful. *Int J Cardiol*. November 1, 2016;222: 1074–1078. https://doi.org/10.1016/j.ijcard.2016.07.213. Epub 2016 Aug 4. Review. PMID:27519521.

285. Hovingh GK, Guyton JR, Langslet G, et al. Alirocumab dosing patterns during 40 months of open-label treatment in patients with heterozygous familial hypercholesterolemia. *J Clin Lipidol*. 2018 Nov - Dec; 12(6):1463–1470. https://doi.org/10.1016/j.jacl.2018.08.011. Epub 2018 Aug 30. PMID:30287210.

286. Shahawy ME, Cannon CP, Blom DJ, et al. Efficacy and safety of alirocumab versus ezetimibe over 2 years (from ODYSSEY COMBO II). *Am J Cardiol*. September 15, 2017;120(6):931–939. https://doi.org/10.1016/j.amjcard.2017.06.023. Epub 2017 Jun 28. PMID: 28750828.

287. HIGHLIGHTS OF PRESCRIBING INFORMATION: PRALUENT (alirocumab) injection, for subcutaneous use. Initial U.S. Approval: 2015. Revised: 12/2018. Available at: http://products.sanofi.us/praluent/praluent.pdf.

288. Sabatine MS, Giugliano RP, Keech AC, et al. Evolocumab and clinical outcomes in patients with cardiovascular disease. *N Engl J Med*. 2017;376:1713–1722. https://doi.org/10.1056/NEJMoa161566. PMID: 28304224.

289. HIGHLIGHTS OF PRESCRIBING INFORMATION: REPATHA (evolocumab) injection, for subcutaneous use. Initial U.S. Approval: 2015 Revised 12/2017. Available at: https://www.accessdata.fda.gov/drugsatfda_docs/label/2017/125522s013lbl.pdf.

290. Kastelein JJP, Nissen SE, Rader DJ, et al. Safety and efficacy of LY3015014, a monoclonal antibody to proprotein convertase subtilisin/kexin type 9 (PCSK9): a randomized, placebo-controlled Phase 2 study. *Eur Heart J*. May 1, 2016;37(17):1360–1369. https://doi.org/10.1093/eurheartj/ehv707. Epub 2016 Jan 12. PMID:26757788.

291. Ridker PM, Rose LM, Kastelein JJP, et al. Cardiovascular event reduction with PCSK9 inhibition among 1578 patients with familial hypercholesterolemia: results from the SPIRE randomized trials of bococizumab. *J Clin Lipidol*. 2018 Jul - Aug;12(4):958–965. https://doi.org/10.1016/j.jacl.2018.03.088. Epub 2018 Apr 3. PMID:29685591.

292. Coles AJ, Cohen JA, Fox EJ, et al. Alemtuzumab CARE-MS II 5-year follow-up: efficacy and safety findings. *Neurology*. September 12, 2017;89(11):1117–1126. https://doi.org/10.1212/WNL.0000000000004354. Epub 2017 Aug 23. PMID:28835403.

293. Montalban X, Hauser SL, Kappos L, et al. Ocrelizumab versus placebo in primary progressive multiple sclerosis. *N Engl J Med*. January 19, 2017;376(3): 209–220. https://doi.org/10.1056/NEJMoa1606468. Epub 2016 Dec 21. PMID:28002688.

294. Voortman MM, Greiner P, Moser D, et al. The effect of disease modifying therapies on CD62L expression in multiple sclerosis. *Mult Scler J Exp Transl Clin*. September 20, 2018;4(3). https://doi.org/10.1177/2055217318800810. eCollection 2018 Jul-Sep, 2055217318800810. PMID:30263146.

295. HIGHLIGHTS OF PRESCRIBING INFORMATION: TYSABRI (natalizumab) injection, for intravenous use. Initial U.S. Approval: 2004. Revised on 1/2012. Available at: https://www.accessdata.fda.gov/drugsatfda_docs/label/2012/125104s0576lbl.pdf.

296. Guo X, Higgs BW, Bay-Jensen AC, et al. Suppression of T cell activation and collagen accumulation by an anti-FNAR1 mAb, Anifrolumab, in adult patients with systemic sclerosis. *J Investig Dermatol*. October 2015; 135(10):2402–2409. https://doi.org/10.1038/jid.2015.188. Epub 2015 May 20. PMID:25993119.

297. NIH: National Library of Medicine at Clinicaltrials.gov Clinical trial; A study to assess the safety and efficacy of elezanumab when added to standard of care in relapsing forms of multiple sclerosis. Available at: https://www.clinicaltrials.gov/ct2/show/NCT03737851?term=elezanumab&rank=1.

298. Agius MA, Klodowska-Duda G, Maciejowski M, et al. Safety and tolerability of inebilizumab (MEDI-551), an anti-CD19 monoclonal antibody, in patients with

relapsing forms of multiple sclerosis: results from a phase 1 randomised, placebo-controlled, escalating intravenous and subcutaneous dose study. *Mult Scler.* February 2019;25(2):235–245. https://doi.org/10.1177/13524 58517740641. Epub 2017 Nov 16. PMID:29143550.

299. Constantinescu CS, Asher A, Fryze W, et al. Randomized phase 1b trial of MOR103, a human antibody to GM-CSF, in multiple sclerosis. *Neurol Neuroimmunol Neuroinflamm.* May 21, 2015;2(4):e117. https://doi.org/10.1212/NXI.0000000000000117. eCollection 2015 Aug. PMID:26185773.

300. NIH: National Library of Medicine at Clinicaltrialsgov Clinical trial; A Phase 3, Randomized, Multi-center, Double-blinded, Active-controlled Study to Assess the Efficacy and Safety/Tolerability of Ublituximab (TG-1101; UTX) as Compared to Teriflunomide in Subjects With Relapsing Multiple Sclerosis (RMS) (ULTIMATE 1). Available at: https://www.clinicaltrials.gov/ct2/show/NCT03 277261?term=ublituximab&rank=3.

301. Connick P, De Angelis F, Parker RA, et al. Multiple Sclerosis-Secondary Progressive Multi-Arm Randomisation Trial (MSSMART): a multi-arm phase IIb randomised, double-blind, placebo controlled clinical trial comparing the efficacy of three neuroprotective drugs in secondary progressive multiple sclerosis. *BMJ Open.* August 30, 2018;8(8):e021944. https://doi.org/10.1136/bmjopen-2018-021944. PMID:30166303.

302. Cadavid D, Balcer L, Galetta S, et al. Safety and efficacy of opicinumab in acute optic neuritis (RENEW): a randomised, placebo-controlled, phase 2 trial. *Lancet Neurol.* March 2017;16(3):189–199. https://doi.org/10.1016/S1474-4422(16)30377-5. Epub 2017 Feb 15. PMID:28229892.

303. Bleecker ER, FitzGerald JM, Chanez P, et al. Efficacy and safety of benralizumab for patients with severe asthma uncontrolled with high-dosage inhaled corticosteroids and long-acting β2-agonists (SIROCCO): a randomised, multicentre, placebo-controlled phase 3 trial. *Lancet.* October 29, 2016;388(10056):2115–2127. https://doi.org/10.1016/S0140-6736(16)31324-1. Epub 2016 Sep 5. PMID:27609408.

304. HIGHLIGHTS OF PRESCRIBING INFORMATION: DUPIXENT (dupilumab) injection, for subcutaneous use Initial U.S. Approval: 2017 Last revised: 3/2017.Available at: https://www.accessdata.fda.gov/drugsatfda_docs/label/2017/761055lbl.pdf.

305. Duggan S. Caplacizumab: first global approval. *Drugs.* October 2018;78(15):1639–1642. https://doi.org/10.1007/s40265-018-0989-0. Erratum in: Drugs. 2018 Dec;78 (18): 1955. PMID:30298461.

306. Peyvandi F, Scully M, Hovinga JAK, et al. Caplacizumab reduces the frequency of major thromboembolic events, exacerbations and death in patients with acquired thrombotic thrombocytopenic purpura. *J Thromb Haemost.* July 2017;15(7):1448–1452. https://doi.org/10.1111/jth.13716. Epub 2017 Jun 5. PMID:28445600.

307. Peyvandi F, Scully M, Hovinga JAK, et al. Caplacizumab for acquired thrombotic thrombocytopenic purpura.

N Engl J Med. February 11, 2016;374(6):511–522. https://doi.org/10.1056/NEJMoa1505533. PMID:26863353.

308. Scully M, Cataland SR, Peyvandi F, et al. Caplacizumab treatment for acquired thrombotic thrombocytopenic purpura. *N Engl J Med.* January 24, 2019;380(4):335–346. https://doi.org/10.1056/NEJMoa1806311. Epub 2019 Jan 9. PMID:30625070.

309. Ataga KI, Kutlar A, Kanter J, et al. Crizanlizumab for the prevention of pain crises in sickle cell disease. *N Engl J Med.* February 2, 2017;376(5):429–439. https://doi.org/10.1056/NEJMoa1611770. Epub 2016 Dec 3. PMID:27959701.

310. NIH: National Library of Medicine at Clinicaltrials.gov Clinical trial; Study of Dose Confirmation and Safety of Crizanlizumab in Pediatric Sickle Cell Disease Patients. Available at: https://clinicaltrials.gov/ct2/show/NCT03474965?term=crizanlizumab&rank=1.

311. Johnson S, Gerding DN. Bezlotoxumab. *Clin Infect Dis.* February 1, 2019;68(4):699–704. https://doi.org/10.1093/cid/ciy577. PMID:30020417.

312. Navalkele BD, Chopra T. Bezlotoxumab: an emerging monoclonal antibody therapy for prevention of recurrent *Clostridium difficile* infection. *Biologics.* January 18, 2018;12:11–21. https://doi.org/10.2147/BTT.S127099. eCollection 2018. Review. PMID:29403263.

313. Simões EAF, Bont L, Manzoni P, et al. Past, present and future approaches to the prevention and treatment of respiratory syncytial virus infection in children. *Infect Dis Ther.* March 2018;7(1):87–120. https://doi.org/10.1007/s40121-018-0188-z. Epub 2018 Feb 22. Review. PMID:29470837.

314. Tripp RA, Power UF, Openshaw PJM, et al. Respiratory syncytial virus: targeting the G protein provides a new approach for an old problem. *J Virol.* January 17, 2018;92(3):e01302–e01317. https://doi.org/10.1128/JVI.01302-17. Print 2018 Feb 1. PMID:29118126.

315. NIH: National Library of Medicine at Clinicaltrials.gov Clinical trial; 155 Studies found for: basiliximab. Available at: https://clinicaltrials.gov/ct2/results?cond=&term=basiliximab&cntry=&state=&city=&dist= .

316. Sun ZJ, Du X, Su LL, et al. Efficacy and safety of basiliximab versus daclizumab in kidney transplantation: a meta-analysis. *Transplant Proc.* October 2015;47(8):2439–2445. https://doi.org/10.1016/j.transproceed.2015.08.009. PMID: 26518947.

317. Rostainga L, Salibab F, Calmusc Y, et al. Review article: use of induction therapy in liver transplantation. *Transplant Rev.* October 2012;26(4):246–260. https://doi.org/10.1016/j.trre.2012.06.002. Epub 2012 Aug 3. Review. PMID:22863028.

318. Kittipibul V, Tantrachoti P, Ongcharit P, et al. Low- dose basiliximab induction therapy in heart transplantation. *Clin Transplant.* December 2017;31(12). https://doi.org/10.1111/ctr.13132. Epub 2017 Nov 3. PMID:28990220.

319. Butts RJ, Dipchand AI, Sutcliffe D, et al. Comparison of basiliximab vs antithymocyte globulin for induction in pediatric heart transplant recipients: an analysis of the

International Society for Heart and Lung Transplantation database. *Pediatr Transplant*. June 2018;22(4):e13190. https://doi.org/10.1111/petr.13190. PMID:29878688.

320. Kutilek S. Burosumab: a new drug to treat hypophosphatemic rickets. *Sudan J Paediatr*. 2017;17(2):71−73. https://doi.org/10.24911/SJP.2017.2.11.   PMID: 29545670.

321. Insogna KL, Briot K, Imel EA, et al. A randomized, double-blind, placebo-controlled, phase 3 trial evaluating the efficacy of burosumab, an anti-FGF23 antibody, in adults with X-linked hypophosphatemia: week 24 primary analysis. *J Bone Miner Res*. August 2018;33(8): 1383−1393. https://doi.org/10.1002/jbmr.3475. Epub 2018 Jun 26. PMID:29947083.

322. Cummings SR, San Martin J MD, McClung MR, et al. Denosumab for prevention of fractures in postmenopausal women with osteoporosis. *N Engl J Med*. August 20, 2009;361(8):756−765. https://doi.org/10.1056/NEJMoa0809493. Epub 2009 Aug 11. Erratum in: N Engl J Med. 2009 Nov 5; 361(19): 1914. PMID:19671655.

323. Zaheer S, LeBoff M, Lewiecki EM. Denosumab for the treatment of osteoporosis. *Expert Opin Drug Metabol Toxicol*.   March   2015;11(3):461−470.   https://doi.org/ 10.1517/17425255.2015.1000860. Epub 2015 Jan 22. PMID:25614274.

324. Deeks ED. Denosumab: a review in postmenopausal osteoporosis. *Drugs   Aging*.   February   2018;35(2): 163−173. https://doi.org/10.1007/s40266-018-0525-7. Review. Erratum in: Drugs Aging. 2018 Mar 9. PMID: 29435849.

325. Gül G, Sendur MAN, Aksoy S, et al. A comprehensive review of denosumab for bone metastasis in patients with solid tumors. *Curr Med Res Opin*. 2016;32(1):133−145. https://doi.org/10.1185/03007995.2015.1105795. Epub 2015 Nov 25. Review. PMID:26451465.

326. Raje N, Terpos E, Willenbacher W, et al. Denosumab versus zoledronic acid in bone disease treatment of newly diagnosed multiple myeloma: an international, double-blind, double-dummy, randomised, controlled, phase 3 study.   *Lancet   Oncol*.   March   2018;19(3):370−381. https://doi.org/10.1016/S1470-2045(18)30072-X. Epub 2018 Feb 9. PMID:29429912.

327. Dugel PU, Jaffe GJ, Sallstig P, et al. Brolucizumab versus Aflibercept in participants with neovascular age-related macular degeneration: a randomized trial. *Ophthalmology*. September   2017;124(9):1296−1304.   https://doi.org/ 10.1016/j.ophtha.2017.03.057. Epub 2017 May 24. PMID:28551167.

328. HIGHLIGHTS OF PRESCRIBING INFORMATION: ILARIS (canakinumab) injection, for subcutaneous use. Initial U.S. Approval: 2009. Last revised 12/2016. Available   at: https://www.pharma.us.novartis.com/sites/ www.pharma.us.novartis.com/files/ilaris.pdf.

329. Katoh M. Multi-layered prevention and treatment of chronic inflammation, organ fibrosis and cancer associated with canonical WNT/β-catenin signaling activation (Review). *Int J Mol Med*. August 2018;42(2):713−725.

https://doi.org/10.3892/ijmm.2018.3689.   Epub   2018 May 17. PMID:29786110.

330. KATOH M, Katoh M. Molecular genetics and targeted therapy of WNT-related human diseases (Review). *Int J Mol Med*. September 2017;40(3):587−606. https:// doi.org/10.3892/ijmm.2017.3071. Epub 2017 Jul 19. PMID:28731148.

331. Department of Health and Human Services. *Food and Drug Administration, Center for Biologics Evaluation and Research (CBER). Guidance for Industry. Revised Preventive Measures to Reduce the Possible Risk of Transmission of Creutzfeldt-Jacob Disease (CJD) and Variant Creutzfeldt-Jacob Disease (vCJD) by Blood and Blood Products*. January 2002. From the US Food and Drug Administration (FDA) website.

FURTHER READING

1. Centers for Disease Control Immunization Practices Advisory Committee (ACIP). Diphtheria, tetanus, and pertussis: recommendations for vaccine use and other preventive measures. *MMWR Recomm Rep (Morb Mortal Wkly Rep)*. 1991;40(RR-10):1−28.

2. Centers for Disease Control. Update on adult immunization: recommendations of the immunization practices advisory committee (ACIP). *MMWR Recomm Rep (Morb Mortal Wkly Rep)*. 1991;40(RR-12), 18,49,70,87.

3. Kretsinger K, Broder KR, Cortese MM, et al. Preventing tetanus, diphtheria, and pertussis among adults: use of tetanus toxoid, reduced diphtheria toxoid and acellular pertussis vaccine recommendations of the Advisory Committee on Immunization Practices (ACIP) and recommendation of ACIP, supported by the Healthcare Infection Control Practices Advisory Committee (HICPAC), for use of Tdap among health-care personnel. *MMWR Recomm Rep (Morb Mortal Wkly Rep)*. 2006;55:1−37.

4. Broder KR, Cortese MM, Iskander JK, et al. Preventing tetanus, diphtheria, and pertussis among adolescents: use of tetanus toxoid, reduced diphtheria toxoid and acellular pertussis vaccines recommendations of the Advisory Committee on Immunization Practices (ACIP). *MMWR Recomm Rep (Morb Mortal Wkly Rep)*. 2006;55:1−34.

5. Snydman DR, Werner BG, Dougherty NN, et al. Cytomegalovirus immune globulin prophylaxis in liver transplantation: a randomized, double-blind, placebo-controlled trial. *Ann Intern Med*. 1993;119:984−991.

6. Bowden RA, Sayers M, Flournoy N, et al. Cytomegalovirus immune globulin and seronegative blood products to prevent primary cytomegalovirus infection after marrow transplantation. *N Engl J Med*. 1986;314:1006−1010.

7. Mair-Jenkins J, Saavedra-Campos M, Baillie JK, et al. The effectiveness of convalescent plasma and hyperimmune immunoglobulin for the treatment of severe acute respiratory infections of viral etiology: a systematic review and exploratory meta-analysis. *J Infect Dis*. 2015;211:80−90.

8. US Food and Drug Administration. *Guidance for Industry Influenza: Developing Drugs for Treatment And/or Prophylaxis*. Silver Spring, MD: US Food and Drug Administration; 2011.

9. Ohmit SE, Petrie JG, Cross RT, Johnson E, Monto AS. Influenza hemagglutination-inhibition antibody titer as a correlate of vaccine-induced protection. *J Infect Dis.* 2011;204:1879—1885.

10. Arnon SS, Schechter R, Inglesby TV, et al. for the Working Group on Civilian Biodefense. Botulinum toxin as a biologic weapon: medical and public health management. *J Am Med Assoc.* 2001;285:1059—1070.

CHAPTER 17

Chimeric Antigen Receptor Therapies

LISA SENZEL, MD, PHD • TAHMEENA AHMED, MBBS • YUPO MA, MD, PHD

INTRODUCTION

Chimeric antigen receptor (CAR) T cells directed against CD19 for advanced acute lymphoblastic leukemia represent the first form of gene-transfer therapy to gain commercial approval by the FDA.[1] CARs are synthetic receptors that retarget and reprogram T cells to target cell-surface antigens independent of HLA.[2] Following the transfer of genes encoding engineered T-cell receptors, the CAR T cells acquire specificity to a cell-surface molecule. CAR T-cell therapy combines the specificity of an antibody with the cytotoxic and memory functions of T cells.[3] CAR specificity comes from the extracellular domain, which is derived from the antigen-binding site of a monoclonal antibody. A single-chain variable fragment is generated by linking the variable region heavy and light chains. A flexible peptide linker is included, and this extracellular domain is fused to an intracellular domain via a transmembrane sequence. The intracellular domain attempts to recapitulate the normal series of events by which T cells are activated.[3] Once infused, each CAR T cell can kill many tumor cells (illustrated in Fig. 17.1). This chapter will discuss the principles of synthetic immunity, efficacy against various tumor types, role of apheresis in manufacturing the product, toxic effects, tumor antigen escape, other challenges, and potential future applications of CAR T-cell therapy.

VEHICLES FOR DESTRUCTION: CAR DESIGN AND T-CELL ENGINEERING

CARs are expressed from a fusion gene that encodes a T-cell activating domain and immunoglobulin-derived heavy and light chains to direct specificity. Chimeric costimulatory receptors enhance proliferation following repeated exposure to antigen and afford antiapoptotic functions. The CAR transgene can be introduced by retroviral or lentiviral transduction and transcribed off of viral or mammalian promoters in the construct.[4] Transduced T cells can be expanded with cytokines and then reinfused into the patient.

EARLY DAYS: TUMOR-INFILTRATING LYMPHOCYTES REPRESENT THE FIRST ADOPTIVE CELL TRANSFER

Adoptive T-cell transfer (ACT) involves the isolation and reinfusion of tumor-reactive T lymphocytes into cancer patients. In 1988, Rosenberg et al.[5] reported the first clinical study using ACT for the immunotherapy of patients with metastatic melanoma. In this study, tumor-infiltrating lymphocytes (TILs) were isolated from cancer samples, expanded ex vivo in the presence of interleukin (IL)-2, and reinfused back into the same patient. Although objective responses were observed in a majority of patients, the tumor regression was not durable because the transferred T cells failed to engraft and persist in vivo.[6] Subsequently, genes encoding tumor antigen-specific T-cell receptors (TCRs) were cloned into a retroviral vector and transduced into T cells isolated from cancer patients. These TCRs were still major histocompatibility complex (MHC)-restricted and thus required antigen-presenting cells (APCs) to process and present the tumor antigen to TCR-transduced T cells. In contrast, CARs directly recognize and target antigen on the tumor surface and avoid the limitations of MHC restrictions.[6] The first CAR T cells were made by the Israeli immunologist Zelig Eshhar in 1993.[7,8]

TRAGEDY, PERSEVERANCE, AND CHANCE: GETTING CARS STARTED

The first published clinical cases described complete remission of refractory chronic lymphocytic leukemia (CLL) following CAR T-cell infusion at the University of Pennsylvania.[9] Because of the efficacy of novel agents such as ibrutinib, idealisib, and venetoclax for CLL, CAR T-cell investigators turned to other B-cell malignancies.[4] However, the CAR T field nearly died from lack of funding until it was reenergized by the survival of Emily Whitehead.[8]

In 2010, 5-year old Emily Whitehead was diagnosed with B-cell acute lymphoblastic leukemia (ALL). After

Immunologic Concepts in Transfusion Medicine. https://doi.org/10.1016/B978-0-323-67509-3.00017-2

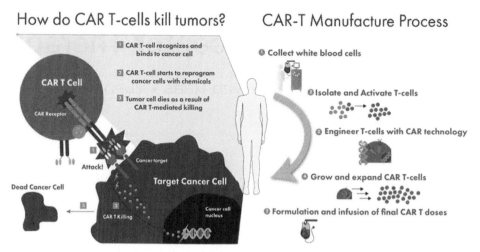

FIG. 17.1 Principles of CAR T therapy and overview of manufacturing process.

two rounds of chemotherapy, necrotizing fasciitis developed in both legs and she barely avoided amputation. Sixteen months later, she had a relapse. One oncologist recommended hospice. Her parents opted to enroll her in a study, and she became the first child to receive CART-19. After receiving her third dose of CART-19, Emily developed high fevers, respiratory failure, and shock necessitating the use of three pressors. Cytokine analysis revealed extremely elevated levels of IL-6. Immunologist Carl June, who had pursued the application of emerging immunologic insights to the development of antitumor therapies following his wife's premature death from ovarian cancer and was overseeing the trial, had an idea.[8] His daughter, who has juvenile rheumatoid arthritis, had recently started taking tocilizumab, a monoclonal antibody that targets IL-6. Within hours of receiving tocilizumab, Emily improved dramatically, and 8 days later, a bone marrow biopsy showed the treatment had worked.

THE FIRST FDA-APPROVED CARS: CD19-DIRECTED CARS FOR B-CELL MALIGNANCIES

FDA approval for Tisagenlecleucel (CTL019, Kymriah, Novartis, Basel, Switzerland) was based on the ELIANA trial in which 68 young patients with refractory or relapsed ALL were treated.[10] Among those, 63 were evaluated for treatment efficacy, with 52 patients (83%) achieving remission at 3 months.[11] At publication of trial results, the median duration of remission had not yet been reached.[11] Axicabtagene ciloleucel (Axi-cel, Yescarta, Kite Pharma/Gilead, Los Angeles, CA) was

approved for adults with refractory or relapsed large B-cell lymphoma based on the ZUMA-1 trial.[12] Of 101 patients who received the drug, 52 patients (51%) achieved complete remission and 21 patients (21%) achieved partial remission. For those with B-ALL, at a median follow-up of 29 months, the median event-free survival was 6.1 months, and median overall survival was 12.9 months.[13] Although CD19 CAR T cells induced initial tumor remission in patients who had failed multiple therapies, relapses occurred in majority of the adults with B-ALL.[6] Tisagenlecleucel gained a second FDA approval for relapsed or refractory large B-cell lymphoma based on the JULIET trial.[14]

LYMPHOCYTE APHERESIS FOR CAR MANUFACTURING

Patients are treated by first collecting autologous T cells via leukocytapheresis, with a goal of around 10^9 T cells, which are then shipped to a manufacturing site. CAR T cells are then manufactured by CD3/CD28 bead stimulation and lentiviral transduction (Tisagenlecleucel) or soluble CD3 antibody/IL-2 stimulation and retroviral transduction (Axicabtagene) with subsequent expansion in a 6–10-day process. An individualized dose (typically $2-4 \times 10^6$ CAR expressing T cells/kg) is then cryopreserved and shipped to the treating facility, where it is infused following a cycle of lymphodepleting chemotherapy consisting of fludarabine and cyclophosphamide.[15] Preinfusion chemotherapy is administered to deplete endogenous T cells that might increase the risk of T-mediated rejection of CAR T cells, and to enhance CAR T expansion in the lymphodepleted host.[16] Preparative lymphodepletion also helps by depleting immunosuppressive regulatory T cells (Tregs), inducing immunogenic cell death and enhancing antigen presentation, and depleting endogenous cells that compete for growth factors or cytokines.[6] Of note, some trials forgo lymphodepletion in patients who are already leukopenic with no evidence of detriment.[17] Fig. 17.1 depicts the process of CAR manufacturing.

Important questions for optimizing T-cell apheresis collections include (1) is there an exact time window for successful collection during the patient's chemotherapy treatment plan, (2) are there tools to ensure or predict an adequate CD3$^+$ collection, and (3) are there effective techniques to isolate T cells from the collected apheresis product.[18] Earlier studies addressing these questions have been published using the COBE Spectra,[19,20] and data using newer apheresis platforms (Spectra Optia [TerumoBCT] and Amicus [Fresenius Kabi]) are anticipated.[18]

TOXIC EFFECTS ASSOCIATED WITH CAR T CELLS: INCIDENTS AND ACCIDENTS ALONG THE ROAD

Many of the toxic effects that are reported with CAR T cells are on-target effects, so they are reversible when the target cell is eliminated or the engraftment of the CAR T cells is terminated.[1] This reversibility contrasts with many of the toxic effects associated with cytotoxic chemotherapy, which are off-target effects. Because of the risk of the cytokine release syndrome and neurologic toxic effects, Tisagenlecleucel and Axicabtagene were FDA-approved contingent with a Risk Evaluation and Mitigation Strategy, whereby the FDA requires that physicians and hospital staff complete training for management of adverse effects.[1]

B-CELL APLASIA

B-cell aplasia occurs with CARs that target B-cell differentiation antigens such as CD19, CD20, and CD22. Clinical experience indicates that the B-cell aplasia induced by CD19 CARs is more complete than that observed after antibody therapy with rituximab. B-cell aplasia is rapidly reversed after CAR T cells are ablated.[1] B-cell aplasia can be managed by periodic immunoglobulin administration.

CYTOKINE RELEASE SYNDROME

In some patients, CAR T cells induce a clinical syndrome of fevers, hypotension, hypoxia, and neurologic changes known as the cytokine release syndrome. In the case of CD19 CARs, the severity of the cytokine release syndrome is associated with tumor burden as measured by blasts in bone marrow at the time of treatment. The cytokine release syndrome manifests with a noninfectious flu-like syndrome and can progress to life-threatening capillary leakage with hypoxia and hypotension. This syndrome is associated with T-cell activation and high levels of cytokines, including IL-6 and interferon-γ. Tocilizumab, an anti-IL-6-receptor antagonist, is usually effective in the management of severe cytokine release syndrome induced by CAR T cells.[1]

NEUROTOXICITY

Neurotoxicity appears to be a class effect with CD19-directed therapies because the same spectrum of toxic effects has been reported with blinatumomab, a bispecific anti-CD19 and anti-CD3 monoclonal antibody. The cause of the neurotoxicity remains unknown; it is usually fully reversible and not related to spread of cancer to the central nervous system. Cerebral edema, sometimes fatal, has been reported some trials.[1] The neurotoxicity syndrome has been termed CAR T-related encephalopathy syndrome.[16]

TUMORS EVADING CARS—THE CHASE IS ON

Despite the high initial response rate with CD19 CAR T cells in ALL, relapses occur in a significant fraction of patients. Relapse with CD19$^+$ leukemia cells can be the result of short in vivo persistence of CAR T cells, either from intrinsic deficiencies of the T-cell product or an immune response to the CAR single-chain variable fragment (scFv). In cases where CAR T cells persist, relapse with leukemia blasts that express little or no surface CD19 molecules can occur. Some CD19$^-$ relapses result from the outgrowth of leukemia cells that express a splice variant of CD19 that lacks the epitope targeted by the scFv.[4] Others involve lineage switch, whereby the evolved leukemic population not only no longer expresses CD19, but also acquires other phenotypic characteristics of myeloid leukemia.[21]

The overall response rate to CD19 CAR T cells in Non-Hodgkin's lymphoma (NHL) is 70%–80%, but the complete remission rate is much lower than that observed in ALL. As with ALL, poor CAR T-cell proliferation and in vivo persistence correlate with incomplete response, and CD19 loss variants have been observed. Additional mechanisms for incomplete tumor eradication are likely operative in NHL. Some tumors express PD-L1 and/or possess cells in the tumor microenvironment that can inhibit the proliferation and effector function of CAR T cells.[4]

ROAD HAZARD: LEUKEMIC CELL EXPRESSES CAR

A case report[22] has described a rare mechanism of fatal relapse following CAR-T therapy. A 20-year-old male patient with B-ALL began to relapse 9 months after receiving the treatment as part of a Phase 1 trial of the then-investigational agent CTL019 (Tisagenlecleucel). The authors excluded several causes of CD19-negativity, including CD19 mutations, CD19 splicing variants, and structural alterations of the B-cell receptor complex. Using a panel of noncross-reactive monoclonal antibodies as well as confocal microscopy, they found that expression of the CAR in *cis* on B-ALL blasts leads to masking of the CAR target epitope. Given that transduction of leukemia cells with a CD22 CAR leads to specific resistance to CD22 and not to CD19 CARs, it is likely that this could be a general mechanism to render any tumor or normal cell specifically resistant to a CAR T cell.

In summary, a CAR gene was unintentionally introduced into a single leukemia cell during the manufacturing process. The cancer cell expressing the receptor was infused back into the patient along with therapeutic CAR T cells, where it multiplied. The CAR expressed by leukemic cells bound the target antigen on the same cells, masking them from CAR-T cells. This conferred resistance, and the patient died of leukemia complications around 20 months after the treatment. The unique case was first reported to a National Institutes of Health advisory committee in 2016. According to a statement provided by Novartis, the company's manufacturing process is different from the academic manufacturing process used in the early trial. Both processes have been improved, and no other such cases have occurred.[23]

OVERCOMING ANTIGEN LOSS

Rather than directing the immune response to a single immunogenic target on B-ALL, the goal of "epitope spreading" is to induce immune responses to coexisting immunogenic targets on tumor cells. It is possible that combining CAR T cells with radiation, checkpoint inhibition, vaccines, or other immune agonists will result in epitope spreading that could help counter immune escape.[21] The CAR molecule itself can also be engineered to recognize multiple antigens. This can be accomplished by linking two binders on a single molecule ("tandem CAR"), which appears, in some cases, to enhance the strength of the immune synapse.[21]

The requirement of high target antigen levels for optimal CAR T-cell activity has limited the efficacy of CAR T cells directed against antigens such as CD22, which is expressed at lower levels than CD19 on B-ALL. One approach to address this limitation is to treat patients with agents that increase expression of the target antigen, such as bryostatin in the case of CD22; alternatively, CARs could be engineered to enhance activity against lower antigen densities, for example by enhancing the affinity of the scFv for its target.[21]

BUILDING A SAFER CAR: SEATBELTS AND AIRBAGS

Modification of the CAR construct to include the inclusion of a suicide gene, such as iCaspase9, or surface tag such as epidermal growth factor receptor, can allow ablation of the CAR T cells in the event of serious toxicity.[24] Ongoing studies aim to elucidate the mechanism of neurotoxicity to design strategies for preventing or treating this complication.[24]

BUILDING A FASTER CAR: SHORTENING THE MANUFACTURING WINDOW

High-grade malignancies do not pause for the several days to weeks needed to expand autologous T cells and engineer them into CAR T cells. One strategy to shorten the window is to target nanoparticles to anti-CD3e f(ab) fragments. Upon binding to CD3 on T cells, the nanoparticles are endocytosed. Their contents, for example a plasmid DNA encoding an antitumor antigen CAR, are directed to the T-cell nucleus via targeting peptides. Inclusion of transposons flanking the CAR gene expression cassette allows for the efficient integration of the CAR vector into chromosomes. This may enable in vivo, nearly instantaneous CAR T-cell production.[25]

TOWARD HIGH-SPEED, ALLOGENEIC CARS: TARGETING A CAR TO THE TCR α-CHAIN CONSTANT REGION

During T-cell development, T cells rearrange gene sequences that encode the TCR so that each T cell expresses a unique TCR that binds a specific antigen. T cells with TCRs that have a high affinity for antigens expressed by the body's own cells (self-antigens) are destroyed to avoid autoimmunity. Attacks on tumors by T cells are usually weak because tumors express self-antigens. When CAR T cells are made by inserting the CAR-encoding gene into T cells without disrupting the resident TCR gene, then the patients' own T cells have to be used to avoid the risk of rejection or graft-versus-host disease (GVHD) when the T cells are transplanted back into the body.[26] This requires collection and processing that can take up to several weeks, which may be too long for some patients to wait.

Eyquem et al.[27] have explored disrupting the resident TCR α-chain constant region (TRAC) sequence when creating CAR T cells, thereby disabling the TCR and enabling a patient to be treated with CAR T cells made from another person's cells. They introduced RNA encoding the DNA-cleaving nuclease enzyme Cas9 into T cells along with an RNA "guide" sequence that targets the TRAC sequence. The Cas9 protein used the RNA guide sequence to create a targeted double-stranded break in the TRAC DNA sequence. A viral vector with a CAR sequence flanked by sequences homologous to the TRAC sequence was introduced into the T cells. The double-stranded break in the TRAC sequence was repaired using the viral vector sequence as a template, resulting in the original TRAC sequences being replaced by the introduced CAR sequences.[26]

Constitutive T-cell activation might cause T-cell exhaustion, a dysfunctional T-cell state characterized by the inability to exert antitumor effects and the expression of some inhibitory receptor proteins such as PD-1. Constitutive signaling might also result in toxicity because of release of immune-signaling molecules such as cytokines.[26] Eyquem et al.[27] demonstrated that integration of a promoter-less CAR into the TRAC sequence results in a more consistent baseline level of CAR expression, more regulated expression of the CAR at both the transcriptional and protein level, and more effective antitumor responses in mouse models of leukemia. CAR expression driven by the natural TCR promoter may avoid constitutive CAR signaling. The targeted nature of their CAR integration might also prove safer than random integration, which carries the potential risk of generating a harmful mutation.[26]

The development of off-the-shelf "universal" CAR T cells is possible with the use of a variety of gene-editing techniques and has been successful in a few children with pre-B-cell ALL with a high degree of immuno-suppression.[28] The major challenge in developing off-the-shelf T cells is avoidance of immune rejection in both host-versus-graft and graft-versus-host directions.[1]

CARS FOR OTHER MALIGNANCIES: NEW TOOLS IN THE CAR TOOLBOX

As mentioned in the Introduction section, the intracellular domain attempts to recapitulate the normal series of events by which T cells are activated. The iterative process of modifying the intracellular domain led to the development of first-, second-, and, third-generation CARs. First-generation CARs consisted of only the TCR complex CD3-ζ chain domain and antigen recognition domains. Second-generation CARs incorporated costimulatory domains, such as CD28 or CD137, to augment CAR T-cell survival and proliferation, leading to increased antitumor activity. Third-generation CARs combined the CD3-ζ domain with additional costimulatory domains.[3] Novel CAR designs, gene editing, chimeric chemokine receptors, chimeric costimulatory receptors, and logic-gated and multispecific receptors represent tools in development for newer generation CAR T therapies.[4] New target molecules include CD30 for Hodgkin lymphoma and anaplastic large-cell lymphoma, SLAMF7 and B-cell maturation antigen (BCMA) for myeloma, and CD123, CD33, Lewis Y, and FOLR2 for acute myeloid leukemia.[2] New costimulatory receptors include PD-1/CD28 and CD200R/CD28.[4]

T-CELL MALIGNANCIES

A challenge with using CARs for T-cell malignancies is the fact that candidate target antigens are also expressed on normal T cells, some of which are used as starting material for CARs. To avoid fratricide, it is necessary to abrogate expression of the target molecule on T cells that are engineered to express the CAR. For example, CRISPR/Cas9-mediated editing has been used to delete CD7 in primary T cells before transduction with a CD7-specific CAR.[29] However, the expected elimination of normal T and NK cells and their progenitors would likely compromise host immunity. Persisting CAR T cells could potentially provide some immune function through their endogenous TCR; however, repertoire diversity would be constrained, and CAR expression may adversely affect TCR signaling.[4]

Fortunately, normal T cells express either one of two TCR β-chain constant regions in a mutually exclusive manner, whereas T-cell malignancies are restricted to one β-chain constant region or the other. CAR T cells can be targeted to only one TCR β-chain constant region, which should leave normal T cells in place that express the alternative TCR β-chain constant region. Maciocia et al.[30] designed CAR T cells that specifically recognized restricted T-cell leukemia and lymphoma cells in xenograft mouse models.

CD37 is present on peripheral T-cell malignancies but does not seem to result in fratricide in CD37 CAR T cells.[31] T cells expressing anti-CD37 CAR showed substantial activity against T-cell lymphomas without fratricide in xenograft models.[32]

MULTIPLE MYELOMA

The tumor necrosis factor receptor family member BCMA is expressed on both plasma cells and myeloma cells but is absent on normal tissues, which distinguishes it from other potential myeloma targets such as CD38 and SLAMF7 that are more widely expressed on blood cells.[4] Early trials have shown promise, despite the observation that BCMA is cleaved by gamma secretase in myeloma cells, leading to variation in surface expression and increased levels of soluble BCMA that can inhibit CAR recognition.

SOLID TUMORS: MANY ROADBLOCKS TO OVERCOME

T cells can eliminate solid tumors, as exemplified by checkpoint therapy and infusions of TILs for advanced cancers, including melanoma, cholangiocarcinoma, and colorectal cancer.[33–35] CAR T therapies are also being tried in the setting of solid tumors.

Brown et al.[36] reported impressive results utilizing IL13R-targeted CAR T cells in a glioblastoma patient. Intracavitary infusion appeared to act locally while intraventricular infusions resulted in a more widespread response. Unfortunately, the initial response was followed by tumor recurrence after 7.5 months at intracranial sites that were different and nonadjacent to the initial tumors. The recurrent tumor had reduced expression of the target antigen, IL13Rα2. Although additional CAR T trials are ongoing in glioblastoma[37] and other solid tumors, challenges abound. One such roadblock is the paucity of suitable cell-surface molecules that are expressed by solid cancers for CARs to target. This can be addressed by engineering T cells with T-cell receptors that recognize tumor-specific antigens derived from intracellular proteins, such as neoantigens arising because of somatic mutations expressed by tumors, which are found in most patients with metastatic epithelial cancers.[38] Other approaches involve modifying the tumor microenvironment.

CAR T CELLS REDIRECTED FOR UNIVERSAL CYTOKINE KILLING

T cells redirected for universal cytokine killings (TRUCKs) are fourth-generation CAR T cells. The goal of the TRUCK concept is to improve control of the tumor microenvironment, which poses more of a barrier in solid tumors than in hematologic malignancies.[39]

TRUCKs can deliver cytokines to kill tumor cells and also recruit an endogenous immune response. CAR T cells have been engineered to express IL-12 through nuclear factor of activated T-cell signaling that is activated upon recognition of the tumor antigen.[40] These CAR T cells deliver IL-12 to the tumor and avoid toxicities that would be caused by systemic IL-12 application. This approach resulted in improved antitumor response via recruitment and activation of innate immune cells, such as antitumor macrophages, to the microenvironment. Infusion of CAR T cells that release IL-18 upon antigen recognition elicited superior tumor control than CAR T cells not engineered to secrete IL-18.[41] IL-18 delivery to the tumor was observed to elicit several antitumor activities, including decreased numbers of immune suppressive cells (Tregs, dendritic cells), increased numbers of antitumor immune cells (macrophages, NK cells), and interruption of immune checkpoint signaling by downregulation of FoxO1 and, subsequently, PD-1 expression on T cells.[39]

The term "armored CARs" similarly refers to CAR T cells that are comodified to express cytokines, ligands, or scFv to elicit an enhanced antitumor immune response through turning a suppressive tumor microenvironment into a proinflammatory one.[42,43] Studies are investigating whether the addition of an IL-12 secretion domain in CAR constructs may also eliminate the requirement for lymphodepletion.[17,44]

DESIGNER CARS: GENOME EDITING

CRISPR-Cas9 has been used to edit CAR T genomes, for example to make CAR T cells less susceptible to the immunosuppressive effects of immune checkpoint by knockout of lymphoid activation gene-3, a negative regulator of T-cell activity.[45] Simultaneous disruption of the endogenous T-cell receptor, β2 microglobulin, and PD-1 resulted in triple knockout CAR T cells with greater anticancer activity and reduced alloreactivity with no evidence of GVHD.[46] Here, stimulated T cells were transduced with lentiviral CAR vectors and then electroporated to deliver Cas9 mRNA and gRNAs. This "hit and run" transient CRISPR-Cas9 approach to disrupt the endogenous T-cell receptor seems to provide a safe means of genome editing, although subsequent T-cell expansion of edited cells was reduced likely due to toxicity of electroporation.[39] The authors caution that deep sequencing of off-target gene disruption should be characterized before conducting human trials, and that careful selection of targeting sequences is essential to minimize the potential of off-target mutations.[46]

In many cases, tumor-specific antigens are intracellular proteins that cannot be targeted by conventional CARs. An approach to circumvent this problem is to use CARs consisting of scFvs to recognize an antigen peptide in association with MHC. Adoptively transferred T cells often suffer from exhaustion and insufficient expansion, in part, because of the immunosuppressive nature of tumor-bearing hosts. Several combinatorial approaches, which include the immune checkpoint blockade, in vivo costimulation, and posttransfer vaccination have been developed.[47,48] One advantage of CARs recognizing the peptide/MHC complex is that there are opportunities for crosspresentation by professional APCs in draining lymph nodes and stromal cells in the tumor, which could facilitate further expansion of transferred CAR-T cells and destruction of stroma in solid tumors leading to more efficient tumor regression. In addition, posttransfer vaccination can be coopted in CAR T-cell therapy targeting peptide/MHC, wherein the forms of antigen and its delivery are of critical importance.[49]

SMART CARS: LOGIC-GATED, REGULATED CARS

Prior strategies to engineer multiinput control of T cells have focused on expressing two CARs in the same cell, each with partial signaling function and distinct extracellular antigen recognition domains.[50,51] Although such cells show enhanced activation when both target antigens are present, success of this approach relies on delicately balancing the same set of coordinated signaling events that occur downstream from the CAR. Thus, behavior is highly dependent on the exact expression ratios and activities of the different receptor chains. Moreover, partial independent function of each receptor inherently limits the dynamic range of this approach—it remains challenging to obtain an AND-gate T cell that is both fully inhibited in the presence of either individual antigen but fully activated in the presence of both antigens.

To construct more reliable multiantigen responses, it would be ideal to have new receptors that function completely independently from the CAR/TCR pathway but that can interface with CAR activity in a controlled manner. Morsut et al.[52] developed a new class of modular receptors called synthetic Notch (synNotch) receptors. SynNotch receptors use an extracellular recognition domain (e.g., scFv) to recognize a target antigen but, different from CARs, binding of the target antigen does not trigger T-cell activation. Instead, ligand engagement leads to cleavage of the receptor and to release of a transcriptional activator domain, which can in turn enter the nucleus and drive expression of user specified target genes. These receptors harness the mechanical activation mechanism of Notch.

Roybal et al.[53] constructed combinatorial antigen recognition T-cell circuits in which a synNotch receptor for one antigen drives the inducible expression of a CAR for a second antigen. These dual-receptor T cells are only armed and activated in the presence of dual antigen tumor cells (AND gate). These combinatorially gated T cells show therapeutic discrimination both in vitro and in vivo—sparing single antigen "bystander" tumors while efficiently eradicating combinatorial antigen "disease" tumors. This type of dual-receptor circuit could lead to precise immune recognition of a larger set of tumors.

SPLIT, UNIVERSAL, AND PROGRAMMABLE CAR: THE SWISS ARMY KNIFE OF CAR

There is a need for a flexible platform that can control T-cell activation with improved precision and tunability to make CAR T-cell therapy safer and more effective. Cho et al.[54] developed a split, universal, and programmable (SUPRA) CAR system composed of a universal receptor expressed on T cells and a tumor-targeting scFv adaptor molecule. The SUPRA CAR is a two-component receptor system composed of a universal receptor (zipCAR) expressed on T cells and a tumor-targeting scFv adaptor (zipFv). The zipCAR universal receptor is generated from the fusion of intracellular signaling domains and a leucine zipper as the extracellular domain. The zipFv adaptor molecule is generated from the fusion of a cognate leucine zipper and a scFv. The scFv of the zipFv binds to the tumor antigen, and the leucine zipper binds and activates the zipCAR on the T cells.

The activity of SUPRA CARs can be regulated via multiple mechanisms to limit overactivation. SUPRA CARs can also logically respond to multiple antigens for improving tumor specificity. The SUPRA CAR system has inducible and logical control capabilities, for example to control cytokine secretion with different zipFv doses and configurations. Their competition-based strategy may improve target specificity by directing the competitive zipFv toward a surface marker for "normal" cells, thus safeguarding them from being targeted by the zipCAR.

USING CARS TO HARNESS THE POWER OF T CELLS IN THE POSTTRANSPLANT SETTING

Therapeutic T-cell administration has been integral to bone marrow transplantation from its inception. Allogeneic hematopoietic cell transplantation (allo-HCT) provides not only hematopoietic rescue following intensive chemotherapy, but also a means to harness the immune system to treat hematologic malignancies in patients who fail to respond to standard chemotherapy. The graft-versus-leukemia effect is primarily mediated by donor T cells present in the graft. The combination of tumor burden reduction and provision of alloreactive T cells can produce remarkable clinical responses, but this intervention comes with a severe risk, that of GVHD. One approach to prevent GVHD is to remove donor T cells from the graft, but at the cost of prolonged T-cell deficiency, increased viral infections, and increased tumor relapse. Many patients with high-risk disease who receive an allo-HCT do not achieve a complete remission posttransplant and, for those who do, the risk of relapse remains high. CAR T cells may help provide a way to access the power of graft-vs-tumor effects while avoiding GVHD.[2]

CARS IN DONOR LEUKOCYTE INFUSIONS

In patients who relapse posttransplant, donor leukocyte infusions (DLI) can be administered with intent to induce an immune-mediated remission. HLA-matched allogeneic CD19 CAR T cells have been infused to patients who relapsed or had not achieved a complete remission after allo-HCT. The donor CD19 CAR T cells were either harvested from the donor or from the recipient. Recipient-derived donor T cells may be expected to carry a lesser risk of acute and chronic GVHD if the CAR T cells are generated from tolerized cells.

Kochenderfer et al.[55] infused donor-derived leukocytes expressing a CD19 CAR to patients with persistent B-cell malignancies following allo-HCT. T cells were administered without additional chemotherapy or lymphodepleting conditioning. Three of 10 patients showed tumor regression without GVHD. In an update to this study, 8 of 20 patients with B-ALL, CLL, or NHL, developed a remission, and few experienced GVHD.[56] In other studies, however, discrepant results regarding GVHD were obtained. Murine studies suggest that different CAR designs providing different strengths of activation may determine whether GVHD develops or not, along with the T-cell subset composition of the CAR-DLI infusion product.[2] GVHD incidence was lower when using recipient-derived rather than donor-derived CAR T cells, suggesting that recipient-derived donor T cells were tolerized. Anwer et al.[57] reported that among 72 patients from seven studies who were treated with donor-derived CAR T cells, only five patients developed GVHD.

CARS IN VIRUS-SPECIFIC T CELLS

Virus-specific T cells directed against CMV, EBV, and adenovirus have been extensively used as prophylaxis or posttransplant antiviral therapy, and EBV-specific T cells have been effective against nasopharyngeal carcinoma and other EBV-associated tumors. Preclinical data with virus-specific T cells suggest that they may serve as an off-the-shelf resource for CAR therapy given that the defined TCR specificity mitigates alloreactivity that could result in GVHD.[58] In a clinical study in which six patients with relapsed B-cell leukemias were infused with donor-derived trispecific virus-specific T cells expressing a CD28-based CD19 CAR following allo-HCT, two of them had an objective antitumor response, whereas the two patients who were treated in relapse remained free of disease.[59]

CAARS: CHIMERIC AUTOANTIBODY RECEPTOR T CELLS FOR AUTOIMMUNE DISEASE

CAR T cells express a recombinant receptor that binds a specific tumor antigen, inducing the cell to kill target tumor cells. Ellebrecht et al.[60] adapted the approach to autoimmune disease. They developed CAAR T cells as an antigen-specific therapy for the autoimmune disease pemphigus vulgaris and showed, both in vitro and in mice, the capacity of the cells to selectively eliminate B lymphocytes that produce autoantibodies to desmoglein (Dsg) 3, the pathogenic mediators of the disease.

Current treatments for autoimmune diseases are based on antiinflammatory and immunosuppressive agents—including engineered biologics; human or humanized monoclonal antibodies; and fusion proteins selective for certain immune cell subsets or signaling pathways—but their effect is transient and not antigen-specific. Chronic administration of these agents leads to the common side effects of general immunosuppression, such as an increased incidence of infections.[61]

Ellebrecht et al.[60] have approached the challenge of antigen-specific therapy by designing a modified form of a CAR that leads T cells to kill autoreactive B cells. A conventional CAR fusion protein consists of an extracellular antibody moiety specific to an antigen of interest linked by a transmembrane domain to an intracellular signaling domain that activates the T cell upon antigen binding. The CAAR design is different in that the extracellular domain includes the autoantigen itself, and the T cell is activated when the autoantigen binds cognate autoantibodies on the surface of pathogenic B cells. Ellebrecht et al.[60] designed a CAAR in which Dsg3, key autoantigen in pemphigus vulgaris, fused to the signaling domains of the T-cell-activating molecules CD3ζ and CD137.

Galy[62] compares their strategy to that of angler fish. In the dark depths of the sea, the angler fish has developed a clever way to lure its prey by dangling a luminous appendix in front of its powerful mouth. Any unfortunate fish trying to eat this bait is quickly eaten in return. For their part, CAAR T cells lure and kill autoreactive B cells by baiting them with their autoantigen.

CAARS FOR WIDESPREAD USE?

Could CAAR T cells be beneficial in other autoantibody-mediated autoimmune diseases? Chatenoud[61] answers tentatively yes, provided that some essential prerequisites are met. First, the pathogenicity of autoantibodies in the disease should be clearly established, as is the case in pemphigus vulgaris. A simple way to approach this question is to consider only autoimmune diseases for which it is proven that autoantibodies can transfer the disease, whether in newborns upon placental transfer during pregnancy or in animal models. Second, the sequence and molecular structure of the autoantigen(s) must be clearly identified to allow engineering of a CAAR expressing the key epitopes recognized by patients' autoantibodies. Chatenoud[61] identifies two diseases that fulfill these conditions: myasthenia gravis and autoantibody-associated neonatal lupus syndrome (also termed congenital heart block), a passively acquired autoimmune condition. This can affect the fetus in pregnant women with various autoimmune diseases, such as systemic lupus erythematosus and Sjögren syndrome. One may hope that significant progress in both defining autoantibody pathogenicity and characterizing the autoantigens will permit the development of new therapies for other autoimmune conditions based on CAARs.

CONCLUSIONS

The genetic modification of T cells to target cancer represents a disruptive new approach to therapy that is now approved for advanced B-cell malignancies. Longer follow-up will determine what fraction of patients achieve durable remissions with current approaches, and ongoing studies of primary and adaptive resistance mechanisms that prevent complete tumor eradication should provide direction for improving outcomes.[4] Although autologous CAR T-cell therapies have immense therapeutic potential, the cost implications and complexity of autologous T-cell therapies remain problematic for broader application. T cells may also be generated from human embryonic stem cells and induced pluripotent stem cells. Thus, the combination of techniques involving induced pluripotent stem cells and synthetic biology may provide an opportunity to generate off-the-shelf T cells that uniquely combine favorable attributes, including antigen specificity, lack of alloreactivity, histocompatibility, and enhanced functional properties.[1]

REFERENCES

1. June CH, Sadelain M. Chimeric antigen receptor therapy. *N Engl J Med*. 2018;379(1):64−73.
2. Smith M, Zakrzewski J, James S, Sadelain M. Posttransplant chimeric antigen receptor therapy. *Blood*. 2018;131(10):1045−1052.
3. Maus MV, Levine BL. Chimeric antigen receptor T-cell therapy for the community oncologist. *Oncol*. 2016;21(5):608−617.
4. Salter AI, Pont MJ, Riddell SR. Chimeric antigen receptor-modified T cells: CD19 and the road beyond. *Blood*. 2018;131(24):2621−2629.
5. Rosenberg SA, Packard BS, Aebersold PM, et al. Use of tumor-infiltrating lymphocytes and interleukin-2 in the immunotherapy of patients with metastatic melanoma. A preliminary report. *N Engl J Med*. 1988;319(25):1676−1680.
6. Ding ZC. The promise and challenges of chimeric antigen receptor T cells in relapsed B-cell acute lymphoblastic leukemia. *Ann Transl Med*. 2018;6(11):235.
7. Kalos M, Levine BL, Porter DL, et al. T cells with chimeric antigen receptors have potent antitumor effects and can establish memory in patients with advanced leukemia. *Sci Transl Med*. 2011;3(95):95ra73.
8. Rosenbaum L. Tragedy, perseverance, and chance - the story of CAR-T therapy. *N Engl J Med*. 2017;377(14):1313−1315.
9. Porter DL, Levine BL, Kalos M, Bagg A, June CH. Chimeric antigen receptor-modified T cells in chronic lymphoid leukemia. *N Engl J Med*. 2011;365(8):725−733.
10. Kuehn BM. The promise and challenges of CAR-T gene therapy. *J Am Med Assoc*. 2017;318(22):2167−2169.
11. Maude SL, Laetsch TW, Buechner J, et al. Tisagenlecleucel in children and young adults with B-cell lymphoblastic leukemia. *N Engl J Med*. 2018;378(5):439−448.
12. Neelapu SS, Locke FL, Bartlett NL, et al. Axicabtagene ciloleucel CAR T-cell therapy in refractory large B-cell lymphoma. *N Engl J Med*. 2017;377(26):2531−2544.
13. Park JH, Riviere I, Gonen M, et al. Long-term follow-up of CD19 CAR therapy in acute lymphoblastic leukemia. *N Engl J Med*. 2018;378(5):449−459.
14. Schuster SJ, Svoboda J, Chong EA, et al. Chimeric antigen receptor T cells in refractory B-cell lymphomas. *N Engl J Med*. 2017;377(26):2545−2554.
15. Boyer MW. Chimeric antigen receptor T-cell therapy hits the market. *Immunotherapy*. 2018;10(11):911−912.

16. Kean LS. Defining success with cellular therapeutics: the current landscape for clinical end point and toxicity analysis. *Blood.* 2018;131(24):2630−2639.

17. Boyiadzis MM, Dhodapkar MV, Brentjens RJ, et al. Chimeric antigen receptor (CAR) T therapies for the treatment of hematologic malignancies: clinical perspective and significance. *J Immunother Cancer.* 2018;6(1):137.

18. Gowda L, Shah NC. CAR-T cell manufacture: snatching victory when defeat is looming. *Transfusion.* 2018;58(6):1335−1337.

19. Allen ES, Stroncek DF, Ren J, et al. Autologous lymphapheresis for the production of chimeric antigen receptor T cells. *Transfusion.* 2017;57(5):1133−1141.

20. Ceppi F, Rivers J, Annesley C, et al. Lymphocyte apheresis for chimeric antigen receptor T-cell manufacturing in children and young adults with leukemia and neuroblastoma. *Transfusion.* 2018;58(6):1414−1420.

21. Majzner RG, Mackall CL. Tumor antigen escape from CAR T-cell therapy. *Cancer Discov.* 2018;8(10):1219−1226.

22. Ruella M, Xu J, Barrett DM, et al. Induction of resistance to chimeric antigen receptor T cell therapy by transduction of a single leukemic B cell. *Nat Med.* 2018;24(10):1499−1503.

23. Abbasi J. Relapses after CAR-T therapy. *J Am Med Assoc.* 2018;320(18):1850.

24. Perales MA, Kebriaei P, Kean LS, Sadelain M. Reprint of: building a safer and faster CAR: seatbelts, airbags, and CRISPR. *Biol Blood Marrow Transplant.* 2018;24(3S):S15−S19.

25. Smith TT, Stephan SB, Moffett HF, et al. In situ programming of leukaemia-specific T cells using synthetic DNA nanocarriers. Nat Nanotechnol. 2017;12(8):813-820.

26. Maus MV. Immunology: T-cell tweaks to target tumours. *Nature.* 2017;543(7643):48−49.

27. Eyquem J, Mansilla-Soto J, Giavridis T, et al. Targeting a CAR to the TRAC locus with CRISPR/Cas9 enhances tumour rejection. *Nature.* 2017;543:113.

28. Qasim W, Zhan H, Samarasinghe S, et al. Molecular remission of infant B-ALL after infusion of universal TALEN gene-edited CAR T cells. *Sci Transl Med.* 2017;9(374).

29. Gomes-Silva D, Srinivasan M, Sharma S, et al. CD7-edited T cells expressing a CD7-specific CAR for the therapy of T-cell malignancies. *Blood.* 2017;130(3):285−296.

30. Maciocia PM, Wawrzyniecka PA, Philip B, et al. Targeting the T cell receptor beta-chain constant region for immunotherapy of T cell malignancies. *Nat Med.* 2017;23(12):1416−1423.

31. Barrett DM. Getting the most from your CAR target. *Blood.* 2018;132(14):1467−1468.

32. Scarfo I, Ormhoj M, Frigault MJ, et al. Anti-CD37 chimeric antigen receptor T cells are active against B- and T-cell lymphomas. *Blood.* 2018;132(14):1495−1506.

33. Postow MA, Callahan MK, Wolchok JD. Immune checkpoint blockade in cancer therapy. *J Clin Oncol.* 2015;33(17):1974−1982.

34. Tran E, Turcotte S, Gros A, et al. Cancer immunotherapy based on mutation-specific CD^{4+} T cells in a patient with epithelial cancer. *Science.* 2014;344(6184):641−645.

35. Tran E, Robbins PF, Lu YC, et al. T-cell transfer therapy targeting mutant KRAS in cancer. *N Engl J Med.* 2016;375(23):2255−2262.

36. Brown CE, Alizadeh D, Starr R, et al. Regression of glioblastoma after chimeric antigen receptor T-cell therapy. *N Engl J Med.* 2016;375(26):2561−2569.

37. Babar Khan M, Chakraborty S, Boockvar JA. Use of chimeric antigen receptor T cells as a potential therapeutic for glioblastoma. *Neurosurgery.* 2017;80(5):N33−N34.

38. Tran E, Longo DL, Urba WJ. A milestone for CAR T cells. *N Engl J Med.* 2017;377(26):2593−2596.

39. Morgan MA, Schambach A. Chimeric antigen receptor T cells: extending translation from liquid to solid tumors. *Hum Gene Ther.* 2018;29(10):1083−1097.

40. Chmielewski M, Abken H. TRUCKs: the fourth generation of CARs. *Expert Opin Biol Ther.* 2015;15(8):1145−1154.

41. Chmielewski M, Abken H. CAR T cells releasing IL-18 convert to T-bet(high) FoxO1(low) effectors that exhibit augmented activity against advanced solid tumors. *Cell Rep.* 2017;21(11):3205−3219.

42. Yeku OO, Purdon TJ, Koneru M, Spriggs D, Brentjens RJ. Armored CAR T cells enhance antitumor efficacy and overcome the tumor microenvironment. *Sci Rep.* 2017;7(1):10541.

43. Rafiq S, Brentjens RJ. Tumors evading CARs-the chase is on. *Nat Med.* 2018;24(10):1492−1493.

44. Kueberuwa G, Kalaitsidou M, Cheadle E, Hawkins RE, Gilham DE. CD19 CAR T cells expressing IL-12 eradicate lymphoma in fully lymphoreplete mice through induction of host immunity. *Mol Ther Oncolytics.* 2018;8:41−51.

45. Zhang Y, Zhang X, Cheng C, et al. CRISPR-Cas9 mediated LAG-3 disruption in CAR-T cells. *Front Med.* 2017;11(4):554−562.

46. Ren J, Liu X, Fang C, Jiang S, June CH, Zhao Y. Multiplex genome editing to generate universal CAR T cells resistant to PD1 inhibition. *Clin Cancer Res.* 2017;23(9):2255−2266.

47. Redeker A, Arens R. Improving adoptive T cell therapy: the particular role of T cell costimulation, cytokines, and post-transfer vaccination. *Front Immunol.* 2016;7:345.

48. Beavis PA, Slaney CY, Kershaw MH, Gyorki D, Neeson PJ, Darcy PK. Reprogramming the tumor microenvironment to enhance adoptive cellular therapy. *Semin Immunol.* 2016;28(1):64−72.

49. Akahori Y, Wang L, Yoneyama M, et al. Antitumor activity of CAR-T cells targeting the intracellular oncoprotein WT1 can be enhanced by vaccination. *Blood.* 2018;132(11):1134−1145.

50. Kloss CC, Condomines M, Cartellieri M, Bachmann M, Sadelain M. Combinatorial antigen recognition with balanced signaling promotes selective tumor eradication by engineered T cells. *Nat Biotechnol.* 2013;31(1):71−75.

51. Wilkie S, van Schalkwyk MC, Hobbs S, et al. Dual targeting of ErbB2 and MUC1 in breast cancer using chimeric antigen receptors engineered to provide complementary signaling. *J Clin Immunol.* 2012;32(5):1059−1070.

52. Morsut L, Roybal KT, Xiong X, et al. Engineering customized cell sensing and response behaviors using synthetic Notch receptors. *Cell.* 2016;164(4):780−791.

53. Roybal KT, Rupp LJ, Morsut L, et al. Precision tumor recognition by T cells with combinatorial antigen-sensing circuits. *Cell*. 2016;164(4):770−779.

54. Cho JH, Collins JJ, Wong WW. Universal chimeric antigen receptors for multiplexed and logical control of T cell responses. *Cell*. 2018;173(6):1426−1438 e1411.

55. Kochenderfer JN, Dudley ME, Carpenter RO, et al. Donor-derived CD19-targeted T cells cause regression of malignancy persisting after allogeneic hematopoietic stem cell transplantation. *Blood*. 2013;122(25):4129−4139.

56. Brudno JN, Somerville RP, Shi V, et al. Allogeneic T cells that express an anti-CD19 chimeric antigen receptor induce remissions of B-cell malignancies that progress after allogeneic hematopoietic stem-cell transplantation without causing graft-versus-host disease. *J Clin Oncol*. 2016;34(10):1112−1121.

57. Anwer F, Shaukat AA, Zahid U, et al. Donor origin CAR T cells: graft versus malignancy effect without GVHD, a systematic review. *Immunotherapy*. 2017;9(2):123−130.

58. Terakura S, Yamamoto TN, Gardner RA, Turtle CJ, Jensen MC, Riddell SR. Generation of CD19-chimeric antigen receptor modified CD8+ T cells derived from virus-specific central memory T cells. *Blood*. 2012;119(1):72−82.

59. Cruz CR, Micklethwaite KP, Savoldo B, et al. Infusion of donor-derived CD19-redirected virus-specific T cells for B-cell malignancies relapsed after allogeneic stem cell transplant: a phase 1 study. *Blood*. 2013;122(17):2965−2973.

60. Ellebrecht CT, Bhoj VG, Nace A, et al. Reengineering chimeric antigen receptor T cells for targeted therapy of autoimmune disease. *Science*. 2016;353(6295):179−184.

61. Chatenoud L. Precision medicine for autoimmune disease. *Nat Biotechnol*. 2016;34(9):930−932.

62. Galy A. Like angler fish, CAARs lure their prey. *Mol Ther*. 2016;24(8):1339−1341.

Index

Note: Page numbers followed by "f" indicate figures and "t" indicates tables.

Printed and bound by CPI Group (UK) Ltd, Croydon, CR0 4YY

03/10/2024

01040300-0010